ANNALS OF THE NEW YORK ACADEMY OF SCIENCES

VOLUME 300

FOOD AND NUTRITION
IN HEALTH AND DISEASE

Edited by N. Henry Moss and Jean Mayer

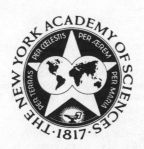

The New York Academy of Sciences
New York, New York
1977

Library of Congress Cataloging in Publication Data

Main entry under title:

Food and nutrition in health and disease.

   (Annals of the New York Academy of Sciences; v. 300)
   "The result of a Bicentennial conference . . . held by
the New York Academy of Sciences in Philadelphia, Pa. on
December 1, 2, and 3, 1976.
   Includes indexes.
   1. Food—Congresses. 2. Nutrition—Congresses.
3. Nutrition policy—Congresses. 4. Nutritionally
induced diseases—Congresses. I. Moss, N. Henry.
II. Mayer, Jean.   III. New York Academy of Sciences.
IV. Series: New York Academy of Sciences. Annals;
v. 300.
Q11.N5 vol. 300 [TX341] 508'.1s [338.1'9] 77–16843
ISBN 0-89072-046-0

PCP
Printed in the United States of America
ISBN 0-89072-046-0

ANNALS OF THE NEW YORK ACADEMY OF SCIENCES

VOLUME 300

November 30, 1977

FOOD AND NUTRITION IN HEALTH AND DISEASE *

Editors and Conference Chairmen
N. Henry Moss and Jean Mayer

Associate Chairmen
Robert I. Henkin and Willard Krehl

Nutrition Advisory Committee
Myron Brin, Sidney M. Cantor, Robin Chandler Duke,
Jonathan E. Rhoads, Howard Schneider,
Bruce Stillings, and Beverly Winikoff

Counsel for the Conference
Harry A. Kalish

CONTENTS

Introduction. *By* N. HENRY MOSS 1

Part I. Global Problems in Food Production

Panel on Food, Nutrition and Population Interactions: An Introduction to the
  Significance of the Conference. *Panelists:* JEAN MAYER, SOL H. CHAFKIN,
  AND ROBIN CHANDLER DUKE 5
Meeting Future Food Needs: The Challenge to Agriculture. *By* SYLVAN H.
  WITTWER 17
Energy Resources and Land Constraints in Food Production. *By* DAVID
  PIMENTEL 26
The Water Potential of the Arid Zone. *By* JOEL R. GAT 33
The How and Why of Climatic Changes. *By* REID A. BRYSON 40
General Discussion. *Moderator:* JEAN MAYER 54

Part II. Global Problems in Food Distribution and Food Policy

Opening Remarks. *By* ROGER REVELLE 57
Access to Food: The Ultimate Determinant of Hunger. *By* C. PETER TIMMER 59
Failure of the Food Distribution System: Dealing with Famine. *By* AARON E.
  IFEKWUNIGWE 69
Beyond 1976: Can Americans Be Well Nourished in a Starving World? *By*
  GARRETT HARDIN 87
Orientation of Domestic and International Food and Nutrition Policies. *By*
  DANIEL E. SHAUGHNESSY 92
Interface Session and Discussion. *Moderator:* ROGER REVELLE 96

* This series of papers is the result of a Bicentennial conference entitled Food and
Nutrition in Health and Disease, held by The New York Academy of Sciences in
Philadelphia, Pa. on December 1, 2 and 3, 1976.

Part III. Technology in Global Food Problems

Increasing Food Production from the Lowland Humid Tropics of Africa and Latin America. *By* D. J. GREENLAND 112

High-Frequency Irrigation and Green Revolution Food Production. *By* S. L. RAWLINS 121

Sources of Protein for Man: The Research Needs. *By* M. MILNER, N. S. SCRIMSHAW, AND D. I. C. WANG 129

The Role of Animal Protein. *By* CHARLES N. DOBBINS, JR. 148

Fortification of Foods with Vitamins and Minerals. *By* WALTER MERTZ 151

The Use and Abuse of Food Technology in the Quality of Our Food Supply. *By* SAMUEL A. GOLDBLITH 161

General Discussion. *Moderator:* SAMUEL A. GOLDBLITH 167

Part IV. Problems and Solutions in Developing Countries

Protein-Calorie Deficits in Developing Countries. *By* M. BÉHAR............ 176

Prenatal Nutrition. *By* E. M. WIDDOWSON............................. 188

Infant Feeding in National and International Perspective: An Examination of the Decline in Human Lactation, and the Modern Crisis in Infant and Young Child Feeding Practices. *By* MICHAEL C. LATHAM 197

Knowledge and Action in the Control of Vitamin A Deficiency. *By* V. RAMA-LINGASWAMI 210

Iron Nutrition. *By* CLEMENT A. FINCH 221

Report from the Club of Rome. *By* W. B. CLAPHAM, JR. AND M. D. MESAROVIC 228

General Discussion. *Moderator:* MYRON BRIN 239

Part V. Nutrition Forum: Nutrition of the American People

Nutrition Forum—Opening Remarks. *By* HOWARD SCHNEIDER.............. 251

Alternative U.S. Food Policies. *By* WALTER W. WILCOX 255

Human Nutrition Norms. *By* GILBERT A. LEVEILLE 259

Ideals and Realities in Food Systems. *By* S. M. CANTOR 262

General Discussion. *Moderator:* HOWARD SCHNEIDER 266

Part VI. Clinical Nutritional Problems in Health and Disease

Early Malnutrition and Subsequent Brain Development. *By* MYRON WINICK AND JO ANNE BRASEL 280

Dietary Fiber: What It Is and What It Does. *By* DAVID KRITCHEVSKY....... 283

Aging, Nutrition, and the Continuum of Health Care. *By* DONALD M. WATKIN 290

Obesity and the Social Environment: Current Status, Future Prospects. *By* ALBERT J. STUNKARD 298

New Aspects in the Control of Food Intake and Appetite. *By* ROBERT I. HENKIN 321

The Nutritional Epidemiology of Cardiovascular Disease. *By* WILLARD A. KREHL 335

Nutritional Carcinogenesis. *By* ERNST L. WYNDER 360

Discussion Paper: Prevention of Atherosclerosis by a Fat-Modified Diet. *By* HAQVIN MALMROS 379

General Discussion. *Moderator:* JONATHAN E. RHOADS 383

Part VII. Contemporary American Nutrition

Contributions of American Industry to the Improvement of American Nutrition. *By* WILLIAM O. BEERS AND JOHN F. WHITE 391

Additives in Our Food Supply. *By* SANFORD A. MILLER 397

Governmental Regulatory Difficulties. *By* JOHN E. VANDERVEEN 406

The U. S. School Food Service Program—Successes, Failures and Prospects. *By* PAUL A. LACHANCE 411

Nutritional Needs of Special Populations at Risk. *By* ARNOLD E. SCHAEFER ... 419

General Discussion. *Moderator:* N. HENRY MOSS 428

Summation and Perspective. *By* MAGNUS PYKE 434

Author Index 439

Subject Index 441

Financial assistance was received from:

- ABBOTT LABORATORIES
- AMERICAN CAN COMPANY
- ARA SERVICES, INC.
- CAMPBELL INSTITUTE FOR FOOD RESEARCH
- ELCO CORPORATION
- FOUNDATION FOR CARDIOVASCULAR RESEARCH
- GENERAL MILLS FOUNDATION
- GERBER PRODUCTS COMPANY
- H. J. HEINZ COMPANY FOUNDATION
- HOFFMANN-LA ROCHE INC.
- KRAFTCO CORPORATION
- MEAD JOHNSON
- MERCK, SHARP AND DOHME
- MONSANTO COMPANY
- NABISCO, INCORPORATED
- SANDOZ, INCORPORATED
- THE SARAH AND MATTHEW ROSENHAUS PEACE FOUNDATION
     INCORPORATED
- WYETH LABORATORIES

INTRODUCTION

N. Henry Moss

Temple University Health Sciences Center
and
Albert Einstein Medical Center
Philadelphia, Pennsylvania 19141

When The New York Academy of Sciences, the fourth oldest scientific organization in America, deliberated its program for the American Bicentennial year, its Committee elected to develop a major international conference on a vitally important scientific issue that was both multidisciplinary and global in scope. A number of topics were suggested. As the list was narrowed to three, it soon became obvious that "Food and Nutrition in Health and Disease" would be the proper and optimum selection.

Considerable planning, broad-based superb advice from an excellent "Blue Ribbon Advisory Committee," and sequential stepwise approval by review committees, the Conference Committee, and ultimately the Board of Governors of the Academy, has brought this Conference to fruition.

This Conference differs somewhat from most Academy conferences which have become increasingly super-specialized. It is not a highly specialized type of conference with in-depth presentation of research data or techniques in a narrow fragment of a limited scientific subject. Rather, it is a broad overview and current assessment of a global, critically important, multidisciplinary field that literally and figuratively involves hundreds of millions of people throughout the world, their well-being, and their lives.

Many papers listed in the program can easily be the subject matter of three-day conferences themselves, and some of them already have so occurred. Numerous inquiries and requests for presentation of papers were received at the Academy and by the cochairmen after the initial announcement was made in July of 1976. Although we are vulnerable to the potential criticism that the program is too broad in scope, we nevertheless could not include some exciting and excellent topics for lack of time. We hope that these seven sessions will encourage and set the tone and stage for future food and nutrition conferences during the next few years to add such topics to our Bicentennial selections.

We have listed a few objectives for the Conference which I shall now enumerate:

1. Present an overview of the world food problem and the role of the United States in it.
2. Identify past abuses and proper uses of technology in meeting food and nutrition needs.
3. Present a current assessment of major clinical nutritional problems and the directions and trends toward solutions.
4. Call attention to the lack of a nutrition policy in the United States and the urgent need to establish a sound national food and nutrition policy in the near future.
5. Provide a panel discussion and dialogue referable to the nutrition of the American people and accessible to the public and responsible consumer representatives.

1

We are deeply grateful to the outstanding speakers on the program from this country and abroad who accepted invitations to participate. We are also most appreciative of corporate and foundation support, which has been most generous.

Finally, I must add a personal note of gratitude for the privilege and pleasure of working with my cochairman, Dr. Jean Mayer. In the midst of accepting and undertaking a complex and most challenging new career as president of a major university, this internationally renowned scientist has been exceedingly helpful in the development of the Conference in detail, very constructive on the numerous occasions of consultation, warm and courteous throughout.

CITY OF PHILADELPHIA

Welcome

Whereas...

With the United States fast becoming the major food supplier to the world, there is a great need for experts in many scientific disciplines to exchange information on the many diverse aspects of the global problems of food and nutrition; and

WHEREAS...

To meet this challenge, the New York Academy of Sciences has convened a Bicentennial Conference to meet in Philadelphia from December 1 through 3, 1976 under the title of "Food and Nutrition in Health and Disease"; and

WHEREAS...

Over fifty world-renowned food, health and nutritional scientists will gather here to explore the global situation regarding food production, distribution, technology, and nutritional problems in health and disease:

Now, Therefore...

I, Frank L. Rizzo, Mayor of the City of Philadelphia, do hereby welcome the members of the

NEW YORK ACADEMY OF SCIENCES

and the participants in this vitally-important conference to our city, and do wish them great success in their efforts because of the increasing significance of food and nutrition to the survival of millions of people throughout the world.

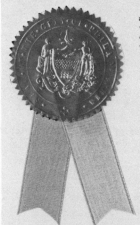

Given under my hand and the Seal of the City of Philadelphia, this first day of December, one thousand, nine hundred and seventy-six.

Scroll presented to The New York Academy of Sciences by the City of Philadelphia.

PANEL ON FOOD, NUTRITION AND POPULATION
INTERACTIONS: AN INTRODUCTION TO THE
SIGNIFICANCE OF THE CONFERENCE

Panelists: Jean Mayer, Sol H. Chafkin, and
Robin Chandler Duke

JEAN MAYER (*President, Tufts University, Medford, Mass.*): Mrs. Duke,
Mr. Chafkin, and I have been asked to set the stage for the conference by
speaking about the general framework of food, population, and institutional
developments in which action on the food problems of the world is likely to
take place in the next few years. The theme that I would like to sound for the
session is that perhaps we have just been through a turning point in the past
two or three years; but it may well be that, as has been true for other great
historical turning points, it is very difficult to perceive when you're right in the
middle of it.

Let me give you a picture which may be very much simplified and might
be slightly overstated. In 1972 or 1973, we hit bottom as far as the world food
situation was concerned. In 1972, we had very bad harvests in China, India,
and the Soviet Union, and that serious drought extending from Mauritania to
Ethiopia across the African continent. Harvests were spotty in Australia and
mediocre in Latin America.

Shortly afterwards the situation was complicated by the outbreak of war in
the Middle East. Also, the Soviet Union went into massive grain buying, not
to maintain their level of calorie and protein consumption, but to continue to
increase the amount of animal products consumed. The oil-producing countries
tripled, then quadrupled, and eventually almost quintupled oil prices, bringing
disorganization of markets in industrialized countries, but much more important, bringing great hardship in the poor countries which do not produce oil.

Meanwhile, the massive phenomenon of population increase throughout the
world continued unabated. World population, which took millions of years to
reach one billion in 1850, reached two billion in 1920, three billion in 1962 or
1963, four billion in 1975, and was predicted to double to eight billion by the
year 2000.

In developed countries, cardiovascular mortality continued to increase
steadily, so we seemed to be making very little progress as regards nutrition
and health. The only point that we seemed to have gained is that in rich countries in general, and the United States in particular, we had filled the scandalous
gap between the levels of consumption of the rich and the poor through a series
of corrective programs. In this country, the number of food stamp recipients
rose from less than 1 million in 1969 to close to 19 million in 1974, with a
great deal of the middle class looking aghast at this situation and predicting
that half of the population of the United States would be on the dole before long.

Since that time a great deal has happened. In our own country some very
important developments have taken place. For three years in a row we have had
a small but quite significant decrease in cardiovascular mortality with a corresponding increase in the length of adult life, a phenomenon which had not been
seen since World War II. The two factors which seem to be most clearly at

work are: first, that we are controlling hypertension in our population much more effectively, and second, that consumption of saturated fats, eggs, and whole milk has decreased. Incidentally, it is very interesting to see that there is a decrease in whole-milk consumption without a corresponding decrease in consumption of non-fat solids, which shows that people really seem to be heeding advice and that changing patterns of consumption are affecting patterns of mortality. A definite effect of changes of patterns of nutrition on health is detectable.

In terms of nutrition of the poor, it is quite obvious that the new corrective measures that were put in place in the early 70's are working as we hoped that they would. As unemployment has decreased, there has been a corresponding decrease in the number of food stamp recipients of about two million in the past year. It seems quite obvious that the food stamp system and other food corrective systems are working to absorb the impact of extreme poverty and are not working simply as a way for people to gouge the government or refuse to work as the pessimists said they would.

Consumer measures are effective in terms of constantly increasing nutrition labeling of an increasingly packaged food supply; the interest of consumers in nutrition, and in nutrition labeling and ingredient labeling is mounting. There is re-examination of the 3,000 chemicals that we have put in our food supply, and the examination is on a more sensible basis, namely the recognition that many of them do offer very serious benefits, but that many, on the other hand, do pose risks which do not seem to be compensated by corresponding benefits. Very slowly we're beginning to do what we ought to be doing, even though we may not be doing it according to a blueprint, with governmental commissions announcing that we are now going to proceed from Step C to Step D.

The World Food Conference signaled itself in the history of mankind by presenting 128 consecutive speeches by 128 consecutive Ministers of Agriculture, surely the most stupefying event in the annals of international meetings. But since that fiasco, serious work really has started getting done, though, again, it is not being done with pomp and circumstance. We've also been luckier as regards the weather, but the net effect is that we are beginning to reconstitute reserves even in countries which, like the United States, officially do not believe in having reserves. The reserves are growing in countries like The People's Republic of China and India, in areas where a few years ago the situation seemed to be desperate and it appeared that they would be living from hand to mouth for a very long time.

This progress does not seem to be particularly dependent on any economic system. The nutrition situation has improved in Red China; it has also improved in Hong Kong, Formosa and Singapore; in India; and in Pakistan; it is even improving in Bangladesh, which a few years ago appeared to be the world's perennial basket-case.

This improvement in nutrition is dependent on two major factors: an improved application of technology and the presence of an administrative structure which permits the development of technology, and a sense of social justice and equity which does not necessarily exist everywhere. Mr. Chafkin and I were discussing this morning, for instance, the case of Brazil, a country with a very steady improvement in gross national product where, however, the nutritional situation, particularly in the cities, is steadily growing worse. Furthermore, there are some areas, like Africa, where the improvement in application of technology is extremely slow, where the population explosion is continuing almost unabated, and where the food situation and dependence on the outside world, particularly on North America, is likely to get considerably worse before it gets better, I would hope around the year 2000. Still, that is better and so is the general projection of population growth for the world as a result in particular of the gigantic work done in The People's Republic of China in curbing the birthrate, and the increasing effectiveness of programs in the Indian subcontinent. The total effect is that the population in the year 2000 is now predicted to be about 6.2 to 6.5 billion, an enormous increase, but certainly a far cry from the 8 billion predicted four or five years ago.

In general, it seems to me that there is cause for optimism in that there is already a demonstration of the fact that if we can maintain the transfer, not just of technology but of managerial capabilities, from developed to developing countries, we can make a considerable dent in the problem between now and the year 2000. Certainly the worldwide famine predicted a few years ago is just not going to take place unless there are cataclysmic changes in the weather.

One very serious problem, however, is whether we will have the continued wisdom to maintain the present momentum, whether we will have: first, institutions which will permit the maintenance of peace in such crucial areas as the Middle East which sits astride the energy supply necessary for the development of the world at large, and second, institutions capable of maintaining pressure for increased agricultural development and increased population control.

Finally, as always, the problem is whether mankind as a whole will continue to have the necessary fortitude, and the new-found enthusiasm for agricultural production which resulted from the near-catastrophe of '72–'73. Agriculture was rediscovered as the single most important occupation of mankind. The questions are whether this will last and also whether the effort to improve the condition of women will continue to be seen as entailing a decrease in the number of children and an emphasis on quality of life rather than quantity of offspring. It seems to me, as we begin the new year, that the signals are favorable and the unrelieved gloom and pessimism that many people exhibited three or four years ago is no longer justified.

I will now call on my fellow speakers either to expand on this optimistic view or to crush it completely.

MR. SOL H. CHAFKIN (*Officer-in-charge, Social Development Programs, Ford Foundation, New York, N.Y.*): Dr. Mayer, the only point I would differ with you on is that I would be inclined to call it a reduction in pessimism rather than an increase in optimism.

You sounded a theme which is worth noting. You referred to small but significant changes here and there, and it suggested to me that what we ought really to be prepared to expect are not great leaps forward but rather significant incremental changes and improvements.

Limited incremental changes may reflect the limits on what governments can in fact do—a point I'd like to touch on in my remarks.

I found a slip of paper in a fortune cookie the other night which said "Action should be the fruit of knowledge." In a sense this is the objective of this conference—an attempt to get action. It's the limits on such action that I'd like to talk about, and I may be a bit more pessimistic than Dr. Mayer's excellent *tour d'horizon*.

I'd like to do this very briefly by illustrating a piece of the title of the panel's concern—food, nutrition, and population interactions—using Brazil, which I visited briefly not long ago as an illustration.

From 1965 through 1975 there was no significant increase in the production of the major food staples in Brazil. In the same period of time the population increased something on the order of 20–30%. The same period witnessed a very sharp price inflation affecting food staples. And, perhaps not surprisingly, infant mortality rates, which had been declining in large cities, began to creep up. This is about as elegant an example of the possible interactions between food nutrition and population as I can think of.

Dr. Moss said that this conference was vulnerable to criticism that it was perhaps too broad. I think it's probably equally vulnerable to the criticism that it's not broad enough. For example, in Brazil, in the same period, 1965 through 1975, the production of soybeans increased from about 500,000 tons in 1965 to close to 10 million tons in 1975. Virtually all of this production is exported, probably for livestock feed. There is a probability that there was a displacement effect—that soybeans were produced at the expense of not producing some other kind of food.

Certain parts of Brazil and certain populations within Brazil suffer from severe nutritional deprivation. But it now becomes necessary to broaden our view to include other interactions affecting the food-nutrition-population syndrome. Brazil carries a heavy foreign debt. It must service this debt every year, so it's quite important to Brazil to maintain as high a level of exports as possible. Lurking behind the already complicated interactions among food, nutrition, and population are many other equally complicated interactions that encompass everything from poverty to environment to international balance-of-payments positions, inflation, and so forth. And, this is where we begin to notice the limits on what governments can do.

All governments face quite serious problems of internal financial stability. All of them are under pressure to keep a lid on budget expenditures as part of their counter-inflationary programs. The softest elements of most of their budgets turn out to be social programs, and here I include nutrition intervention programs, health programs, and so on. Health ministries typically are the weakest ministries in most governments in developing countries, and what begins to happen is the exercise of what I'll call the iron laws of international financial survival and internal financial stability.

There are problems that are more important to governments than nutrition and health. Governments are directly responsible for their international financial survival, for national defense, for economic development, for doing something about domestic prices, unemployment and so on. Those of us who are interested in actions flowing from knowledge have to recognize that employment levels may take first priority over health and nutrition and, indeed perhaps should. There are few things I can think of that are more important to health and nutrition status than a job and income.

There will be, from this conference and others, proposals coming forth which are in the nature of calls for "more"—more money for health, more money for nutrition, and so on. I suspect that in the next 10 years this country and others are going to have to be far more ingenious in getting more results from the same quantum of resources than we have ever had before. This is going to be the challenge. It is no trick for governments to give things away. Of course there are logistical problems and administrative problems, but the trick is to find alternative ways of solving problems that would produce the same stream of benefits at lower costs or a higher stream of benefits at the present cost.

To turn to another theme, I want to congratulate the organizers of this conference for doing something that most other conferences do not do in dealing with this subject and this is to break away somewhat from the conventional "we-they" reference points, i.e., "we," the industrialized countries view with alarm the problems "they," the developing countries face; "they" need help and "we" are the ones to give it. In fact, as most of you know, many of the developing countries are way ahead of us in certain areas of social and cultural polices and way ahead of us in a number of areas of health-nutrition research. Some of the leaders of this research are in this room.

I think we need to recognize that nutritional status is a pan-human problem. For example, concern for iron deficiency anemia is not limited to poor countries. In the United States we have, what seems to me, a startling high incidence of such a phenomenon. As our uses and abuses of food technology proceed and are exported to less-industrialized countries, I suspect that we will see them begin to wonder about the nutritional and health effects of this increasingly sophisticated technology. There will be more conferences to exchange information on another set of problems. So, the "we-they" distinction is rapidly disappearing and becoming "us," whether it be iron deficiency anemia or what we learn about the effects of energy deficits in poor countries that might help us understand the mechanisms affecting obesity.

I would like to close with a suggestion for those of us at this conference. As the findings are presented and the proposals and solutions are offered, we ought to subject these to a couple of simple tests: (1) Is what is being offered in the way of a finding or in the way of a proposed solution consequential for low income groups in the particular place for which this is being proposed? Somehow the health, agricultural, and other breakthroughs don't quite hit the problems of the lowest income groups. Health programs in many countries somehow don't quite make it. The coverage isn't broad enough, transportation obstacles are not overcome, and this failure to reach those who most need services most is really the heart of the problem. We are essentially concerned with populations that are by any measure disadvantaged in terms of income and other ways. So, the first test is does the proposed solution make a difference to such population groups?

The second test is whether what is being proposed can in fact be done and is it manageable. Dr. Mayer referred to this point with respect to the existing institutional arrangements in the places that we're talking about. The landscape is littered with pilot programs of one kind or another that somehow never leave the pilot stage. One reason is often financial. Another reason is that the program is simply not susceptible to scaling up. You cannot scale it up because you don't have the right people and you don't have an adequate institutional infrastructure that can handle it. And so the application of knowledge from science and technology is severely limited because of failure on the part of governments in many countries to face up to the kind of painful tasks that are associated with institutional rearrangements, redeployment of resources, and reordering of priorities.

The last observation I'd like to make is in connection with Dr. Moss' remarks about getting a sound national food and nutrition policy in the United States. I'm in favor of it, but I'm a little worried about doing it wrong. It often happens that "when all else fails, make a policy." But don't let the policy-making substitute for actions which may require budgetary commitments of needed money.

Thinking in terms of a "single and coherent" national policy troubles me if it overlooks the flexibility and the pluralism that characterize the U.S. We should pay attention to finding approaches that work before locking ourselves into a "single and coherent policy" that's made in an office in Washington.

I would pay close attention to the kind of policy that leaves the door open for a variety of actions, including actions at community levels. Increasingly, developing countries are recognizing that highly centralized intervention programs often don't work as planned unless something is happening at local levels—local initiative or energy that converts what is an interesting but not quite successful idea into something that benefits the lives of the people there.

MRS. ROBIN CHANDLER DUKE (*National Co-Chairperson, Population Crisis Committee/Draper World Population Fund, New York, N.Y.*): I would like to expand on this discussion to take in the rights of humans, the rights of women specifically, and bring in more about population.

I have just come from one of those remote parts of the world where occasionally they eat people, and there is a story going around of a father and son who were walking through the jungle when they saw a beautiful girl leaning against a palm tree. The son said to the father, "Gosh, she's beautiful. Let's take her home and eat her." And the father said to the son, "I've got a better idea. Let's take her home and eat Mom."

Well, Mom, dear old Mom, has had her problems with bad jokes. But as I've worked with Mom here and abroad, I realize how few rights she has, *really*. Maybe this is not Mom's fault, but I wonder if you've ever thought of the life of a woman in some of the underdeveloped areas and how little it has changed over the centuries. Here is a woman who gets up at 5:00 a.m., puts her baby on her back and goes out into the fields where she sows and she plows and she pauses to feed her baby and she pauses to placate her child. On her way back to the village at night, she has to collect firewood. Then she may have to walk a mile to a well, unless she's lucky enough and has a well for water in her village. Then she pounds her grain, cooks supper and everyone else eats. She, of course, eats last.

In Bangladesh, she will have 11 pregnancies, and 6 children will survive. She'll live to be 50. She was probably given in marriage when she was about 14. She has no basic rights. Any little bit of money or resources that she may have belongs to her husband. This same woman's life, with a few variations on the theme, is like that of the woman in, let us say, Africa. When seeds and tools were brought in even as recently as during the tragic drought in the Sahel, automatically, those seeds and those tools went to the men, even though women do over 50% of the farming and certainly have the entire responsibility of preparing food.

We've learned, working in population, trying to bring to every woman the knowledge of how to control her fertility, how to control her own body, how to make her own decisions about the numbers and spacing of her children, that we must also bring to this woman some kind of decent nutrition and health care. This is why, really, I am here today. I'm here because everything we deal with in what we hope is development toward a decent quality of life must be a totally integrated concept of food, nutrition, education, and the rights of human beings to know. The knowledge is what we want to bring to the village level all over the underdeveloped world.

And what of the developed? How many women in the United States know much about what is good, healthy, and nutritious for their families? Aren't we sold junk food almost every day? I'm so conscious of it when I return to the

States after having been away for a long stretch and turn on my television. I'm told, and worse, my children are told, that all this junk food is the thing they should eat. Jump on your motorcycle or bicycle and get down to wherever it is and buy junk food. Why don't we merchandise good food? This seems pretty basic. We have the knowledge, and yet we don't even disseminate this knowledge within our own country to the degree that we should. Corporately, we do not assume the responsibility that we should regarding what we and our children should eat.

Well, this same knowledge for a woman in a village in Pakistan, Bangladesh, Indonesia, the Philippines, wherever you want to choose, is the knowledge she deserves to have. She deserves it because the right kind of diet, the right kind of nutrition, will obviously produce for her healthier children. And so it comes down to the rights of the whole family, and this is what we deal with. Who helps this woman whom I described?

Well, you know all your agencies for assistance from the private agencies of International Planned Parenthood Federation, the United Nations Fund for Population Activities and our own Agency for International Development (AID). Each kind of agency, government and private, is involved, not in just coming in and saying, "Madam, you must have fewer children." This is not the way it's done. It's "Madam, we want to help you in terms of helping yourself." And so, through village leaders, we take people into the village, and those leaders tell their own people about nutrition, health, contraception. Contraception should be a household word like soap or toothpaste.

It's incredible that in our own country, until very recently, you would never see contraceptive devices sitting out in a drugstore. Two weeks ago in Pakistan a minister of family planning said to me, "You know, we have to find some nice words, Mrs. Duke, for all these ugly things." "Ooh," I said, "are they ugly things?" "Well," he said, "you wouldn't understand because in the United States you take a very broad-based view of this. You talk about condoms and IUD's and pills." "Oh no," I said, "I have a son 30 and another 28 and another 14, and I would wager my older sons went into the drugstore once and looked at the ceiling and the four walls and said, "I'd like to buy some condoms." And I'm sure they were embarrassed, since condoms are not items sitting out on the shelf. In other words, in many ways we are no more advanced about this than many less-developed nations. We did have 60,000 unwed pregnant teenagers in New York City last year.

We fight for sex education in the public school system, and mothers look at me and say, "That's out of the question." Yet, girls are becoming pregnant younger and younger. How ridiculous! So, indeed, we have the same problems here.

Last night we were discussing the problems of many emotional sicknesses and so many sicknesses of the body that relate to the kind of food one eats. So, in our programs in family planning, worldwide, we work hand in glove with people in health and nutrition. No program goes into a village that isn't tied into giving the family advice. Women have often said to me that they didn't know; they didn't understand.

I left Manila just 5 days ago and went through a clinic in the urban areas where women were bringing in malnourished children. They didn't understand. They explained that they had been giving the child the diet that they assumed was perfectly adequate. There was no protein in this diet at all, and the child was critically malnourished. Right there, while children were being fed a sound and nutritious lunch program, the mothers were given advice and told something about what to feed their children. And these were women who, with the knowledge, were able to obtain some of the protein foods to give these children. So, it was basically a question of ignorance, and it seems to me, like the policeman who stops you when you make a wrong turn and you indicate you didn't know, he says, "Well, lady, ignorance is no excuse." Well, it really isn't because we know so much, and I think one of the important roles of people who do know is to disseminate the knowledge they have. And if one wonders—how do you use this around the world?—how do you make this kind of thing work?—what are the agencies that can get the word out and tell people? Well, there is no one simple technique for this, but I do know one thing: every country in the developing world with a leader who has the political will can implement a powerful program integrating family planning, health, and nutrition. This you will see, and I can cite one example in Indonesia.

Indonesia is one of the most populated countries of the world. The Chief of State, Suharto, has determined that unless he is able to control the exploding population and feed his people, Indonesia will not get ahead. And so, with the assistance of a strong AID mission there and with private agencies constantly beating the drum with innovative approaches, village programs exist today in Indonesia that are working and bringing to people knowledge of nutrition, knowledge of health, of child-maternal care and giving every woman the right to know how to space and how to control the number of her children. It is essential that this kind of program be taken to the rural areas, interpreted to the people—Indonesians telling Indonesians. We can come in with the knowledge and the conviction and the understanding of what to do, but it must be reinterpreted by the people to their own people. Every single program must be tailored to the particular idiosyncracies of a given part of the world. A thing that works in Indonesia won't necessarily work in South Korea. I've been in areas where the pill is impossible—they tell me. People understand getting an injection in the arm when you are speaking of female contraception. They understand it because they are conditioned to the early health programs where they had a vaccination or an injection. Therefore, the injectables work in a more satisfactory way. At the same time, one shows a woman that she can slow down birth, space her children, and she sees that with certain kinds of food her existing children are in better health, she begins to learn to value a better quality of life.

The same is true in every village program when we deal with them on the basis of what they're growing. As you probably know, there are many countries of the world where they grow many things we don't need—things that don't help the lot of mankind, but indeed, they are good cash crops and so they continue to grow them. And, they are even grown in countries where they have starving people.

I feel as though it is important to cite some of the optimistic notes in this concept of integration of food and health and education, development and family planning, because too many people speak of the impossibilities. The Draconian methods of Madame Gandhi in India have racked the nerves of lots of liberals. She's facing a very difficult situation. With incentives—25 rupees or whatever it is—a man can have a vasectomy; and they've done the same thing in Bangladesh. Well, now it's not an option in India. Apparently, one has no option after two children. But what is India to do—have children she cannot feed?

China is constantly cited as having great programs. They are able to feed their people, and their family planning programs work. We don't have any hard and fast statistics on China, but from all the best guesswork it is working—late marriages, sensible planning and spacing, really remarkable and good agricultural programs. All of these things are being effectively employed to the best of our knowledge.

There is one more point I should like to make and it is this: No matter how the crop potential improves—and indeed, it's an improved year for India; it's an improved year for Pakistan; Pakistan will be able to export some of her long-grain rice—the input and increase of population in India and Pakistan immediately absorb this remarkable new production. So, unless you take into account the concerns of population, you cannot catch up. You are running standing still. There is just no way to reach out. So, basically, even though you have a good crop year—let's say you don't have flooding in Bangladesh, let's say you're fortunate enough that there is no drought in the Sahel, you have the remarkable tools of Western medicine and therefore, lower mortality rates—but tragically enough, people then are born only to die of starvation.

So, I think what is terribly important to accent, and I know this is a large and vast subject, we must move the knowledge out into every area. We ought to be able to help every citizen with information and understanding, if nothing else. There is one note on which I will close—and that is *waste*.

I ordered my breakfast this morning at the Hilton. I said I wanted a poached egg on toast. The waitress said, "We have only two poached eggs on toast." I said, "But I only want one poached egg." "But," she said, "the menu requires that you have two." I replied, "I can't eat two eggs—too much cholesterol. Let me pay for two but send me one egg." "That's not possible," the remote voice of Room Service replied. That, Ladies and Gentlemen, is an example of America's efficient waste of food. Thank you.

DISCUSSION

DR. DONALD WATKIN (*HEW, Washington, D.C.*): This is directed principally to Mr. Chafkin. On a recent trip I made to South America I was struck by the tremendous amount of land available for grazing animals—land that I'm told is not being effectively utilized. This is particularly pertinent to ruminants because they have the ability of converting cellulose into something that is edible by man.

I wonder if any of you have had any thoughts on how we might make more use of the available land areas in the world for animal food production.

MR. CHAFKIN: I don't have any bright ideas on the question you posed. I am struck by two things. First, is the debate that may go on with international lending institutions as to whether they could invest their capital in projects for cattle in those countries that have choices on land utilization for food crops or for cattle. Where there is no choice, it's simple. Where the choices exist, then the decision becomes somewhat more complicated. The second thing that strikes me as a non-expert is that those who advocate a shift from investment in cattle to growing more food crops may be overlooking the possibility that a cattle industry, under certain circumstances and in certain places, can serve as a stabilizer for grain markets to ensure continued high production. A cattle industry might help make more efficient other sectors of the agricultural economy.

DR. MAYER: Mr. Chafkin, I think the emphasis that you placed is one which should be underlined, that one can justify cattle production in areas where there is no direct competition with man and to absorb surpluses of certain cereals. The demonstrated slowness of shifting from grain production for cattle to grain production for man was certainly one of the major factors in the crisis in '72–'73–'74. It appears reasonable that if we had large enough reserves to start with, we could use the cattle industry as a way to absorb the ups and downs and smooth the bumps, but where we are very low in reserves we no longer have that flexibility.

A dominant factor, I think, in the world food situation is the gigantic amount of grain which is stored every year by the Soviet Union, possibly as much as 100 million tons. The stocks are changed on the average of every two years because of deterioration of quality, and the wheat is fed to cattle in what must be one of the most gigantic wasteful operations as far as the world food picture is concerned. While everybody looks at the errors of the system, very little attention has been paid to the maintenance of what must be enormous war stocks by the Soviet Union.

DR. HOWARD SCHNEIDER (*University of North Carolina, Chapel Hill, N.C.*): Mr. Chafkin pointed out that the drive for a single policy left him somewhat uneasy because he felt more comfortable with pluralism. We now have as a matter of national policy clean air as a goal. It's not levels of different kinds—we are striving for clean air. We are striving for pure water—I don't find any pluralism there. Might I ask Dr. Mayer whether, instead of trying to develop laundry lists, we might think of developing a mechanism as a matter of policy which would in a dynamic way continue to accommodate itself to these changing tides?

DR. MAYER: Clean air is not a policy, it is a goal. One of our serious problems is that we have not had a clear national goal. For example, if we have certain goals in preventive medicine, like knocking down the average blood cholesterol of American males by 50 mg. per 100 c.c. or some such figure, we can then start developing policies in order to try to achieve this goal. The cattle industry is employed in converting complex carbohydrates into fat and essentially into saturated fat. In the process it upgrades somewhat the quality of protein, but at the cost of 80% of the vegetable protein being chewed up and made unavailable.

The reversal of such an operation, which has gigantic economic implications, is going to be extremely difficult. For instance, three years in a row the McGovern committee tried to put together hearings on nutrition and cardiovascular health, and three years in a row the hearings were cancelled because of the opposition, not of the more reactionary or conservative elements in the Mid-West or the Old South, but of some of the most liberal Senators in the country, who were under pressure from the dairy industry in their states.

Until we can get the whole health establishment and, in particular, the entire medical profession, to agree that knocking down blood cholesterol is going to be a national goal, we don't even have to worry about policy and mechanisms. Now, once we have a national goal then I think we need a multiplicity of mechanisms with some loose form of coordination.

Similarly, we define clearly what it is that we want to do abroad—the sort of objectives that Mrs. Duke so eloquently expounded—and really try to put some figures to the sort of effort that is needed, then I think we should ask whether our institutions and our AID program, our various governmental institutions to carry out those objectives, are in fact adequate. My perception is that we don't have adequate institutions at this point to do technical assistance effectively.

But, I see the problem, Dr. Schneider, as much deeper than the one you are discussing. What worries me is that at this point we have not defined our national goals, and the hope is that a conference like this will bring us nearer to some sort of a consensus as to what we ought to be doing, and then we can worry about how to do it.

MR. CHAFKIN: Before we formulate a single coherent national policy we need an understanding of what works—what makes a difference. The amount of assessment or measurement of the nutritional and health effects of food stamps, of school eating programs, is practically zero.

So, the writing of policies with respect to "there ought to be this and we have to have more of that" without some kind of firm basis as to what works, what kinds of payoffs you get from what kind of investment, seems to me to be a bit premature.

DR. V. RAMALINGASWAMI (*India Institute of Medical Sciences, New Delhi, India*): I was tremendously intrigued by the comments that Madame Duke has made with reference to knowledge on the part of women. I think it's perhaps most crucial to all our discussions. Perhaps we really ought to be concerned more about functional literacy rather than literal literacy—how to bridge this gap is one of our most critical areas.

May I refer to a development that's taking place now in the State of Kerala, India, which according to classical economic parameters, is the poorest state in India? The female literacy rate in that state is the highest in the country, and population dynamics in that state are extraordinarily interesting. You now have a rapid decline in birth rate taking place in that state, with the poorest of the poor. It seems to me if we can, in this conference, channel this human energy it doesn't matter if oil energy drains out.

MRS. DUKE: The crux of all this is political will—a governor of a state who is strong, who believes and does not make political appointees a major factor in his health and educational programs, who looks for quality people who will carry out and implement programs.

MR. ARTHUR IBERALL (*General Technical Services, Inc., Upper Darby, Pa.*): Both the currents of institutions and the processes that they are engaged in rise from some kind of a generalized homeostatic regulation of the entire society. Without some clear understanding of these interrelations, the notion that this can be regulated simply by reason or "policy" is just too far off. To what extent are you going to examine the integrative relations that exist in the entire system as a whole—whether it be a nation or the world?

MR. CHAFKIN: In this country, it's generally well understood how the system works with respect to making political decisions. One way or another every four years something happens called a presidential election, and some of it is highly visible and some of it is not. Large numbers of people understand the pressures that are at work on the decision-making process in government and elsewhere. I personally have some doubts about the benefits that flow from the continual poking away at all the possible relationships including that between the banana and the Democratic party and how it operates.

The system in the U.S. that produces decisions about investments of large sums of money from government sources for nutrition education programs or for a national health insurance scheme is visible enough so that those who want to climb into that system can choose among the various ladders that are lying around. This probably is the case in other countries.

While I appreciate the importance of studying all the complex interrelationships, policies may be evolved more efficiently by learning through small actions. Somebody once told me that when Napoleon was asked, in his heyday, what his battle strategy was, he said, "On s'engage, puis on voit."—"You get into it and see what happens."

DR. GENE CALVERT (*American Public Health System, Washington, D.C.*): I would like the panel members to comment on the potential role of nutrition in lowering population growth rates.

MRS. DUKE: When nutrition is combined with family planning—that is, when you deal with a mother's spacing of children and at the same time give her nutritional advice, I believe it is all designed to bringing down fertility rates. This is also combined with the health factor. Her present children would have access to parasite control and other health programs which she can see. In simple wayside villages I've seen jars of formaldehyde with hookworm in them, and the children know what this is; they've seen this; they've passed it; they understand it, and when they know they must have their various injections and pills, they again grasp the significance of this. All these programs are ingrained with family planning—health, nutrition, child-care, et cetera—and these programs do reduce the fertility rate.

DR. MAYER: The important thing to remember is that at the village or barrio level experience shows that the same agencies can do maternal and child nutrition, preventive medicine and population control, but none of these is going to work unless there is a real understanding on the part of the population as to what the aims and the methods of those three programs are.

MEETING FUTURE FOOD NEEDS: THE CHALLENGE TO AGRICULTURE*

Sylvan H. Wittwer

*Agricultural Experiment Station and
College of Agriculture and Natural Resources
Michigan State University
East Lansing, Michigan 48824*

INTRODUCTION

The world's greatest challenge is to provide adequate food for an expanding population. Jean Mayer's projection of a year ago is appropriate: "We will have to find in the next 25 years food for as many people again as we have been able to develop in the whole history of man 'til now." [1]

The immediate solution to meeting world food needs lies in all-out agricultural production, improved nutrition, and in education. There are now significant technological, financial, and organizational opportunities for effective action. For the first time in history we have the capability to relieve mankind from the scourge of malnutrition and hunger. The reality of a rapidly growing world population with rising international affluency and demand discourages a policy of no action. Never before has a nation produced so much food. Never before has it been done on so few hectares. Never before has any nation exported so much food abroad. And never before has any nation exercised such a monopoly on the world's surplus.

Assuring our food supply, however, is more than production technology. It involves removal of a host of socio-politico-economic and institutional constraints, and effectively dealing with food policy issues. It involves research in post-harvest handling, processing, storage, transportation, and consumer acceptance. Food is truly a high technology export.

That people today are malnourished or starving is a question of food distribution, resources and economics, not agricultural production limitations. Enough food is now produced to feed the world's hungry. We are producing more food per capita than 20 years ago. The problem is delivery. It's putting the food where the people are, and providing an income so they can buy it. Only poor people have a problem in meeting their food needs.

Only scientists develop new technologies. Only farmers produce food. Motivation and incentives are important both for scientific discovery and food production. The time between a basic research discovery and its first application averages 13 years. The time from introduction of a new technology until its adoption reaches the expected ceiling is 35 years. It now takes 6–10 years to train scientists to do research. We must force the pace of agricultural development. New technologies must be tailored to each local condition. This can best be done by scientists who also know how to farm—a commodity that is becoming rare, indeed.

There have been many recent assessments of technologies that are available or that can be developed for increasing plant and animal resources for human

* Michigan Agricultural Experiment Station Journal Article No. 7882.

consumption. One is impressed by the number of studies as well as alternatives.[2] Others are in progress and have been initiated by Congress through a Food Advisory Committee of the Office of Technology Assessment, by the Office of Technology and Policy of the White House through a Food and Nutrition Subcommittee, and by the World Food and Nutrition Study of the National Academy of Sciences National Research Council.

The intent of all these efforts is to identify agricultural technologies that would result in an enhancement of food production, stability of supplies at high levels, and improved nutrition. All recommendations focus eventually on the cereal crops, the seed legumes, forages for livestock, the roots, tubers, sugar crops, fruits and vegetables, ruminant nutrition, better feeding practices, animal health and genetic improvement, improved utilization of byproducts, management of resources, and reductions in resource inputs and losses.

An increase of investment in research relating to the biological processes that control or limit crop and livestock productivity is a common theme. There is the consistent undertone that we know far more than is being put to use— the ever present challenge to make operational the knowledge we already have. To know is not enough.

Plants provide directly, or indirectly, up to 95 percent of the world's food supply. Increased production of crops can come from a combination of three approaches: (1) bring more land into production; (2) enhance yields per unit land area, and (3) increase the number of crops produced per year. With livestock, increased output relates to improved nutrition, genetic gain, and better environment and disease control. Enhancement of output per unit land area, per unit time, and for each increment of water, energy, fertilizer, and chemical added must be sought after. The productivity of the individual farmer must be increased. This can be achieved by the development of new technologies, by teaching farmers how to use them, and by providing incentives for farmers to put them to use.

Stating it differently, we must now seek food-producing technologies and farming systems that result in stable production at high levels; that are scale neutral; with the least possible inputs of land, water, energy, fertilizers and chemicals, with achievable minimum environmental impacts, and accompanying improvements in nutritional quality. Such technologies can be created. We will address ourselves to some of these. What is food for man and where does it come from?

Chief among the major food crops, in approximate order of importance are the cereal grains—rice, wheat, maize, barley, sorghum, millet, oats and rye; the seed legumes—field beans, peanuts, chick peas, cowpeas, pigeon peas, soybeans, mung beans, and broad beans; the roots and tuber crops—potatoes, sweet potatoes, and cassava; the sugar crops—sugarcane and sugar beets; the tropical crops—bananas and coconuts. A variety of fruits and vegetables are secondary staple food crops. Processed and fresh, they add personal enrichment and pleasure to eating, and essential dietary nutrients. Hundreds of millions of people depend primarily on what is produced in gardens or small holdings at or very near the point of production. These are seldom considered in world food inventories. Several crops a year may be grown. Greater scientific inputs for increasing the stability and productivity of food and its storage and preservation on small holdings are the world's most urgently needed agricultural technology. Hay, forages, pasture crops, and shrubs provide most of the feed units for flocks and herds. Wastes and byproduct utilization figure strongly in the production of swine and poultry.

Cereal grains constitute the most important food group on earth. They provide 60 percent of the calories and 50 percent of the protein consumed by the human race. Twenty percent of the protein comes from seed legumes. Other sources of protein are animals (25 percent) and fish (5 percent).

FRONTIERS IN FOOD PRODUCTION

The first relates to the biological processes that control productivity of economically important food crops. These include greater photosynthetic efficiency, enhancement of biological nitrogen fixation, regulation of plant development processes (including use of bioregulators and cellular approaches to plant breeding), improved nutrient uptake, greater resistance to environmental stresses, and protection from other biological systems.[2-4]

Three of these—photosynthesis, biological nitrogen fixation, and plant genetic manipulation—have been put together in a funable package.[5] The message is simple. For significant future progress in research for enhancement of food crop production in any one of the three areas, there must be a simultaneous input with programs for each of the other two. Progress in one is mutually dependent upon what happens with the other two. Special containment facilities for recombinant DNA may be required. Equipment needs must be met and manpower requirements outlined.

There is a second message: Improvements in photosynthesis, biological nitrogen fixation, and genetic materials, and greater recovery of applied fertilizers by crops would add to the resources of the earth, be nonpolitical, with no defined limits, and be non-polluting and without noise. Finally, all of the above technologies can potentially increase the energy influx/energy outflux ratio in the production of food. Agriculture is basically a solar energy processing machine, the efficiency of which could be greatly improved with modest research investments in these basic biological processes that control productivity.

The future of the world's food supply and much of the energy rests squarely at the door of photosynthesis and subsequent partitioning into harvested parts. It is a travesty of all times that with the billions of dollars currently being expended in the U.S. on energy research scarcely $10 million can be accounted for with photosynthesis or biological solar energy conversion. The relative simplicity of the approach belies its credibility!

There is another grossly neglected researchable area in food production and delivery. It relates to the effects of changing climatic and weather patterns on agricultural productivity and what can be done about them.[4] Weather and climate are still the most determinate factors in food production. We should no longer ignore the potential, through research, for precipitation enhancement and the alleviation of droughts in the corn belt and for making our crops more climate proof.

The collection, preservation, and utilization of genetic materials of food crops are vital for alleviation of genetic, climatic, and chemical vulnerability.

Remarkable progress in food crop productivity has been achieved through genetic manipulations utilizing standard plant-breeding techniques. These techniques have provided the means for crop improvement in the past, constitute the chief approaches today, and will likely predominate for the foreseeable future. They have ranged from selection based on phenotypic expression, to the management of food crop gene pools, controlled hybridization, and heterosis identification of the genetics of yield components, including plant architecture, yield physiology, biochemistry; and finally selection for super nutritional qualities. Great progress has been made with maize, rice, wheat, sorghum, millet, barley, and some legumes.

There are still many frontiers with food crops for greatly improved production efficiency, and improvement of nutritional factors. Cassava and sweet potatoes are basic sources of energy for over 400 million calorie-deficient people in Africa, South America, Asia, and the Far East. Developmental programs with cassava and sweet potatoes, for the tropics, are only 5–8 years old. Cassava is now in a position similar to that of wheat and rice prior to the spectacular yield increases ushered in with the green revolution. There are many other undeveloped tropical food plants.

Improvement programs are just beginning for most of the seed legumes—chick-peas, cowpeas, pigeon peas, mung beans, and dry field beans. They are all soil-improving crops.

Oil crops deserve special mention. Cottonseed oil accounts for 10 percent of the world's edible oil. A milestone that yet remains to be exploited was the development of a glandless variety free of gossypol. The recent introduction of the F_1 hybrid cotton in India provides a crop that is labor intensive with twice the productive capacity of ordinary cotton. Soybean oil accounts for $\frac{1}{3}$ of the world's edible vegetable oils. The residue approximates $\frac{1}{2}$ of the world's oil seed meal production. Any significant breakthrough for increasing productivity of soybeans would profoundly affect the food and feed industry of the U.S. and the world. The sunflower is becoming an important source of edible oil. F_1 hybrids with superior yielding abilities have been developed. Seventy-five percent of the U.S. oilseed acreage was planted to hybrids in 1976. We had a half million hectares.

African oil palm has emerged as a major competitor for soybean, cottonseed, and sunflower. It will produce up to 5 tons per hectare per year of oil over a 20–30 year life span. This compares with 600–800 pounds of oil per hectare per year for soybeans. Palm oil imports have risen tenfold in 5 years. That used in shortenings and margarine approximated 11.5 percent during 1975.

Many indigenous high-protein and potentially important food crops have been neglected. Good examples are two legumes, each with built-in nitrogen sources. One is the pods and seeds of the desert mesquite; the other, the winged bean of the tropics. All plant parts of the winged bean may be harvested for human food.

Progress in raising levels of protein and critically deficient amino acids with cereal grains has been singular. Rice, wheat, and barley selections have been identified with higher protein levels. Both the biological value and the level of the protein of maize have been enhanced using the opaque-2-recessive gene, and, more recently, in corn of normal genetic background. Triticale, the new synthetic species, with its improved nutritional contributions, great adaptability, and high yields is now receiving limited commercial acceptance.

There is the strong suggestion that the world's food problem, from the standpoint of a balanced diet, is not one of protein deficiency but caloric adequacy. If sufficient calories are provided through conventional cereals and grain legumes, and the biological values of the proteins of these same crops are genetically upgraded, there would be no protein problem. Indeed, it has been demonstrated that much of the clinically observed "protein malnutrition" is the secondary consequence of a calorie inadequacy that occurs with people whose diets contain sufficient protein but which they are unable to assimilate when caloric uptake is inadequate. The dietary merits of a predominantly vegetarian diet based on use of new improved cereals and grain legumes should be experimentally evaluated.

Fertilizer manufacture is the most important industrial input into agricultural productivity. Yet, only 50 percent of the nitrogen and less than 35 percent of the phosphorus and potassium applied as fertilizer in the U.S.A. are recovered by crops. The recovery of fertilizer nitrogen in the rice paddies of tropics is only 25–35 percent. The balance is lost to the environment. Nitrogen is lost to the atmosphere by denitrification. Nitrification encourages losses in the soil from leaching. Food production could be greatly improved if these enormous losses, particularly of nitrogen, in the warm soils of the tropics could be only partially alleviated. Much of the loss of nitrogen occurs from bacteria-induced nitrification and subsequent denitrification. Both synthetic and natural nitrification inhibitors have been identified and are being introduced.

An important approach to better recovery of soil-applied fertilizer and also to increased crop productivity in marginal soils is a further microbiological one. In sharp contrast to the action of nitrifying bacteria, which greatly reduce fertilizer nitrogen utilization, other microorganisms—the mycorrhizae (specifically the endomycorrhizae)—may result in large increases in the uptake of phosphorus and other poorly mobile ions. Most all food crops respond. Mycorrhizae can be viewed as fungal extensions of root systems. There are super strains of mycorrhizae, and crops can be inoculated with them. Mycorrhizal fungi are known to increase yields of food crops by as much as 20–120 percent.

There is now great excitement after a dormancy of interest for 30 years as to the potential of non-root (foliar) absorption of nutrients. It comes from a remarkable increase in the productivity of soybeans when nutrients are sprayed on the foliage at appropriate developmental stages.

Losses of food from other biological systems have been estimated at one-third the total world harvest. Crop protection technology becomes obsolete at an alarming rate. Reasons include appearance of genetic resistance in many pest species, breakdown of natural control mechanisms (the average useful life of new crop variety is only 5 years), and ever more stringent regulations in chemical controls. Potentials ahead for protecting plant and animal resources include insect viruses and bacteria and juvenile hormones—so called third generation chemicals—that interfere with reproductive cycles. Egg and larvae parasites, pheromones, and resistant varieties are viable alternatives.

Allelopathy for weed control is an emerging technology. It is defined as mutual harm, where chemicals produced and released by one plant species inhibit the growth of another. There will still emerge new ways to fight pests with less chemical and energy inputs.

Bioregulators can be expected to have exciting impacts on agricultural productivity. They often duplicate genetic effects. There is new hope and interest in improvement of yields of agronomic crops prompted by the use of chemical ripeners that enhance sugar yields by as much as 10 percent on sugarcane. Better test methods and low-volume application will open new frontiers for useful application.

MANAGEMENT OF RESOURCES

Food adequacy is first one of calories or energy. Most protein deficiencies occur in parts of the world where caloric intake is short. Fossil energy, land (which is often equivalent to water in irrigated areas), and human labor are primary resources used for crop and livestock production. They are interrelated, and one can be partially interchanged or substituted for the others. The decrease in the output/input ratio resulting from new energy technologies in crop production in the U.S. has resulted in land freed from corn production to produce soybeans.

More efficient land, water, and energy use patterns can be designed. Examples include drip or trickle irrigation. This new system of water management has now been installed in excess of 65,000 hectares of high-value crops in the U.S., with a worldwide total of over 125,000. One quarter of a million hectares for the U.S. is projected for 1980.

Another example is reduced or zero tillage. For the U.S. corn belt, zero tillage has proven the most effective management practice ever developed for the control of wind and water erosion. It offers an improved system of land use for highly erodible and difficult to manage tropical soils. The technology conserves soil, water, energy, and soil organic matter.

Controlled environment agriculture offers stable production at high levels. Enclosed cropping effectively conserves water in arid lands and extends growing seasons in temperate latitudes. Year-round production is possible where only one crop per year is now produced. Enclosed atmospheres can also be enriched with CO_2. This will greatly enhance crop productivity. Associated with controlled environment agriculture is the Nutrient Film Technique. It is the first real breakthrough in a completely automated feeding system for the production of food crops. It eliminates evaporation losses from soil surfaces and drainage losses, and reduces transpiration losses. Controlled environment agriculture, however, is a food-producing system that demands a maximum of capital, management, and energy resources. Its economic viability for substantial contributions to world food needs has not been established.

It has been estimated that losses of energy and waste and effluent in food processing could be reduced by 35 and 80 percent, respectively. Food losses between harvest and consumption could be reduced by 30 to 50 percent. All this could increase the available food by 10–15 percent without more land or increasing yields. Annual production of crop and animal wastes in the U.S.A. exceeds 800 million tons of dry matter. The U.S. produces 1.2 billion pounds of seafood waste and 35 million tons of fruit and vegetable-processing wastes. Globally, approximately 150 pounds of cellulose is produced daily for each of the earth's 4 billion inhabitants. Economic incentives as well as inadequate technologies are not yet conducive to improved utilization of these vast resources in food production systems.

Forage and range production is not a direct food source for man, but indirectly provides a food supply for approximately 2.5 billion ruminant animals useful to man. It is technically and economically feasible to double this production. Land and water resources for forage production in the tropics are enormous. There are three distinct areas that extend from the Tropics of Cancer to Capricorn remarkably adapted for forage production—the lowlands, the high elevations and the Cerrada or Savannah. Tremendous productivity is possible in the tropics, with yields approaching 60 tons of dry matter/hectare/year. There are at least four frontiers of technology for improvement of forage crops for livestock: higher yielding types, increased nutritive values, improved harvest techniques, and the merger of production and utilization systems.

Livestock numbers of the earth are double the human population. Domestic animals produce meat, milk, and eggs from nutrients derived from crops, forages, and byproducts that have less value elsewhere. Food resources produced by animals fall into two categories: Those derived from ruminants (dairy, beef cattle, water buffalo, sheep, goats, llama, alpaca) and the monogastric (swine, poultry, guinea pig, rabbits). Ruminants provide foods of the highest quality from range and grassland, forages, plant byproducts, crop residues, and browse. Swine and poultry are providers of food derived from consumption of many products not edible by man. Animals serve as important sources of food, dietary improvement, income, power, fuel, and fertilizer. They also constitute a living food reservoir that exceeds the commercial reserves of grain and is far better distributed, not being concentrated in a few nations with surpluses.

Future strategy for enhancement of livestock productivity must include simultaneous emphasis in three interrelated and interdependent areas: better feeding, genetic improvement, and animal disease control. Little progress in better utilization of feeds can be achieved without timely inputs for disease control and genetic improvement. Similarly, research emphasis on improvement of animal health would be of little value unless accompanied by better feeding and incorporation of genetic resistance to disease. Again as with photosynthesis, nitrogen fixation, and cellular biology in food crops, progress in these three areas resulting in greater animal productivity would add to the resources of the earth and be sparing rather than demanding of non-renewable resources.

Finally, there are the new farming systems technologies—the most promising of all approaches for enhancement of the supply, dependability, and nutritional quality of our food, and also the most complex and difficult. Research management for farming systems is contrary to the traditional disciplinary approach. Special and expanded administrative skills are required. Future progress in increasing crop and livestock productivity from research must come from packages that articulate simultaneous efforts on several frontiers.

The number and array of subsystems at the farm level are enormous. There are diverse systems for land, water, energy, fertilizer, mechanization, labor, waste, pests, and climate. There are cropping systems, livestock systems, and tillage practices that bridge all the above resource systems. There are many alternative systems for managing beef cattle operations and dairy herds, and in the production of corn, cotton, soybeans, or sugar beets. Farming systems technologies must be broken down into local geographical and ecological areas, and to site-specific socioeconomic, institutional and political conditions.

Food systems must extend beyond the farm gate. There are diverse processing, handling, storage, transportation, packaging, and marketing systems. Domestic and international trade and port facilities are involved. There are regulatory inputs; taxation of inputs and products; availabilities of credit and subsidies; institutions to serve and create new technologies; a complex of public and private support; and an infrastructure to provide supplies and services—to supply food for people everywhere.

CONCLUSIONS

We are in the midst of an agricultural revolution, but we can record only the initial stages. Most of the dramatic developments in food production in the western world have occurred in this generation. Hybrid corn has been commercialized scarcely more than 40 years; grain sorghum only 20, and primarily in the U.S.A. Most scientific achievements for increased agricultural productivity have occurred during the past 20 years. Many have originated during the past 10 years. Dramatic changes have occurred in many agricultural and food events during the last 5 years (TABLE 1).

TABLE 1

MAJOR AGRICULTURAL AND FOOD EVENTS, UNITED STATES, 1971–76 *

Item	1971	1972	1973	1974	1975	1976 (est)
Set aside land (10^6 acres)	37	62	20	0	0	0
Grain stocks (10^6 metric tons)	51	69	42	31	27	33
Agricultural exports (10^9 $)	8.5	13	21	22	22	22
Prices paid by farmers for nitrogen ($\cent$/lb.)	4.8	4.9	5.4	11.2	16.2	11.6
Yields of corn (bu/acre)	88	97	91	71	86	86
Milk production per cow (10^3 pounds)	10.0	10.2	10.1	10.3	10.4	10.6
Price of corn ($/bu.)	1.08	1.57	2.55	3.03	2.55	2.30
Price of wheat ($/bu.)	1.34	1.76	3.95	4.09	3.52	3.00
Price of soybeans ($/bu.)	3.03	4.37	5.68	6.64	5.00	6.25
Price of sugar, U.S. raw duty paid equivalent, N.Y. ($\cent$/lb.)	8.5	9.1	10.3	29.5	22.5	15.0
Wholesale price index of fuels and related products and power (1967=100)	114	119	134	208	245	261
Income for food (%)	16.4	16.3	16.3	17.0	17.1	16.7
Enrollments, colleges of agriculture (10^3 students)	60	65	73	82	91	98
Gross agricultural income (10^9 $)	61	70	95	100	98	105
Federal funding of agricultural food and nutrition research						
Cooperative State Research Service (payments to states)	60	63	67	68	85	98
Agricultural Research Service	179	192	208	205	224	251

* Data provided with the assistance of John N. Ferris, Professor of Agricultural Economics, Michigan State University.

Modern food production technology has touched only a few geographical areas and commodities. Major food crops such as seed legumes, sweet potato, cassava, the millets, and most fruits and vegetables have received thus far only token attention. Modern technologies adapted for small-scale agricultural units are noticeably lacking. No one has yet designed for enhancement of livestock production a fundable research strategy for simultaneous efforts in better feeding, genetic improvement, and disease control. The greatest of all opportunities abroad may reside with farming systems that are labor intensive, scale neutral, with stable production at high levels and those that require a minimum of resource, capital, and management inputs.

REFERENCES

1. MICHIGAN AGRICULTURAL EXPERIMENT STATION & CHARLES F. KETTERING FOUNDA-
   TION. 1976. Crop Productivity—Research Imperatives, Proceedings of an International Symposium. 399 pp. East Lansing, Mich.
2. WITTWER, S. H. 1977. Increased Crop Yields and Livestock Productivity, *In* World Food Prospects and Agricultural Potential. The Hudson Institute. N.Y., N.Y.
3. NATIONAL ACADEMY OF SCIENCES. 1975. Agricultural Production Efficiency. Board on Agricultural and Renewable Resources of the Commission on Natural Resources, National Research Council. 199 pp. Washington, D.C.
4. NATIONAL ACADEMY OF SCIENCES. 1975. Enhancement of Food Production for the United States. World Food and Nutrition Study. Board on Agriculture and Renewable Resources of the Commission on Natural Resources, National Research Council. 174 pp. Washington, D.C.
5. OFFICE OF TECHNOLOGY ASSESSMENT. 1976. Assessment of Alternatives for Supporting High Priority Basic Research to Enhance Food Production. U.S. Congress. Washington, D.C.

ENERGY RESOURCES AND LAND CONSTRAINTS IN FOOD PRODUCTION

David Pimentel

*New York State College of
Agriculture and Life Sciences
Cornell University
Ithaca, New York 14853*

For 990,000 years of the more than one million years that humans have been on earth, the total population of the United States numbered less than 200,000 (about the population of Providence, Rhode Island). During this period people were hunter-gatherers and were exclusively dependent on solar energy for food. Each hunter-gatherer needed about 10 square kilometers of the natural ecosystem to sustain his needs. Using this type of food system, a maximum population of about 750,000 (about the population of Boston, Massachusetts) could be supported in the United States.

As population numbers increased above 750,000 many years ago, people were forced to turn to simple "slash and burn" agriculture. In "slash and burn" or "cut and burn" agriculture, the trees and shrubs are cut and burned on-site to let the sun in, kill weeds, and add nutrients to the soil. Crop production on the cleared land is adequate for about 2 years before soil nutrients are depleted by the plantings. After the depletion of soil nutrients, it takes about 20 years for the regrowth of the forest and shrubs and renewal of soil nutrients. Using "cut and burn," a maximum population of 10 million could be supported in the United States.

"Cut and burn" crop technology required only an ax and hoe, which were initially made of stone, later of metal. Obviously, this type of agriculture requires large inputs of human labor. For example, in a section of Mexico where "cut and burn" corn culture was investigated, a total of 1,144 hours of labor was required to raise a hectare of corn (TABLE 1). The yield of 1,944 kg/ha provided a yearly food supply for about four persons eating primarily vegetables and grains. If instead of the vegetarian diet, the family desired the high-protein/calorie diet of the United States today, then about 4,000 hours of labor using "cut and burn" technology would be required to feed the family of four.

Energy use is essential to U.S. food production because of the food-land-population equation. The current high-protein/calorie diet of the U.S. requires about 0.5 hectare (1.3 acres) of cropland and 1.2 hectares (3 acres) of pastureland per person. From our agricultural land we must produce 4,800 kg of grain, 114 kg (250 lbs) of meat, 129 kg of milk, 285 eggs, and a quantity of fruits and vegetables per person per year. Energy inputs in the form of fertilizers, pesticides, etc., are essential if this much food is to be produced from the available crop and pastureland in the United States.

In the United States today, with our high-energy technology, about 350 hours of labor is devoted to producing, processing, and distributing food (assuming 17% of one's income is for food). The use of fossil energy in the U.S.

high-energy-intensive food system substitutes for the work of more than 79,000 man-hours * or more than 30 times our current labor input.

The work of 10 persons is about the equivalent of 1 horsepower-hour (hp-h). One hp-h is defined as the ability to do 22,000 foot-pounds of work per minute for 1 hour, which is based on the ability of an average horse to do 22,000 foot-pounds of work per minute for a 10-hour day. One hp-h of work is equal to 641.56 kcal. A person working a 10-hour day can produce an equivalent of nearly 1 hp-h or about ⅒th of the work of a horse, or put another way, one horse can accomplish the work of 10 persons.

Fossil fuels (petroleum, natural gas, coal) represent a tremendous concentration of energy and ability to do work. For example, from a gallon of gasoline (36,000 kcal) used to operate a mechanical engine, we can obtain 7200 kcal of work (assuming 20% efficiency in converting heat to mechanical energy). This is the equivalent of 11.2 hp-h of work. Hence, a single gallon of gasoline has the work equivalent of 1 horsepower for an 11-hour day or about 11 men for one 11-hour day. In other words, one gallon of gasoline produces the equivalent work of a person working an 8-hour day, 5 days a week, for 3 weeks!

TABLE 1

ENERGY INPUTS IN CORN PRODUCTION IN MEXICO USING ONLY MANPOWER *

Input	Quantity/ha		kcal/ha
Labor	1,144	hrs	
Ax & hoe	16,500	kcal	16,500
Seeds	10.4	kg	36,608
Total			53,108
Corn yield	1,944	kg	6,842,880
kcal return/kcal input			128.8
Protein yield	175	kg	

* After Pimentel.[19]

The use of fossil fuels enables us to produce food on limited land, improve public health, and provide other services we desire for our comfort. During the past two decades the consumption of fossil energy supplies has been increasing faster than population numbers. For example, while the U.S. population doubled during the past 60 years, its energy consumption doubled within the past 20 years. More alarming is the fact that while the world population about doubled its numbers during the past 30 years, its energy consumption doubled in the past decade. Since our world population is currently 4 billion and there seems to be no way to prevent it from reaching 6–7 billion during the next 25 years, the effect this growth will have on energy supplies is cause for concern (FIGURE 1).

The energy used in food production has been increasing faster than energy use in many sectors of the world economy. For example, energy inputs in U.S.

* About 330 gal of fuel equivalents is employed to produce per capita food. Assume 20% efficiency of converting this fossil energy into work—hence 79,000 man-hours.

corn production have more than *tripled* since 1945.[1] By 1970 the total amount of fossil energy used to grow a hectare of corn averaged about 660 liters of fuel (TABLE 2). Since 1945, the quantity of energy used for the production of nitrogen fertilizer has risen sharply because of increased nitrogen use to increase crop yield. In 1970 the energy input for nitrogen fertilizer about equalled the total energy inputs for corn production in 1945. At present, the energy inputs of nitrogen plus machinery and fuel total almost two-thirds of all the energy inputs in corn production.

Using energy-intensive production techniques, the return in food energy per input of fossil fuel energy is about 2.7 (TABLE 2). In contrast, raising corn

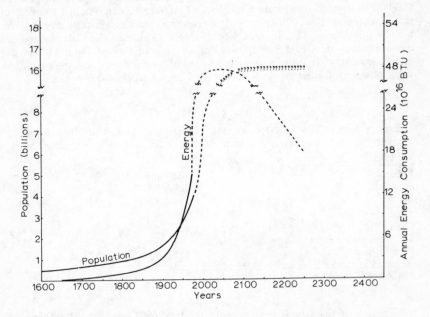

FIGURE 1. Estimated world population numbers (———) from 1600 to 1975 and projected numbers (- - - - -)(?????) to the year 2250. Estimated fossil fuel consumption (———) from 1650 to 1975 and projected (- - - - -) to the year 2250. (After Pimentel *et al*.[5])

by hand (cut and burn) gives a return of 129:1, or about 50 times greater (TABLE 1). Based on current economic values, however, U.S. corn production profits are greater from corn produced with large inputs of today's cheap fossil fuels than from corn produced by expensive human labor.

Although we have been emphasizing the use of fossil energy in crop production, the solar energy input is far greater than the fossil energy inputs. During the growing season about 5 billion kcal (about 500,000 liters of gasoline equivalents) of light energy reaches 1 hectare of corn.[2] The corn plant captures 1.26% of this light energy reaching the field. Therefore, about 90% solar energy and only 10% fossil energy are used in U.S. corn production today. Fossil energy is a nonrenewable resource, so our concern is with the 10%.

TABLE 2

ENERGY INPUTS IN U.S. CORN PRODUCTION (in kcal/ha)*

Input	1945	1970
Machinery	539,000	1,078,000
Fuel	1,400,000	2,060,000
Nitrogen	121,440	1,897,500
Phosphorus	25,600	112,000
Potassium	13,200	147,400
Seeds for planting	77,440	147,840
Irrigation	103,740	187,000
Insecticides	0	82,790
Herbicides	0	82,790
Drying	9,880	296,400
Electricity	39,500	380,000
Transportation	49,400	172,900
Total inputs	2,379,200	6,644,220
Corn yield (output)	7,504,640	17,881,600
kcal return/kcal input	3.15	2.69

* After Pimentel.[19]

U.S. energy accounting is complicated by the fact that most of our corn and other cereal grains is fed to livestock. Of the estimated 1,000 kg of grain per capita produced in the United States, only about 100 kg is consumed directly by humans.[3, 4] Most of the cereal grains are fed to livestock. The livestock population in the United States outweighs the human population by more than fourfold (FIGURE 2), and the per capita animal protein consumption is one of the highest in the world. In 1974, annual per capita meat consumption was 114 kg (250 lb) or about 312 g of meat per day.[4] Beef consumption amounted to 53 kg; pork, 30 kg; chicken and turkey, 23 kg; fish, 6 kg; and veal and lamb, 2 kg. Per capita milk and milk product consumption was 129 kg, and an average of 285 eggs were consumed.[4]

The conversion of vegetable protein to animal protein has substantial "costs."

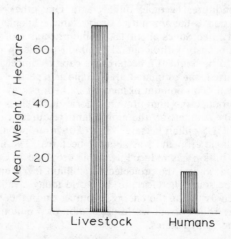

FIGURE 2. Livestock biomass significantly outweighs human biomass in the United States.[5]

Thus, about 5 kg of grain and fish protein are fed to livestock (plus a large amount of forage) to produce 1 kg of animal protein,[5] or translated into energy inputs, about 10 times as much fossil energy is used to produce a unit of animal protein as to produce a unit of plant protein. One of the highest energy costs is for beef protein produced under feed-lot conditions, which requires about 78 kcal of fossil energy per kcal of beef protein.[5] In milk protein production, 36 kcal of fossil energy is expended per kcal of milk protein. For egg protein, the ratio is 13:1.

Yearly in the U.S. about 6 million metric tons of animal protein is produced by feeding an estimated 26 million metric tons of plant and animal protein to animals.[5] If only grass-fed livestock were produced, livestock protein production would decline from 6 to an estimated 2 million metric tons. (This assumes an effective shift in animal protein consumption from swine and poultry, which cannot be grass-fed, to more milk, beef, lamb, and goat.)

Therefore, based on the specific high energy costs of our high-protein/ calorie diet, plus needs of our energy-intensive food production, processing, distribution, and preparation systems, an estimated 15% of the energy utilized in our economy is used in the food system. Compared with the energy costs of other sectors of our economy, 15% may not appear much, but in gasoline equivalents this is about 1,250 liters per capita per year, or a total of 262 billion liters annually.

If we were to feed the current world population of 4 billion on a U.S. diet employing U.S. food system technology, the energy requirement would be 5,000 billion liters of fuel annually. To estimate the energy needs of the future, let us assume the use of known petroleum reserves solely for food—none for transportation, heating, or cooling. Then our known reserves could feed 4 billion people for a mere 13 years.[5] Unfortunately, we are faced not only with the need to supply food for 6 to 7 billion people by the year 2000, but also with the energy needs of diverse sectors of the world economy other than those involved in food production.

Today an estimated 25% of the world's energy (including wood) is used for the food system.[6] Based on the projection of population growth, we estimate that current energy inputs in the food system will have to be increased threefold if the food needs of the human population are to be met.

Thus, the interdependence of food supply, population numbers, and energy expenditures becomes quite clear. One other vital, interrelated factor in this equation is the amount of arable land available for agricultural production. In the United States about 160 million hectares of arable land currently is planted with crops. With about 212 million people in the United States, this averages out to be about 0.7 hectare per capita. Since about 20% of our crop yield is exported, the estimated arable land per person drops to about 0.5 hectare (1.2 acres). This amount of land plus a high-energy agricultural technology are used to produce the high-protein/calorie diet that is consumed in the United States.

By comparison the arable land resources of the world are estimated to be about 1.5 billion hectares. In 1650 with a population of 500 million, per capita available cropland was about 2 hectares. The increase in the world population to 4 billion has reduced available cropland to about 0.4 hectare (0.9 acre) per capita; and at the projected 6–7 billion level, only 0.2 hectare will be available per person. Therefore, in the world today, available arable land is not sufficient (even assuming the energy resources and other technology were also available) to feed the current world population of 4 billion a diet similar to that consumed in the United States.

Arable land resources might be expanded to about 15% of land area (2.0 billion hectares) without great costs and effort. If marshlands are drained, some arid land is irrigated, and other lands are altered by technological inputs, the physical potential of land that might be cultivated is about 25% or 3.4 billion hectares.[7, 8] At a population density of 16 billion that might be the maximum, land satisfactory for cultivation per capita would only be 0.1 hectare. Thus, on a worldwide basis, land suitable for cultivation is an important constraint.

The 0.1 hectare per capita assumes no degradation of the land. Unfortunately, arable land is being degraded at an alarming rate. For example, in the United States from 1945 to 1970 over 29 million hectares has been lost to highways and urbanization, about half of which had been cropland.[9, 10] Another estimated 80 million hectares has been either totally ruined for crop production by soil erosion or so seriously eroded that it is only marginally suitable for production.[11-13] In developing countries the rate at which land is lost due to soil erosion is estimated to be nearly twice that in the United States.[14]

Erosion seriously reduces the productivity of land. The rate of soil erosion per hectare of cropland in the United States is estimated at 27 metric tons annually.[15, 16] This relatively high rate of soil erosion has resulted in removing at least one-third of the topsoil of cropland in use today.[17]

The reduced productivity of U.S. cropland due to soil erosion has had to be offset by increased quantities of fossil energy in the form of fertilizers and other inputs.[16] An estimated 47 liters of fuel equivalents per hectare is being used to offset the soil erosion loss on U.S. cropland.[13]

Soil erosion also degrades reservoirs, rivers, and lakes by depositing annually about 1.4 billion metric tons in these water bodies.[18] Soil sediments, the associated nutrients (N, P, K, etc.), and pesticides have an ecological effect upon stream fauna and flora.[13]

Certainly the next 25 years will be crucial for humanity. Land resources are limited; fossil energy, a finite resource, is dwindling rapidly; food shortages already exist; and to compound the problem human numbers are growing rapidly. Advances in science and technology should help us overcome some problems, but the real solution to most of the shortages and problems facing humanity is effective control of human numbers. If we do not control our numbers, nature will.

REFERENCES

1. PIMENTEL, D., L. E. HURD, A. C. BELLOTTI, M. J. FORSTER, I. N. OKA, O. D. SHOLES & R. J. WHITMAN. 1973. Food production and the energy crisis. Science **182**: 443–449.
2. TRANSEAU, E. N. 1926. The accumulation of energy by plants. Ohio J. Sci. **26**: 1–10.
3. USDA. 1974. Agricultural Statistics. U.S. Dept. Agr. Gov. Print. Off. Washington, D.C.
4. USDA. 1975. National Food Situation. U.S. Dept. Agr. Econ. Res. Serv. NFS-151.
5. PIMENTEL, D., W. DRITSCHILO, J. KRUMMEL & J. KUTZMAN. 1975. Energy and land constraints in food-protein production. Science **190**: 754–761.
6. PIMENTEL, D. *et al.* 1975. Unpublished manuscript.
7. KOVDA, V. A. 1971. The problem of biological and economic productivity of the earth's land areas. Soviet Geogr.: Rev. Trans. **12**(1): 6–23. *In* Land and Water. A. Orvedal & D. Peterson. Natl. Acad. Sci. Draft Rept. Study Team 4B.

8. Buringh, P., H. D. J. Van Heemst & G. J. Staring. 1975. Computation of the Absolute Maximum Food Production of the World. Agr. Univ., Dept. Trop. Soil Sci. (Wageningen).
9. USDA. 1971. Agriculture and the Environment. U.S. Dept. Agr. Econ. Res. Serv. No. 481.
10. USDA. 1974. Our Land and Water Resources, Current and Prospective Supplies and Uses. U.S. Dept. Agr. Econ. Res. Serv. Misc. Publ. No. 1290.
11. USNRB. 1935. Soil Erosion—a Critical Problem in American Agriculture. U.S. Natural Resources Board, Land Planning Comm. Suppl. Rept.
12. Bennett, H. H. 1939. Soil Conservation. McGraw-Hill. New York.
13. Pimentel, D., E. C. Terhune, R. Dyson-Hudson, S. Rochereau, R. Samis, E. A. Smith, D. Denman, D. Reifschneider & M. Shepard. 1976. The effects of land degradation on food and energy resources. Science 194: 149–155.
14. Ingraham, E. W. 1975. A Query into the Quarter Century. On the Interrelationships of Food, People, Environment, Land and Climate. Wright-Ingraham Inst., Colorado Springs, Colo.
15. Wadleigh, C. H. 1968. Wastes in Relation to Agriculture and Forestry. U.S. Dept. Agr. Misc. Pub. 1065.
16. Hargrove, T. R. 1972. Agricultural research: impact on environment. Spec. Rept. 69, Agr. & Home Econ. Exp. Sta., Iowa State Univ. Sci. & Technol. Ames, Iowa.
17. Handler, P., Ed. 1970. Biology and the Future of Man. National Academy of Sciences. Oxford University Press. New York.
18. USDA. 1968. A National Program of Research for Environmental Quality. Pollution in Relation to Agriculture and Forestry. Report, USDA Research Program Development and Evaluation Staff. Washington, D.C.
19. Pimentel, D. 1976. The energy crisis: its impact on agriculture. In Enciclopedia della Scienza e della Tecnica, Annuario della EST. Mondadori, Milan.

THE WATER POTENTIAL OF THE ARID ZONE

Joel R. Gat

Department of Isotope Research
Weizmann Institute of Science
Rehovot, Israel

INTRODUCTION

A desert is defined as an arid area, with insufficient moisture to support widespread vegetation.* In the context of the present conference, Meigs' definition of the arid zone as an area in which rainfall is not adequate for regular crop production [1] seems most relevant. Emphasis is on the inadequacy and irregularity of rainfall on the one hand and on the lack of regular or widespread natural vegetation, on the other. However, when water sources such as groundwater or river water are available for irrigation an oasis may be formed in the arid zone; from the ecological point of view such an area is then anything but arid and hostile.

There are widespread desert areas with suitable soils and plenty of sunshine which could be transformed into flowering oases, provided that water for irrigation is available. This paper addresses itself to the availability of water resources in the desert for such a purpose. One should, of course, also consider the importation of water from outside the arid zone or the desalinization of sea or brackish waters; the problems that arise then are predominantly economical rather than hydrologic and beyond the scope of this review.

DESERT WATER SOURCES

As all desert dwellers know there are a variety of water sources in the desert: water holes in the bottom of dry riverbeds, seasonal springs issuing from crevices in rocky areas, shallow groundwater beneath the sands which at times drains uselessly into depressions to evaporate and form salinas. Here and there, gushing perennial springs transform the arid landscape into a local paradise. Moreover, deeper drillings (often performed for the sake of oil exploration) have struck water at varying depths. Notable is the widespread occurrence of potable water in the sandstone formation of the North African, Egyptian, and Negev deserts.

Another important source of water is the sporadic flash floods that are one of the surprising and impressive features of the desert hydrology. By diversion, damming, and storing of this water, modern and ancient desert dwellers skillfully augmented their precarious water supply. Justly famous are the surface flow-control systems of the Nabateans,[2] which have been copied in modern times for impressive achievements in irrigated agriculture.[3]

These desert water sources suffice for the domestic needs of a sparse popula-

---

* *Random House Dictionary of the English Language.* This definition excludes alpine and high-latitude deserts from the discussion, where low temperature rather than lack of moisture are to blame for the absence of a vegetation cover.

tion * on a primitive level, for drinking water of cattle and domestic animals, and for limited irrigation of local vegetable patches and small orchards of fruit trees. Larger scale agriculture based on local water sources can be found in association with the larger spring systems, such as in the oases of Jericho and of Palmyra, or based on wells that tap deep aquifers, such as in the Arava Valley in the Negev or the New Valley project in the Western Desert.[4] Irrigation programs that are based on a river flowing through the arid zone (e.g., in the Nile Valley or the Imperial Valley of California) do not, *sensum strictum*, belong to this discussion.

The average water requirement for growing one crop under arid conditions (based on the climate of the Negev Desert) is given as between 0.5–1.0 m^3/ yr·m^2 (G. Stanhill, private communication), equivalent to a water depth of 500–1000 mm. When one then intends to use the local groundwater sources for irrigated agriculture (or large-scale domestic and industrial use), two related questions arise: How large are the available (exploitable) quantities? Are these waters replenished or do they represent fossil sources? Other questions relevant to their use as irrigation waters concern the salinity and water quality in general.

ORIGIN OF THE DESERT GROUNDWATERS AND RECHARGE ROUTES

A direct meteoric origin of groundwater seems improbable at first sight, since the amount of precipitation in the desert is insufficient for even wetting the soil enough to nurture a plant cover. In the semiarid zones at similar latitudes it is accepted that only precipitation amounts in excess of a certain minimal value can drain through the soil column and recharge the groundwaters. Smaller rain amounts are predominantly intercepted by the soil cover and used up by the transpiring plants. The minimum amount depends on the climate condition, the type of vegetation, distribution of rainfall, and in particular the season of rain (winter rains are more effective in recharge than rains falling during the period of peak moisture demand). For northern Israel a value of 360 mm, on the average, has been established[5] and can serve as a guideline.

The arid zone boundary is usually drawn in the midlatitudes around an isohyet of less than 350 mm. More conservative authors take 100 mm as the arid zone boundary.[6] In most of the desert areas discussed here the annual precipitation is as little as 50 mm, with as large fluctuations in the yearly rain amounts. Under desert conditions, then, recharge would be expected to be minimal, and groundwater of meteoric origin should be a rarity. Yet groundwater sources are widespread, if not plentiful.

The frequent occurrence of desert water sources and oases in low-lying depressions and in dry riverbeds (wadis) suggested an indirect recharge mechanism through the intermediacy of floodflows; flash floods in desert wadis are a quite common feature of desert hydrology. It has indeed been suggested by

---

* Actually, the availability of water is the limiting factor that determines the natural population density; larger population centers that can nowadays be found in the desert areas for the sake of oil or mineral exploitation, as tourist sites, harbor facilities, or for political and miltary reasons, must rely to a great extent on "expensive" water sources, such as the desalinization of seawater, or on freshwater brought in by overland trucking or pipes.

Schoeller [7] and others [8] that recharge through wadi beds is the dominant mechanism of groundwater recharge under desert conditions. The origin of other desert groundwater was claimed to be outside the desert region proper, on mountainous fringe areas with more abundant rainfall.[9]

The geographic association with wadis seems, however, on closer scrutiny, to be an insufficient guide as to the nature of the recharge route; in many instances water sources located in riverbeds are fed by larger regional aquifers or conduits which happen to be exposed in the river bed as a result of its cutting through the terrain. The oasis in Wadi Feiran in the Sinai Desert is one such case where recharge does not primarily occur from the occasional floodflow in that wadi.[10]

In the arid zone piezometric data and subsurface geological information are usually insufficient to establish the boundaries and flow characteristics of aquifer systems. Isotopic dating and tracing methods [11] have then been a major source of information. In particular, the distinction between recent (local) and fossil or distant water sources can be made on the basis of dating with the help of the tritium and ^{14}C content of the waters.

In a study that utilizes these techniques for the characterization of water sources in the Sinai Desert,[10] we found a wide spectrum of ages. On the young end of the time scale were springs emerging from the igneous rock complex, many of these at topographically elevated sites, so that a local origin by direct rain infiltration on the outcrops of these rocks is indicated. Other young waters are shallow aquifers in wadi beds where direct recharge from surface flows occurs. In sand dune areas surface flows cannot happen, and the fact that the groundwaters are young is evidence for direct imbibition on the sandy surface. Similar evidence for widespread occurrence of recent recharge (through the utilization of tritium analysis) has been presented for the case of the Sahara,[12] where direct intake of water takes place through thick sand layers, up to 10 m deep, or through exposures of limestone. The same is true for the case of the Kalahari Desert.[13]

On the other end of the time scale (>10,000 years) are fossil water sources in Nubian sandstone formations (dubbed paleowaters), which appear to have been recharged during a period of less arid climate in the last stages of the Pleistocene. In other desert areas, e.g., the Northern Sahara, waters of old age are not necessarily fossil but may be related to rain-recharged aquifer systems from faraway areas, for example in the Atlas Mountains. In these cases the age is an indication of a lengthy underground route.

Both the occurrence of flash floods and the widespread groundwater recharge following small rain events are surprising anomalies when judged by the yardsticks of the hydrology of temperature climate zones. These phenomena can be explained by the absence of a plant and soil cover, in itself a result of aridity. Rainwaters run off the surface of bare rocks and impermeable loess layers or infiltrate into exposed cracks and into the loosely structured sand cover. Recharge by means of fractured rocks actually takes place through a combination of local surface flows and infiltration processes from local depression. In the absence of deep-rooted plants that would pump back (transpire) the infiltrated waters, any water that manages to penetrate to a depth of a few tens of centimeters may escape reevaporation and drain downward with great rapidity. Under arid conditions the field capacity of the top layer is small (N. K. Guirski, in Schoeller [7]), and apparently the finer grained material, whose holding capacity is larger, is bypassed in the recharge process.[14]

The relative contribution of the direct rain infiltration route compared to that occurring through the intermediary of surface flows is difficult to establish. One normally distinguishes between surface waters and precipitation [15] on the basis of the enrichment of the heavy isotopic species (^{18}O and deuterium) in surface waters subject to evaporative water loss; in contrast the isotopic composition is invariant in waters of the soil column (water loss from the soil through evapotranspiration does not fractionate between stable isotopes). Under desert conditions such a distinction was found difficult to apply.[10] Apparently, there is little evaporation during the course of a flash flood; conversely, there appears to be some enrichment of the heavy isotopes in rainwater as it percolates through sand [16] as a result of vapor transport through the wide pores of the sandy layers. To distinguish between the two recharge mechanisms we have then to fall back on age determinations (groundwaters recharged through regional subsurface drainage network are older than those fed locally through the wadi bottom) and on direct measurement of the hydraulic response of the groundwater to the flood event. As already stated, there is evidence that both recharge mechanisms occur.

The isotopic and dating methods give less ambiguous information concerning the origin of fossil water sources or those originating in faraway geographic localities. The stable isotope composition of paleowaters is radically different from the present-day precipitation. More depleted in the heavy isotopes in all cases,[17] its isotope composition stands out relative to the meteoric waters in the eastern Mediterranean area due to its position on the $d = 10‰$ meteoric water line.[15] These findings are interpreted as evidence for recharge having occurred during a period with less arid climate conditions.

QUANTITIES OF WATER AVAILABLE IN THE DESERT

Whereas one can in most cases specify the origin and nature of waters found in the arid zone, there are almost no reliable data on the quantitative aspects. We have to consider the yields of surface flows and efficiency of groundwater recharge as well as the size of fossil groundwater reserves. The surface sources are most immediately available, whereas access to deep fossil reserves may be difficult to achieve and require expensive drilling operations. On the other hand, the latter will be the most stable supplies, as surface flows are most fickle. Spottiness (in time and space) is a basic characteristic of desert precipitation,[18] and the recurring lengthy periods of "no rainfall" contribute as much as the low mean annual precipitation amounts to the aridity. As an example one recalls the years-long droughts in the Brazilian Nordeste and in the Sahel. Consequently, any permanent agricultural development based on surface flows requires availability of standby groundwater resources or water-storage reservoirs.

The runoff yield in the Negev Desert has been estimated by Hillel [19] to be about 5% under favorable conditions. The agricultural value of this runoff is in the areal concentration into smaller plots in which sufficient water depth for crop production can be achieved. The natural runoff process, as exploited and channeled by the ancients, enabled crops to be grown on 1:20 to 1:30 of appropriate desert areas.[20] Modern inducement of runoff by artificial treatment of surfaces [19] is claimed to yield up to 80% of the precipitation in small-scale experimental plots: "The importance of runoff inducement is possibly greater than the mere increase in total runoff yield which it may produce. Effective inducement of runoff can also lower the runoff threshold, that is, the minimal rainstorm needed to start runoff. This decrease of the threshold may correspondingly increase the probability of obtaining adequate runoff a sufficient number of times during the season and thus effectively decrease the incidence of drought." [19]

It is difficult to establish the possible scale of runoff farming, since no widespread surveys of soil and surface conditions suitable for such an application have been performed. Undoubtedly, the practicality of such schemes decreases with decreasing rain intensity. At a precipitation level of about 100 mm/yr (where under optimal conditions a 1:10 ratio of cultivated to runoff area would be required for modern crop requirements), the scheme may not be too attractive from an economic point of view; where precipitation exceeds 250 mm annually, one can foresee a considerable potential for this method.

Guirsky (in Schoeller [7]) has estimated an average annual groundwater recharge rate of 1–2 mm for the world's deserts, with somewhat higher values along riverbeds, in which recharge rates of 10 mm/yr have been claimed. A similarly low value of recharge of 1 mm/yr was estimated by Kafri in the central Sinai from drainage measurements.[21] These estimates appear too low to supply the known desert water sources. Dincer et al.[16] interpreted the tritium profiles measured in the sand dunes of Saudi Arabia in terms of an infiltration rate of 20 mm annually for a total precipitation of 70 mm, ca. a 30% yield. There seem to be no corresponding estimates for the recharge rates in the rocky terrain. In both cases, however, recharge is most effective following an occasional heavy shower.

From quite general considerations it follows that the recharge to groundwaters through the intermediary of floodflows is less effective: taking a liberally high figure of 10% for the streamflow yield and supposing all this water to infiltrate, then this recharge route falls behind the 30% imbibition efficiency of sandy areas. Actually, the groundwater recharge along a riverbed is much less than 100%, owing to direct evaporation from the wet soil and the evapotranspiration by vegetation that grows along the riverbeds because of the more steady supply of water. The annual water loss in such a well-watered riverbed has been found to be 920 mm,[22] 68% of this due to transpiration.

The largest water reserves in the desert are fossil water sources. Issar et al.[21] estimated the quantities stored in the Nubian sandstone aquifer beneath parts of the Negev and Sinai at several hundred billion cubic meters (10^{12} m^3). These waters appear under confined conditions at depths of up to 1000 m. Similar aquifers of pluvial origin have been discovered under large parts of the North African, Libyan, and Egyptian deserts.[4] The present rate of replenishment of the Negev-Sinai aquifer (through the outcrops of the sandstone formations in the central Sinai) has been estimated by Issar [21] to be very small, of the order of 10^6 m^3/year. Any exploitation beyond this recharge rate must be considered a "mining" operation. How much of these waters can be extracted in an economical way is not well known. Issar gave a conservative figure of $20 \cdot 10^6$ m^3/yr over a period of 30 years, based on the storativity of the aquifer. Figures that are one to two orders of magnitude higher would deplete the reservoir by only 10%, and may be technically feasible in the future.

In the final analysis it is found that flood diversion techniques, direct groundwater recharge, and the pumpage of fossil water sources can each contribute about equal quantities, based on unit area of desert land. As a very rough estimate, appropriate for the Negev and Sinai deserts below the 100 mm isohyet line, it would be possible to bring about 1% of the total desert area under regular crop production. In an area where flood diversion or continuous deep aquifer exploitation is feasible, it may be possible locally to cultivate to the order of 10% of the land. The pumped waters are expected to have an advantage due to the greater reliability of continuous supply. All these figures must be viewed as quite tentative and not based on any cost analysis.

WATER QUALITY, SALINITY AND LONG-RANGE PROBLEMS

The problem of water and irrigation in the arid zone is not only one of quantity but also of salinity.[23] Owing to the slow rate of water movement (long contact times) and the reevaporation of most of the waters within the desert areas and the absence of flushing, the desert water sources accumulate salts to varying degrees and often beyond levels acceptable for normal agricultural use. Even surface floods are often surprisingly saline, e.g., in the Brazilian Nordeste,[24] because of the dissolution of salt accumulations near the surface. The paleowaters, in particular, show chloride concentrations in excess of 500 mg/l.

Agricultural usage of such waters requires suitable crops and soil conditions. Over the years the accumulation of salts in the top soil may endanger further use of the land. Moreover, the exploitation of fossil paleowater sources is necessarily possible only over a limited time period; an estimate of 30–50 years has been given.[21] During such a period, plans for alternative and fresher water sources must be made to make up for decaying water sources and to counteract (by flushing of the soil) the effect of salinity accumulations. The native water sources of the desert can give short-range solutions for the development of agriculture, but imported or treated waters have to be provided in the not too distant future.

Possible changes in microclimate and of precipitation patterns due to the process of aforestation and verdanization have been discussed. Charney[25] has speculated about increases in precipitation triggered by the changes of albedo. In favorable locations, such an effect might push back the arid zone boundary. On the other hand, an increased plant cover and soil formation is expected to affect the desert recharge process adversely and endanger some of the groundwater sources. The information is of too preliminary a nature to express a firm view on these future developments, except for the need of further study and careful, widespread monitoring of the environmental effects that accompany large-scale irrigation schemes in the desert areas.

REFERENCES

1. MEIGS, P. 1953. World distribution of arid and semi-arid homoclimates. Rev. Res. Arid Zone Hydrol. **1:** 203–210. UNESCO.
2. KEDAR, Y. 1967. The Ancient Agriculture in the Negev Mountain. Bialik Institute Publication. Jerusalem, Israel.
3. EVENARI, M., L. SHANAN & N. H. TADMOR. 1968. Runoff farming in the desert. Agron. J. **60:** 29–32.
4. PALLAS, P. 1972. Water resources in the Northern Sahara. Nat. Resour. **8**(3): 9–17.
5. GOLDSCHMIDT, M. J. & M. JACOBS. 1958. Precipitation Over and Replenishment

of the Yarkon and Hanal Hateninim Underground Catchments. Hydrol. Pap. No. 3. Hydrol. Serv. Jerusalem, Israel.

6. DROUHIN, G. 1953. Problems of water resources in N.W. Africa. Rev. Res. Arid Zone Hydrol. **1:** 9–42. UNESCO.

7. SCHOELLER, H. 1959. Arid Zone Hydrology: Recent Developments. UNESCO Series on Arid Zone Research. No. 12. Paris, France.

8. GOLDSCHMIDT, M. J. 1961. On the mechanism of the replenishment of aquifers in the Negev. *In* Groundwaters in the Arid Zone. IASA Pub. No. **57:** 547–550.

9. SLATYER, R. O. & J. MABBUT. 1964. Hydrology of arid and semiarid regions. *In* Handbook of Applied Hydrology. V. Techow, Ed. **24:** 1–46. McGraw Hill. New York, N.Y.

10. GAT, J. R. & A. ISSAR. 1974. Desert isotope hydrology: water sources of the Sinai Desert. Geochim. Cosmochim. Acta **38:** 1117–1131.

11. HARPAZ, Y., S. MANDEL, J. R. GAT & A. NIR. 1963. The place of isotope methods in groundwater research. *In* Radioisotopes in Hydrology : 175–190. IAEA. Vienna, Austria.

12. CONRAD, G., A. MARCE & P. OLIVE. 1975. Mise en evidence par le tritium de la recharge actuelle des nappes libres de la zone aride Saharienne. J. Hydrol. **27:** 207–224.

13. VERHAGEN, B. T., E. MAZOR & J. P. F. SELLSCHOP. 1974. Radiocarbon and tritium evidence for direct rain recharge to groundwaters in the northern Kalahari. Nature **249:** 643–644.

14. ELBOUSHI, I. 1975. Amount of water needed to initiate flow in rubbly rock particles. J. Hydrol. **27:** 275–284.

15. GAT, J. R. 1971. Comments on the stable isotope method in regional groundwater investigations. Water Resour. Res. **7:** 980–993.

16. DINCER, T., A. ALMUGRINAD & U. ZIMMERMAN. 1974. Study of the infiltration and recharge through the sand dunes in arid zones with special reference to the stable isotopes and thermonuclear tritium. J. Hydrol. **23:** 79–109.

17. MUNICH, K. O. & J. C. VOGEL. 1962. Untersuchungen an Pluvialen Wassern der Ost-Sahara. Geol. Rundschau **52:** 611–624.

18. SHARON, D. 1972. The spottiness of rainfall in a desert area. J. Hydrol. **17:** 161–175.

19. HILLEL, D. 1974. Artificial inducement of runoff as a potential source of water in arid lands. *In* Infiltration and Runoff as Affected by Soil Conditions. Final Report to USDA on Project 10–SWC–75. Hebrew University Faculty of Agriculture. Rehovot, Israel.

20. TADMOR, N. H., L. SHANON & M. EVENARI. 1960. The ancient desert agriculture of the Negev. VI. The ratio of catchments to cultivated area. Isr. J. Agric. Res. **10:** 193–222.

21. ISSAR, A., A. BEIN & A. MICHAELI. 1972. On the ancient water of the upper Nubian sandstone aquifer in Central Sinai and Southern Israel. J. Hydrol. **17:** 353–374.

22. HELLWIG, D. H. R. 1973. Evaporation of water from sand, 3: The loss of water into the atmosphere from a sandy river bed under arid climate conditions. J. Hydrol. **18:** 305–316.

23. GAT, J. R. 1975. Elucidating salinisation mechanism by stable isotope tracing of water sources. *In* Proceeding International Symposium on Brackish Water as a Factor in Development : 15–23. Beer Sheva, Israel.

24. GAT, J. R., E. MAZOR & A. MERCADO. 1968. Potential application of isotope and geochemical techniques to the hydrological problems of N.E. Brazil. Report to B.A.E.C. and Sudena.

25. CHARNEY, J. 1975. Dynamics of deserts and drought in the Sahal. Q. J. R. Meterol. Soc. **101:** 193–202.

THE HOW AND WHY OF CLIMATIC CHANGE

Reid A. Bryson

Institute for Environmental Studies
University of Wisconsin
Madison, Wisconsin 53706

I'm sure you all remember the climatic events of 1972, with the Russian wheat failure, the Sahelian drought, and unfavorable agricultural conditions in dozens of countries. In the following years the climate continued to have a large number of odd patterns, with crop failures here and there, frosts in some places, too much heat in others, drought and flood. Since 1972 there has been a lot of discussion as to whether the climate is changing and how it is changing. One recent book, called *The Cooling,* says that the earth is getting colder; another one, *Hothouse Earth,* tells how the earth will get hotter and burn up. But on a topic like climate and its impact on food production we can't afford to engage in "hand waving" and speculation. We must be realistic and factual, and base our estimates on sound science. I would like to outline some of the important facts about climatic variation, and some results of careful scientific analysis that bear on future prospects.

First, let's take a look at some graphs and see in a long perspective how the climate has changed over the last 13,500 years. I want you to first look at the right-hand curve on FIGURE 1, which shows how the temperature has changed century by century over the last 13,000 years in a place in the North American corn belt: southeastern Minnesota. Now you will notice that at about 10,800 years ago there was a sudden and considerable change—the end of the Ice Age. But you will also notice that since then the temperature hasn't changed very much, except for a slight tapering off starting about 2,500 years ago. If you look at the middle curve, which is the number of hours of sunlight per year, you will notice that back during the Ice Age, more than 11,000 years ago or so, Minnesota was cloudy. It became less cloudy, with more sunlight, but there was a period back about 5 or 6,000 years ago when the sunlight diminished a bit but came back before getting more cloudy in the last 2,500 years. The length of the growing season over that same period of time shows changes even more dramatically. A period of a couple thousand years, 5,000 to 7,000 years ago, was somewhat different. If you look at rainfall during the growing season on the right of FIGURE 2 you will see that even more clearly, and the snowfall shows still more dramatically these periods of change in climate.

Now what do these facts show us? Certainly that dramatic climatic changes can occur very rapidly, as indicated by the end of the Ice Age. The change from a glacial climate to a post-glacial climate took about one century, and that's about as dramatic a change as you can ask for. But even in the post-glacial period you see that the climate can change significantly, and rapidly, and stay changed for a couple thousand years—it does not just fluctuate around some average value. You cannot count on the so-called "law of averages" that the climate will soon return to what you think of as normal. It can change rapidly, and it can stay changed for a long period of time.

Not only in North America do we see this: we also see it in Asia. FIGURE 3 shows a 10,000-year record of the amount of monsoon rainfall in northwestern India, right on the edge of the major wheat area of India. Again, 10,800 years ago you see a dramatic change, a change from essentially no monsoon rainfall to sufficient rains to produce fresh-water lakes in the region. That's a very dramatic change. Before that time, northwestern India was a desert of drifting sand dunes. After that time the monsoon rains came and lakes formed. Farmers moved into the region 9,400 years ago and planted crops, and a vast agricultural

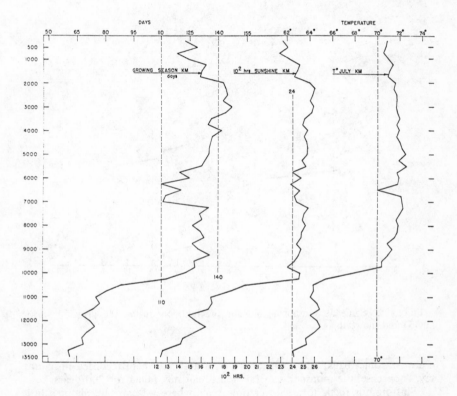

FIGURE 1. 13500 years of climatic record for Kirchner Marsh, south of Minneapolis, Minnesota reconstructed from fossil pollen data. Years are before 1950.

civilization developed about 5,000 years ago—the Indus civilization. Then about 1700 B.C. the fresh-water lakes turned salt, dried up, the Indus civilization disappeared, and for 700 years the region was unoccupied and was once again a desert of drifting sand dunes. Some 2,500 years ago (a significant date if you remember the pattern from North America) the rains came back a little bit so that the Aryan people could move into northwestern India. The lakes reformed in part about 2,000 years ago. So even in the monsoon land where some scientists have said "The monsoon is the monsoon, you know, it is reliable,

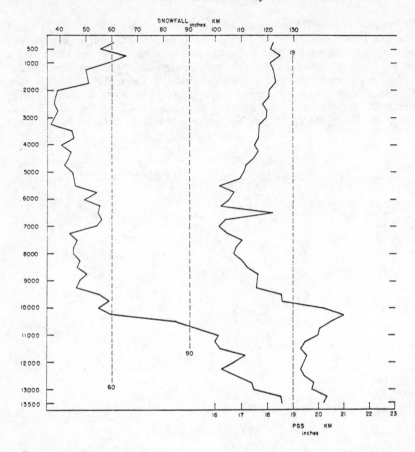

FIGURE 2. Same as FIGURE 1, but for precipitation during the growing season (PGS) and snowfall.

it always comes back," the facts, as we have observed them recorded in nature, say, "nonsense, the monsoon can fail and it can stay failed for 700 years."

Shifting our focus to a shorter time scale where we can talk about a little more detail, we have in FIGURE 4 a record of temperature for the last 1,000 years, by 20-year periods, for Iceland.

Now you all know Iceland is a very small nation, and, really, who cares, because there isn't much agriculture. Well, the reason for paying attention to this record is that Iceland happens to be in a key location—it is located in the region where the center of maximum climatic change occurs, and the pattern of climate over the rest of the hemisphere is related to what goes on in the far north Atlantic sector. In fact, within the last months my research group has shown that the pattern of circulation over the whole northern hemisphere can be related rather neatly to the temperature level in the far north Atlantic.

So look at this 1,000-year record and you find that a thousand years ago when the Vikings first settled in Iceland it was warmer, but then about 1200

A.D. there came about a 200-year period of lower temperature. That 200-year period was a period of great distress in European agriculture. There was too much humidity, but mild temperatures, and great outbreaks of the ergot blight of the grain—whole districts in western Europe were wiped out by the presence of this disease on the plants and the toxic byproducts of that blight in the food eaten by the people. In North America there was a quite different pattern which we will get back to in a moment. But notice that very cold period that started about 1600 A.D. and goes up to the beginning of this century. That is known as the 'Little Ice Age" because glaciers in the Alps and the Rocky Mountains advanced, and northern regions were too cold for agriculture. There were changes all over the major agricultural regions of the hemisphere during that time. You will notice that it was not very long ago and it lasted for 300 years. Now, look at the present century, at the time that you and I have been alive, and what do you see? You see a phenomenal rise of temperature, and a short period of high temperatures. That little stitchery on top shows what

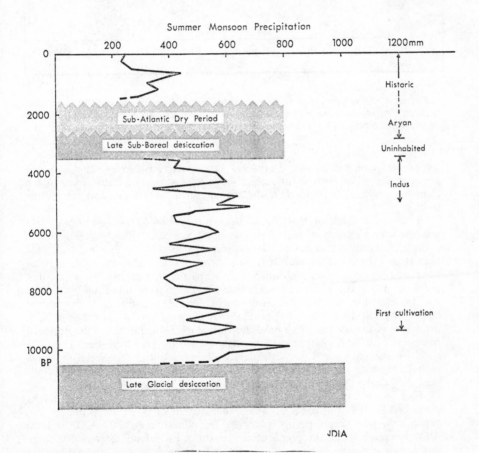

FIGURE 3. Reconstructed history of monsoon rainfall in northwestern India (Lunkaransar, Rajasthan). BP indicates "before present."

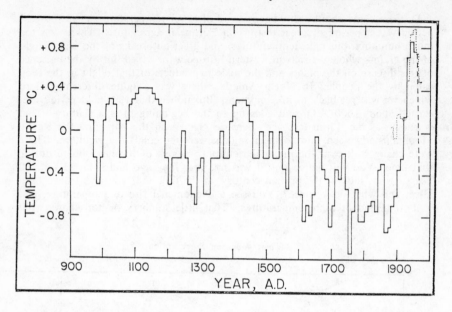

FIGURE 4. 1000 years of average annual temperature in Iceland derived from drift ice data by Bergthorsson. The dotted line indicates the average temperature variation of the whole Northern Hemisphere.

the average temperature in the northern hemisphere has been. You see that it goes parallel to the pattern for Iceland but not as strongly because most of the change is in high latitudes and the temperatures don't change much in the tropics.

You and I think of that high-temperature period as being normal. Our weather services think of that period as being normal. The population of the earth tripled during that period. It is during that period that our patterns have been frozen the way they are. It is during that period that most of the agricultural industry of the world has established its particular pattern. But notice that by hindsight, in the perspective of history, that is a most abnormal period. If you are a gambler, will you bet on the outside chance that *that* short period will be the shape of the future? I think that is not a good bet. As a matter of fact, the events of the last few years have shown that the temperatures of the northern hemisphere and the weather patterns associated with them have been changing back towards the pattern of the Little Ice Age. Statistically speaking, the most probable climate for the next few decades is more like that of the mid-1800's than the pattern that you and I have been exposed to most of our lives.

FIGURE 5 is a pattern which is engraved in my mind because this is a pattern developed in the course of ten years of research on what happened to the North American corn-farming Indians in the period from 1200 A.D. to 1400 A.D. Remember that the graph of temperatures in Iceland showed that there was a change starting about 1200 A.D. and lasting through 1400 A.D.—200 years. This figure shows the corresponding pattern of rainfall change in the United States at the beginning of that time.

We have done the work to establish what happened in that period in North America. Prior to 1200 A.D. there were thousands of villages occupied by corn-farming Indians scattered across the plains of the United States. Starting in 1200 A.D. nearly all of that agricultural enterprise disappeared, and the reason was that a drought in the United States started about 1200 A.D., with this pattern, and continued off and on for 200 years. A 200-year drought in the spring wheat and corn belt regions of the United States *is* possible because it has happened.

Now look carefully at this diagram because the pattern shown here is quite similar to the pattern of 1974 and 1976. We need to decide in North America whether this pattern is now over and will go back to something else or whether this is the shape of the future. With this pattern of 25 to 50 percent reduction in summer rainfall, we would cease to be a food-exporting nation. It is possible for such a drought to last off and on for 200 years. If it happened again it would totally change our economy.

For a little detail of what has happened, FIGURE 6 shows, on the left side, winter temperatures at various latitudes. You will notice that the temperature changes have been mostly in winter, and mostly at very high latitude. But the atmosphere of the earth is a unit, and you cannot change one part without changing the pattern of the rainfall over the whole hemisphere. So the question is "Why did this happen?" Once we know why this happened we might be able to figure out what will happen in the future.

You know that the sun drives the atmosphere. How can you change the sun? You don't have to; all you have to do is change the transparency of the atmosphere, and in that way you change the amount of energy available at the

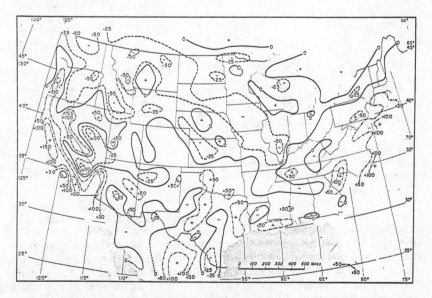

FIGURE 5. July precipitation change to be expected when the westerlies shift southward into the United States. This appears to be the pattern of change that took place about 1200 A.D. Numbers are percent change, dashed lines indicate decrease.

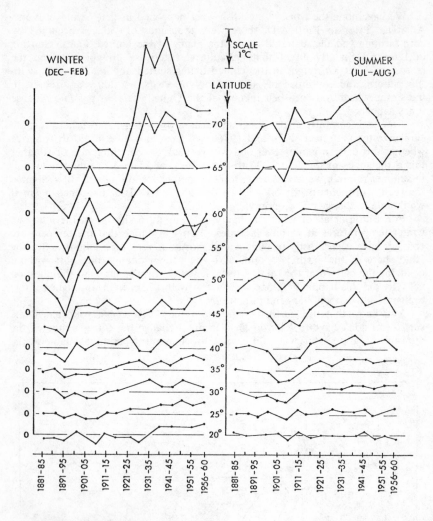

FIGURE 6. Yearly change of average temperature at various latitudes of the northern hemisphere, according to Russian sources.

ground to drive the atmosphere, which in turn makes agriculture possible. One
thing that changes the transparency of the atmosphere is volcanic activity. Now
all of you have flown in jet aircraft and know that at 39,000 feet the sky above
you is beautifully deep blue—but not when there has been a volcanic eruption!
Over Bali, just after the eruption of Agung, the sky was brown because of the
great amount of volcanic ash in the air. Volcanos reduce the amount of sunlight
that reaches the ground. The numbers of volcanos in the world changes from
time to time. FIGURE 7 is a graph of the changes in transparency of the atmosphere derived from data on volcanic activity. You see a transparency change

from not very transparent, around 1904–20, to very clean during most of our lifetime. The higher atmosphere was pretty clean. It didn't have much volcanic "ash" in it during the lifetime of those of you who are my age. There was not much volcanic activity during that time, but in recent years the number of volcanos in the world has been increasing, sharply but irregularly increasing, since about 1955. That increase has continued just about to the present time. Right now there are many volcanos active and spewing volcanic ash and gases into the atmosphere, where they reduce the atmospheric transparency and in turn reduce the amount of sunlight reaching the ground.

There are other sources of "dirtiness" of the atmosphere that can reduce the amount of sunlight. One, of course, is industry—but it is not industry alone because just as much material is put into the atmosphere by non-industrial human activities in the form of the smoke from slash-and-burn agriculture, and in the form of dust from the farming of marginal dry lands. That activity, industrial and otherwise, has been increasing rapidly in recent years. There are more people than ever before, and FIGURE 8 shows the effect of that on the transparency of the atmosphere. The lower atmosphere was quite transparent until after World War II because the world as a whole had not yet reached the industrial revolution, nor had antibiotics and other things made the abrupt explosion of population possible. So we see that man and his activities have been decreasing the transparency of the atmosphere also.

Man, by his use of fossil fuels, has also been increasing the carbon dioxide content of the atmosphere (FIGURE 9). This has an effect upon the transparency of the atmosphere by keeping radiation from the earth from going out to space. The interplay of sunlight coming in and heat being lost back to space determines

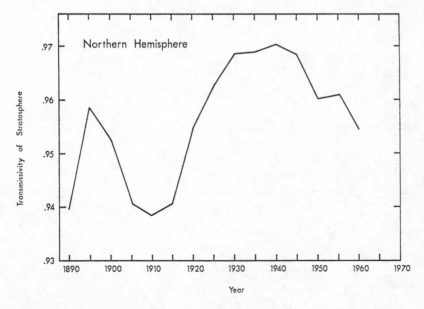

FIGURE 7. Variation of the transparency of the high atmosphere (stratosphere), due to variations in volcanic activity.

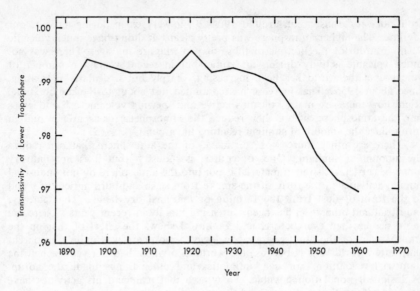

FIGURE 8. Variation of the transparency of the lower layers of the atmosphere, due to human activities.

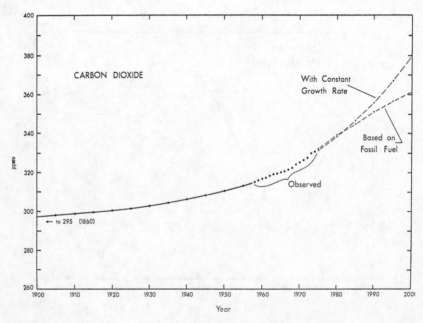

FIGURE 9. Variation of the carbon dioxide content of the atmosphere. This is generally attributed to increased consumption of fossil fuels.

what the temperature of the earth will be, and in turn what the distribution of rainfall will be. We can put together all of this in an equation (which I won't bother you with), put it on a computer, and calculate what the temperature of the earth should be as it depends upon the transparency of the atmosphere, in other words, as it depends upon volcanic activity and on human activity. FIGURE 10 shows that we can do it.

What does the future hold? Well, we are pretty sure what people are going to do. We know that people are going to continue to produce children, and we know they are going to continue to use marginal lands. We can't stop them without having them starve. They will continue to burn brush to clear fields in the tropics. We cannot stop them; they would starve. They will continue to

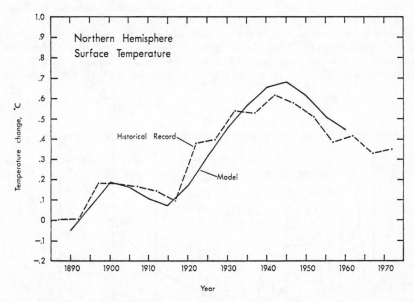

FIGURE 10. The observed average temperature of the Northern Hemisphere compared with the values computed using a computer model that responds to volcanos, man-made dust, and carbon dioxide.

use fossil fuels as long as they are available. And so we know how the man-made pollution of the atmosphere will proceed for at least the next few decades. What we don't know yet is what the volcanos of the world will do. However, we can suggest several possibilities. We can suppose the volcanos turn off as fast as they turned on, that the volcanic activity decreases at the same rate that it has increased, and calculate the result. We calculate that the hemispheric temperature would return to the 1940 level in a decade or so; 1970 would appear to be near the bottom. However, this year volcanic activity has increased, and so we can delay the warming at least, and that suggests that the next five years or so will be more or less like the last five years. Now think of the last five years—a severe drought in Europe, two Russian crop failures, two droughts in the corn belt, frost in Brazil, failure of the rains at the right time in Australia, floods in East Asia, drought in China—it is not a pleasant prospect to say that the next five years will be like the last five years, climatically speaking.

Another possibility is to say, "Well, suppose the volcanos just stay the way they are for the next ten years or so." The cold period lasts longer, and the period of climate different from what we think of as normal continues to the end of the 1980's. But if we say, "Suppose the volcanos continue to increase until they are twice as active as the last decade?" Then the temperatures go very low indeed. In fact, if this analysis is correct, such a circumstance would probably change the climate into an ice age climate. It doesn't mean that glaciers would push down New York City in ten years. But it would mean severe climatic problems around the world.

Well, why do we care? One of the reasons we care is because there are a lot of people who depend upon the pattern of rain. Turning to northwestern India we see that at the turn of the century failures of the monsoon were rather common (FIGURE 11). Then, in the period of benign weather that we had, the monsoon became very regular. But in recent years the frequency of drought, in northwestern India at least, has started to increase, and we have excellent

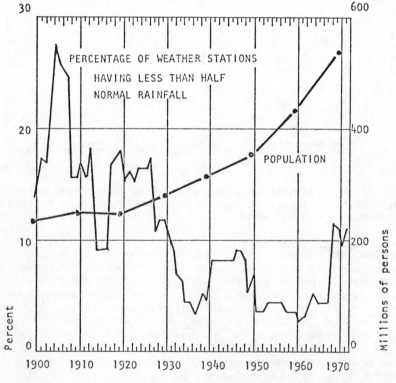

FIGURE 11. Frequency of drought in northwest India, 10-year averages, and population of India.

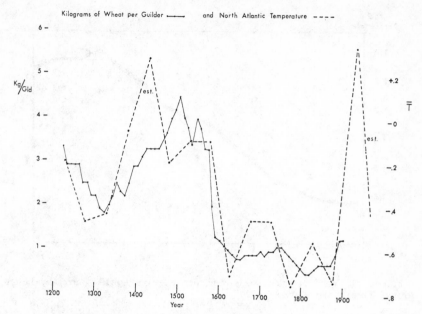

FIGURE 12. Price of wheat in England and Holland compared with North Atlantic temperature (as indicated by Icelandic temperature).

reason to believe that if the hemisphere continues to cool the monsoons of south Asia will become less reliable. If we look at European agriculture, we see that over the last few hundred years, as the temperature of the north Atlantic has gone up and down with the warmer spell of 1400 A.D. or so to the lower temperatures of the Little Ice Age, the price of wheat in western Europe has gone up and down with it (FIGURE 12). When it's warm, wheat is cheap; when it's cold, wheat is expensive in western Europe. I didn't put on the price in the century because you all know that in that warm period back in the 1930's wheat was very cheap but in the cooler period of the 1970's wheat was more expensive. We know what that means. As the temperature goes down, European agriculture becomes less productive and prices go up. In terms of business in general it can be shown that a 1° Celsius change in the average temperature of a country will affect its gross national product by 2½% (assuming constant energy use). That is an enormous amount of money. Now, what has happened since 1971 or 72? Worldwide crop yields have been diminishing—not going up—according to this data from the U.S. Department of Agriculture (FIGURE 13). Try as we can, and agriculture is trying, the yield per acre has been going down, and that is important because the population has been going up.

The heavy solid line in FIGURE 14 shows the increase of population since 1961. The light broken line shows the number of people that could be fed each year with the grain produced in that year plus all the reserves of grain that we had including the potential of idle U.S. cropland.

From 1961 to about 1968 the general level of population that could be fed, using everything, rose slowly—more slowly than the population. This is shown

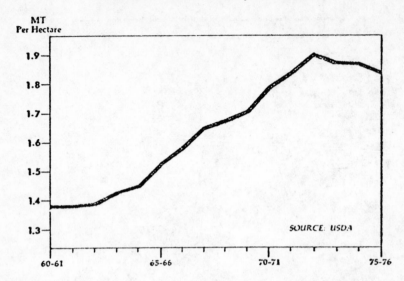

FIGURE 13. Yield of grain, world-wide, derived from USDA sources by Lester Brown. Three-year averages.

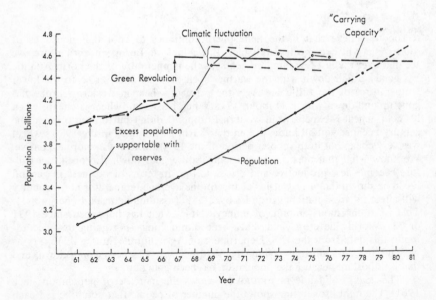

FIGURE 14. Population and food reserves. Population (solid curve) and population supportable by each year's production plus reserves (dash-dot). Locally held reserves are unknown, but unless trends change it appears that production plus carryover will soon be inadequate. Based on USDA figures.

in the figure by the heavy broken line, which we can call the "carrying capacity" of the earth. I think the slow rise was largely due to increasing fertilizer use. Then came the "Green Revolution"—the introduction of high-yielding varieties of wheat and rice—which was the culmination of a heroic 20-year development period. As a result the carrying capacity of the earth jumped higher. At the same time, however, the climatic change of recent years began to be evident, so that the carrying capacity has stayed constant, or declined slightly, since about 1970. Whether the reserve figures are exactly correct or not, they are of the right order of magnitude. What this shows is that we are approaching a crisis unless there is a new Green Revolution within the next couple of years—but I know of none that is imminent. Climatic fluctuations could move the crisis a year or two sooner or delay it.

Clearly we must produce either fewer new mouths each year, or more food—soon. Peace, health, happiness, and human dignity hang in the balance. Will we change the shape of the future?

GENERAL DISCUSSION

Jean Mayer, *Moderator*

Tufts University
Medford, Massachusetts 02155

MR. WILLIAM W. GORDON (*Ted Klein & Co., Brooklyn, N.Y.*): Dr. Wittwer, I wonder if you would expound, sir, on what you meant by the term "scaled neutral."

DR. SYLVAN WITTWER: The reference here is to technologies that are adapted to varying sizes of farm operations. In other words, many technologies that have been created in this nation are adapted to large-scale agriculture only: mechanization, water management systems, soil management systems, cropping systems. I was speaking of "scaled neutral" agriculture as being technologies that are adapted to any scale of operation. We have not addressed ourselves to this type of technology in this nation effectively.

DR. RICHARD ELLIS (*University of California, Santa Barbara, Cal.*): Dr. Pimentel, in your calculations of energy costs, did you include the costs of agricultural research?

DR. DAVID PIMENTEL: No, I did not include that as a factor in the estimates. It's obviously an important one.

UNIDENTIFIED SPEAKER: If the ratio of livestock to humans is estimated at about 2½ to 1, on a global basis, if my arithmetic is correct, by the year 2135, using that same ratio, we will have about 45.5 billion mouths to feed. What is the solution to this problem?

DR. PIMENTEL: It's obvious that if the human population continues to increase, based relative to the energy resources, the land resources, the water resources, that the standard of living will have to decline on a per capita basis. We already see this occurring in the United States, in Europe, and in the rest of the world. That's what's related to the inflation. The standard of living is declining, and the more humans you add on earth, the poorer the standard of living will be.

MS. ANN POTTMAN (*Simon Fraser University, Vancouver, British Columbia*): Dr. Bryson, you mentioned the effects of the intensity of the sunlight which reaches the earth if volcanos stop erupting at certain times in the future. This seems to me, although interesting, somewhat futile because we have no control over whether or not the volcanos erupt. Have you done similar calculations for the effect of controlling the level of man-made dust and pollutants in the air on the intensity of the sunlight which reaches the earth?

DR. BRYSON: Yes, we have. I doubt very much if we can, within the rest of this century, control, in any significant way, the amount of dust put into the atmosphere by man. If you go to the Cambodian farmer or the Congolese farmer, or the Syrian farmer and say, "Don't burn that field. You're making smoke which affects the climate of the world." He'll say, "I've got to eat this year. I'm going to burn it." If you go to the Sahelian farmer and say, "Don't run your goats around on that desert, they're kicking up too much dust." He'll say, "I'm sorry, but I have to eat."

So, nothing is going to happen, really, in terms of controlling dust. We're

54

not going to control the industrial input either, because while we do it to a certain extent here in the U.S., there are other nations where they say, flat out, "It is our turn to pollute. We don't have time or resources to control it." So the world-wide input of industrial pollutants is going up, not down, in this age of environmental concern. I don't think we're going to control it at all. We're not going to control the amount of carbon dioxide put in the air. Every scholar I know agrees with what the rest of the next century will look like in terms of carbon dioxide.

Volcanos are the unpredictable variable, and that's why I gave three scenarios, if they do this, if they do that, if they do something else. There we don't even know how to predict what they're going to do.

DR. ARNOLD SCHAEFER (*University of Nebraska Medical Center, Omaha, Nebr.*): Dr. Pimentel, you used a figure that I really have to question: 21,000 kilocalories of fossil fuel to yield 270 calories of beef. Are you sure you meant fossil fuel, or were you talking about calories that cattle get from roughage which fundamentally comes from solar fuel? That's one question. Now the other: Your statement of 2,000 pounds of excess grain per capita is the highest figure I've seen. Are you taking into account the fact that we export roughly 50–55% of all grain? Secondly, you said the 2,000 pounds of excess grain went basically to cattle—that I would dispute. If you think it takes 2,000 pounds of grain to make 125 pounds of beef, you should come out and take a look at feed lots in Nebraska, where it takes 20 pounds of hay and roughly 4 pounds of supplement, of which half of is not grain—half is by-products, to make a pound of beef.

DR. PIMENTEL: First, it takes roughly 78 kilocalories of energy to produce 1 kilocalorie of beef protein. So, if you multiply 80 times about 270 it ought to work out pretty close. Second, that 2,000 pounds of excess grain per capita in the United States is not my figure—it is USDA's, and several others have these numbers and that is exclusive of exports. And the quantity of grain— it's not 125 pounds of meat that we consume per capita but 250 pounds, about 116 pounds of beef. That's close to half.

In addition to beef we consume 285 eggs, 130 pounds or more of milk and dairy products, and I've forgotten what some of these other numbers are, so the animal protein is not insignificant. Per capita consumption of protein in the United States is roughly about 100 grams a day, and two-thirds of that is animal protein. When you get a yield of only six pounds of beef from 100 pounds of protein, you can burn that 2,000 pounds quite rapidly.

DR. MAYER: May I add that there are some unexpected energy costs. We have done some calculations on the energy cost of fish and fish products. Actually the energy cost of shrimp is even higher than the energy cost of feedlot beef, by the time you calculate the energy cost of building the trawlers and of trawling, refrigeration, transportation, and storage. No matter how we look at it, the energy cost of animal products is extremely high. The one thing that can be said is that you use less energy at home to cook steak than to cook rice or vegetable dishes, but unfortunately that doesn't make up for the energy costs at the initial production level.

DR. S. L. RAWLINS (*U.S.D.A., Riverside, Cal.*): My question is to Dr. Gat. I have heard it said that the extensive planting of trees in some of the arid areas of Israel has caused a change in the climate by attracting increased precipitation. Would you care to comment on that?

DR. JOEL R. GAT: I don't think this is true. It certainly may have changed very locally the type of climate. I've heard no claim of increased precipitation, but I think the problem there is one of the size. The results may be very different in a small area compared to the whole Sahara Desert. I think it's a matter of the microclimate. It certainly affects the amount of runoff retained in the soil—so it has very dramatic effects on the water in the lakes and so on, on a local scale, but not on the climate in general, not in that area.

OPENING REMARKS

Roger Revelle

Center for Population Studies
Harvard University
Cambridge, Massachusetts 02138

This is the second session of this Conference on Food and Nutrition. This morning we talked about global problems in food production. This afternoon, we shall discuss Global Problems in Food Distribution and Food Policy.

This afternoon we are dealing with short-range problems—problems of immediate urgency and desperate concern. These are problems of food distribution because, at the present time at least, there's plenty of food in the world for everybody, enough to provide everyone on earth with a diet a good deal better than they obtain now. But, in fact, many people, certainly several hundred million, are badly malnourished at the present time. This is primarily a problem of food distribution.

The desire of most countries, no matter how small or how poor or how disadvantaged, is to attain food self-sufficiency; these countries are concerned that their people will not be able to obtain sufficient food unless they can grow it themselves. Self-sufficiency in a rational world would be a will-of-the-wisp, a chimera which doesn't have any real justification, but perhaps in our irrational, one might almost say insane, world of nation-states self-sufficiency in food production may be temporarily, at least, a desirable goal because of the problems of distribution.

These problems of distribution, as far as I can see them, are of three kinds at the present time. In such areas as North Africa, south of the Sahara, one of the main problems is simply inadequate transportation—a very, very high cost and extreme difficulty of transportation of anything let alone food from one part of the region to another. In most of the world, however, problems of food distribution are closely related to problems of poverty and ignorance: poverty as far as distribution between families, between classes, or between social groups is concerned, and ignorance about distribution within the family or within groups where the total food supply may be quite adequate but ignorance causes serious problems of maldistribution.

I hope this afternoon some of our speakers will talk about the necessity for a food reserve—a food reserve not to make sure that starving people can be given food but a food reserve simply to stabilize prices.

The characteristic thing about food is that the demand for it is what the economists call "extremely inelastic." The most important thing in the lives of most people is getting enough to eat, and the demand for food hardly varies no matter what else varies. On the other hand, the supply is also extremely inelastic—you can't increase the supply in short run by raising prices or at least can't increase it very much. The result of these inelasticities of supply and demand is that whenever there is a very, very small shortfall in world food production compared to world food demand the prices go through the roof. For example, in 1972 there was about a 5% shortfall in food supply with respect to food demand on a worldwide basis, and the prices of cereal grains went up from 200 to 400% with this very slight difference in supply and demand.

On the other hand, whenever there's a slight excess of a few percent in food supplies with respect to food demand, prices fall through the floor, and this is happening right now because of the bountiful harvest in several different countries. Prices of staple foods are falling so low that farmers may not be able to make ends meet, i.e. to actually pay their costs.

The need for a food reserve in my opinion, therefore, is primarily the need for a device for stabilizing prices at a level which will provide incentives to farmers. One of the things which we mustn't forget is that farmers can't grow, cannot and will not grow, food at a loss. They must make a profit. They must have return which is greater than their costs. At the same time, we must also have fair prices for consumers, which means that the prices should be within the range that most people can pay. And this combination of problems of incentives for farmers, fair prices for consumers is perhaps one of the major problems, if not the primary problem, of food distribution.

ACCESS TO FOOD: THE ULTIMATE DETERMINANT OF HUNGER

C. Peter Timmer

Department of Nutrition
Harvard University
Boston, Massachusetts 02115

How can the productivity gains in agriculture generated by modern farming techniques and the application of scientific breakthroughs likely in the next several decades be translated into meaningful gains in nutritional status for the 500 million individuals most in need? This was the central question for the Nutrition Overview Study Team of The National Academy of Science's World Food and Nutrition Study. Even rough familiarity with global food production patterns and individual nutrient requirements is sufficient to indicate that present conditions of hunger and malnutrition are not due to a shortage of food in global terms. Total grain production is currently about 1.3 billion metric tons relative to a global population of 4 billion people. If evenly distributed, this grain would provide over 65 grams of protein and 3000 kilocalories of energy per day for every person on earth, before any nutritional contributions from pulses, fruits and vegetables, fish, or forage-fed animals.

Crude as the calculation is, it provides justification for the Nutrition Overview Team's decision to search beyond present gaps in knowledge of agricultural science and of nutritional biochemistry as the primary causes of hunger and malnutrition. Important as research in these areas will be, especially in the longer run, it must not be allowed to divert scientific attention and funding priority from the more pressing factors that are the proximate causes of malnutrition.

Despite substantial gray areas of ignorance about the long-run significance of under- or over-consumption of most nutrients and of the impact of many nutrient-nonnutrient interactions, diets can be devised that have extremely low probabilities of doing nutritional harm. Countries politically committed to eliminating overt malnutrition, with populations willing to consume the prescribed diet, need no further research in biomedical aspects of nutrition. Very few countries answer to this description, however, and the many that do not frequently require quantitative evidence that, at the margin, policies and programs aimed at reducing malnutrition are worth their cost in scarce resources. It is to this vast majority of the world's governments that the research program outlined by the Nutrition Overview Team—summarized in the Appendix—is addressed.

The extent to which scientific knowledge can substitute for political commitment to eliminate basic hunger is less than complete. Like most substitutions, this one becomes less and less perfect at either extreme. A considerable amount of political commitment is needed, even when the scientific issues of how much of what to feed to whom are clarified. Similarly, this basic scientific work can have a high payoff for countries already heavily committed to feeding their people adequately because more knowledge will narrow the range of uncertainty and permit much more careful allocations of financial and scarce food resources to those programs and people where it will do the most good. The nutrition research program proposed by the NAS Study Team is organized by this logic of government needs and is propelled by a concern for understanding the factors that determine access to satisfactory nutritional status.

Why should societies put resources into food and nutrition research when it is already possible to specify diets that will do no nutritional harm? The answers are several. First, food habits are strongly ingrained, and many people will not voluntarily adopt the recommended diet. What cost are they and society incurring? Second, the prescribed diet necessarily errs on the side of liberality for nearly all nutrients. In a world of increasingly scarce resources and a narrower and narrower margin of food surpluses, such a diet may not be feasible in the future. For many areas of poor countries it is not feasible now. The research directly addresses the issue of how finely the reference diets can be tuned. Third, many governments regard investments in adequate nutrition as a political sop without the benefits of, say, a road or even a fighter plane. This attitude reflects an existing distribution of economic and political power that feeding the poor may threaten. But scope exists for using the political sop effectively or ineffectively. One goal of research on individual and social costs of malnutrition is to use funds channeled into nutrition as effectively as possible.

Even with this knowledge in hand, however, the most fundamental issues in understanding the causes of hunger and malnutrition remain to be addressed. Despite how little we know about the gray areas of malnutrition, we do know that if everyone had access to over 3000 kilocalories and 65 grams of grain protein every day—the present per capita output of the world's agriculture— that most of the world's 500 million malnourished would be substantially better off. Campaigns to eliminate the remaining malnutrition would be on a par with campaigns to eliminate malaria or schistosomiasis.

To understand why some families have that access while others in the same village do not; why some villages do and others do not; why some regions do and others do not; why some countries do and others do not, is to understand a society's political economics. It is to understand the causes of the distribution of income and the foundations of social and political power. It is to understand why some are hungry and some are not.

What does scientific analysis have to offer in this most intractable of research areas? Primarily it offers knowledge about the nutritional impact of government policies and of programs of income redistribution, in the hope that knowledge will expand the scope for rational choice between positive and negative nutritional impact, even when that is not a costless choice. More importantly, with this analysis the productivity breakthroughs promised by the agricultural scientists can reach their most important target, those half billion people presently suffering from hunger and malnutrition.

Analysis of the fate of the Green Revolution demonstrates the importance of understanding the factors that determine access to food. The major nutritional problem in the world is inadequate energy intake from normal food sources. TABLE 1 indicates that nearly two-thirds of total caloric intake is provided by cereals in West Asia, China, South and Southeast Asia, an area that contains over 70 percent of the total undernourished on the planet. The productivity potential of the Green Revolution, based as it is on higher yields for wheat, rice and maize, has enormous promise for solving most nutritional problems in poor countries by increasing the amount of grain available. If the hungriest parts of the population had access to the increased grain supplies, their energy deficits could be satisfied and the worst of the obvious malnutrition eliminated. In some countries the Green Revolution *has* solved most of the problems of hunger and malnutrition in just this fashion.

The question is why this promise has not been translated into reality in more countries. The answer is complicated and depends on varying factors unique to each country. The answers are not available because the research is not done. But the questions can be set in an analytical framework that organizes them into a set of potentially researchable topics.

The "generational problems" of the Green Revolution have become common knowledge to physical and social scientists working in this field. Falcon [1] summarized three generations of problems in the following categories:

1. First Generation: Great Production Successes, but Important Limitations.
2. Second Generation: Problems of Marketing, Markets and Resource Allocation.
3. Third Generation: Social Forces and Uncertain Consequences.

TABLE 1

IMPORTANCE OF CEREALS IN ASIAN DIETS *

Region	Daily Per Capita Calorie Intake			Percentage of Total Calorie Intake from:	
	Total	From Cereals	From Pulses, Nuts and Cocoa	Cereals	Pulses, Nuts and Cocoa
West Asia	2316	1480	91	63.9	3.9
China	2045	1383	134	67.6	6.6
South Asia	1975	1300	176	65.8	8.9
Southeast Asia	2121	1589	78	74.9	3.7

* Source: The World Food Situation and Prospects to 1985. ERS–USDA, Foreign Agr. Econ. Rep. No. 98, March 1975.

Since these three generations were identified in 1970, several others have been suggested, the most important of which would be the energy-intensive nature of the Green Revolution and the drain on depletable resources implied by widespread adoption of its modern technology.

Rather than pursue higher generations, the nutritional impact of the Green Revolution should be examined in terms of four levels of effects: (1) The direct impact; (2) the indirect impact; and (3) the roundabout impact. The fourth level might be termed the "way out" impact.

DIRECT IMPACT

The direct impact measures the effect on the nutritional status of a peasant household that adopts the package of Green Revolution technology and directly consumes the greater part of the higher yield. At first sight this would appear to be far and away the most important aspect of any nutritional impact from the Green Revolution, and in China it has been. But in most other countries this direct impact has probably been quite small. The evidence is now reasonably strong that in market-oriented countries the *first* users of Green Revolution technology are larger, commercial-minded farmers whose increased cereal output will mostly be sold in the market. The nutritional status of these commercial farmers and their families is seldom cause for concern. The most pressing cases of hunger are to be found among the smaller subsistence farmers, the landless rural workers, and urban slum dwellers. The *direct* impact of the Green Revolution on these groups is slight because they do not have access to the resources—land and money—needed to use it. Any impact, positive or negative, must come through other mechanisms.

The situation in China is quite different. If nothing else, the emerging story of China's solution to her food problem underscores the potential of the Green Revolution technology for eliminating basic hunger. Sterling Wortman, chairman of a National Academy of Sciences delegation of agricultural scientists, which visited the People's Republic of China, summarized the findings in this manner: "The most populous nation appears to have achieved the objective of producing enough food for all its people. It has done so largely by the adoption of improved strains of rice and wheat." [11]

The available evidence does not suggest that food grain production has risen markedly faster in China than in a number of other poor countries where malnutrition remains a serious problem. The secret of the Chinese success is a more even diffusion of the new cereal technology, coupled with much more direct and equitable access to the resulting output.[8] China has managed to avoid urban bias in its food policy, a bias which Michael Lipton [4] argues "has led [in other countries] to inadequate, ill-directed and maldistributed farm inputs. Planning in particular has been directed, by normal processes of politics and not by malice, towards eliminating not hunger but food imports, and towards unbalancing output structures to meet rich townsmen's growing demands —milk before millet." By rationing food in the cities and providing incentives and productive inputs for agriculture in the rural areas, China has apparently succeeded in guaranteeing access to adequate cereal supplies to all members of the population.

INDIRECT IMPACT

Indirect nutritional effects of the Green Revolution also have an impact on the farm households which experience the direct effect through their own use of the new technology, but they are secondary for this population group. All other population groups must rely entirely on the indirect effects—through price and income changes—to improve their nutritional status. With all other things equal, the new cereal production should make possible lower food grain prices, as demonstrated by the falling rice prices in international trade from 1968 to 1971. In most cases, lower prices mean greater consumption, which leads to improved nutritional status (although there are some fallible points in this chain).

Similarly, the improved productivity made possible by the Green Revolution leads to higher real incomes. These higher incomes can then be used to purchase a more adequate diet. The indirect nutritional effects of the Green Revolution should be positive and, on balance, they probably have been. But reliance on the market as the mechanism to translate greater cereal production into improved nutritional status opens several possibilities for individuals to miss out on the potential.

First, the flow of goods through markets is determined almost entirely by purchasing power, raising the opportunity for what Lyle Schertz calls food imperialism.

> For example, economic growth can improve national nutrition averages but at the same time, make the low income people worse off. One reason for this potential whiplash on the poor is that, as people's incomes rise, they desire more animal products. They bid the grain off the plates of the poor for use as livestock feed. Whether these are the rich of the developed countries or the better off people of developing countries makes little difference to the poor. They only know the resulting hunger.[5]

A second important market effect of the Green Revolution is the tendency of cereal-importing countries to substitute increased domestic grain production for imports. The roundabout effects of the saved foreign exchange may have important productivity and distributional implications, but the immediate effect is to neutralize any gains. In his recent survey in *Science,* Nicholas Wade concluded that "because of population growth and substitution for imports, the Green Revolution has probably not made any great difference to average diets." [9]

ROUNDABOUT IMPACT

The extent and complexity of the various roundabout effects of the Green Revolution on nutritional status stretch as far as the imagination. One path in particular concerns nutritionists; a second, economists and political scientists. The first is the increased profitability of new technology cereals relative to vegetables and pulses, which are the traditional sources of vitamins and high quality (or complementary) protein in poor people's diets. Martin Forman and Byron Berntson were among the first to express this concern, in the following fashion:

> Ironically, however, the same Green Revolution which offers promise of closing the world's calorie gap may be causing a reduction in the supply of low cost protein products in some areas of the world. This is occurring due to a shift in land use away from growing food legumes (one of the lowest cost sources of good quality protein) to growing the new higher yielding varieties of cereals. The incentive to the farmer is the higher income that he may now derive from the sale of increased cereal crops. This may have a deleterious effect on total protein availability in a country, but far more serious is the effect it may have on the people living in the immediate farming area who may have heretofore consumed portions of the food legume crop as a regular practice. Their diets, often nutritionally marginal to begin with, may now suffer a critical drop in protein as they switch from legumes to cereals because of their greater availability and lower price.[2]

In view of the evidence reviewed by Waterlow and Payne [10] that cereal diets provide adequate protein so long as the cereal protein is not burned to supply energy, the displacement of legume acreage does not appear as serious as it did 5 years ago. In any respect, it was a trend established well before the Green Revolution, at least in India.

The roundabout effect that most concerns economists is the changed technology of farming which is frequently stimulated by the productivity potential of the Green Revolution. The extent of change varies widely from region to region and country to country, and its occurrence and impact depend critically on the nature of land tenure and existing technology. With all the provisos, however, the Green Revolution has set in motion some very unfortunate changes in some rural areas. One effect noticed in India was for absentee landlords to return to their farms in order to take over cultivation themselves because of the greater economic return made possible by the Green Revolution. Consolidation of land holdings and mechanization permitted landowners to evict their tenants, who then joined the rural landless work force. In the first instance this meant that the former tenants no longer had access to the direct impact of the Green Revolution. This impact, it was argued earlier, had the potential for doing the most to improve nutritional status in the rural areas. The roundabout effect that works through changed farm technology actually runs the direct nutritional effect in reverse.

Changed farming technology need not displace tenants to have an important roundabout nutritional impact. The indirect effects via prices and incomes can also run in reverse if the changed technology reduces employment opportunities for landless laborers. This would reduce their income and hence lower their purchase of cereals from the market, almost certainly resulting in lower nutritional status. Although a number of nutritional anthropologists have argued that higher incomes often do not lead to better nutritional status, none seem to argue the reverse, that lower incomes might improve nutritional status.

"WAY OUT" IMPACT

The "way out" effects of the Green Revolution on nutritional status involve the broader impact of the new cereal technology on the interwoven social and political fabric of poor societies. The argument, in essence, says that the emergence of one revolution in the countryside may well foment others. Static societies frequently require a major stimulus to break the traditional bonds that maintain the status quo. The Green Revolution may do this either by succeeding or by failing. Success may set up new patterns of wealth that eventually buy out the old ruling cliques, as in the English agricultural and industrial revolution. Failure, on the other hand, may set up inescapable tensions between what is and what might be. This, in the colorful popular press, is the contention that if the Green Revolution turns brown, it will ultimately turn red. Whatever the color, Gershenkron [3] has made a strong argument that the tensions of backwardness relative to what is possible often determine the strength of economic and political response when change finally comes. And radical change carries important nutritional implications. Among poor countries, Cuba and China have probably done more to eliminate basic malnutrition than any other in the world.

CONCLUSIONS

Three important lessons emerge from the above discussion. First, for a primarily rural society with substantial malnutrition, the most important nutritional aspect of the Green Revolution is its direct potential to raise cereal consumption of small farmers' households. Planners should aim at extending these direct effects as widely as possible. This means bringing access to the Green Revolution to the very smallest of farmers—those on less than a third of a hectare on Java, for instance. These farmers must be given access to the credit needed to use purchased inputs. In some regions the direct impact can be significant only if land reform creates access for many small farmers. These are difficult tasks, and considerable research and experimentation will be needed to find out how to do them effectively. But this is where the most fruitful opportunities to have a major impact on nutritional status exist.

Second, the indirect effects from prices and incomes must be planned to avoid negative nutritional effects on one hand and negative production incentives on the other. Steering this course involves some very narrow roads (and possibly no roads at all within some institutional settings). Designing financial incentives for farmers while maintaining access to food grains on the part of the poorest groups in a society is one of the most difficult tasks for modern political economies. Recent research efforts have just begun to grapple with the issue in a serious intellectual fashion.[6, 7]

The third task is to anticipate some of the roundabout effects of new agricultural technology before they happen. This is especially true of changed profitability of new farming systems, either for crop mix (cereals vs. legumes) or, more importantly, for new mechanical technology. Planners should be prepared with productive rural employment programs if the new farming technology is deemed desirable. Alternatively, research might show that a social accounting would seriously question the desirability of rapid and widespread tractorization and displacement of tenants, for example. In such cases, planners should be prepared with policies to prevent the development of the new farming system. These might involve removing existing interest rate or foreign exchange preferences for tractors, or they might involve limits on the amount of land one man can farm. Whatever the means, anticipating the problems makes them easier to resolve than after the new systems are entrenched.

It is precisely to anticipate these problems and to know how to deal with such complex effects of policies that research and analysis must be done. Greater production of cereals alone will not solve nutritional problems, any more than present cereal production, unless the mechanisms of food access change. There is little hope for changing these distribution mechanisms at an international level, and most progress must of necessity come from the countries themselves. How to do this within existing political realities is a black art. Success stories exist, but they are undocumented, unanalyzed, and not understood. Research that gains this understanding will have enormous payoff in terms of improving access to food for the most disadvantaged.

REFERENCES

1. FALCON, W. P. 1970. The Green Revolution: Generations of Problems. Am. J. Agr. Econ. **52**(5).
2. FORMAN, M. J. & B. L. BERNSTON. 1971. The nutritional impact of the Green Revolution: I. Paper prepared for the 162nd National Meeting of the American Chemical Society. Washington, D.C.
3. GERSHENKRON, A. 1965. Economic Backwardness in Historical Perspective. Preager. New York.
4. LIPTON, M. 1975. Urban bias and food policy in poor countries. Food Policy. November 1975.

5. SCHERTZ, L. P. 1973. Nutrition Realities in the Lower Income Countries. ERS-USDA. June 1973.
6. TIMMER, C. P. 1976. Food and fertilizer policy in LDC's. Food Policy. February 1976.
7. TIMMER, C. P. 1975. The political economy of rice in Asia: Lessons and implications. Food Res. Inst. Stud. XIV(4).
8. TIMMER, C. P. Food policy in China. Food Res. Inst. Stud. XV(1).
9. WADE, N. 1974. Green Revolution (I): A just technology, often unjust in use; and (II): Problems of adapting a Western technology. Science 186.
10. WATERLOW, J. C. & P. R. PAYNE. 1975. The protein gap: A review article. Nature 258: 117.
11. WORTMAN, S. 1975. Agriculture in China. Sci. American. June 1975.

APPENDIX

SUMMARY OF RESEARCH PROPOSED BY THE NUTRITION OVERVIEW TEAM OF THE NATIONAL ACADEMY OF SCIENCES WORLD FOOD AND NUTRITION STUDY

The team attempted to identify those research topics that would complete a nutritional overview of all the other primarily production-oriented research topics. The issue was how to translate productivity gains in agriculture into meaningful gains in nutritional status among those most in need. Addressing that issue required a conceptual framework that placed heavy emphasis on the interdependencies among nutrition as a biomedical science, nutrition as a human activity involving highly personal decisions within the context of individual, family, and social constraints, and nutrition as a social concern for the well-being of a population. The gaps in knowledge in all three dimensions of nutrition were treated as equally legitimate claimants for research attention.

The research topics have been organized around four basic themes. The first, and in many ways the fundamental, theme directs research toward understanding the individual and social costs of malnutrition. The costs are to be measured in several dimensions—work performance, disease resistance, learning and behavioral adaptation, fertility and infant death rates, and so on. The focus is on identifying priorities for nutritional intervention programs. Is energy the critical factor in a sub-population's food intake, or should resources be devoted to iron or vitamin A supplementation? Hence the purpose of this research is to define malnutrition in terms of the degree of impairment of biological, social, and economic functions associated with different degrees of deficit.

Because societies and individuals constantly face tradeoffs in how to allocate their resources, the scientist is asked to phrase his research questions in such a manner that the results will provide individual and social decisionmakers with guidance about the gains and losses at the tradeoff point. For which nutrients is it critical to provide 80, 90, or 100 percent of recommended allowances, at what period of development, and for how long? What is the long- and short-term functional cost of providing only 60 or 70 percent? Or 120 or 150 percent? At what stage or degree are the effects irreversible?

The second major research theme shifts from individual nutrient-individual host interactions to a concern for insuring the quality, safety, and adequacy of the diet as actually consumed. Understanding the many complex interactions among nutrients and non-nutrients such as toxins and fiber, among nutrients and various diet-borne contaminants or additives, and among nutrients and the physiological state of the consumer, occupies the first half of the profile. This research will have a heavy biomedical and biochemical orientation and can draw on extensive findings presently available for individual foodstuffs. The new concern in this area is understanding individual diets as they are consumed, rather than isolated foodcrops as they are grown and marketed.

The second half of this theme extends the quality and safety issue to a concern for dietary adequacy. This research area has important components in both the biochemical sciences and the social sciences. First, a set of alternative, satisfactory patterns of all recognized nutrients in diets needs to be established for various age/sex/environmental groups. Second, a much fuller understanding is needed of the determinants of dietary patterns among these various groups. The roles of income and relative prices are obviously important but need to be much more carefully specified, especially in the context of a host of important and interacting social and cultural food needs and habits. Food preparation and distribution patterns within households are especially critical determinants of individual nutritional status, but very little is known about them even descriptively. Important methodological and measurement problems must be resolved for this research to be successful, but they should be resolved in the context of field research efforts.

Research in the first two areas is designed to further our understanding of what people need to eat and why they eat what they do. This information will provide a much firmer base than presently exists for intervention programs designed to improve the nutritional status of selected groups. Such programs have a long history and some notable successes. But many have failed because of inadequate understanding of what was needed, lack of sensitivity to the real factors that cause people to eat what they do, and/or a serious lack of comparative experience on the types of interventions possible and how they can be effectively implemented. The next research topic is addressed to the last issue.

Three major subareas have been identified where research is essential to improving the efficiency and effectiveness of resources used in nutritional interventions. Benefit-cost methodology needs to be developed to aid planners in formulating effective interventions. Part of the methodological bottleneck lies in measurement of benefits, a topic given priority above. But part of the problem also lies in knowing what to measure, when to measure it, and how to compare benefits in widely different forms. The benefit from improved physical work output may be immediately measurable in financial terms. Improved learning abilities may have such payoff after 10 or 20 years. Improved receptivity to family planning may be more important than both in the long-run, and yet *measuring* its impact and incorporating the result into evaluations will be extremely difficult and complex. Failure to do so, however, will seriously undervalue the social utility of a nutritional intervention and hence bias the decision making against it.

The two other subareas involve evaluating interventions of increasingly broader scope. Direct food interventions such as school feeding programs, food stamps, rationing, introduction of new foods, and nutrition education are popular with many governments precisely because of their directness. Such popularity should not obscure the fact that relatively little is known about the nutritional effectiveness of such programs or of how to implement the program in a cost-effective manner.

Direct but nonfood interventions, especially in the public health environment, can have important nutritional benefits. Research in this area would recognize that malnutrition is frequently not a disease of food deficiency but has causes rooted in the physical, biological, and social environments in which people live. The most directly relevant and important environmental areas of concern are water supply and sanitation; the prenatal environment of both mother and fetus; the newborn infant's environment, especially the relationships between infection defense mechanisms and breast feeding; and the two-way interaction between infection and nutrition. Interventions in these aspects of the environment may allow sparing of food for growth and development within the body rather than diverting the nutrients for defense and repair functions or having them pass unutilized through a diseased gastro-intestinal tract. Quantified understanding of these savings and the interactions that generate them will make the design of integrated programs easier, cheaper, and more effective.

The last research area seeks an even broader reach than the previous profiles in searching for the roundabout and usually haphazard nutritional impact of general government policies. Most countries do not have coherent food and nutrition policies and thus end up with "nutrition by happenstance." Methodology presently available for agricultural sector analysis and development planning would increase knowledge about the potential nutritional impact of existing policies (or non-policies) or proposed changes if the questions were asked, the data gathered or organized, and the analysis performed.

Within the range of food and agricultural policies are a number of areas of concern. What are the nutritional effects of the agricultural production strategy, of resource use, and of attempts to reach food self-sufficiency? Somewhat more broadly, what are the effects of the basic price policy, of marketing structure and technology, and of international trade? And most generally, what are the nutritional effects of income redistribution measures, of the budget process, of the policy-making process, and of the nutritional "ad hocery" found in virtually every country of the world? The research asks whether we can do better if we are better informed. Doing better may be very costly, but it may also cost very little. Until the research is done, no one will know.

FAILURE OF THE FOOD DISTRIBUTION SYSTEM: DEALING WITH FAMINE

Aaron E. Ifekwunigwe

Charles R. Drew Postgraduate Medical School and
University of California
Los Angeles, California 90059

INTRODUCTION

Adequate supply of food to an area depends as much on the adequacy of food production as on a system of food distribution that can convey food from the areas of production to the areas of need. The area of need could represent a whole country, when the country depends on supplies across international boundaries for items of food, or it could be a region of the same country, which depends on other regions for part or all of its food supply. The morning session should have covered food production, and the previous speaker would have dealt with food availability, which includes distribution.

I shall, therefore, consider briefly the factors that might lead to a failure of the food distribution system, and then the measures that should be adopted in dealing with famine.

Food distribution will be impaired by any event that disrupts transportation, food storage, marketing system, or cash availability, or by situations that encourage speculation, leading to hoarding, and inflation, or by physical and/or economic blockade.

Shortage of food in an area leads to hunger, and particularly when prolonged, hunger becomes synonymous with *"famine"* defined by the Oxford English Dictionary as "extreme and general scarcity of food in a town, country, etc.; also as want of food, hunger; hence starvation."

CLASSIFICATION OF CAUSES OF FAMINE

Famines are usually due to disasters, which are brought about by a variety of causes, and affect food production and/or distribution. Disasters can be classified according to their origin or duration or relative to the area's baseline conditions and problems.

Origin

Natural. Under this heading fall droughts, floods, earthquakes, hurricanes, tidal waves, and locusts and other pests.

Man-made. This heading includes wars, revolutions, civil upheavals, religious/social persecutions, blockades, defoliation, and crop destruction.

Duration

Short-term. The disaster and interruption of food supplies are short-lived and expected to last for a few weeks, before normal supplies resume. This type of disaster usually gives no warning and involves only a limited area. Examples are earthquakes, volcanic eruptions, floods, hurricanes, tidal waves, large fires in cities, and stoppage of food supplies to cities by strikes or riots.

Medium-term. The disaster is such that the food shortage continues until the next harvest season, usually a period of 6 to 12 months, when, hopefully, the cause is no longer operative. In general, there is a warning period, and the disaster affects a larger area than the first type. Crop failures resulting from such disasters are commonly due to drought, excessive rains (leading to extensive flooding), plant disease, and animal pests such as locusts.

Long-term. The food shortage produced by this type of disaster lasts for a year or more and is usually a national problem, involving the entire country or a significant part of it. An example of this category of disaster is the disruption of food supply by war and blockade, as in Biafra and Bangladesh. Another example is due to failure of two or more successive rainy seasons, as in North China in 1876–79 and in the Sahel region of West Africa and Ethiopia in 1969–74. A final example is long-term feeding programs of large numbers of refugees, who cannot be resettled for years, as the East Pakistan refugees in India in 1971–72 or even for decades, as the Palestinian refugees in the Middle East.

Relative to the Area's Baseline Conditions or Problems

In many instances, the degree of food shortage that constitutes a famine is a relative judgment, based on the pre-existing food and nutritional conditions. For example, the daily per capita energy supply of the population in Asia and the Far East is only about 1,900 kilocalories, whereas the figure for North America is over 3,000 kilocalories. The people of Asia and the Far East accept this as the "normal" way of life, yet if, for some reason, the daily per capita energy supply of the population of the United States were restricted to even 2,500 kilocalories, this would constitute a national emergency. Therefore, based on the baseline food situation, disasters can be divided as follows:

Acute. The disaster produces an unaccustomed shortage of food in an area previously self-sufficient. However, these are usually countries with substantial resources, economically stable and technologically more advanced, hence facilitating relief measures and rehabilitation.

Chronic. Many developing countries, dependent on subsistence agriculture, have such a precarious food/nutritional balance that the specter of famine is never far away. In fact, it is recognized as the norm to have the "hungry" season of the year, between the planting and harvesting seasons. Nevertheless, it is this very state of chronic under-nutrition that is partly responsible for the countries being trapped in the vicious circle of poverty: Decreased economic production → Poverty → Undernutrition → Decreased economic production, *ad ifinitum.* The plight of such countries is further aggravated by the unabated rapid increase of population, galloping inflation, increased cost of food production and possible fall in food production, due mainly to rising cost of agricultural equipment and fertilizers. With the worsening situation, a stage may be reached in these areas when it becomes a fine point of argument as to when a chronic disaster qualifies for emergency assistance.

Acute-on-Chronic. Even more significant for the areas just described, any disaster, even those that would normally produce only a limited effect or short-term disorganization, will upset the precarious balance in these chronic disaster areas and precipitate a long and major crisis. Ironically, developing countries are situated in locations where natural disasters are frequent, and they are also more prone to man-made disasters. Furthermore, a single disaster may set off a chain reaction of secondary disasters, which can be avoided in richer countries.

NECESSITY FOR PLANNING IN FAMINE RELIEF

Although famines, resulting from disasters and requiring emergency assistance, have occurred throughout history, the assistance, in most cases, is still rendered on an "ad hoc" basis, without planning, assessment, or coordination. The "emergency nature" of disaster relief has been taken too literally in the past, but it is possible in most cases to anticipate the famine, even if not the precipitating disaster. Unfortunately, the increasing vulnerability of much of the world indicates that the frequency and severity of disasters are rising, further emphasizing the necessity for planning.

Concern for the haphazard nature of emergency assistance led to the convening of an international symposium at Saltsjobaden, Sweden, in August 1970, by the Swedish Nutrition Foundation. Two cf the recommendations made by that meeting called for the establishment of an International Disaster Relief Organization (IDRO), as well as the creation of a permanent National Disaster Relief Organization (NDRO) in each country. These organizations will increase international cooperation, avoid wasteful competition and duplication, place the authority and control of relief operations in the hands of the national government, and can indicate possible directions for national development, so that the problems of disasters and famines can be tackled in a more fundamental way, with the emphasis on prevention.

The meeting in Sweden recommended that the IDRO have a permanent secretariat, to keep up-to-date records on available relief resources and continuously collect data relevant to disaster prediction and for emergency assistance. In the event of a disaster, this secretariat would coordinate and serve as the liaison between international governments and agencies and the NDRO of the affected country. In March 1972, the Office of the United Nations Disaster Relief Coordinator (UNDRO) was established, with a mandate covering some of these recommendations.

It was recommended that the NDRO be directed by a NDR Coordinator— an influential person at Permanent Secretary level or above, working out of the Cabinet Office. He would be responsible for planning and maintaining a state of preparedness in the pre-disaster period, coordinating emergency assistance in the event of a disaster, and establishing close liaison with relevant ministries, voluntary agencies, and international organizations. The NDRO would be the focal point for all emergency operations in the following three phases:

I. Before a Disaster: State of Preparedness
II. During a Disaster: Deliberate, Decisive and Directed Action
III. After a Disaster: Rehabilitation and Reconstruction Programmed into Long-Term Development

BEFORE A FAMINE: STATE OF PREPAREDNESS

Every country should have a national plan to deal with disasters and famines in a prompt, effective, and coordinated manner. Ironically, it is those countries that are most prone to disasters and famines that are least prepared for them. Efforts should, therefore, be made at the international and national levels to encourage and assist these countries to plan for such inauspicious events.

National Policy Provisions for Famine Relief

It can be assumed that governments normally feel obliged to bring relief to their citizens when striken by a disaster, except possibly in politically-generated disasters like civil disturbances and wars. Even in these circumstances, governments should be encouraged to provide relief to the innocent victims and noncombatants in the dispute. Constitutional provisions should be made and enabling legislations passed to facilitate relief operations, especially in the following areas:

The government should have the power to declare an area a disaster area and impose a state of emergency. Such a step will give the NDRO extraordinary powers for speedy, effective relief operation.

Disasters of medium or long-term duration, especially, tend to engender fears of severe food shortage. As such, hoarding, profiteering and black-marketing of foodstuffs are widespread. The government should be able to impose price controls on all or selected items, when indicated and provisions made for enforcement.

During a disaster, the demand for food may so outstrip the supply that rationing of some or all food items may be the only means of equitable distribution. Adequate arrangements need to be made for its administration.

In an emergency, some relief personnel may be the only ones in a position to render a particular service that is traditionally outside their scope; for example, nurses performing doctors' tasks. It is necessary to have legislation waiving such restrictions in an emergency.

For a smooth relief operation, it should be possible to circumvent bureaucratic red tape and have visas issued free and expeditiously to "bona fide" relief workers.

Inasmuch as relief materials to a disaster-stricken country are usually free, it is only fair that the recipient country grant them tax and customs duty exemption.

Special treatment should be given ships carrying relief materials as regards expeditious berthing and customs clearance.

Cash given as relief aid should be given a realistic and favorable exchange rate since it is to the advantage of the country.

Warehouses and stores should be provided free to relief agencies, and the government should be able to commandeer such facilities, if necessary.

Top priority should be given to relief supplies and personnel in allocating transport and communications facilities, such as vehicles, fuel, telegraphic, telex and telephone services.

Short-wave radios may be the only means of quick communications between the control headquarters and the command posts in a remote disaster area; therefore, radio frequencies and licenses should be available to "bona fide" relief organizations.

Establishment of the National Disaster Relief Organization

Central control at the national level is crucial to effective famine relief. The NDRO should have complete coordinating authority over the relief activities of all governmental, civilian and military, and private voluntary agencies. The NDRO should not usurp the internal authority of any of these bodies but reserve the right of delegation and assignment of functions. The NDR Coordinator should be an influential high-ranking official directly responsible to the President or Head of State or Prime Minister.

The NDRO, in its pre-planning, should include all existing governmental, civilian and military, and private agencies. Appropriate senior officials from these ministries, departments, or organizations should be closely involved in planning. In the inter-emergency periods, these officials will be engaged in their regular duties, but as soon as a disaster strikes, they will be automatically fully seconded to the NDRO.

The NDRO is organized into operational divisions or directorates to be responsible for specific areas and functions. Each directorate is headed by a director who should be a senior official with policymaking powers.

A sample organizational chart is shown below (TABLE 1). The individual directorates will be responsible for each phase of famine relief. Prior to a famine, each directorate will organize itself and work collectively with the other directorates as follows:

1. Compile the information necessary for its operation, including lists of personnel who might be available for relief work.
2. Understand clearly its role in the relief operations and also the roles of voluntary and international organizations.
3. Develop administrative procedures for its staff and, under the guidance of the NDR Coordinator, means for effective communication with the other directorates.

Functions of the National Disaster Relief Organization

The NDRO, through its Directorates, will undertake the following:

1. *Identification of disaster-prone areas.* The geographical zones where natural disasters like earthquakes, droughts, floods, cyclones, hurricanes, and tidal waves occur are predictable. These zones should be identified in the country and disaster plans focused on the localities. Climatic data, including drastic reduction or increase in rainfall, should be monitored.

   Agricultural data should be collected through regular monthly reports by agricultural extension and field workers on the condition of crops, factors that may prevent or have prevented planting or harvesting, and factors that may reduce yields seriously, e.g., crop destruction. The Food and Agricultural Organization (FAO), at the international level, has instituted such a monitoring system.

   Other useful data in identifying disaster prone areas are migration patterns and sudden and large population movements and the causes, e.g., food shortages, wars, natural disasters, trend of food prices (especially a sudden rise) and the causative factors.

   Man-made disasters, e.g., war and civil upheavals, develop more slowly, and there is usually time for plans in anticipation of the disaster. In Biafra, malnutrition did not become a public health problem until about six months after the outbreak of hostilities.
2. *Setting up and coordinating early warning systems.* The impact of most

TABLE 1

NATIONAL DISASTER RELIEF ORGANIZATION—ORGANIZATIONAL CHART

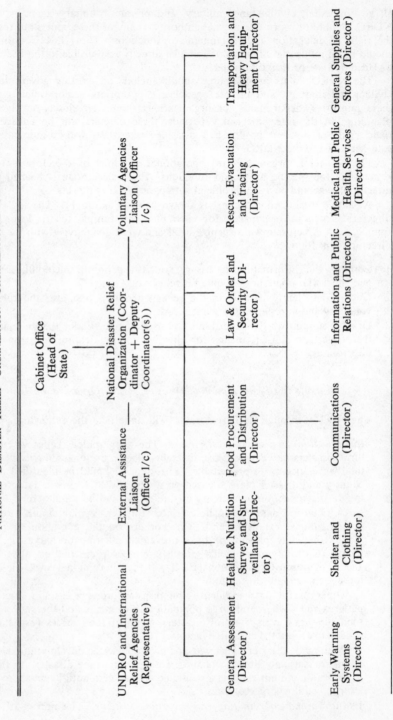

natural disasters can be minimized, if it were possible to warn the potential victims, so that they could take defensive actions. Sophisticated instruments are now available for predicting some disasters, e.g., seismographs, weather satellites, and hurricane warning stations. However, these are too expensive for most developing countries, but they can benefit by international cooperation and coordination.

Often, even when such a warning is made available to the country at the central level, the communications systems in the developing countries are not adequate to disseminate quickly the warning to the specific area. The NDRO should devise an effective early warning system, particularly for the disaster-prone regions of the country. It might include placing radio sets in each village under the charge of a responsible person, and educating the villagers on the significance of the various warnings and the protective actions indicated. When the warning of an impending disaster is received, the responsible person through the local Civil Defense body and appropriate medium communicates the message promptly to the inhabitants.

3. *Background information on local conditions.* Information on local conditions should be gathered and documented by the NDRO. This would assist planners and international organizations in rendering the most appropriate and realistic relief effort and materials.

The types of information needed would include food availability, consumption patterns, food habits and taboos, clothing worn during different seasons, types of shelter and construction materials, health facilities, nature of common health problems, transportation and communication facilities, administrative structure, institutions and organizations of potential value in emergency assistance, and socio-cultural traditions relevant to assistance needs and operations.

It would be extremely useful to prepare grid maps of the country showing the following: topography; areas vulnerable to disasters and the nature of anticipated disaster; service establishments, air force, navy, police, civil defense, fire-fighting installations, voluntary agencies, seaports and harbors, airports, railway stations and depots, public transport depots, commercial vehicle depots; construction plants—mobile cranes, bulldozers, excavators, trucks, etc.; construction material stocks; ambulance stations; mobile cooking and food distribution centers; utilities networks—electricity, drinking water, gas; fuel depots—for vehicles, cooking, heating; television stations; radio stations and mobile radio equipment; telephone exchanges; hospitals; blood banks; drug warehouses and large stores; administrative boundaries; towns and villages; sites suitable for temporary housing and mobile hospitals; permanent buildings likely to be suitable as emergency shelters, first aid and feeding centers—schools, churches, colleges, cinemas, etc.

4. *Health information and surveillance.* The NDRO should collect information from such sources as the Ministry of Health, universities, institutes of child health or special health surveillance units. Such information should include deaths and their causes, prevalence of infections and other diseases, medical facilities, drug supplies, health personnel and their availability.

A particularly sensitive indicator of the health status of any developing country is the information on the mortality and morbidity of the young child. A system for collecting this type of data would be very desirable, but some countries would need technical assistance in establishing it.

5. *Nutritional information and surveillance.* Available sources, including institutes of nutrition, should be tapped by the NDRO for nutritional information. It is possible to collect data based on attendances at the hospitals and outpatient clinics. These would, however, neglect those who are too ill or malnourished to leave their homes, or those not used to the health facilities. Therefore, a realistic nutritional assessment can only be done by special units, using clinical assessment and physical anthropometry, especially on young children.

A surveillance system collecting this type of information is a very sensitive indicator of the population's nutritional status and can provide an early warning system of an impending famine. Again, many developing countries will need technical assistance in establishing it.

6. *Contingency plans.* Based on the information thus collected, the NDRO would make plans for effective relief operations, including the following:

   a) *List of likely requirements.* The supplies, personnel and logistical support necessary for each region of the country and for specified disasters are listed in order of priority.

   b) *List of possible sources.* The possible sources of the requirements listed should be identified. First preference should be given to local sources, and domestic preferred over foreign sources. The items identified will include food supplies; transportation facilities, e.g., vehicles by number, type and make, spare parts, maintenance facilities and personnel, railways, aircraft and airport facilities; professional and skilled personnel by number, categories and location, e.g., doctors, nurses, engineers, etc.

   c) *Stockpiling of essential supplies.* Ready availability of supplies will permit rapid response to an emergency. It may not be necessary, nor indeed desirable, to have physical possession of the supplies, but prior negotiations should be made with the sources, so that the pre-pledged items could be called on immediately when they are needed. Within a country, this would likely mean a redistribution of resources, e.g., transferring food from an area of surplus to an area of scarcity. Care has to be taken, however, so that shortage is not created and inflation produced by diverting too much food from an area of surplus to an area of shortage.

   d) *System of food distribution established.* Food rationing is often necessary and plans for this, including printing of coupons, should be made in advance. Price control may be needed and plans for enforcement made. Full use should be made of existing institutions and facilities, such as schools, churches and health centers. In Biafra, for example, the most effective channels for food distribution were the religious agencies, particularly the World Council of Churches and Caritas Internationalis. These agencies had a network of organizations that extended to practically every village and through their indigenous missionaries were particularly effective in reaching most communities.

   e) *Planning for logistical options.* A disaster relief operation often is as good as its logistical support. The need to move large quantities of supplies quickly poses a big problem. Therefore alternative plans for modes and routes of transportation should be made, e.g., the use of waterways or animals, such as camels in the desert.

7. *Publication of disaster (famine) manuals.* The NDRO should prepare and distribute a Disaster Manual for the country, giving administrators and others the procedures for an emergency. It should reflect regional varia-

tions and the different types of disasters and their peculiarities. The manual should be frequently revised. A good example is the "Famine Code" of India, first published in 1913, which has been extremely useful during crises.

8. *Training for emergencies.* There is clearly a need for a cadre of people to be trained in disaster relief operations in each country. The trainees return to their normal occupations but constitute a reserve of trained personnel to be mobilized in an emergency. The NDRO should be responsible for the training, although technical assistance from international agencies may be necessary.

9. *Holding mock disaster maneuvers or drills.* In order to maintain a state of preparedness, the NDRO should organize mock disaster maneuvers at regular intervals, to test the operability of the disaster plan. The drill should test the facilities, relief personnel, and reactions of the mock victims.

10. *Coordination and liaison.* The NDRO should serve as a liaison between the national and the international relief agencies.

DURING A DISASTER: DELIBERATE, DECISIVE AND DIRECTED ACTION: ADMINISTRATIVE CONSIDERATIONS

Coordination

The national government of the affected country, through the National Disaster Relief Coordinator, should assume ultimate control and responsibility for the conduct of the relief operation. Governmental, international, and voluntary agencies should conform with the plans and directions of the Coordinator.

The international relief agencies will thus be under the direction of the NDR Coordinator, and they should regard themselves as donors and technical advisers, their actions supporting, not competing with, indigenous efforts.

Authority will need to be delegated to the field personnel from the headquarters. Good and accurate records of projects, the type, quality, quantity and location of supplies are crucial. The maintenance of good relations between the relief workers and the recipient population is vital to success. In the past, agency administrators and relief workers have been criticized for extravagance and high standards of living in the midst of misery and starvation. Sensitivity and prudence demand the exercise of as much frugality as possible.

When a disaster strikes, there is often a convergence of many relief agencies on the affected area. The agencies involved may wish to retain autonomy and resist interagency division of labor, which results in competition, wastage, duplication, and chaos. The NDR Coordinator, through an External Assistance Liaison Officer, should establish an information pool for the agencies and ensure cooperation and coordination.

Maximum use should be made of the local expertise, skills, and labor, and expatriate relief volunteers limited to the required minimum. Often, expatriates are sent for too short a time—4 to 6 weeks—which is nearly the time it takes them to adjust to the local conditions. They should be sent for 6 months or longer, whenever possible.

All too frequently the wrong balance of expertise is made available. Thus, in some cases, there are too many doctors, since much of the medical relief work can be undertaken by paramedical personnel properly trained and directed. Equally, surgical teams are not always a high priority in natural disasters, as doctors trained in tropical medicine, child health, and epidemiology are more useful. However, the main requirement will usually be for technicians, nurses, sanitarians, engineers, communications experts, and the like.

Logistics

For relief supplies, maximum practical use should be made of local and domestic resources, e.g., for foods and building materials (although without provoking inflation). These are usually much cheaper, more appropriate and acceptable, and moreover local purchases stimulate the economy. Goods imported into the disaster areas must be acceptable to the community and suitable for the local climatic and cultural conditions, and, if possible, foods with a high black market value should be avoided. Relief materials should therefore be screened for appropriateness for the local conditions, and only essential supplies should be sent into a disaster area. The long-term effects of imported relief goods to a community must also be considered. It is a fact of life that bureaucratic red tape, delays, and corruption rear their ugly heads, and in reality a judicious balance between reasonable efficiency, use of limited resources, and social justice will have to be struck.

Relief supplies are best channeled through existing institutions, e.g., schools and health centers, but special efforts must be made to reach the needy in their homes. A reliable survey can define the vulnerable groups and establish priorities, e.g., patients with overt malnutrition, infants, young children, pregnant and lactating women, older children, elderly people.

Transport and communication, often already poor and further disrupted by the disaster, pose the most difficult problem. Relief supplies have to be moved quickly and in large quantities. The suitability of various modes of transportation—air, rail, road, water—needs to be examined and the payoffs assessed, and supplies in transit must be accompanied by a reliable person to guard against theft. Vehicle donations by agencies must be coordinated in order to limit the number of different makes, so that parts are interchangeable and maintenance easier. Fuel, spare parts, and skilled mechanics are essential and should be given high priority.

Operational Aspects

Assessment and Surveillance

It is essential that very early in an emergency a team of qualified personnel make a rapid, simple, but objective assessment of the situation in the affected area.

The exercise of field assessment, even in short-term disasters, is necessary to allay anxiety, clarify needs, identify areas of greatest need, permit more realistic planning, and assign priorities. Later, a more detailed assessment should be made, in order to establish a baseline for judging future trends and evaluating relief operations. The information from the assessment is useful for briefing the press, donor groups, and interested governments. Also, keeping the affected public informed of current developments is very important to alleviate fears, dispel rumors, curb panic, and boost morale.

After processing, the information should be transmitted to field workers, as this feedback assists coordination and serves as an incentive for continued field reporting. A relief program should be able to respond rapidly and effectively to needs detected by the surveillance team.

A multidisciplinary team is needed and should include experts with appropriate field experience in epidemiology, tropical medicine, nutrition, agriculture, public health, logistics and possibly anthropology. The NDRO assembles the team and preference should be given to nationals. If there is already a national surveillance unit, it may only be necessary to strengthen it, and some of the information may already be available.

The team, even if expatriate, should be under the direction of the NDRO. All information from surveys is the property of the government and only released to the public at its discretion. The data should be standardized by using standard forms, questionnaires, and diagnostic criteria.

The initial rapid survey should focus on areas of greatest concern to the victims: shelter, food, and health hazards. The techniques employed would depend on the type of assessment, the team, nature of disaster, and what is available. However, they must be rapid, simple, reasonably accurate, objective, reproducible, and inexpensive. Sample sites must be carefully selected, and measurements made not only in clinics and feeding centers, but also in homes. The sample size should be about 10% of the target population, in order to be statistically valid. Processing of large volumes of data would be facilitated by the use of computers for analysis, banking, and retrieval. Computers are now available in many large cities in the developing countries and are not used to capacity. Even if a computer is not available, it is now possible to have a teletype connected to a computer terminal elsewhere, at short notice.

The data and the methods for obtaining them will vary in different situations. The data will be classified by geographical regions into the following categories:

- —Prevalence of malnutrition: determined by clinical signs, anthropometry (e.g., weight, arm circumference, fatfold thickness) and possibly simple biochemical tests.
- —Food: availability, consumption patterns by age groups, production, size and location of stocks, storage facilities.
- —Prevalence of "conditioning" infections, which further decrease the nutritional and health status of the population and decrease the effectiveness of dietary intervention, e.g., measles and diarrheas.
- —Health: deaths and their causes, prevalence of the common diseases, medical facilities, drug supplies.
- —Water supply and environmental health: source of water, wells, rainfall, sanitation.
- —Shelter from exposure: types, availability of shelter, clothes, blankets.
- —Transport: capacity of various modes and routes, number and types of vehicles, fuel availability, spare parts, maintenance facilities.
- —Supplies: requirements, allocation, delivery, location, distribution.
- —Personnel: types, training, experience, availability.
- —Relief programs: types, personnel, progress.
- —Types and extent of social and economic disruption: extent of family

disruption and possible methods of identification and tracing systems for reunification; extent and possible uses of public information system; extent and possible uses of employment and welfare schemes; availability, disruption and possible uses of market system, currency system, etc.; conditions of and need for public works programs (roads, bridges, etc.); number of lives lost, houses destroyed, homeless people, crop losses.

Food and Nutrition Relief

—Foods used should be, as far as possible, from local and domestic sources, provided this does not provoke inflation.
—The number of items should be limited to the basic essentials.
—Foods must be palatable, acceptable, and conform with food habits, taboos, and religion.
—They should be nutritionally compact, with high caloric and nutritive value.
—They should be well packed, easy to transport and store, with a long shelf life.
—The foods should be simple to distribute, and, if possible, be in dry form and prepacked ration units.
—Whenever possible, the foods should be wholly or partially precooked.
—The uncooked foods should be easy to prepare and require a minimum of utensils, and if special equipment or ingredients are needed for preparation, they should accompany the food packages.
—Clean drinking water is often an even more pressing need than food.
—A field nutritionist to offer advice on diet, nutrition and the preparation of foods is very desirable.

In disasters of short duration, "something to eat" is often more important than a balanced diet, and the nutritional value of the relief food is of secondary importance.

If the crisis is of moderate or long duration, a more carefully formulated food program, based on accurate field assessment of nutritional status and specific deficiencies is essential.

It should be emphasized here that protein deficiency cannot be fully corrected unless caloric demands are also satisfied, because during starvation, proteins are preferentially metabolized for energy.

The relief foods should include these categories:

—General foods, e.g., cereals, legumes, preserved animal protein (powdered or evaporated milk, dried fish, tinned meat), vegetable oil, salt, sugar.
—Special foods, for specific age groups and needs, especially the severely malnourished and most vulnerable groups. Examples are specially formulated weaning food mixtures, such as C.S.M. (corn-soya-milk); powdered milk-based formulas for artificial feeding; and preparations designed for the treatment of malnutrition, such as Kwashiorkor Food Mix (K-Mix), preferably packed with vegetable oil required for preparation. If available, cheaper, locally made nutritious vegetable multi-mixes, should be used.
—Supplements, vitamins and minerals in areas of known deficiencies, such as vitamin A in parts of Asia and Latin America and iron in most countries.

Rations should be determined on the basis of nutrient requirements and issued in simple, easy-to-use familiar domestic measures and units. The amounts of food issued will depend on decisions by NDRO on the availability of food and the need for food relief—"emergency subsistence," "temporary maintenance," treatment or rehabilitation. Calculations of the actual quantities of ration would then be based on the nutrient composition of the local and imported foods.

On rare occasions, enough resources are available to feed the entire population; otherwise, selective distribution will be necessary. Nutritional status will be assessed by simple methods. A decision is made on which categories require feeding as inpatients in institutions, in feeding centers more than once daily, several times weekly, or only weekly supplements.

Any distribution system must be based on the priority of certain groups:

—Physiologically vulnerable: overtly malnourished subjects, young children, pregnant and lactating women, older children, the sick, the aged, others.
—The main work force, whose effort will be needed for reconstruction, future food production, etc.
—The relief workers, administrative staff, the police.

It is necessary to exercise great flexibility and adapt distribution to local situations. Ration cards, if culturally acceptable, may be used. When appropriate, it is preferable to issue food as "dry" rations to be taken home. However, under certain circumstances the foods should be prepared and consumed under supervision in feeding centers, run by respected community leaders. These include imported foods requiring special preparation to be locally acceptable, foods that need qualitative selective distribution, such as to young children, to avoid the risk of the foods not reaching them.

The maximum use should be made of the feeding centers for health and nutrition education, and for immunizations, as was the case in the multipurpose clinics in Biafra. Every effort should be made to reach the vulnerable groups, who do not attend the feeding centers, in their homes.

Health and Medical Relief

Health and medical relief, particularly disease control, deserves the same priority as food and nutritional relief. This is because of the well-known synergism between malnutrition and infection and the fact that infectious diseases may directly cause more morbidity and mortality than starvation *per se*.

The diseases encountered in an emergency in any place are largely the same as in normal times, but their frequency and severity are greater in malnourished subjects. Furthermore, the disruption leads to a breakdown of the already poor sanitation and overcrowding, thereby increasing the risk of food-and-water-borne epidemics, respiratory and contagious diseases.

Most of the diseases in developing countries are preventable by public health measures, which should receive the most attention. Also, the vast majority of the population has no access to health services, and there is an acute shortage of trained personnel.

The health survey and surveillance will provide a direction for the services. Health care is best provided by local doctors, nurses, nutritionists, administrators, and auxiliaries. Local manpower is usually inadequate and needs to be supplemented by staff from outside and paramedical workers trained to assist.

Health facilities, equipment, and drugs should be as simple and versatile as possible. Sophisticated field hospitals and foreign surgical teams have a limited place in disasters. Mobile clinics may be the most useful and practical way of delivering health services to dispersed or mobile populations, such as refugees, and for mass immunizations, as in Biafra.

Communicable diseases should be controlled through surveillance, together with treatment of individual cases and immunization of contacts. The provision of clean water, sanitation facilities, and control of pests and vermin should receive a high priority in health programs.

Emergency Shelter

In an emergency, protection from the elements should receive very urgent consideration, since death from exposure to adverse weather conditions occurs long before death from starvation. Thus, in certain weather conditions, there may be immediate need for blankets and protective clothing. If construction of shelters is necessary, it is preferable to use low-cost, local building materials and labor; any imported materials should be cheap, lightweight, and compact. The shelters should be quick, easy and cheap to assemble, needing a minimum of trained personnel and equipment.

The structural design should be as similar as possible to the traditional housing and its utilization should conform with the local practices. The shelter should be suitable for the climate, with adequate insulation.

Finally, it is important that emergency shelters should not be permanent enough to become slums, but sturdy enough that, when the emergency subsides, they could be used for other purposes, e.g., for storage or animal housing.

Peculiarities of Wartime Famine Relief Operations

The problems of relief operations are further compounded in disasters produced by military conflict.

—One of the combatant groups may not have an internationally recognized legal status, and thus cannot directly appeal to other nations for assistance. Also, the group with international recognition may use its political influence to block attempts at relief for the civilian population.

—A state of blockade might be imposed, making it very difficult for communications and relief supplies.

—There is usually disorganization of even essential services, and social disruption, including breakup of families and separation of young children from their parents, posing the problem of reunion.

—The population is very mobile in response to the movements of the war fronts, making it very difficult to organize services.

—The relief workers and the recipient civilian population may be in constant physical danger from military attack by land or air.

—Crop destruction may take place, as in the defoliation campaign in Vietnam. In wars lasting longer than a few weeks, planting or harvesting of crops may be obstructed, leading to the need for long-term relief, even after the end of the war.

—Each side in the conflict may exaggerate or play down the extent of the disaster, for political reasons, thus making planning very difficult.

—There might be interference by the army with the relief operations, and relief supplies intended for the civilians may be commandeered by the army, or they might try to influence the distribution of supplies.

During hostilities, international organizations should provide assistance to noncombatant victims on all sides, regardless of political loyalties. The organizations should be free of political influence and establish their credibility as truly unbiased humanitarian agencies.

External relief organizations, through the NDRO, should be given immediate access to a disaster area, in order to assess relief needs. They should be permitted to establish contact and negotiate with all sides in the conflict, if they are to function effectively.

The force of world opinion can play a role in strengthening the international organizations in their impartial role in relief operations.

Concern for the use of famine as an instrument of warfare led to a recommendation, by the Saltsjobaden Symposium in 1970, calling on all nations of the world for an agreement on its ban. The preface to the recommendation stated that bacteriological warfare has been renounced through international convention as a legitimate instrument of war, because it was considered indiscriminate and may kill or harm bystanders as much as armed enemies. Starvation, even more so, should similarly be outlawed as a measure of warfare on the grounds that it is worse than indiscriminate—it preferentially affects the noncombatants: children, pregnant women, nursing mothers, and the elderly. It also stated that, historically, the following methods directed to causing famine have been ineffective as military tools: food blockade and destruction of crops and food stores.

The recommendation was then made that any use of starvation as a means of pressure or punishment against individuals or small or large population groups is a violation of the rights of man and should be outlawed. However, no action on it has as yet been taken.

Concurrent Evaluation System

In disaster relief operations, it is essential to have a concurrent assessment by an independent body not directly involved in the operation. It is necessary for testing the efficiency of the information-gathering systems, the activities and rapidity of feedback needed for any immediate revision of operational procedures.

The evaluation could be done by a designated section of the assessment and surveillance unit. The data collected during the initial assessment would provide the baseline for evaluation of the operation. Then, surveillance, on a continuing basis, provides the data on the various aspects of the relief operation, and monitoring of the trend of each indicator will furnish information on the progress of that aspect.

The results of evaluation would indicate the reasons for success or failure in a relief operation. The lessons thus learned will be useful in the planning and operation of future disaster relief.

AFTER A DISASTER: REHABILITATION AND RECONSTRUCTION PROGRAMMED INTO LONG-TERM DEVELOPMENT

Planning for Rehabilitation

Rehabilitation and reconstruction should be regarded as a continuation of relief operations and planned for at the start. The rehabilitation phase should smoothly and imperceptibly follow relief efforts.

The NDRO again should provide the leadership, with support and technical assistance from international agencies. The administrators need to recognize the long-term implications of relief efforts and plan to coordinate them with rehabilitation and development plans. Rehabilitation should not be just a practical "make-work" activity, but purposeful and aimed at the long-term improvement of the affected people and country. Some examples of such activities are provision of tools to carpenters, boats and nets to fisherman, livestock and ploughs to farmers. These items could be issued free or on loan for future payment or sold at reduced rates.

Types of Activities in Rehabilitation

Return of Displaced Persons

This activity is of prime importance, not only because it is humanitarian, but also because it is a morale booster. The first step is reunion of separated family members, and the next is return and resettlement of the family to its home.

Reunion of family members can be a very difficult problem, especially for separated young children. The following are some of the methods used to tackle the problem in Biafra:

—Parents and relatives were notified, through various information media, of the location of the centers housing the children, and called to identify and claim their children.
—Children old enough to furnish details of their homes, were grouped according to their areas of origin, transported in batches, and delivered to their addresses.
—Very young children (usually under 4 years) presented the biggest problem, but, by displaying them or their photographs in public places, many of them were identified and claimed by their families. It would be very helpful for family tracing, if plans were made, at the beginning of a disaster, for affixing durable identification labels on young children, bearing their names, parents, and places of origin.
—A related problem was that of orphanages in Biafra after the war. It is important that relief measures are culturally acceptable and should not, even unintentionally, destroy the indigenous social structure and cultural mores. Many well-meaning humanitarian organizations, immediately after the war, planned the establishment of orphanages for the homeless children. The idea was vigorously opposed because it ran counter to the closely knit family units in the extended family system. Under this system, no child is left uncared for. The responsibility for a child who has lost his parents, or whose parents are incapable of caring for him, automatically fell on the

next-of-kin. Orphanages would have encouraged people to shirk their traditional responsibilities; children would have grown up in institutions, without family roots. A home, even if poor, is preferable to a comfortable orphanage, in the long-term interests of a child. Therefore, the proposed orphanages were used as temporary holding centers for children, until they were reunited with their families, or failing that, placed with foster families, or legally adopted.

Restoration of Essential Services and Production

—Agriculture and food production must be encouraged, if necessary by replacing farm implements and providing seeds and livestock.
—Schools, health facilities, and other social services need to be rebuilt, reequipped, and reestablished.
—A system will be needed to assist people rebuild their homes, for instance, by setting up a loan scheme with favorable terms or providing building materials at subsidized prices.
—Roads and communications systems need to be rebuilt and reestablished, and broken bridges repaired.

Use of Food-for-Work Programs

These programs have the advantage of providing incentives for community action and fostering self-help and pride. They can be used for reconstructing homes, schools, roads, bridges, amongst others. However, great caution must be exercised, especially with limited food supply, not to divert food to such programs from the vulnerable groups.

Timing of the Phases

The phases should be so well integrated that it becomes difficult to tell when relief ends and rehabilitation begins. However, relief supplies should not be continued beyond the period of demonstrated need, in order to discourage the dependency syndrome. On the other hand, premature cessation of relief or rehabilitation efforts might result in a deteroration of the situation. Thus, to consolidate gains, the timing has to be right, with guidance provided by the surveillance reports, which continuously monitor the operation.

Cashing In On the Psychology of Disaster Relief

Disasters are often dramatic and catch attention, and it is possible to cash in on this psychological climate by using relief measures and projects as a leverage for long-term development. In an emergency, many new projects and techniques are introduced, and some of them should become permanent. Some examples are the loosening of bureaucratic red tape, enabling things to be done quickly; some traditions are relaxed and people are more willing to accept changes; the concept of self-help and pride may be fostered and local initiative and motivation engendered for development; paramedical workers and multi-purpose village-based health and nutrition clinics are accepted by the people and incorporated into the health system.

The confidence and rapport, which develop between the local inhabitants and relief workers, both national and international, facilitate acceptance of development projects. The attention that is focused on a country during a disaster often exposes neglected conditions and areas of need. These attract attention and assistance, which may otherwise never have occurred.

Prevention of Recurrence of the Disaster

A part of rehabilitation programs should be directed at measures that will prevent future disasters. For example, construction of tube wells and an irrigation system will mitigate the effects of drought, and construction of embankments, planting of trees, and building of resistant shelters will help in areas prone to cyclones and earthquakes.

REFERENCES

1. BLIX, G., et al., Eds. 1971. Famine: Nutrition and Relief Operations in Times of Disaster. Swedish Nutrition Foundation. Stockholm.
2. IFEKWUNIGWE, A. E. 1974. Priorities in Child Nutrition. Vol. IV. Emergencies. Harvard University School of Public Health.
3. IFEKWUNIGWE, A. E. 1977. Organization of Emergency Assistance. Food and Nutrition, Food and Agricultural Organization. Rome. In press.
4. MASEFIELD, G. B. 1969. Food and Nutrition Procedures in Times of Disaster. Food and Agriculture Organization. Rome.
5. IFEKWUNIGWE, A. E. 1975. Treatment of large numbers of people with severe protein-calorie malnutrition. Am. J. Clin. Nutr. Jan. 1975.

BEYOND 1976: CAN AMERICANS BE WELL NOURISHED IN A STARVING WORLD?

Garrett Hardin

Department of Biological Sciences
University of California, Santa Barbara
Santa Barbara, California 93106

Many will find the title question threatening: it suggests scenarios of the future that end in disaster, or that unacceptable sacrifices must be made to avoid disaster.

There are three principal ways to avoid attacking a psychologically threatening question: (1) censor it; (2) deny it (in the Freudian sense); or (3) smother it with facts. The first means seldom works in our culture. The second may work more often than we think, but it is not available in this instance because the title question has already been asked by many people. It is the third tactic—smothering with facts—that is the most popular and effective in our time. For a conspicuous example, consider the Warren Report on the Kennedy assassination, a report that ran to some 20 volumes and effectively put an end to inquiry, though there are millions of people who are still not satisfied that truth has had its day in court.

Smothering is also the method of choice in the food/population complex. Several things favor this technique. First, there is no end of data. Second, the data have a pleasingly low degree of reliability: censuses are infrequent and incomplete, births and deaths are not always recorded, and the imports and exports of food published by the United Nations Food and Agriculture Organization (FAO) are the unaudited figures reported to the FAO by the member states, which have a variety of reasons for bending the truth.

Third, in trying to deal with the future of populations, demographers have long emphasized that whatever figures they turn out are only projections (of present trends), not predictions. The result is a plethora of statements beginning with the words, "The data suggest that . . .," a phrase that suggests that something is about to be said, but leaves no grounds for criticism should the implication later prove false.

To guard against the temptation to smother a threatening question with data in the following discussion, I shall go to the opposite extreme and present almost no data. The factual statements made will be on a par with the statement that "Apples fall to the earth." Such statements need no documentation at this late date, and any qualifications that need be attached to them are obvious enough to require no saying. I adhere to this spartan simplicity in the hope of focusing attention on fundamentals that are all too often lost sight of in the food/population area. The simple approach should also facilitate criticism.

What should be the most obvious principle is that all shortages are relative to demand. We say there is a shortage of food: why do we not say instead that there is a "longage" of people? One is as accurate as the other. The choice is determined by the magnitude of our courage in facing the truth, and by the action we are willing to commit ourselves to. By saying there is a shortage of food we commit ourselves to a program of increasing the food supply and spare ourselves the necessity of facing the implications of exponential popula-

87

tion growth and the political difficulties of controlling it. To say there is a longage of people is to imply that we are going to tackle the problem of population control. This, for most of us, is too frightening a prospect, and so we continue to speak of food shortages.

Yet it should be obvious that a food shortage cannot be solved by producing more food. In the short term this may be possible, but in the long term more food produces more people, which then results in a greater shortage. The principal defense for seeking to produce more food is that it "buys time" in which to look for a more fundamental attack. Unfortunately, people who buy time generally throw it away.

A curious myth has been propagated in recent years to the effect that a bountiful supply of food will, if long enough maintained, somehow quench population growth. It is not claimed that it will diminish fecundity (the inherent ability to produce children)—that would be too blatant a contradiction of animal data. It is claimed that abundant food will ultimately diminish fertility (achieved family size) to the point where zero population growth (ZPG) is achieved. There is no place where this hypothesis is explicitly stated, but it is implicit in countless calls for inaction by influential voices. These inaction calls are most commonly based on what is called "development theory" or "demographic transition theory." A few words should be said about these theories before going further.

Two forms of the demographic transition theory need to be distinguished, the weak and the strong. The weak form says only the following: If the ZPG condition is changed by a reduction in the death rate first (thus producing population growth) this will ultimately be followed by a corresponding reduction in the birth rate, reestablishing ZPG at a higher population level. (This ignores the alternative of a secondary rise in death rate; but this approach is historically justified by the actual increase in carrying capacity brought about by technology.) Demographic transition theory implicitly acknowledges that there are limits to growth. It assumes a finite world. In its weak form the theory must be regarded as true.

The strong form of the theory can be called the "benign demographic transition theory." It is an application of the attitude of *laissez-faire* to population. This form of the theory asserts that there is something automatic about the secondary fall in the fertility rate, that under conditions of increasing economic development, prosperity and comfort, fertility will automatically and painlessly fall to the level necessary for ZPG. The past 200-year history of Europe is cited as evidence.

Unfortunately, it must be admitted that the European demographic transition is not complete. The population is still growing. Some of the eastern European nations are momentarily in the ZPG condition, but observers agree that this is due, more than anything else, to a severe housing shortage. This is hardly a benign form of population control. No instance can be cited of a people who are well fed, adequately housed, and who feel secure in the future who have voluntarily reduced their fertility on an individualistic basis to the level needed for ZPG.

China is often cited as a success story in population control. Her history fails to corroborate the benign demographic transition theory on several grounds. First, the country is at a low stage of "development," as that term is understood in the industrial West. Second, China is far from being at ZPG: the lowest estimate of her population growth rate is 1.7 percent per year. (No census has been taken for 20 years.) Third, and most important, the individualism of John Locke does not hold sway in China. Whatever success China has in population control she achieves by pressure of the community on the individual of an intensity not envisaged or approved of by the supporters of the benign demographic transition theory.

Let us be blunt: there is no substantial evidence for this theory. We must, therefore, take it as given that a food shortage cannot be solved by producing more food. Attempts to do so merely postpone the day when painful decisions must be made, and increase the number of people who will be affected by hard decisions. More importantly, making food production the primary consideration creates shortages of other kinds. Technology has created a large degree of interconvertibility of substances on the one hand, and of forms of energy on the other, and of substances into energy. In a finite world, we can maximize the production of the particular substances we call food only by reducing our production of other substances and energy. We can convert wood into sugar, petroleum into carbohydrates, and use gas to produce fertilizer to grow more food. We can sacrifice national parks to agriculture. We can destroy wilderness to produce more energy to produce more food. As regards the quality of food we can forego meat to free grain to nourish more people. Luxury-energy can be almost wholly converted to energy for necessities. Art can make way for bread. The decision to maximize the quantity of human life is a decision to minimize the quality of life, by any person's definition. Is that what we want?

I submit that it is not. Though the exact level of the quality of life desired is difficult to agree on, I am sure that the vast majority of mankind would prefer a life considerably above the level of minimal subsistence. It has been estimated that Americans use at least 150,000 kilocalories per day for non-food purposes versus 3,000 for food. No doubt we could be quite happy with much less, but how much less? Would we (or anyone else) find 6,000 kilocalories per day adequate for the good life? I doubt it. If we want to control the quality of our life we must some time decide, and that means we must set a limit to population and enforce it, by direct or indirect means.

Decisions of this sort are difficult enough on the national level; they are impossible on the international. There is no prospect of the establishment of a supranational sovereignty soon enough to deal effectively with our urgent populational problems, therefore we must face the question "Can Americans be well nourished in a starving world?" We would, of course, rather be surrounded only by people who are equally well nourished, but since that is not in the cards we must face the less pleasant question. I think the easiest way to show the necessary conditions for national survival—of our's or any other nation—is to lay out the conditions under which we will fail to be well nourished. The most important of these are 13 in number.

1. We will fail to survive in a well-nourished condition if we permit our population to grow up to the maximum that can be supported by our current food-producing ability. The weather between 1950 and 1970 was the most favorable for agriculture of any weather in the past thousand years. It seems highly improbable that such favorable weather will continue. When productivity declines there will be no other country in the world that can supply us, for the U.S. now furnishes more than half of the world's grain in export trade, and other countries will be adversely affected by the same unfavorable weather.

2. We will fail if we do not bring immigration nearly to an end. Net legal immigration into the U.S. is about 400,000 per year; the illegal is difficult to

determine but it is generally agreed that it is at least twice as much and growing. This means that immigration is approximately equal to natural increase; and it is growing. Lowering our fertility will not produce ZPG if immigration more than makes up for the diminution.

3. We will fail if we accept the Marxist thesis that need creates right. "To each according to his needs," said Marx in 1875; this is the guiding philosophy of those who propose a world food bank. The same voices assert that the production of more people is a national right. Rights unmatched by responsibilities produce havoc. A world food bank run on Marxist lines would be a food siphon, creating a common store without control, and ultimate ruin for all.

4. We will fail if we do not acknowledge that carrying capacity is a higher ethical principle than the sanctity of life. There is no country so poorly endowed that its people could not enjoy a happy, even gracious, existence at some level of population. (India has three times our population on only a third as much land. With only 70 million—instead of 600 million—people she could be prosperous.) Failing to accept carrying capacity as the primary ethical reality results in measures that destroy the environment and diminish carrying capacity in the future. Hillsides are deforested to save human lives today, causing soil erosion, loss of timber-producing capacity, destructive flooding of lowlands, siltation of dams, and other effects that diminish the land's ability to support human lives in the future. In the catalog of ethical goods, carrying capacity must come first in the making of national policy.

5. We will fail if we mistake mutualism for isolationism, and reject it. Countries that exceed their carrying capacity ask for free gifts. The proper relationship between sovereign and responsible nations is one of mutualism, of *quid pro quo* trade. Those who want gifts call the insistence on mutualism "isolationism." It is not. Trade is not isolationism, and deserves no condemnation.

6. We will fail if, in our foreign aid, we fail to distinguish between crisis and crunch. An earthquake hitting a country that is generally living within its carrying capacity creates a crisis that can be alleviated by external aid, which continues for only a short period of time and does not increase the need for aid. But a country (like Bangladesh) that is overpopulated is in a crunch situation: foreign aid in the form of food merely increases the need for aid. (The population of Bangladesh is increasing at nearly 3 percent per year.) Contributing food in a crunch is like pouring gasoline on a fire.

7. We will fail if we do not insist that every claim of food shortage in a crunch situation is *ipso facto* acknowledgment of overpopulation, and that therefore the phrase "food shortage" should be systematically replaced by the phrase "people longage" before proceeding with the search for remedies.

8. We will fail if we forget that parasitism, long continued, harms the parasite. Operationally speaking, charity (viewed from one side) is parasitism (viewed from the other). It is a biological truism that abilities that are not exercised are lost. This is true also in the human realm. For the good of all we must neither be parasites ourselves nor encourage parasitism in others.

9. We will fail if we base policy on the fear that a modern war can be started, or waged, by a hungry people. Causation is a tricky concept in history; multiple causation is the rule. But there is no credible sense in which it can be said that hunger caused the Vietnam War, the Korean War, the Second World War, or the First World War. The fear of a war caused by hunger is a

poor justification for embracing the Marxist position and supporting further population growth in irresponsible and overpopulated nations.

10. We will fail if we build a new foreign policy on massive grain diplomacy. Half of the grain we produce we sell abroad: it is our principal source of foreign exchange. As we enter a time of increasing food shortages our ability to sell or not to sell grain becomes an increasingly valuable diplomatic weapon. But all diplomatic weapons are potential boomerangs. As the world becomes more dependent on Arab oil, the position of the Arabs becomes increasingly more powerful and at the same time more hazardous for those possessing the power. So also will it be for us if we seek to control others with our grain. It is to our long-term interest to decrease the dependence of the rest of the world on our agriculture.

11. We will fail if we assume that intervention equals aid. For an example of the error that this equation leads us to, consider the parallel cases of India and China. Half a century ago these two countries were equally poor, and their futures looked equally bleak. For the past quarter of a century we have intervened with so-called "aid" on a large scale in India. China has received no "aid" from us, and precious little from anybody else. By all accounts China is better off today, and her prospects are better. We must conclude that intervention is not necessarily aid. Overall, well-intended intervention usually harms, occasionally is neutral in its effects, and very rarely really helps. What we are up against is the limitation of human knowledge and power in political and social matters.

12. We will fail if we strengthen the hands of beggar-politicians in needy countries. A nation is not an organism: it has no voice. The "demands" of needy countries are really only the demands of self-elected spokesmen. When we accede to such demands we strengthen beggar-politicians in their own countries, and set the stage for another round of demands. There is no end to this circle. Refusing such demands results in a short-term vilification of us, but a long-term strengthening of more independently minded politicians in the needy countries, who may find ways of making their nation's population match its carrying capacity.

13. We will fail if we do not distinguish amiability from charity. As human beings we want to help others if we can. Acceding to unwise demands is amiable, but if the results are a lessening of the ability of others to take care of themselves, and a diminution of the carrying capacity of their land in the future, our actions do not deserve the name of charity.

For Americans to remain well nourished and at the same time to work toward the day when all people will be well nourished we must have the courage to reject amiability for the stricter virtue of true charity.

ORIENTATION OF DOMESTIC AND INTERNATIONAL FOOD AND NUTRITION POLICIES*

Daniel E. Shaughnessy

Office of Food for Peace
Agency for International Development
Washington, D.C. 20523

The subject of this discussion, "The Orientation of Domestic and International Food and Nutrition Policies," deserves some explanation. In this context, the word "orientation" presupposes some favorable or consistent relationship between domestic and international approaches to food and nutrition. For the United States, many believe that, at least, this means we should be prepared to do domestically what we ask others to do internationally. It also means that some policies do exist; that there is not a complete void in guidance or direction on what to do about the world's food and nutrition concerns, and that coordination of various policy approaches is essential.

Obviously, orienting or coordinating any phase of policy development is a difficult and complex process. Furthermore, effective policy development in food and nutrition activities is probably more difficult than in many other areas of human concern, since it ultimately will focus on very personal and individual needs.

At the onset, it is essential to remember that policy development is usually responsive to specific needs and circumstances or particular actions. It is rarely anticipatory, particularly in fields such as food and nutrition, where it may often respond to a very specific base of concern. Identification of these concerns is an obvious, but difficult, first step, and in United States food and nutrition matters, this identification process has had such wide-ranging policy results as the establishment of a Food Stamp program, agricultural production subsidies, regulatory controls on food processing, and Federal involvement in school feeding, nutrition education, and care for women, infants, and children.

Internationally, current U.S. food and nutrition policies provide (among other things) for substantial foreign assistance to improved agricultural production, support to international organizations such as the UN Food and Agriculture Organization, and food aid valued in excess of $1 billion annually.

Therefore, there is not so much a lack of food and nutrition policy direction in the U.S. as there is a need to better refine, coordinate, and orient what already exists. To accomplish these objectives, I believe that those who are involved in and care about the world's food and nutrition must recognize that they are dealing with a political as well as a technical situation. Activities such as Federal involvement in school lunches, the WIC program, and food stamps (as well as all the others) did not come into existence simply because they were needed: they were also politically attractive. For it is possible to find situations where the origin of food and nutrition policies were not necessarily based on specific food and nutrition concerns. Often the development of a specific food and nutrition policy that may have an extremely beneficial result

* The views expressed in this paper are those of the author alone and do not represent official views or policy of the Agency for International Development.

may well be based solely on political opportunity. While significant technical progress has been achieved in the improvement of human nutrition over the past quarter century, the practical application of that technology is often dependent on political decision-making. The applied aspects of food and nutrition improvement are as complex and difficult as the technical efforts usually necessary to achieve those gains. In this context, those involved with food technology, nutrition research, nutrition planning, or various phases of food and nutrition work must become more involved in the political process.

In many developing countries, where significant progress has been achieved in the development and application of food and nutrition policies, such progress has been primarily achieved in the political forum. The Indian five-year plan, which devotes substantial attention to food and nutrition objectives is, of course, a political document. However, the specific nutrition objectives that one finds in the plan are the work of interested technical individuals who not only knew nutritional requirements but also knew how to translate those requirements into basic political objectives for their country. Time and again, major aspects of policy development relating to food production or nutritional improvement have in one way or another been linked to the attainment of political objectives. In most countries, ministers of agriculture and health are politicians not agriculturists, or medical doctors. While there are often exceptions to this rule, the decision-making process in most ministerial hierarchies is a process that involves politics.

In the U.S., some of the major U.S. policies dealing with international food and nutrition concerns have focused on what can be essentially described as a political situation. An excellent example is the PL-480 Food for Peace program. Originally enacted in 1954, Public Law 480 was in direct response to U.S. domestic political concerns relating to excess supplies of grain and concerns about surplus disposal. The very fact that what has become a major part of U.S. development aid abroad began in response to a domestic political situation, provides a lesson that can be replicated over and over again.

Policies relating to food and nutrition must also be realistic. If we are to suggest or develop food and nutrition policies for international concerns, it is very appropriate for us to question whether or not, in a political context, we are suggesting policies that may require others to do what we would not do ourselves. In addition, the practicality that is required in food and nutrition policy development often translates very simply and basically to astute political assessments. In short, proper implementation of food and nutrition policies is usually dependent upon good use of the existing political system.

For example, the application of knowledge from food and nutrition activities abroad here in the U.S. or the application of experience in the U.S. to the overseas situation sounds good in the abstract. Nevertheless, the actual implementation of such knowledge transfer is usually through some political process, such as multilateral or bilateral aid activities, or officially sponsored activities in which country leaders and technicians deal with and consult one another.

Another excellent example is nutrition planning, an activity that has achieved greater (and well-deserved) attention in recent years. Nutrition planning is extremely important; nevertheless, its initial stages may often be based on very practical and existing activities. While the need for nutrition planning is evident in many countries throughout the world, the ability to initiate planning activities and to actually see results from such activities will depend on political decisions and vary considerably from case to case.

In most countries, nutrition planning has to be attractive to planning commissioners and ministers of finance. This means two things: (1) There has to be some visible payoff or immediate results evident in order to undertake planning activities; and (2) it is and becomes a part of the political process.

This latter emphasis on nutrition planning as a part of the political process is extremely important, yet often overlooked. We must remember that any action rendered by a government is a political action. Nutrition planning is no exception. One of the more popular terms making the rounds in the development lexicon these days is the term "agent for change." I like this term; however, in the context of nutrition planning, it really means nothing more than the political action necessary to make the decisions that are needed and achieve the results that are desired.

For those concerned with food and nutrition policy, I also believe there are two other areas of influence that are either neglected or improperly employed. Here, I refer to the private sector and the media.

With regard to the latter, food and nutrition advocates either find themselves faced with nearly unlimited opportunities to influence public policy or they are faced with extremely formidable obstacles to any widespread embracing of a particular point of view. The media today do an excellent job of identifying food and nutrition problems, pointing out deficiencies in existing programs, and drawing attention to what needs to be done. However, it is still an unfortunate fact of life that pictures of bloated bellies and dying children attract far more attention than major research accomplishments in food and nutrition. Obviously, the successful coordination, development, and orientation of food and nutrition policies, both at home and abroad, requires the support of today's media, with its wide range of influence capability. However, it is equally important that the media acquire a sense of perspective that might diminish the sensational and emphasize the substantive. I doubt that such a change will come from within; it is, in my opinion, the role and responsibility of the would-be food and nutrition policy maker or technical expert to make the substance of policy attractive to the media.

In discussing the private sector, we are dealing with the single, most important element in worldwide food and nutrition delivery. If I read the program of this conference correctly, it will last 3 days and include 30 speakers; yet it has devoted the grand total of 35 minutes to hear from individuals representing the private sector! Are we deluding ourselves? The food we eat does not come from government, foundations, universities, or hospitals. Obviously, here and in most countries, it comes from private, industrial, and free-enterprise trade channels, which, as a simple fact of life, have a major influence on domestic and international food and nutrition policy development because they have a major influence on political processes. It is very fashionable these days to blame inadequate distribution of food and nutrients on those who control the production processing and marketing systems. Yet, I wonder how much attention has been devoted to the domestic and international policy framework within which these systems operate? If there are to be improvements in adequacy of supply and distribution, most of those improvements will be achieved by the private sector. And for those who believe that improvements are necessary and desirable, closer relationships and coordination on food and nutrition policy matters between the private sector and the rest of the "food and nutrition community" is essential. I further believe that the burden of effort to initiate such improved relationships does not rest with the private sector.

Finally, there is an additional factor in the world food situation that is unique to our times. This is the sheer magnitude of food production, availability, and need. With world grain production at 1.3 billion tons for 1976–77, domestic and international food and nutrition policies must take into account the quantitative effects of such large amounts of food. These effects are already noticeable in commercial trade transactions, the U.S. commodity market, government food aid programs, and the related areas of food production, processing, and storage. All of this translates to a situation where policies must be developed to cope with a situation in which quality of food and nutrients and the ability to pay for such essentials is dependent more and more on quantity alone.

Make no mistake about it: in facing the world's food crisis (and I believe there is one), political concerns over total quantities of food and the use of political systems to orient resulting domestic and international policy approaches, are as much an ingredient for survival as improved food quality or technical knowledge.

And so, to the "food and nutrition community" I would offer the following advice on policy development:

—Pay a little less attention to your by-lines and stop talking only to each other; you have good ideas and many of the answers; do some influencing, cajoling, forcing if necessary, to ensure that those ideas are translated to public and political action. Get to know as much about the corridors of Capitol Hill and board rooms of major corporations as you know about the complexities of hunger and human nutrition.

—Learn to use the media; they certainly know how to use you! It is probably the most effective way of quickly influencing food and nutrition policy development and coordination.

—Seek ranges or levels of policy commitment. Nothing in food and nutrition happens immediately, particularly when the objective is to be more consistent in domestic and international approaches.

—Try to anticipate the effects of policy suggestions or changes. The food and nutrition requirements of the world will not wait for continued trial and error approaches or endless experiments. Food and nutrition policy development, both domestic and international, must be realistic and attainable.

Finally (and I repeat again), know your politics—it is probably the best way to get things done!

INTERFACE SESSION AND DISCUSSION

Roger Revelle, *Moderator*

Center for Population Studies
Harvard University
Cambridge, Massachusetts 02138

Ms. EMMA ROTHSCHILD (*Yale University, New Haven, Conn.*): Well, I have a brief comment and question for Garrett Hardin having to do with Bangladesh. Dr. Hardin is extremely critical of U.S. food aid to Bangladesh. I wonder whether Dr. Hardin has.any views as to how his judgment on the value of U.S. food aid to Bangladesh would hold up under a different set of circumstances. What I mean by that is change: I can think of several ways in which the situation of Bangladesh might change rather dramatically and suddenly. On the political side, imagine for example, that Bangladesh in the next 10 years adopted a fiscal system leading to distribution of income and food similar to that in China. On the resource side, imagine that the search for natural gas as presently going on in the Bangladesh region which has, so far, been quite successful suddenly becomes dramatically successful and that Bangladesh, 10 or 15 years from now, becomes as rich as Saudi Arabia.

It's my view that under certain circumstances the situation in Bangladesh, 10 or 15 years from now, could be different as regards population and capacity to feed itself, including buying food from abroad.

I would like to ask Dr. Hardin whether he thinks that the possibility of such a changed set of circumstances would alter the moral character of a judgment to stop food aid to Bangladesh now—a judgment that he's against buying time.

DR. BEVERLY WINIKOFF (*Rockefeller Foundation, N.Y., N.Y.*): Several of the speakers today brought up the point either implicitly or explicitly that, in fact, there is no shortage of food, that we have what is categorized as a distributional problem. In connection with this, I have a question originally addressed really to Dr. Wittwer but since he's not here then I address it to anybody who would care to answer it and some associated questions about the implications of the nature of technological expertise at this point. It seems to me that many people involved with high levels of technology in agriculture suffer from a "don't blame us" syndrome in which they say "Well we know how to do it—we already have the answers so why are you bothering us with the fact that there are malnourished people."

Coming out of a medical background, this sort of reasoning has never been accepted from people working with medical technology. They have never been permitted to say "Well, we have a vaccine—don't worry us with the fact that the disease is still around."

I'd like to know exactly how we should reassign responsibility for utilizing technology, for managing technology. We've heard that we have a balance between the number of people, quality of life, and type of diet, and these variables can be changed but they are dependent upon each other—choices in one affecting ultimate outcomes in the other. Who is going to decide exactly what level of which variable we will ultimately accept? It's quite easy, I think, to discuss these as interrelated in that we have choices but nobody has answered the question of where the decision will lie and how we can go about moderating or changing the circumstances so that the decision comes out to be what we are implicitly considering equitable.

Also, in this context, we talked about modifications in climate and uses of resources. Who is going to decide which technologies will be acceptable—which technologies will be employed and which costs we can afford to bear and who will give up which technologies because of their overall effect on the total picture on the globe?

DR. REVELLE: Those all sound to me like leading questions. Should we attempt to give one answer to them? Who is going to decide? Timmer must have some ideas about it.

DR. WINIKOFF: Well, I think there are many possible answers. I'm just not sure the different speakers have made all possibilities explicit. There are some societies that, of course, will be fundamentally political. There are other societies based on equity goals, and there are other societies that seem to say "Well, we farmers produce food and industries refine and distribute the food, and we have to leave it to the people who do the producing. There are still others that are in charge of technological research to make the choices.

DR. REVELLE: I didn't understand your question about the balance between the quality of life and the number of people in the world on any given type of diet to which people have access. Now the question is who will decide about that balance. Would you like to say something, Dr. Timmer, about the question Mr. Rensberger asked about whether the Communist system is the only system that we can expect to work in the less-developed countries?

DR. C. PETER TIMMER: I hope that's not what I said. I think the fact that Cuba and China have probably done better in meeting basic food needs for virtually everybody in their society is not coincidental with the type of distribution system, that is the Socialist distribution, that they have. The fact is that there aren't other examples around of countries of similar levels of real income that are anywhere close to having as well-fed a population as those two societies. Most governments are based on urban preferences. In fact, that's where most of the well-educated people are; it's where the workers are—they're organized and have a significant political base, it's where the government workers themselves live, it's certainly where the high government officials live.

And so it takes something fairly dramatic to turn that around. The Chinese Revolution and the Cuban Revolution—they both came out of the countryside and changed that whole way of looking at the world. I think that's terribly important. I don't think that it's necessary that you be a Communist to think that what's going on in the countryside is terribly important when 70% of the population is in the countryside. It just so happens that the first two times that it's been done were done under Marxist philosophy. Whether there's going to be anything in the future to substitute for that, whether we should be afraid of it or whether we should encourage it—that's obviously something that we can only speculate about.

DR. REVELLE: I would like to give another answer which is a more long-term answer. That is that we have really two choices. We have a choice of putting everybody in the poorhouse at a very poor level of diet but an equitable one—one that really isn't very satisfying for human beings in any way except that it provides them with enough calories and enough protein—or we have the possibility of a real agricultural revolution in which there would be so much production, so much food produced, and such an increase in the incomes of the poor that the whole population would be much better off. The characteristic thing, I think, about both Cuba and China is that in terms of economic growth they're doing badly. They're doing very well in terms of equity, in what ethicists call distributive justice, but not particularly well in terms of production.

For example, if you look at the Chinese production it looks very impressive until you realize that there are 950 million people in China and that their figures are compiled in a different way than they are in, let's say, India. They include not milled rice but paddy, unmilled rice. They include potatoes in their food grains, and if you actually make a realistic appraisal of the figures, I think it shows that their production per capita is not much more than 10% higher than it is in India. But there's no question about the fact that it is much better distributed. The real question is—can you get food production up to the point where distribution is not quite such an obvious concern? In other words, a really adequate food supply. And, I think that is possible and possible under systems other than the Communist one.

MR. BOYCE RENSBERGER (*New York Times, N.Y., N.Y.*): Doesn't that run counter to what you said earlier? You said that science cannot completely replace politics in serving as a solution for the food shortages.

DR. REVELLE: But there are all kinds of politics.

DR. TIMMER: We've been accused of saying that there's no production problem, that there is merely a distribution problem. I don't think that anybody has said that it was merely a distribution problem. I think the distribution issues are almost certainly more difficult to solve, at least for academics like myself, who are not experienced in politics. We are not used to walking in the halls of Congress but are a little more comfortable in front of a blackboard in a class.

So, I think the distribution problems are the more difficult ones, that's all, but it may well be, as Professor Revelle argues, that the easier way to do this is not to solve the distributional problem at all but simply to work via the production side of things. I don't think the Chinese had that option. The Chinese started from higher yield base than did India, from heavier population pressure. With 950 million people they have less arable land than India does with 600 million people, they did not have the choice of dramatically increasing yields and total output quickly. If they are going to have a well-fed population they had to go right now in the short run with the distribution measure. And, they've done it.

On the other hand, I think, they have a very respectable growth in agricultural output especially if you look at their agricultural output for 1974 where in the face of some very adverse climatic conditions, they have at least stabilized agricultural production at a high level—at a level that is adequate.

The other thing that I would quarrel with is the fact that the people are really suffering from this monotonous starchy diet. Anybody who's eaten traditional Chinese food would realize that even a diet that's 80% carbohydrates can be very interesting and certainly varied and quite tasty.

DR. REVELLE: Well, it depends whether you're living in Shanghai or living in some remote district.

DR. TIMMER: Well, even out in the Mountains with corn base diet they do some very, very remarkable things. We were served 21 different varieties of dumplings in different kinds of soups. But, I don't think monotony is going to be the downfall of the Chinese regime.

DR. REVELLE: Dr. Hardin, would you like to respond to Ms. Rothschild's question?

DR. HARDIN: Yes, I think the point she brought up was quite important because in answering it I can remedy a deficiency in my talk.

What we call in the human situation the carrying capacity has to include all sorts of things that you would not include if you were studying some other animal. But, I would say as a practical matter, we should always regard the carrying capacity of a country as its carrying capacity at this moment. In other words, not try to meet today's demands with tomorrow's supplies. Now that's a curious sort of accounting if you do that.

Now, if Bangladesh does indeed discover rich sources of gas that she can bottle and market then at that moment her carrying capacity becomes immensely greater because one has to define human carrying capacity as the population that can be supported directly and also by trade. If Bangladesh has something she can trade in great supply then the carrying capacity becomes greater. So, from moment to moment, year to year, you determine the carrying capacity of a responsible country. If it had a policy and if it could enforce it, it would at every moment try to keep its population within the carrying capacity of the moment and not trade on an unknown future.

Ms. ROTHSCHILD: Just to come briefly back: I may have misunderstood this but I thought that one element in your argument against food aid was that by stopping providing food to countries in, as you put it, a crunch situation now you are preventing a greater evil sometime in the future. Now, if the carrying capacities of countries can change as much as that, as you seem to agree with me that they can, perhaps that situation puts a different light on the moral aspects of the judgment to not provide food aid now to prevent starving more people later.

DR. HARDIN: Well, what you're going to try to deal with in the future I question. For example, do we know by the year 1981 how many BTU's of gas Bangladesh will be producing. You see, that's the unknown future. I think the conservative intelligent way is always to deal in terms of present reality; to hope for the future but don't write the future into your account books.

MR. RENSBERGER: You don't think the distribution system had anything to do with China?

DR. HARDIN: I wouldn't say that, but whatever she's done about the distribution system, she has done. We could not have done it. We could not have moved into China and enforced a just distribution system. See, these are the limits of power, and we should accept it. So, whatever a country does about it's distribution system, it has to do—we cannot do it.

DR. WINIKOFF: Would you clarify another aspect of this carrying capacity concept? It seems to me that if you try to define carrying capacity in numbers you run into an immediate block because you have to define what level of diet and what level of quality of life you're talking about, and I don't see how a country can actually calculate a carrying capacity, first of all.

Second of all, does this imply that, if you see an advantage or way of increasing your carrying capacity by taking the next 15 square miles of your neighbor's territory which has certain resources and thus enlarging your carrying capacity, does that become a moral imperative then to increase carrying capacity in any way possible?

And, does this situation in turn suggest that perhaps the idea of carrying capacity, as defined by national boundaries, is an artificial construct and that we are back with the idea of the carrying capacity of the globe, which I think everybody is trying to grapple with—not defined by national boundaries and national moral imperatives?

DR. HARDIN: Thank you. First of all, with respect to defining the carrying capacity of a country, we have a very simple operational method. If the country is asking for aid, not trade, they thereby acknowledge that they are past the carrying capacity by their own standards, and having so defined it we accept it and, of course, according to my standards we would do them harm by giving them that for which they ask.

Second, as a matter of taking something from other countries, this has, of course, for thousand of years been a way of enlarging the carrying capacity of a country. From here on out, I think this is a dangerous method. Now, if country A does do this to country B, the question is—should we interfere? I don't know. This is a tough one. You know, the threat of a Third World War and so on—at what point do we try to become policeman for the world? I think we can express our displeasure at A taking from B and say this should not be a legitimate way from here on out.

As for the national boundaries, these are, of course, an accident of history, but I know of no way to redraw the lines of the nations of the world and enforce it or even perhaps to improve them. I think we'd better accept the ones that exist and simply assert that there is no nation so poorly off that it cannot exist at a comfortable level of living within the real estate that it happens to have. That means that some areas of the world will have a lot of people, say Indonesia; other areas will have very few, say the Sahara; but I see no point in trying to gerrymander the Sahara and Indonesia into one new country.

MR. RENSBERGER: Could I just ask whether Britain has now exceeded her carrying capacity and should be cut loose?

DR. HARDIN: If she's hurting, she's exceeded the carrying capacity. Some of Britain's troubles, I think, are due to rather unfavorable political affairs, and so on. But, that's part of the problem too.

DR. REVELLE: I think we might now turn to questions from the audience. I see one hand raised there.

UNIDENTIFIED SPEAKER: Perhaps I can try to help Ms. Rothschild try to illuminate the question by putting a question, in a semi-rhetorical fashion, to Dr. Bryson and that is: What was the batting average among meteorologists when they used that "conservative kind of prediction," which is to predict tomorrow on the basis of what you have today?

And perhaps, he would illuminate the issue by discussing the kind of modeling in meteorology which is going on at present which has managed to untangle these complexes where weather changes from day to day. He has to ask himself the question—how would he manage the weather? Would he use such issues as triage?

DR. REID A. BRYSON: This question of carrying capacity is one that I have given some attention to, and it can be defined. There's no question but what you can write down an equation which defines the number of people that a country can support at a defined level of technology and a defined level of production of either food or tradable substances, brains, whatever. You can do this, but then you have to take account of different lag times. The doubling time of human population, though it is dangerously short in terms of how fast you can really accomplish something, is quite different than the lag time of productivity variations, for example, due to climate.

The worst thing that could happen to us, and it has happened to a certain extent already, is for the climate to vary slowly—slower than it does right now. Suppose we did have a return of the superb weather that we had in the 1960's where there just weren't any bad years in North America and there weren't any bad years in South Asia. Suppose we had that for 20 years, so that there would be more food and the population would grow—double let's say. And then, the climate changed—that's much worse than if the climate changed every couple of days, or every couple of years. You'd be aware of the limits before the limits ever caught up with you. The big problem in discussing carrying capacity is whether you mean carrying capacity in terms of this year or carrying capacity of, let's say, a generation, because the carrying capacity in terms of people cannot be defined in terms of how many you can feed this year—it must be determined in terms of how many can be fed in the worst sequence of years. And that's where reserves come in.

All of this can be modeled in the sense that you're talking about, putting it together in a computer model and coming out with an answer, but somebody has to decide at what level of consumption this will happen.

I personally don't think that we're ever going to see the time when we have 7 billion people. I don't think this is going to be because of failure to distribute things at all; because, looking at the world situation in a broad sense, I think the carrying capacity of the earth with our present technology, with our present levels of consumption, is not as much as 7 billion.

DR. JOHN OPPENHEIMER (*Johns Hopkins University, Baltimore, Md.*): A question for Dr. Bryson and also for Dr. Pimentel: Trying to bridge the gap between your two talks—Dr. Pimentel was talking about the actual energy required to produce a certain amount of grain and then, of course, how much energy is needed to support an individual per capita—can we come up with the actual amount of additional energy that would be needed, to maintain that amount of food per capita with a one degree change in temperature, plus or minus? In this case we are concerned with the minus.

DR. BRYSON: That's a calculation that hasn't been made yet, so I'll just give you some very vague hints as to the sort of magnitude you're talking about.

If you look at the nations of the world the GNP per capita varies 2½ % per one degree centigrade that the temperature of that nation changes. That's a big number. So, that's one kind of answer that can be done on a gross scale. To put it right down to the food level, a one degree centigrade change in temperature in the upper Great Plains area, the spring wheat region of the United States and Canada, a one degree change there in the temperature of the summer, increase of temperature, would cost the farmers about $170 million in gross income from reduced production of food. Now divide that by $3.00 (I assumed that it was $3.00 wheat) and you get some idea of how much extra wheat you would have to produce. Multiply that by Pimentel's number and you have the answer.

DR. GENE CALVERT (*American Public Health Association, Washington, D.C.*): I have the suspicion that we've been talking about national nutrition policy this afternoon, in fact, all day with limited consistency, precision, and clarity. I have three reasons for this suspicion.

One, beginning this morning there seemed to me to be some slight disagreement between two very distinguished participants in this conference, Dr. Mayer and Dr. Schneider, as to what a health policy is. You recall that Dr. Schneider referred to clean air as a national health policy, and Dr. Mayer responded to that by saying, "No, that is a goal—that a policy has to do with how you reach a particular goal; that goals precede policies."

The second reason for my suspicion is that no one today has defined what is a national nutrition policy.

And the third reason has to do with my own struggles to define it for myself.

I would like to invite any of the panel members that would care to identify and define the basic components of a national nutrition policy.

DR. REVELLE: Maybe we should ask Mr. Shaughnessy that question.

MR. D. E. SHAUGHNESSY: Well, I'm not sure that a single basic national nutrition policy is either possible, appropriate, or desirable. The range of variables that we deal with in this country that carry the label "food and nutrition" is considerable. It covers everything from production to consumption to processing of food shipments—the whole spectrum of the entire food cycle. I am not sure that it really is possible to define a single nutrition policy.

I mentioned in my talk, for example, that I question whether it's appropriate for us to talk about this in terms of what other countries do when we really can't do it ourselves. We've gone so far as to ask for some description of a nutrition policy or strategy from the countries that we assist, and I find this a little hypocritical, quite frankly, because I'm not sure we can do it ourselves. I guess what I'm saying is that in order to define the nutrition policy I think we've got to first of all look at what we would want to include in that policy and then make the definitions accordingly, and I'm afraid that I can't give much of a better answer than that.

DR. CALVERT: I'm sorry—I didn't ask how many nutrition policies we have but what a nutrition policy consists of.

MR. SHAUGHNESSY: In my opinion, I think it has to consist of approaches and procedures that a nation would follow in order to attain the objectives that it's looking for, whether these are production, betterment of the human condition, or controls on production and processing. Perhaps some of my colleagues here have some better ideas.

DR. TIMMER: It seems to me that we want to distinguish a food policy from a nutrition policy in the first instance, and I don't have too much difficulty in thinking that a food policy ought to have as one major goal at least that everybody should have access to whatever we think is the recommended allowance of the various nutrients—that access is really the goal at the issue of food policy. Nutrition is a different thing, though, because we know from U.S. experience and other experience around the world that simply having access to food isn't going to solve all the nutritional problems. We may eat too much because we've got unlimited access to food. We may eat the wrong things. We may eat things that are going to cause all kinds of problems—lack of fiber, too much cholesterol, whatever it is, these are nutritional concerns that have to be dealt with in something other than the basic access fashion.

Education is the thing we always fall back on, and it obviously hasn't worked very well in the past and I don't see any evidence that it's going to work any better in the future. I was impressed by how much of the goal of the National Heart Association in reducing cholesterol intake was accomplished, not by education programs of the American Heart Association, but by high prices for beef.

I think you'll find that one of the reasons cholesterol intake has gone down and heart disease has gone down in the past three years is almost certainly associated with high meat prices, and with meat prices coming down we may well see those heart disease rates go right back up again. Economics, in other words, is a very powerful factor here. Education hasn't seemed to work right off. But, it's those kinds of issues that we then have to deal with in the context of the nutrition policy. We can't keep them separate.

DR. GLEN KING (*Columbia University, N.Y., N.Y.*): I would like to ask Dr. Shaughnessy or someone at the panel table how we can get integrity in transferring what we know in the science of nutrition to the consumer in an effective way? It seems to me we're bedeviled, not by a lack of food, but by misinformation or no information on the part of the public. Now, unless the public is adequately informed they're in no position to manage the political machinery, as Dr. Shaughnessy urged. It seems that we have no adequate method yet of either controlling, guiding, or limiting the press. We have no effective means of keeping a lot of fakers off of the lecture platform. We have no way of keeping them out of the daily press, books, publications. We have to find some way to get the public informed and with confidence to make use of the resources that we have. If you can suggtst something to us I think it would be very helpful.

DR. TIMMER: I'm wrong in one thing I said earlier—that we don't know how to do nutrition education. We do know how to do bad nutrition education in the sense that anybody who's watched Saturday morning television will realize how very effective the commercials are for the incredible variety of cereals, snack foods, junk foods, whatever you like—how incredibly effective that advertising is on children!

The point is that the technology is there—the knowledge is there to communicate. One obvious way to make a quantum jump in consumer understanding of good nutrition would simply be to ban all food advertising on television. That would do probably more than anything else.

MR. SHAUGHNESSY: I'm not sure I can add too much to what I said earlier. The media are a fact of life—they're there—we've got to find better ways of getting the right messages across. I'm not sure that the extreme of banning certain types of advertising because of detrimental effects is really the answer because I think this could lead to an awful lot of results we really wouldn't want, but I'm afraid that other than saying that we've got a situation where the media are very influential, we do have people like yourselves who know many of the right answers—we've got to find better ways to simply again and again keep putting the right messages across. And I think the answer is to find ways to make those answers and those approaches both desirable and economic, and once you've done that I think you've probably achieved your goal.

MR. RENSBERGER: As an employee of one medium I would like to point out that there are other media, other mass media, than the ones we conventionally think of as radio and television and the newspapers, and perhaps one of the most powerful mass media that we have in this country is the school system.

Schools and educational systems: I remember when I went to school there were charts on the walls describing the basic seven kinds of food, and we were taught that you should eat one of each of these every day. I later found out that that's nutritional nonsense put up by the various producer groups who had interest in making sure you ate some of their product every day and that one really doesn't need to eat seven different types of food daily.

I wonder whether much has been done through the school systems. I don't see that newspapers are a reasonable medium except through advertising in which to do this. It doesn't seem an appropriate role for the newspapers or television, which is primarily an entertainment medium—almost exclusively an entertainment medium. I don't think that those mass media are going to be very responsive and very helpful in this matter.

DR. WINIKOFF: I just want to ask Mr. Shaughnessy if he might try to relate this issue on food advertising back to his point on the role of the food industry in nutrition because it seems to me that in your presentation you were very, perhaps overly, optimistic about the potential role of the private sector in promoting nutritional goals. It seems to me that as a basic motivating factor one at least has to take cognizance of the fact that both on the individual level and on the corporate level the prime mover in industry and the private sector in general is making a profit and that to nourish people is an incidental by-product.

DR. REVELLE: I'm a little bit puzzled by this use of the word private sector. What you really mean is private business interests.

MR. SHAUGHNESSY: I think what I said in my address was that what I call the food and nutrition community, those who know what is right about food and nutrition, need to be more involved with and have better relationship with the private industry and the processed food industry, the people who do make the food available. I think that there's not enough of that kind of relationship between people who are here today and the people who have something to say about how foods are produced and processed. Secondly, I think I also mentioned in response to a question earlier that if we can find ways to make human nourishment and betterment economic, then that is going to be very attractive to the food industry, and I think that's the type of thing that needs to be done.

DR. AARON IFEKWUNIGWE: I think it was about a week ago in Los Angeles, there was a motion that came before the unified school district to ban the slot machines that sold junk food in the schools. There had been an ongoing battle over the past year about this because the people who taught nutrition or who felt children should be taught good nutrition in school felt that there was no point teaching them about good nutrition if when they go off on their breaks there are all kinds of machines that sell junk food, and the best way to deal with it is to actually replace these by selling fruit and other more desirable and better and nutritional items than the current usual items such as potato chips.

This came up for full debate and it very nearly passed but, in fact, as of yesterday just before I left I heard that it had been struck down, and the reason for this was that the school district realized over $1 million a year out of these machines which, in fact, went into the school revenue. It goes to the question of economics. This is, in fact, just one aspect of it, and I'm sure Los Angeles is no different from most other school districts in the country.

The other point is the question that Mr. Shaughnessy raised about the utilization of mass media for nutrition education. I think we certainly have the technology available. We also have the knowledge to impart, but as those who are responsible for the Saturday morning programs and others that advertise breakfast cereals and the like know it costs money. Who would pay for this? I think this is probably the biggest single problem facing those in nutrition education.

DR. JOHNSON: I'd like to get back to this question of a global policy that we're discussing today and come back to the question whether it should be a nutrition policy or food policy or whether it should be in terms of goals, which was the question discussed this morning by Dr. Schneider and Dr. Mayer. I think that one of the things we have to answer is: do we accept or to what extent do the people in the United States accept the goals and the specifics set forth by Dr. Hardin this afternoon. He set forth many specific ways in which he felt that the nutrition policy of the country should be conducted in regard to global nutrition; that we should only give away food under these conditions, we should do these things under specific conditions, and, I think, until conditions such as these are defined and accepted or rejected it's impossible for people to go to meetings on an international basis, on a political basis, and either speak in favor of things that the farm bloc wants to sell more food or other groups want to do other things or whether Congress wants to appropriate monies to support McGovern's types of distribution of food within this country. I think it's a list of things of this sort which might be called goals which must be defined and put together in some way and then on the basis of this draw up the several policies taking into account the change in policies depending upon various conditions of climate and amount produced, etc. But, I think something along these lines has to be done in this way.

DR. MICHAEL LATHAM (*Cornell University, Ithaca, N.Y.*): I'm also concerned like a number of others about this question of a national food and nutrition policy. Personally I was a little alarmed this morning to hear Jean Mayer backing a little bit away from a commitment or even a feeling that we needed a national food and nutrition policy when he chaired the White House Conference on Food and Nutrition in Health. I think one of the very strong things that came out of that was the need for not only a national food and nutrition policy but more the mechanisms that would allow sensible decisions to be made that could look at the nutritional and food implications of different policies. And, I think that's really what we need.

Howard Schneider responded to that. He and others here did serve on a small committee that advised the Carter-Mondale ticket. For the first time a Presidential candidate really wanted a statement on food and nutrition. I think for the first time we have a possibility of the mechanisms being set up for a national food and nutrition policy. This does not need to be a closed door policy. It can be flexible, it can be open door, it can follow the very laudible principles on which this country functions, but at least have the mechanisms there by which we can make rational and sensible decisions about a national food and nutrition policy.

How this mechanism is set up and where it fits, I think, those are difficult questions. I think all four speakers this afternoon, in some kind of a way, called for these kind of policies: Professor Timmer in the need for research policies, which I think are very important; Dr. Ifekwunigwe for policies for countries that are likely to face disasters but this also affects U.S. policy; Dr. Shaughnessy talking about food aid and Garrett Hardin, who is perhaps the only one who tried to actually state his views on a food and nutrition policy.

I personally think that we need to support very strongly as nutritionists and as people concerned about food the setting up of the correct or appropriate or desirable mechanisms that could meet this. I can't leave the platform or the microphone without saying that though Garrett Hardin was the only one who tried to express his views on a policy, that to me I thought by December 1, 1976 we would have gotten past a debate on triage or the lifeboat ethics, a philosophy that I think is unacceptable to 95% of human beings. But, if that philosophy is our philosophy it surely must hold true here in the United States as well as our policy towards other countries. It's possible that Garrett Hardin has an elderly relative, perhaps a father or mother. Maybe they're parasites—should we aid them? We have people who are insane in this country—they also are parasites. They're not productive—should we support them? If this kind of philosophy becomes the philosophy of a country such as this then I think, and I think you, Mr. Chairman, have expressed this very well previously, we really don't deserve to be taken seriously and all respect for us will certainly be lost.

Our free education system is providing assistance to those who can't afford to pay for their education. I just don't think that we can get along with this kind of philosophy, and I really don't believe it deserves serious thought in this day and age.

MR. CHARLES HOMER (*University of Pennsylvania, Philadelphia, Pa.*): I've two questions. The first one would be to Dr. Hardin.

Your arguments, which I think were well addressed by Dr. Latham, pointed specifically against direct food aid—direct aid in terms of giving goods, which is a concept which has been attacked by developing nations as well at the World Food Conference who consider such things as production disincentives and that can be debated as to whether that was actually an intentional policy in the anti-poor program. The question which comes up now—what about development aid and what about changing things like carrying capacity by our funds. Where do you stand on that, Dr. Hardin?

DR. HARDIN: I'm often misunderstood in these matters. I'm not against aid. I don't think anybody is against aid, but I am for a very serious critical look at every intervention. In other words, all that we knowingly do in any other country is intervene, and we have to ask—is this intervention aid or is it dis-aid? Is it something that hurts the country? And we know so many examples in the past.

For example, in agriculture, obviously it's better to teach people how to grow their own food than to send them food. Unfortunately, most of the poor countries of the world are tropical countries. We don't know much about tropical agriculture. All of our splendid work in our agricultural experiment stations is working with temperate zone agriculture, and you simply cannot translate the means used one place to another, particularly to the very delicate areas of the semi-desert. So, with the best will in the world our intervention has often turned out to harm the country. I think we have to be very dubious about what we're doing.

If I could recommend anything at all that we do for the poor countries it would be this: that we help facilitate and even pour a great deal of money into the establishment of tropical agricultural experiment stations run in the countries themselves and ultimately run by their own people. Initially, we might have to help them with some personnel but phase ourselves out as fast as possible. That, I think, is a good program to take part in, but as you heard this morning or the afternoon, the lag time, the time before you reap the benefits of that, is very long, roughly 25–50 years. That's no reason for not starting it. We should start it but bear in mind that this will have no effect on what is viewed as the food crisis. That would be doing something for the long-term, and that I would recommend. Most of the short-term things we want to do have, in the past, I think, turned out to be disastrous and we should stop this.

DR. REVELLE: I can't resist commenting on this point. I think that's complete nonsense. The fact of the case is that right now there are something like

12 international agricultural research institutions working very effectively in tropical countries. Every one of them, so far as I know, was started by either the Ford or the Rockefeller Foundations or both; and the green revolution, the increase in food production in the tropical countries, certainly has benefited greatly by the results obtained by these research institutions which are interventions right now. It's quite right that they are working with agricultural research institutions in the countries themselves. For example, in India, the Indian Council of Agriculture Research has an elaborate and effective agricultural research establishment which works very closely with these international research institutions. The countries where, in fact, food production has greatly increased are countries such as Korea and Taiwan and Sri Lanka and Pakistan and India, not so much per capita, but something like 40–50% overall, and in every case one of the important elements here was American aid intervention— intervention in helping with agricultural colleges, with package food programs, with the introduction of the high-yielding wheat varieties, new concepts in irrigation. Many aspects of the development of Pakistan depended directly upon not necessarily American aid but foreign aid—aid which involved the United States, Great Britain, France, Japan, Mexico, in that case under the leadership of the World Bank. So, it's just not true that American aid has been disastrous. For the most part it's been quite beneficial. The food aid program was criticized because it tended to encourage countries to industrialize rather than to develop agriculture. Unfortunately, that was the recommendation of American economists at the time, and if we have anybody to fault it's the international economics community who thought that industrialization was the royal road to development following the Soviet model. But that turns out now to have been not the correct model. This is a learning process—the problem of technical assistance and financial and other kinds of aid.

DR. HARDIN: Right, may I speak to that, Roger? It is a learning process, but remember this is a learning process at the expense of the developing countries themselves. The attempt to industrialize some of these countries beyond the wise level which was carried out in the 50's at the advice of the economists we now see was badly advised, so now we have different advice. How do we know the advice that we're giving today is any better? We can see our errors in the past, but what about the future? The people living in the Equatorial Highlands are about 10% of the world's population, and Eric Ekholm says what they do affects 30% of the world's population. Unfortunately, in this context the populations are increasing in those equatorial highlands and the people are deforesting their country at a tremendously rapid rate, which is followed by essentially irreversible loss of soil and degradation of the environment. In other words, every increase in population has a very bad effect on the carrying capacity of their own land as well as on the lands below them in the lowlands.

You see, the point is that if you set out to maximize the number of human lives, you will necessarily minimize many of the measures of the quality of life.

DR. SHAUGHNESSY: Dr. Revelle, I too can't resist making an intervention here. As an official of our foreign aid program, as an administrator of our food aid program, I couldn't agree more with what you just said.

Secondly, on the point of intervention, we do not walk around the world throwing our aid around. The process of assessing the needs, of responding to requests, of looking at what is needed and making our aid available, is a slow, deliberative and very analytical process. It isn't something that occurs overnight. We aren't just jumping in and intervening in the affairs of other governments. To leave that impression with you would be totally wrong.

MR. HOMER: I agree with Dr. Shaughnessy completely that scientists must become more directly involved in the political process. But simply saying that is not enough without dealing with the economic realities.

For example, in the case of heart disease, which is one of the areas where scientists have made strong inroads into public communications, we were still unable to get governmental change. For example, the National Heart Institute never came out with a policy of recommending any dietary change. The Army, in particular, continued to serve butter, fried eggs, specifically because of the dairy lobby.

Another instance is sugar and dental disease. The National Institute of Dental Health carefully and brilliantly researched the role that sugar plays in the origin of dental caries. Yet the NIDH has invested very little money in the public area and has been dissuaded, primarily because of the sugar lobby. So what I'm saying is that simply advocating scientific involvement in politics is begging many of the major points.

DR. SHAUGHNESSY: Very briefly I agree with you. I'm not saying the job is easy, but I'm saying it has to be done. The influence that needs to be brought to bear to compete with other forms of lobbying and influence just has to be generated. And I think if people like yourselves are really concerned and interested in what occurs in the food and nutrition affairs of the world, you've got to find ways to do it. And having said that, I know it's a very difficult thing to do.

DR. REVELLE: Dr. Pyke, could I get you to say something before you leave? We have a distinguished Englishman here, the Secretary of the British Association for the Advancement of Science, one of the great nutrition experts of the United Kingdom. Perhaps he might make a comment.

DR. PYKE: I hadn't intended to say anything now since I was reserving my thunder until Friday. But since you have invited me I wonder whether I might just give an inkling of the way, if I were asked to do it, I would edge my way towards answering the question.

I strongly agree with the point that nutrition policy and nutrition as applied to benefit in the human condition is a political act. The question was asked and we've just been dealing with it now, to what extent scientists, and people who apply that science, should be politicians.

I have very mixed views about this. I don't very much like the idea of rule by scientists, and my blood has run a little bit cold today as I've heard, in this center of freedom in the United States, people recommending that freedom of the press is a dangerous thing, that the media should be muzzled, and that education in the schools should control the information that's disseminated, although, poor, weak, ignorant creatures that we are, we really don't quite know about nutritional policy because things interlock in such a complex way.

If, as scientists, we know something, we should make that claim, and make it as plain as we can.

What we know I think we should clearly make plain to each other, because one specialist scientist is often very obscure to another. Microbiologists are sometimes totally misunderstood by engineers. We should make this plain. And I think then we should try to look at our fellowmen as if we were all God's creatures. And when I talk about fellowmen I am including in that category people who work on television stations, journalists, and I'm even including those most denigrated people, the politicians.

Mr. Ralph Flood (*National Public Radio*): I have a question about the demographic transition, whether it's a myth or a reality. It seems to me that the failure to discuss it is part of the double bind that I sense at the conference.

Dr. Hardin, in the printed version of his talk, said "Let us be blunt. There is no substantial evidence for this theory." That is the theory that development leads to population control, which is, I take it, the semiofficial position of the United Nations in the Seventh Special Session on New Economic Order, and various other statements they've made.

"We must therefore take as given that food shortages cannot be solved by producing more food."

Now, most of the undeveloped countries, I think, agree with that position too. Technology is simply not the solution for population control and feeding people. Yet most of the talks at the conference are devoted to the technology of increasing food production. And I think Mr. Revelle, you speak in the *Scientific American* article in September of the technological possibility of feeding up to 40 billion people on the planet. And that's sort of out of phase with Dr. Hardin's views of what could or should be.

The idea that politics may enter into the control of population and the adequacy of food has been touched on. But the Club of Rome's recommendation of a transformation of values necessary to both the East and West, particularly in the Western countries, I don't think has been dealt with directly. I would wonder if anyone wants to address the statement by Dr. Hardin that there is no substantial evidence for the theory that development leads to population control.

Dr. Revelle: I'll try to answer that one since I'm supposed to be a quasi-specialist on population. Dr. Hardin's statement I think is not borne out by the facts. The fact is that in the Western countries, so-called "rich" countries or developed countries, more than half of them are now at a net reproduction rate of less than one, including the United States. Our total fertility rate is now about 1.8, which means that the average woman is less than reproducing herself.

In West Germany—the most prosperous country in the world right now— the birthrate is 10 per thousand, so far below the net reproduction rate that in fact they have achieved zero population growth even though that is very difficult in terms of the age distribution. In all the Scandinavian countries the net reproduction rate is less than one. It is also probably true of England at the present time.

If you look at the Russian part of the Soviet Union, it also has a net reproduction rate of less than one. It worries the Soviet government no end because all those "wogs" in the Eastern part of the Soviet Union, the Muslims, are out-reproducing the Russians. And it's going to change the character of the country. My opinion is it serves them right. This was the greatest imperialist power in history for 300 years. They expanded their frontiers 100 km every 10 years for 300 years. They're taken in all these lesser breeds without the law, and now they're getting their comeuppance.

If you look at developing countries at the present time, there are at least a dozen where the birthrate is dropping very fast. In every one of these you've had two things: a considerable improvement in the life of poor people, and a considerable equalization of income. Nobody has any idea what's happening in China, except that the evidence is pretty good that no one is starving there. But what the birth or death rate is, nobody really knows. There aren't any statistics.

But in Sri Lanka, in Korea and Taiwan, Hong Kong, Singapore, Mauritius,

Costa Rica, Trinidad and Tobago, all together about a dozen countries, birth-rates are coming down faster than they ever came down in the democratic transition in the early part of this century in the Western world. In every case there has been a considerable improvement in the life of the ordinary person, much more than simply meeting animal needs—that is, meeting the needs for minimum dietary level, something like that.

So, in fact, the evidence is pretty clear that what you need to do in order to bring down birthrates is to meet human needs. Now, the key word there is "human." What are human needs? They are much more than just getting enough to eat. They're having some kind of realizable aspirations, some hope for the future, some security, some sense of participation, some sense of remembrance or immortality which doesn't depend upon having children.

Sri Lanka, for example, has a per capita income really no greater than that of India. But it is a much better distributed income. Most everybody in Sri Lanka can read and write, there is no discrimination against women, there are very good health services, a life expectancy well over 65 years—all these together seem to be directly related to a decline in the birth rate. The statement that development leads inevitably to population decline is, itself, a doubtful statement. But the statement that birth rates are lowered by giving people some other reason for living than having children is not a doubtful statement. It seems to work, and the empirical evidence is very clear.

DR. MAX MILNER (*Massachusetts Institute of Technology*): Thank you, Mr. Chairman. I'm fascinated by the frequency with which the question of nutrition policy, presumably U.S. style, keeps coming up—and the apparent inadequacy of answers, because it keeps recurring all the time.

I would like to refer you to the extremely wise point that Dan Shaughnessy made several times. And that is, get with the political system. What I'm saying is that Congress gets more advice than it needs, more advice than it wants. And in this point what I wish to refer to is the fact that I was involved with the Office of Technology Assessment for some number of months this year, precisely on this question which we received from the Congress on what are the elements of nutrition policy.

Now, one thing I would like to contend, Congress marches to the beats of a number of drums. Congress has to know many things. They have to be extremely wise people.

But the point I'm trying to make is that we in the Office of the Technology Assessment did not advise Congress, did not recommend to Congress, what policy and legislation they should be concerned with. It was our job to define the issues upon which Congress could arrive at policy and legislation.

And I may say that in this context, using the talents of many people in this room as a matter of fact, that we went ahead and defined a number of issues which will shortly be brought to the attention of Congress, whose prerogative it is to develop policy and legislation. Some of these, I think, when you take that point of view become quite clear.

What are the public health impacts, is one issue. What are the public health impacts of U.S. dietary patterns, which are very bad and which are root causes of cardiovascular disease, diabetes, and so forth. That is an issue. What about nutritional surveillance, which we lack so badly in this country? To know what is going on nutrition-wise in relation to public health, that indeed is an issue. What about nutrition awareness? We talked about that in terms of education. What about the quality and safety of the food supply? What indeed is it that consumers are so very nervous and concerned about? Need they be? This is an issue. What about the impact of our foreign food policies that Dan Shaughnessy spoke about, on the welfare of U.S. consumers? These are just some of the issues which were identified and which will be brought to Congress' attention, from which they themselves will decide what the policy shall be.

This is more sophisticated than the definition of Mr. Butz who said, "Of course we have a food policy in the United States. We have unlimited production, unrestrained production at maximum prices to the producer, and we have reasonable prices and reasonable qualities for the consumer. Now, that is a food policy" he said.

I contend it has to be a little more sophisticated than that. We don't advise Congress on policy. We advise Congress on the issues upon which policy and legislation are made.

Ms. ROTHSCHILD: Yes, I guess I do have something I'm burning to say, and I'll say it very briefly. It refers closely to Dan Shaughnessy's very interesting presentation of the political aspects of it.

This is really the rather dramatic changes that have in fact taken place in U.S. food exports in the 1970's. I think very much the tendency today has been to talk as though U.S. foreign food policy was a matter of food aid policy. In the period up to 1972 to a significant extent this was the case, as with regard to developing countries. But the situation has in fact changed almost beyond recognition in that up to 1972 more than half of all U.S. food exports to developing countries went under U.S. Government-financed Aid programs. Since then only about 15% of all U.S. exports to developing countries are aid-financed. So the bulk of this trade, 85%, is in fact going under commercial conditions paid for with cash or with private credit, and to give a sort of particular example a country which has been talked about today, Bangladesh. In 1974, the year of the recent famine in Bangladesh, the country bought commercially all U.S. food aid aside, something like $100 million of U.S. wheat, leaving out any kind of food aid whatsoever.

And I think this change and this sort of utterly new policy question that it raises is something that should not be left entirely out of the discussion—the question of how the U.S. government should control these food exports, if at all. It hasn't up to now had much control over commercial food exports.

INCREASING FOOD PRODUCTION
FROM THE LOWLAND HUMID TROPICS
OF AFRICA AND LATIN AMERICA

D. J. Greenland

Department of Soil Science
University of Reading
Reading, Berkshire, England
and
International Institute of Tropical Agriculture
Ibadan, Nigeria

INTRODUCTION

In spite of successful population planning, it is probable that food production in the year 2000 will need to be twice what it is now if present nutritional levels are to be maintained. During the past 10 years, food production in developing countries has barely kept pace with population increase; in tropical Africa it has not done so.

In the lowland humid tropics, taken to mean those areas of the tropics below 1,000 m where precipitation exceeds evaporation for 5 months or more each year (roughly, areas with more than 1200 mm of rain per annum), there is, nevertheless, very considerable scope for substantial increases in food production. The lowland humid tropics include large areas of Africa and Latin America and parts of the tropical Asian and Pacific areas. Only in Nigeria and Asia are population densities high. In Asia the extreme dependence on rice production creates a situation different from that in Africa and South and Central America, and is not discussed here. In Africa and Latin America the relatively widely distributed population is dependent on agricultural production obtained by cultivating areas seldom larger than 3 hectares per family and in Africa often much less. As long as population density remains low, the farms are cultivated intermittently on a shifting cultivation or natural fallow rotation basis, normally with longer periods of fallow than cultivation. As population increases, land pressure develops and the fallow period is shortened. Consequently, soil fertility and production decline. If methods can be found to enable continuous food production to be maintained in these areas, without a decline in crop yields or soil fertility, a very substantial addition to world food resources will become possible. This arises partly from the difference between actual and potential crop yields, and partly from the low proportion of the land available for arable agriculture which is actually in production at any one time. The production capabilities of soils within the humid tropics differ considerably, and the highly acid Oxisols of low or very low fertility [1] are probably less dominant than has been thought. Certainly, in the areas where rainfall is less than 2,000 mm per annum, Alfisols are relatively common, and maize yields on research stations in these areas commonly attain 5 tons per hectare, and in breeders' trials reach 8 to 10 tons per hectare.[2] By contrast, the national average yield in Nigeria in 1974 was less than 1 ton per hectare, and in Brazil was 1.5 tons per hectare (FAO statistics). For cassava, research station yields of 40 to 50 tons per hectare are not uncommon, whereas national average yields are generally below 10 tons per hectare.[3] For grain legumes, 2 tons per hectare of cowpeas are attainable in pure stand, and 1.5 tons where intercropped with maize. Because they are almost invariably grown in complex mixtures,[4] quoted average yields are not particularly meaningful, but figures of 100 to 300 kilograms per hectare would be of the right order.

In spite of difficulties in assessing national average yields, and although research station yields may reflect the fact that the stations were established on better quality soils, it is clear that through better management and the availability of improved varieties there is great scope for increasing yields. This is borne out by the results of trials conducted on farmers' fields in Nigeria by the National Accelerated Food Production Program of the Nigerian Federal Department of Agriculture. Using local varieties but improved practices, yields in 298 trials averaged 1.6 tons per hectare, whereas improved varieties averaged 2.5 tons per hectare. For cassava, where yields of local varieties were severely depressed by the incidence of diseases, improved varieties gave yield increases of several fold.[2]

In addition to production increases associated with better yields, the cultivated land area in Africa and Latin America can be expanded substantially. Hopper[5] estimates that the proportion of arable land in Africa under cultivation is 22%, and in Latin America it is only 11%. These are overall figures and refer to subhumid as well as humid areas, and the areas of uncultivated land do of course include more of the poorer quality land. Nevertheless, even on many of the better soils, natural fallow cultivation systems are followed, in which the land is abandoned to regenerating forest for periods substantially longer than those for which it is cultivated. If farming systems can be developed that enable the land to be used more continuously, a major increase in production and productivity will result.

Unlike Asia, wet lands in Africa and Latin America have been little exploited for rice production. A further potential for increased food production exists in proper development of these areas together with the dry lands.[6] The present paper, however, is limited to discussion of the ways in which food production in the humid tropics may be increased, omitting reference to the important but special topic of rice production.

The dominance of root crops in the diets of people in many parts of the lowland humid tropics has given rise to concern that there is a problem not only of the quantity of food which can be produced, but also of quality. The question of quality is therefore also considered very briefly.

CONSTRAINTS ON FOOD CROP PRODUCTION IN THE LOWLAND HUMID TROPICS

A characteristic of crop production in the humid tropics is the rapid decline in yields of crops planted immediately following forest clearing. At the International Institute of Tropical Agriculture (IITA), Ibadan, Nigeria, in the first year after clearing secondary forest, yields of an improved cultivar of maize (TZb) grown without fertilizers or weeding were close to 5.0 tons per hectare.[2] After 4 years, yields fell almost to zero. With proper inputs, particularly of fertilizers, yields could be maintained between 5.0 and 7.0 tons per hectare. Similar results have been obtained on several soil types in southern Nigeria and in Uganda.[2, 9] This and earlier work establishes the major importance of nutrient supply and weed competition in limiting productivity in these areas.

Soil erosion is another major constraint. Under the high erosivity of the rainfall of the lowland humid tropics, it may attain catastrophic dimensions.[10] Even when it does not result in more obvious effects, the loss of nutrient elements when the surface soil is removed by erosion, causes a substantial loss of production potential, as the nutrient elements tend to be strongly concentrated in the immediate surface of soils developed under tropical forest. Exposure of large areas of land by mechanized production systems even when conducted using contour ploughing, and other methods developed for erosion control in less erosive climates, is particularly liable to be accompanied by erosion of surface soil. Inadequate attention to this fact, or translation of erosion control methods from areas of lower erosivity, has led to failure of many otherwise well conceived development schemes. The difficulties of extending large-scale mechanical farming to the lowland humid tropics appear to be still not fully appreciated. If forest is to be cleared, and crops grown in monoculture and managed as crops are in the temperate zone, there is an extreme erosion hazard. For food crops, the value of the crops is not normally sufficient to justify the cost of conventionally designed erosion control measures. At the heart of the problem is the danger of exposing soil without a vegetative or mulch cover to direct rainfall impact, especially if large areas are involved, as they must be for mechanization projects. In these areas long-term arable food crop production is confined to valley bottom soils used for sugar cane and rice, and to terraces built to withstand the high erosivity, and whose construction is not an economic proposition in present circumstances. The successful development schemes in these areas have all involved perennial tree crops (rubber, oil palm, cocoa) which maintain a permanent protection for the soil. No scheme for increasing food crop production from the humid tropics can hope for success unless it takes proper account of the erosion hazard.

A third major problem is the incidence of serious plant diseases in areas of constant high humidity and high temperature. This may be illustrated by the disease problem of cassava (*Manihot esculenta*).[12] Cassava mosaic disease (CMD) is almost universal throughout Africa. In recent years cassava bacterial blight (CBB) has reached epidemic proportions in parts of Zaire and Nigeria and has been found in many other parts of West Africa. Other root crops, most grain legumes, and rice and maize are also seriously affected by diseases.[2]

Insect pests are another major constraint to increased food production. They attack all of the major food crops of the humid tropics and pose serious problems in relation to storage of crops. They are also important disease vectors.

Apart from soil fertility and pest problems, further constraints are imposed by the fact that hand labor restricts the areas that can be cultivated and maintained. This of course has its advantages in terms of prevention of serious erosion, and buildup of pests and diseases. The system in much of Africa is in fact a relatively sophisticated adjustment to the problems of production in the tropical forest region.[7, 13] However, it is important to recognize the severe restraint on productivity imposed by the high labor demand at planting time when weeding is critically important, and at harvest.[14] There are, of course, also major economic constraints arising from lack of organized distribution services, marketing and storage facilities, credit provision, and advisory services.[15]

OVERCOMING THE CONSTRAINTS

In developing methods to overcome the physical constraints it is essential to bear in mind that they must be such that long-term productivity of soils is maintained.[16] It is also important that they should be capable of adoption rapidly by farmers who are accustomed to using only hand labor, working areas of about 1 hectare, and usually without access to monetary credit, nor experience of management. The problems posed by poor roads, poor communication services, and poor marketing and service facilities must also be recognized.

Maintenance of Soil Nutrient Levels

The need for long-term stability of the system requires that primary consideration be given to soil fertility.[16] Ecologically, the lowland humid tropics are adapted to forests and tree crop production. The soils are also of low intrinsic fertility, although, as mentioned above, a distinction should be drawn between the Alfisols of areas with less than 1500 mm rainfall per annum of modest fertility, and the Ultisols and Oxisols of the very high rainfall areas of low or very low fertility.[17] On all soils of the humid tropics, however, phosphorus and nitrogen deficiencies are very common,[18] and response to potassium and sometimes trace elements arises when cultivation is prolonged.[19]

The need for inputs in terms of fertilizers is unavoidable, but the amounts required can be minimized by ensuring that all crop residues are returned to the soil, and that nitrogen is obtained as far as possible from the atmosphere by inclusion of legumes with appropriate N-fixing rhizobia in the cropping system.

Characteristics of the legumes, as well as those of the rhizobia, are important in determining nitrogen fixation. Legumes that fail to grow well will not provide good hosts for rhizobia. The competition between yield of grain and nitrogen fixation should also be recognized, since there may be competition between root nodules and seeds for photosynthate.[23] Much remains to be done in screening both legumes and rhizobia with regard to their potential contribution of nitrogen to different cropping systems. The existing rhizobial population in the humid tropics has been little studied, and some interesting discoveries are possible. For instance, in highly acid soils in southeastern Nigeria, highly active indigenous nitrogen-fixing rhizobia have been found; these nodulate freely on cowpeas when these are planted. This is contrary to expectation for soils with pH close to 4.0.

Another observation worthy of mention is the intense colonization of the roots of cassava, cowpeas, and maize grown at Ibadan, Ikenne, and Onne, Nigeria, by *Endogone* mycorrhiza (Sanders, private communication). The mycorrhiza are believed to improve growth by effectively extending the root surface, so that the plant becomes a better collector of phosphate and other slowly diffusing ions in short supply. Similar mycorrhiza appear to be widespread on crop plants in Nigeria. In pot experiments responses to inoculation with selected strains of mycorrhiza have been obtained (Mosse, private communication), which suggests that utilization of existing or added phosphate fertilizers may be improved cheaply, provided that the introduced mycorrhiza can compete effectively with indigenous strains, and are superior to them.

Contributions to plant nutrition from appropriate conservation of plant residues, and encouragement of contributions to plant nutrition from microorganisms, can only help to alleviate the problems of crop nutrition. For most soils of the humid tropics it is absolutely essential to provide additional plant nutrients both to raise the level of potential yield and to make good the inescapable losses of nutrients that accompany continuous food crop production.

Soil acidity is often considered to be a major constraint to crop production in the humid tropics.[20] Where lime is readily available, it normally helps to solve acidity problems. Questions have, however, been raised about its efficiency in the humid tropics, because of the rate at which it is likely to be lost due to leaching, and negative responses to liming that have sometimes been observed. Recent results [21] have indicated that in fact effects can persist for 6 years or more, and the negative responses to be due to induced deficiencies of trace elements such as zinc and copper present at marginal levels.[22, 2] Such induced deficiencies can be avoided if the lime is used in small dressings, sufficient to correct calcium deficiency and reduce aluminium solubility, but not to increase pH by more than one unit.

In much of West Africa and other parts of the humid tropics, lime is not readily available. Thus, acidity which inevitably develops if continuous arable cultivation is practiced, remains a major problem to be solved. In the indigenous system of shifting cultivation the loss of bases is restored by cycling of cations from the subsoil in the forest fallow vegetation, and their release together with micronutrients when the forest is felled and burnt prior to planting.

Stable and economic continuous arable production systems for these areas will probably require the involvement of trees in some manner. They will not necessarily have to be grown on the same land that is used for arable production, provided that they are able to exploit the subsoil to bring basic cations into their vegetation. Either the vegetation itself, or the ash from it, will need to be used as an amendment for the arable land. If leguminous trees are grown and unburnt vegetation used as an amendment, a substantial contribution to the nitrogen status of the soil may be obtained. Leguminous shade trees have long had a place in plantation farming in the tropics, and there are indigenous farming practices in Nigeria in which shrubs are planted and coppiced and used in the way described above for maintenance of soil fertility.[4] The species planted (*Acioa barteri, Anthonota macrophylla* and *Gliricidia sepium*) are not all legumes, and the rooting habit and ability to accumulate bases are probably the factors determining their selection.

A final important point regarding acidity in soils of the humid tropics is the accentuation of the problem that is bound to occur as fertilizers are used increasingly. The most rapid effects come from production of acidity by nitrification of ammonium or urea, but accelerated cation depletion due to increased removal by crops, and enhanced leaching because of higher soil nitrate levels, will also contribute. Unless a long-term solution to the acidity problem is found, no stable increase of food crop production in the humid tropics is possible.

Prevention of Soil Erosion

Techniques of erosion control are well established for the temperate zone. They generally involve rather extensive mechanical constructions to control runoff water. For small-farmer conditions such mechanical construction work is seldom feasible because of the highly fragmented land holdings. Fortunately, zero tillage methods, in which weeds are killed by herbicides, together with crop residues used as a mulch, have been found successful as a method of minimizing erosion in southern Nigeria.[24] High yields of maize and other crops have been obtained together with almost complete elimination of soil loss. While this work was initiated on small plots, it has now been demonstrated to be equally effective as a production technique for areas of 10 hectares or more, and with slopes up to 15%. Comparisons made at the International Institute of Tropical Agriculture of zero-tilled maize with crops on conventionally contour-bunded areas, planted after ploughing and harrowing, show that zero-tillage methods are advantageous in economic as well as erosion control terms.

In general, erosion control methods developed for the less erosive rains of the temperate zone appear to be unsatisfactory in the lowland humid tropics, and even methods such as tied-ridge contour ploughing have severe disadvantages in terms of work involved in construction, and effects on plant growth. The advantages of zero-tillage methods are that they enable a cover of crop and weed residues to be maintained on the soil. Further, it is found that soil fauna under zero-tillage is much more active than when the soil is ploughed and comparable to that present under standing forest. If the forest is hand-cleared prior to crop production by zero-tillage methods, the natural porosity of the soil is preserved, as well as the soil population, and high rates of water infiltration are maintained.[25]

Control of Pests and Diseases

Chemical control of most pests is possible but can be expensive and requires some sophistication in understanding concentrations of pesticides to be used, time to use them, and which to use. They are not well suited to the small farmer. For many insect and disease problems it is possible to produce resistant varieties, and achieve substantial yield increases without requiring any additional inputs. This is notably true with cassava in Africa, where mosaic disease and bacterial blight can be devastating.

Highly resistant cassava cultivars have been selected at IITA, and crossed with South American material to provide high-yielding varieties of good root characteristics. These materials are now being distributed through national programs in Nigeria, Zaire, and other parts of Africa.[2]

In legumes very important successes have been obtained at the international institutes in selecting materials with multiple resistance to insects and diseases. These materials are now being distributed widely to national programs for use as the parents for crossing with local material to produce varieties with desired characteristics related to local consumer preferences. By establishing large collections of breeding material, the international institutes have an essential and important role to play in breeding of cultivars with wide resistance, but must collaborate closely with national and regional programs, to ensure proper utilization of these materials.

Breeding of resistant materials is not the only economic method of reducing pest attack. Growing crops in mixed stand rather than in monoculture also reduces pest incidence, and similarly mulches reduce weeds and some insect pests. Insufficient information is available on the changes in pest ecology associated with the change from mixed to monoculture. Thus, Trenbath[26] comments: "Although very few experiments . . . have been performed to test the point, a consensus of opinion is developing which maintains that mixtures have a generally greater tolerance of disease and pest attack." His review of the literature and analysis of physical and biological factors affecting crop performance in mixed and inter-cropping experiments, indicate that "pathogen escape" and reduced incidence of insect pests are frequently factors contributing to "overyielding," by which is meant the production of yields in excess of those that would be obtained by growing the same crops on the same proportion of the total area of land but as a sole crop. Much further work is needed on this topic.

Reducing Labor Constraints

Increase in productive capacity requires development of the means for one man to manage larger crop areas. Weeding is one major bottleneck. Dead mulches and zero-tillage techniques may help. "Live mulches" of prostrate legumes that maintain a good cover are a further possible aid.[2] Herbicides used with "controlled droplet application" (CDA) sprayers may be an economic proposition, as they can reduce the amount of herbicide needed by a factor of 2, the amount of water that has to be carried by a factor of 20, and the cost of the sprayer by a factor of 4. Again more work is needed, but they appear to be an attractive proposition. Their introduction substantially increases the area that one person can manage. Similarly, small tools and power sources for ploughing wet rice land, or for drilling zero-tilled land, can substantially increase the area with which one man can deal.[2]

IMPROVING THE QUALITY OF THE FOOD PRODUCED

Root crops constitute the major part of the diet in all parts of the lowland humid tropics outside the great rice-producing areas of southern Asia.[3] In southern Nigeria the white yam, *Dioscorea rotundata,* is the major staple; elsewhere in Africa and in South America it is cassava and in the Pacific region it is taro, *Colocasia esculenta.* In the less humid areas sweet potatoes, *Ipomea batatis,* are frequently the major staple. All of these are often considered to be unsatisfactory in nutritional terms because of their low protein content. However, although cassava often contains less than 2 percent of protein, the other root crops are more satisfactory. In particular, the white yam often contains 5 to 8 percent of protein, of good nutritional quality.[27] Further, the hybrid yams recently produced[28] not only show vigorous growth and disease resistance, but some contain over 10 percent of protein (Sadik, private communication).

Where cassava provides the major staple a quality problem may exist, in spite of changes in viewpoint regarding "the protein gap."[29] Trypanosomiasis is a major obstacle in developing animal production in the humid areas of Africa, and even when it is overcome, the reeducation of the people that will be required to bring animals into farming systems will take much time. Probably the most practical method of improving the diet in the short term is to encourage grain legume production. Although severe problems exist due to insect pests and diseases, recent work has shown that there is considerable scope for improvement of cowpeas (*Vigna unguiculata*) and lima beans (*Phaseolus lunatus*) (see Annual Reports of the Grain Legume Improvement Program, IITA, 1973, 1974 and 1975), as well as possibilities for extending the cultivation of species such as the winged bean (*Psophocarpus tetragonolobus*). Further exciting possibilities arise from the fact that it has been shown that interspecific crosses in the genus *Phaseolus* can be made, and that these produce viable seed (Maréchal and Le Marchand, private communication).

Conclusions

Although very serious constraints exist to increasing food production from the lowland humid tropics, at least potential methods for removing these constraints exist. Some of them are already moving into practice through collaboration between national agricultural programs and the international institutes; others require further research.

The food problem facing the world is grave, but given the right approach I believe that it can be solved and that the efforts of the peoples and governments of the countries of the lowland humid tropics will make a significant contribution to it, aided by support through the international institutes.

References

1. AUBERT, G. & R. TAVERNIER. 1972. Soil survey. *In* Soils of the Humid Tropics: 17–44. National Academy of Sciences. Washington, D.C.
2. International Institute of Tropical Agriculture, Ibadan, Nigeria. Annual Reports, 1974 and 1975.
3. COURSEY, D. G. & P. H. HAYNES. 1970. Root crops and their potential as food in the tropics. World Crops: 261–265.
4. OKIGBO, B. N. & D. J. GREENLAND. 1977. Mixed intercropping and related cropping systems in tropical Africa. Am. Soc. Agron. Spec. Pub. In press.
5. HOPPER, W. D. 1976. The development of agriculture in developing countries. Sci. Am. **235** (3): 197–205.
6. ABEYRATNE, E. F. L. 1956. Dryland farming in Ceylon. Trop. Agric. (Ceylon) **112**: 191–212.
7. NYE, P. H. & D. J. GREENLAND. 1960. The soil under shifting cultivation. Tech. Comm. No. 51. Comm. Bur. Soils. Harpenden.
8. RUTHENBERG, H. 1971. Farming Systems in the Tropics. Oxford University Press. London.
9. JONES, E. 1972. Principles of using fertilizers to improve red ferrallitic soils in Uganda. Exp. Agri. **8**: 315–332.
10. GREENLAND, D. J. & R. LAL. 1977. Soil Conservation and Management in the Humid Tropics. J. Wiley & Sons. Chichester, England. In press.
11. SIOLI, H. 1973. Recent human activities in the Brazilian Amazon region and their ecological effects. *In* Tropical Forest Ecosystems in Africa and America: A Comparative Review. B. J. Meggers, E. S. Ayonsu & W. D. Duckworth, Eds. Smithsonian Institution Press. Washington, D.C
12. LOZANO, J. C. & R. H. BOOTH. 1974. Diseases of cassava (*Manihot esculenta* Crantz). Pans Pest Artic. News Summ. **20**: 30–54.
13. ALLAN, W. 1965. The African Husbandman. Oliver and Boyd. Edinburgh, Scotland.
14. FLINN, J. C., B. M. JELLEMA & K. L. ROBINSON. 1975. Problems of increasing food crop production in the lowland humid tropics of Nigeria. Z. Ausland. Landwirt. **14**: 37–48.
15. BUNTING, A. H. Ed. 1970. Change in Agriculture. Duckworths. Letchworth, England.
16. GREENLAND, D. J. 1975. Bringing the green revolution to the shifting cultivator. Science **190**: 841–844.
17. SANCHEZ, P. A. & S. W. BUOL. 1975. Soils in the tropics and the world food crisis. Science **188**: 598–603.
18. GREENLAND, D. J. 1973. Soil factors determining responses to phosphorus and nitrogen fertilizers in tropical Africa. Afr. Soils **17**: 99–108.

19. GREENLAND, D. J. 1974. Intensification of agricultural systems, with special reference to the role of potassium fertilizers. Trans. 10th Congr. Int. Potash Inst. Budapest: 311–323.
20. KAMPRATH, E. J. 1972. Soil acidity and liming. *In* Soils of the Humid Tropics: 136–149. National Academy of Sciences. Washington, D.C.
21. DE FREITAS, L. M. M. & B. VAN RAIJ. 1975. *In* Soil Management in Tropical America. E. Bornemisza & A. Alvarado, Eds. : 300–307. North Carolina State University. Raleigh, N.C.
22. SPAIN, J. M., C. A. FRANCIS, R. H. HOWELER & F. CALVO. 1975. *In* Soil Management in Tropical America. E. Bornemisza & A. Alvarado, Eds. : 308–329. North Carolina State University. Raleigh, N.C.
23. HAM, G. E., R. J. LAWN & W. A. BRUN. 1976. Influence of inoculation, nitrogen fertilizers and photosynthetic source-sink manipulation on field-grown soyabean. *In* Symbiotic Nitrogen Fixation in Plants. P. S. Nutman, Ed. : 239–254. Cambridge University Press. London.
24. LAL, R. 1974. No-tillage, soil properties and maize yield. Plant Soil **40:** 129–143, 321–331, 589–606.
25. WILKINSON, G. E. & P. O. AINA. 1976. Infiltration of water into two Nigerian soils. Geoderma **15:** 51–60.
26. TRENBATH, B. R. 1974. Biomass productivity of mixtures. Adv. Agron. **26:** 177–210.
27. SPLITTSTOESSER, W. E. 1973. Amino acid composition of five species of yams (*Dioscorea*). J. Am. Soc. Hortic. Sci. **98:** 563–567.
28. SADIK, G. & O. U. OKEREKE. 1975. Sexual propagation, a new approach to improvement of yam, *Dioscorea rotundata*. Nature (London) **254:** 134–135.
29. WATERLOW, J. C. & P. R. PAYNE. 1975. The protein gap. Nature (London) **258:** 113–117.

HIGH-FREQUENCY IRRIGATION AND GREEN REVOLUTION FOOD PRODUCTION

S. L. Rawlins

U.S. Salinity Laboratory
Agricultural Research Service, USDA
Riverside, California 92502

Although only 15 to 20% of the world's cropland is irrigated, it produces a far greater proportion of the world's food because the yield per unit area is about twice that for nonirrigated land.[1] The reason is not always fully recognized. Where the farmer controls the quantity of water and its timeliness of delivery, he can plan other operations to increase production. Assured of an adequate water supply, he is more willing to invest in the needed fertilizer and seeds of high-yielding varieties. For this reason, irrigation has played an essential role in the remarkable gains in productivity obtained with the so-called green revolution technology package. This package includes new varieties that produce abundantly when they are grown in dense plantings with adequate fertilizer, pesticides, and water.

Typical of the experience of many countries adopting this green revolution package in the early 1960's is that of Mexico.[2] In the 1930's and 1940's, Mexico's growth in food production was stagnant. Imports accounted for 15 to 20% of the food required to feed its 22 million people. With green revolution technology, the food deficits were erased by 1960, and from 1963 to 1968, Mexico exported food even though its population had increased to over 43 million. But in the late 1960's, growth in food production began to lose momentum. By the early 1970's, population had once more outstripped production, and Mexico was again importing 15 to 20% of her food.

Wellhausen[2] concluded that the green revolution technology package had succeeded in Mexico in the early 1960's primarily among the larger, more commercial farmers, particularly where full-scale irrigation could be practiced. These farmers were in a better position than small farmers to afford the fertilizer, pesticides, and other inputs necessary for the new high-yielding varieties to reach their full potential. And irrigation eliminated much of the risk of these expensive inputs being wasted by a drought. The third of Mexico's farmland that is irrigated produces more than half of its food. But by the late 1960's, Mexico began to run out of clients for this specialized technology package. Practically all the water resources in the areas adaptable to full-scale irrigation were being used. In some cases, groundwater aquifers were being overdrafted. Future gains in food production by putting additional land under full-scale irrigation will be extremely costly in Mexico.

Wellhausen[2] suggested two approaches to bring about Mexico's second agricultural revolution: One is to intensify production on the full-scale irrigation projects. In areas subject to frost, winter wheat could be grown. With ideal management, present yields could be doubled. In frost-free areas, improved management could permit three or even four crops to be grown instead of two. The other approach is to bring the green revolution to the large rainfed areas practicing traditional agriculture. Wellhausen commented that supplemental irrigation is the key to this development. In humid areas, it takes away the risks so that investment can be made in fertilizer and other inputs. And it extends modern production techniques to areas with less rainfall.

Both of these approaches will be necessary in other countries also. But, a key to their success will be the development of irrigation systems that give individual farmers control over their water supply. A farmer's capability of withholding water during harvest or land preparation and applying it precisely when it is needed to germinate a new crop can make a big difference. Irrigation timing is crucial for multiple cropping. A few days can often mean the difference between growing an additional crop and having to allow the field to lie idle for a season.

Most of our present full-scale irrigation systems do not give the farmer the water control he needs. Too often, large irrigation projects consist of spectacular structures and canals that end at main outlets serving 40 to 200 hectares. The individual farmer is usually denied the facilities for effective water control and is forced to resort to taking water whenever it is available, whether he needs it or not. In attempting to insure against the prospect of not having sufficient water when he does need it, he often applies more than the soil will hold. The extra water percolates below the root zone to the water table. Not only does this waste water, but it also causes extremely serious damage. In the 10 million hectares irrigated in the Indus Plain, for example, deep percolation and canal seepage have caused the water table to rise to within 3 meters of the surface in over half the area. Waterlogging and salinity are severe in well over 1 million hectares. The problem is worsening and threatens to eliminate agriculture in large areas if the pace of remedial steps is not quickened. Egypt, which produces all its food on irrigated land, is even more threatened by encroaching waterlogging and the resulting soil salinity. High water tables contribute to soil salination by permitting capillary movement of water from them to the soil surface. As the water evaporates, salt contained in this water is left on the soil surface. The magnitude of the problem of poor water management is underscored by a recent survey by the International Commission on Irrigation and Drainage,[1] which showed that only 25% of the water diverted into continuous flow canal systems was beneficially used by crops. Pipeline systems increased this efficiency to 50%.

In addition to farmers not having control over irrigation timing, another reason for this poor record of water use is that most farms are irrigated with surface distribution systems. Surface irrigation imposes two fundamental constraints on irrigation management: (1) it depends on flow over the soil surface to distribute water from one end of the field to the other, which requires a minimum depth of water simply to achieve coverage; and (2) a fixed labor cost is associated with each application.[3] Both of these constraints tend to make it advantageous to decrease the number of irrigations required in a season. This is done by storing as much water as possible during each irrigation and then using as much of this stored water as possible before the next. Irrigating just to fill the available soil storage capacity, and no more, requires a knowledge of soil properties and conditions that practically no farmer has. Add to this the fact that both water-storage capacity and infiltrability (the rate at which the soil absorbs water when supplied freely to its surface) can vary widely from place to place in a single field, and it is obvious that surface irrigation is prone to supply far too much water to some areas of a field before others have enough. This extra water percolates below the root zone and all too often is either wasted, or worse, creates serious waterlogging or salinity problems. This waste of both water and productive land must be prevented if we are to intensify food production in present full-scale irrigation projects.

The use of closed conduits to distribute water within a field can eliminate nonuniform infiltration caused by nonuniform soil properties by transferring control from the soil to the irrigation system. This occurs as the direct result of eliminating surface flow. If water is applied uniformly to the soil from a closed-conduit system at a rate less than the soil infiltrability, the infiltration rate will equal the application rate, and every portion of the field can receive the same quantity regardless of soil nonuniformity. Because the closed-conduit system effectively delivers water to each plant, no minimum depth need be applied to attain uniform distribution. As a consequence, water can be applied in small enough quantities that the storage capacity of the soil is not exceeded in any part of a field. In fact, if irrigations are made frequently enough, the storage capacity of the soil is of such little importance that one can farm extremely coarse-textured soils that would otherwise be useless. Uniform, frequent irrigation made possible with closed-conduit irrigation systems can, therefore, drastically reduce the quantity of water lost by deep percolation, and can permit this saved water to be used on marginal lands that otherwise could not be farmed.

Irrigating frequently can also optimize soil conditions for crop growth.[3] For one thing, it maintains the soil water content at a high level. The reason for this lies in the fact that with frequent irrigation, infiltration occupies a significant portion of the time. Crop roots can then absorb the water as it goes by. With infrequent irrigation, a large quantity of water is stored during a short time. For this stored water to be used, it must be brought into contact with active roots. The only way this can take place is for the soil near the roots to dry sufficiently to establish a sizable hydraulic gradient. But, as the soil dries, hydraulic conductivity decreases precipitously—as much as several thousandfold. (See Rawlins[4] and Rawlins & Raats[3] for a detailed theoretical analysis of this process.) The larger the quantity of water stored in the soil profile, the deeper it will extend beyond the active roots, and the longer and more severe the drying period must be to bring it back to the roots. This drying can seriously reduce crop growth. If the soil is not permitted to dry long enough to allow this water to be pulled back to the roots and used, the remaining water is simply flushed out the bottom of the root zone when the soil's water storage capacity is refilled by the next irrigation. By supplying the crop's water needs on a frequent basis, water need not be stored deep within the profile, and the long extraction process can be avoided. As a consequence, the average soil water content remains far higher, even with very low deep percolation, than it does with infrequent irrigation. This constantly high soil-water content is ideal for maximum growth of most crops. It eliminates drought-induced yield reductions and keeps solutes contained in the irrigation water diluted.

Whether water is actually saved with high-frequency irrigation depends on how closely the irrigator matches the quantity of water applied to the crop's needs. Considerable progress has recently been made in the use of climatological data to schedule irrigation on a wide area basis. With experience, the error in estimating seasonal water use can be kept small, but short-term errors are appreciable. To compensate for these short-term fluctuations in demand and to make maximum use of rainfall, the storage capacity of the soil profile needs to be used effectively. In rain-fed agriculture, water stored in the soil profile is often the only source for a growing crop. The quantity of water that can be withdrawn from storage, in such cases, is often not limited as much by the quantity stored as it is by the rate at which it can be withdrawn by the growing crop. Once this rate drops below the crop's needs, for reasons explained above, growth begins to decline, and in severe cases, the crop dies. Often this occurs with considerable stored water left in the soil profile. But, it is at depths too great to be moved to the crop's root surfaces fast enough to sustain life. By supplying part of the crop's water needs with frequent, light irrigations, the remainder can be withdrawn from deep storage at a sustained, but much slower, rate without reducing crop growth. Fischbach et al.[5] have used this method of gradually depleting stored soil water during the growing season to make soil storage capacity available for winter rains, and to reduce the maximum required capacity of a center-pivot sprinkler system. High-frequency irrigation goes a long way toward meeting the conflicting demands of maintaining the soil wet enough for maximum yield while providing sufficient capacity to store erratic rainfall, or short-term mismatches between the quantity of water applied as irrigation and that required by the crop.

Yet another advantage of irrigation systems capable of metering water precisely, uniformly, and frequently to the individual plants regardless of topography or soil properties deserves attention. Soluble fertilizers, primarily nitrogen, move with the soil water, and are often lost by deep percolation. Reducing deep percolation by uniform and precise irrigation keeps applied nutrients in contact with roots longer, increasing the proportion taken up by the crop. But, the chance always exists that intense rainfall will leach nutrients below the root zone. By applying soluble nutrients frequently in small amounts with the irrigation water, little is stored in the soil, which drastically reduces the quantity that can be lost in a single incident. Rawlins and Raats[3] cited an extreme case where efficient irrigation could save over 300 kg of N per hectare annually compared to current use. Particularly as energy for nitrogen fertilizer production becomes more scarce, this saving alone may play a significant role in determining how water is managed on the farm.

Any irrigation scheme certainly must have some disadvantages, and high-frequency irrigation is no exception. The two primary closed-conduit water-delivery systems capable of high-frequency irrigation that are now being used commercially are sprinkler and drip. Both can deliver any desired quantity of water directly and uniformly to each plant. But, because pressure is required to distribute water uniformly with sprinklers, and to force it through filters to prevent clogging of drip emitters, the water saved by increased uniformity of application is often at the expense of increased energy required for pumping. And continued supplies of low-cost energy for agriculture are not assured. Continued expansion of food production by expanded use of fossil energy is risky. We should not be comfortable with a food production system that ignores future stability. Any system that depends on fossil fuel energy has a finite life. And although we certainly cannot afford to abandon such systems, we need to consider their potential to produce food in the future, and come to grips with the question of how the population that survives because of them will be fed when they fail. It's no longer enough to blithely exclaim "Hang the cost, if people are hungry, let's feed them," for, in reality, we are being generous with someone else's resource. The fossil energy we expend belongs not only to us, but also to future generations.

Failure to count the energy cost is not a unique failing of irrigation system designers. American agricultural scientists often take pride in the tremendous increase in farm productivity they have achieved. But, most gains in productivity have resulted from huge expenditures of energy, not from sheer scientific genius. In a permanent sense, this expenditure has not solved our problems. It has simply bought time, delaying the day when we must plan for permanent solutions. We now face a problem that cannot be solved by simply spending more energy. Sooner or later, we must learn to live on our energy interest, not our capital.

Although it is true that green revolution agriculture now requires high energy inputs in terms of fertilizer, water, and pesticides, the relevant question is what is the possible return in food per unit energy input when the whole technology package is put together with a goal to conserve energy. It's not enough to extrapolate energy efficiencies from a past where the cost of energy has been ignored. Putting the technological package together elegantly, in a way that does not leave out some critical input that causes all others to be wasted, will be necessary to maximize food output per unit energy input. Inefficient irrigation that increases the quantity of water necessary to be pumped, wastes energy-intensive fertilizer by leaching, and reduced production by waterlogging and salination cannot be a part of this package.

FIGURE 1 shows a sixfold increase in rice production per unit area as farming intensity in Japan increased. More than half of this increase was the consequence of technical innovation and structural reforms in the rural economy. These reforms established the full range of institutions and infrastructures needed to support high-productivity agriculture. Evapotranspiration tends to be rather constant per unit of cropped area, and therefore, these reforms greatly increased crop yield per unit water consumed. Particularly if the high level water management possible with high-frequency irrigation were practiced, it is entirely possible that the highest yields with many crops could be obtained with as little as half the water now being used. Because fertilizer and water are usually the two highest continuous energy inputs, if by efficient water management these could be kept at an adequate level with minimum inputs, the one-time energy inputs represented by structural reforms that yield such high increases in production have the potential of raising the energy efficiency of high-intensity farming systems above that of low-intensity systems. Of course, without adequate fertilizer, water, and other necessary inputs, little gain from structural reforms can be expected.

Thus, relatively high energy input into irrigation may often be justified by its catalytic effect on other inputs. But we should not stop looking for less energy-intensive ways to irrigate efficiently. Aside from their energy requirement, sprinkler- and drip-irrigation systems are rather complicated, requiring many different kinds of parts to be stocked and maintained. To some extent, both, but particularly drip systems, require diligent maintenance by skilled personnel. What is obviously required, if the benefits of high-frequency irrigation are to accrue to the nations that need to increase their food production most urgently, is an inexpensive, simple system, that requires a low level of energy and skill to operate. Particularly if supplemental irrigation is to be brought to farmers practicing traditional agriculture on small holdings in humid areas, the systems must be simple to install and operate.

I have recently developed a system that shows promise of meeting these requirements.[7] It delivers water through inexpensive, 76- or 102-mm ID, buried corrugated polyethylene pipe laterals. Water is delivered from the lateral

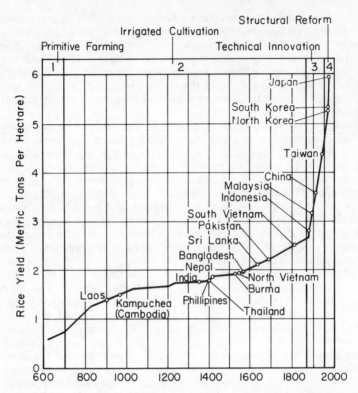

FIGURE 1. Intensification of farming on land now being farmed is the other way to grow more food. This means moving farming in developing regions to higher stages of development, in effect recapitulating the historic progression exemplified here by the case of Japan. Kunio Takase of the Asian Development Bank found that typical rice yields in Japan increased as Japanese agriculture moved from the traditional stage through the advent of irrigation to scientific agriculture and finally to structural transformation. Current yields in most Asian countries, where less than 50% of the rice land is cultivated, place them still in second stage, as plotted. (From Hopper.[6] By permission of *Scientific American*.)

to fill a small basin (for example at the base of a tree) through 9.5-mm ID, smooth-wall, polyethylene hose. Because of their low cost the lateral pipes can be sized large enough to reduce friction to the point that the system can operate from a water supply less than 1 meter above the field. In many cases, the existing canals could supply this pressure without pumps. Outflow is precisely regulated from each hose by fastening its outlet to a stake or a tree trunk at the proper elevation. In addition to the pipe and hose described, the field distribution system consists of only two other parts: a plastic, barbed-tee connector stapled to the stake or trunk of each tree, and a simple O-ring coupler to join the 75- or 100-meter lengths of corrugated pipe. By eliminating pumps, filters, sprinkler heads, or emitters, and by keeping the smallest diameter opening larger than 9 mm, the system operates with less attention than most surface irrigation systems—and, where the water source is sufficiently elevated, at no more energy cost.

Capital costs for materials at Riverside, Calif., were approximately $620/hectare where 76-mm ID laterals were used, and $740/hectare where 102-mm ID laterals were used. This cost is considerably less than solid-set drip or sprinkler systems that include pumps and filters. Because the system is buried, labor costs for installation would be greater than for drip systems, but probably less than for a buried-line sprinkler system. The increased life expectancy of the buried system over that of a surface drip system (approximately 20 vs. 10 years) should more than repay the additional labor cost. The fact that the system can be installed with simple tools and the flow regulated without instruments, may make this closed-conduit, gravity system an attractive alternative for developing countries. Once installed, water is precisely delivered to the field with an emission uniformity greater than 97% by simply maintaining water at the source at the proper level. A similar buried lateral system designed to fill short furrows for row crops [8] also shows promise.

These simple systems that have precise water control designed into them may be only the beginning of what can be accomplished if energy conservation and ease of operation are made valid strategies for irrigation system development. But, any closed-conduit system can operate at its full potential for controlling water precisely only if the farmer has water available on demand. The most easily operated and ideal water supply providing this is a pipe distribution system resembling a municipal water system. In this regard, Maletic and Langley [9] stated:

> Operation of an irrigation water supply system on a demand basis rather than on a conventional scheduled basis provides the water user additional flexibility in his efforts to improve irrigation efficiency. Pipe distribution systems, resembling municipal water systems, more readily provide this capability than do open canal systems. . . . When the source of supply for a distribution system is a canal, a frequent adjustment of the canal flow and its control structures is required to match the variation in flow created by automatic operation of the distribution system to meet the water users' demand.

The capital cost for closed-pipe systems exceeds that of open canals, and closed-conduit distribution systems cost more than surface systems. But, we need to bear in mind that even though capital is short in developing countries, it will be easier to supply these one-time inputs than it will be to provide the highly skilled technicians needed to operate open supply and distribution systems efficiently. Even in the United States with the highly skilled operators and sophisticated communication and automated controls available, open canals and surface distribution systems always end up with water that cannot be used efficiently. If the continuing cost of drainage and land reclamation required as the result of poor water management is considered, these closed systems may be far more competitive.

Closed water conveyance and irrigation water distribution systems are elegant engineering solutions to the water management problem in the sense that control is built into the system. (Anyone can operate a water tap to draw a glass of water.) A one-time investment replaces the continuous investment of energy, labor, and capital required with open conveyances and surface irrigation systems. The most highly skilled operators of open systems can seldom approach the water management efficiency that unskilled operators can attain with closed systems.

If we are serious about solving the world food problem, and I think we are, we need to opt for the possible solutions. Water is a necessary input before other inputs can help. Doubling our irrigated land area at present irrigation energy efficiencies to meet sustained food needs, with present fossil fuel reserves, is not possible. Training the required number of skilled water managers to gain the level of water control necessary to intensify food production sufficiently with the present irrigation systems is only slightly more likely to be possible. Developing the capital to install inherently efficient water-delivery systems that will give farmers independent control is expensive in the short run, but possible. It's a matter of choosing this investment over alternative ways we can spend our capital. The catalytic impact that efficient water control could have in permitting multiple cropping, taking the risk out of investing other inputs, saving valuable nutrients, reversing the alarming rate of waterlogging and salination, and permitting new lands that were previously useless to be irrigated with the saved water by high-frequency irrigation may be more than worth the one-time cost. Closed-conduit supply and distribution systems not only have inherent capability for efficient water control, they also save energy by conserving gravitational potential energy in the form of pressure required for efficient irrigation. In an energy-short future, systems that operate without additional energy input for pumping should be given high priority.

REFERENCES

1. DOORENBOS, J. 1975. The role of irrigation in food production. Agric. Environ. **2:** 39–54.
2. WELLHAUSEN, E. J. 1976. The agriculture of Mexico. Sci. Am. **235**(3): 128–150.
3. RAWLINS, S. L. & P. A. RAATS. 1975. Prospects for high-frequency irrigation. Science **188:** 604–610.
4. RAWLINGGS, S. L. 1973. Principles of managing high frequency irrigation. Soil Sci. Soc. Am. Proc. **37:** 626–629.
5. FISCHBACH, P. E. & B. R. SOMERHALDER. 1974. Irrigation design requirements for corn. Trans. ASAE **17**(1): 162–165, 171.
6. HOPPER, W. D. 1976. The development of agriculture in developing countries. Sci. Am. **235**(3): 196–205.
7. RAWLINS, S. L. 1976. Uniform irrigation with a closed-conduit, gravity distribution system. Agricultural Water Management. In preparation.
8. WORSTELL, R. V. 1975. An experimental buried multiset irrigation system. Am. Soc. Agric. Eng. Pap. No. 75–2540.
9. MALETIC, J. T. & M. N. LANGLEY. 1971. Experience and trends in automation of project and farm irrigation systems. "Experts Panel on Irrigation." Tel Aviv, Israel. Sept. 6–13, 1971.

SOURCES OF PROTEIN FOR MAN:
THE RESEARCH NEEDS

M. Milner, N. S. Scrimshaw, and D. I. C. Wang

Department of Nutrition and Food Science
Massachusetts Institute of Technology
Cambridge, Massachusetts 02139

A study at M.I.T. on behalf of the National Science Foundation has examined in detail the status and potential of various protein resources in order to identify priorities for research to increase their availability and acceptability in relation to U.S. national needs and international commitments. Among the resources studied were grain crops including cereals, soybeans and food legumes, cereal proteins, oilseed proteins, livestock animals, dairy products, meat, poultry and eggs, aquatic proteins, non-photosynthetic and photosynthetic single cell proteins, leaf proteins, and chemical synthesis. Problems common to all protein resources such as nutritional requirements, safety, political and regulatory constraints, processing technology as well as economic considerations, were taken into account. Research support was recommended for unconventional approaches for increasing agricultural and fisheries productivity, as well as development of new protein resources for animal feeding and direct human use. The latter includes single cell protein produced from plant and animal wastes and hydrocarbon derivatives, plant protein isolates, fresh- and salt-water aquaculture, and economical utilization of krill, the Antarctic crustacean.

BACKGROUND

It is clearly unnecessary to review for this informed audience the dramatic developments on the U.S. and world food scenes during the past four years, which have sharply intensified interest in research aimed at increasing food supply. Suffice it to say here that as a consequence of these events, questions have been raised about the longer term capability of U.S. food and protein production capacities to fill domestic needs, to sustain major export demands, and to respond to urgent international emergency feeding programs.

In this context, the National Science Foundation found itself receiving, primarily from U.S. universities, requests to finance projects for research in an array of unconventional and novel protein sources. It quickly became evident that there was a lack of information which would permit adequate critical judgment of the relative priorities for such funding requests. It was clear, furthermore, that in the foreseeable future the bulk of U.S. and world food supplies would have to come from traditional agricultural sources. Logically, therefore, fundamental and applied research for improving the productivity of conventional agriculture would have to have the greatest emphasis, and priorities assigned to unconventional proteins would need to be judged in this context.

Late in 1974, with these considerations in mind, NSF proposed to the Department of Nutrition and Food Science at MIT a study to analyze, in some detail, the status and potential of all relevant protein resources, and to provide recommendations for carefully selected projects and priorities worthy of research support. It may be worth noting that at precisely the same time, the National Academy of Sciences received from President Ford, as a consequence of Mr. Kissinger's commitments to the World Food Conference a few weeks earlier, a request to develop specific recommendations for how the nation's agricultural research and developmental capabilities could be applied to world food supply problems. This and other initiatives in the National Academy, as well as those of the Agricultural Research Policy Committee of the National Association of State Universities and Land Grant Colleges and USDA, have already been referred to by other speakers.

The MIT study recognized that many aspects of protein resources research are already receiving attention, principally from the U.S. Department of Agriculture, from the state universities and Land Grant colleges with their associated experiment stations, and from industry. Nevertheless, we believe that important areas of research vital to strengthening U.S. food and protein productivity are either inadequately funded, or are entirely neglected, in terms of available research support. Also, in the decades ahead, there is likely to be a need to supplement conventional agriculture, and some resources should be directed toward research on possible unconventional protein sources, as well as innovative areas of agricultural research not now receiving adequate attention and support. These are the primary areas which this study has delineated and recommended for NSF research emphasis.

ORGANIZATION OF THE STUDY

Various groups of specialists, organized into committees or working groups, developed the information needed to evaluate problems affecting protein production, and the status of various resources and their research needs. Problems that were analyzed as affecting proteins generally included nutritional quality and its assessment, toxicology and food safety, processing technology, energy constraints, plant genetic potentials, nitrogen fixation, marketing of protein foods, and legal, regulatory, and political constraints that may influence introduction of novel proteins. Protein resource areas for which status analyses and research recommendations were prepared included grain crops, cereal proteins, oilseeds, food legumes, livestock production, dairy products, meat, poultry and eggs, aquatic proteins, potatoes, nonphotosynthetic single-cell protein (SCP): photosynthetic SCP, leaf proteins, and chemical synthesis of nutrients.

Significant Determinants of Research Recommendations

Review of the extensive documentation prepared for this study suggested that there were a number of significant conclusions or hypotheses which had considerable relevance when identifying research recommendations and priorities. The following are pertinent:

1. U.S. agriculture will continue in the foreseeable future to supply in abundance the protein foods and feeds to which this country has become accustomed, but it will obviously do so with rising costs and increasing pressure on our land, energy, and environmental resources.

2. Appropriate research and technological development must be pursued more vigorously to achieve increases in productivity, protein quality, and pro-

tein quantity of primary food crops and aquatic resources, to meet both domestic demand and export opportunities.

3. A strengthening of U.S. food and agricultural research capabilities will be necessary to ensure continued growth of food export, a major contributor to the maintenance of favorable U.S. trade balances. With adequate research support, and if other appropriate policies are adopted, U.S. food export capacity should, at least until 1985, increase at a rate following the trend established prior to 1972.

4. The food and feed demands of affluent industrial countries will continue to increase and will exert growing pressure on food resources available in international markets.

5. Even with probable improvements, the agricultural production capacities of some major food-deficit developing countries will not soon be adequate to feed their growing populations. They will need to import food for many years to come, and the U.S. will play a leading role in supplying these needs, largely on regular commercial terms.

6. When food-deficit countries improve their own agriculture and food production capacities, not only will the nutritional status of their populations be increased, but, experience has shown, they will also tend to increase their commercial food purchases in the U.S.

7. In the foreseeable future, the relative cost of proteins (e.g., meat, soybeans) for human and animal feeding is likely to increase more rapidly than the cost for staple sources of food or feed energy (e.g., corn, wheat).

8. The foreseeable domestic and world demand for U.S. soybeans as a primary protein resource, notwithstanding increasing production in other countries such as Brazil, will grow faster than for other food or feed crops. While a major breakthrough in soybean yields may occur, it is not likely to be effective in the next 10 years. This will stimulate interest in alternative protein sources of both conventional and unconventional types.

9. It is likely that new and more productive grain crops will be developed, particularly from intergeneric crossing of cereals, of which triticale is a prototype.

10. The marketplace must reflect the increased value of crops with improved protein quality and quantity if farmers are to be persuaded to produce them. Incentives may also be needed to encourage commercial initiatives by the seed industry and others directed toward more rapid development of improved food crop varieties.

11. The increasing costs of agricultural food production may eventually encourage the use of unconventional techniques for protein production which are not now commercially competitive.

12. The reclaiming of organic wastes of all kinds for food and feed use is a major priority.

13. The development and application of innovative food-processing techniques and of new science and technology to the production of protein foods will require fair and objective regulatory standards and procedures on the part of the Food and Drug Administration, the U.S. Department of Agriculture, and the Environmental Protection Agency.

14. Acceptance by the U.S. consumer of novel protein foods to any significant extent will require innovative marketing and promotional approaches which, to be effective, must go beyond emphasis on nutritional benefits.

15. Adoption and enforcement by many countries of a 200-mile offshore fishing limit will remove some prime fishing areas from free international exploitation and thus may affect protein supplies and prices in international markets. Over 30 countries including the U.S. have already adopted this limit.

COMMON PROBLEMS AND ISSUES REQUIRING RESEARCH

Nutrition

Adequate assessment of the protein problem is handicapped by lack of knowledge in two fundamental areas: (1) human requirements for protein at different ages and physiological states, and (2) the evaluation of protein quality of foods. These issues are further complicated by increasing evidence that both are greatly affected by caloric excess as well as caloric deficit.

It is apparent that the present FAO/WHO recommendations for protein requirements and, similarly, those of the National Academy of Sciences/National Research Council's Food and Nutrition Board do not provide an adequate basis for determination of a safe practical allowance for either individuals or populations, especially under adverse environmental circumstances.

There is an urgent need to develop and apply improved methods of protein quality evaluation that are sufficiently rapid and inexpensive to be used by the food industry, by regulatory agencies, and by plant breeders seeking to develop new crop varieties of high nutritional value. These methods should be feasible with the extremely small samples likely to be available. For novel protein sources in general, and in particular for novel or conventional sources subject to extensive processing, evaluation of protein quality is especially important.

Toxicology

Toxic factors, which even in small amounts may pose a threat to animals and humans, occur in many widely used foods unless the foods are specially processed, or restricted in use. A group of inhibitors of protein-digesting enzymes—e.g., the hemagglutinins (lectins) and trypsin inhibitors, which are themselves protein in nature—occur widely in food legumes (peas, beans) and oilseeds (soybeans). Fortunately, most of these inhibitors are deactivated by heat during processing. Cyanogens (glucosides containing hydrocyanic acid) occur in significant quantities in foods as diverse as lima beans, almonds, cassava, and sorghum. Saponins are toxins occurring in over 400 species of the plant kingdom—including sugar beets, spinach, and asparagus. Gossypol is a toxic pigment found in cottonseed (*Gossypium*). Favism is a genetically linked disease caused by ingestion of a toxin in broad beans (*Vicia faba*). Lathyrism can be severely debilitating and even fatal in humans ingesting the legumes of the *Lathyrus* (sweet pea) species. Goitrogens, usually in the form of thioglucosides, are present in the *Brassica* species (cabbage, turnips, and mustard). A variety of antivitamins also occur in plant foods.

In addition to natural food toxins, substances that are potentially hazardous to man and animals may be added to foods as preservatives or coloring and flavoring agents. Some toxicants may be introduced unintentionally through the use of pesticides or fungicides. Food-safety problems associated with incomplete removal of mycotoxins and other microbial toxins are well-recognized.

In many cases, studies on experimental animals alone are not sufficient to eliminate all possibilities of adverse reactions in man, since symptoms that may appear in human trials may not arise in experimental animal tests.

The need for toxicity studies is particularly evident with such proposed new protein sources as single-cell protein from both photosynthetic and nonphotosynthetic organisms, forage and leaf protein concentrates, and new legume and oilseed sources.

Innovative Technology for Protein Utilization

Traditional techniques for isolating proteins for processing into food are based mainly on extraction of a primary product, e.g., oil from oilseeds, with little concern for the integrity of the protein. As a result, the byproduct proteins may become unsuitable for many useful functional applications. New technology should be developed for more effective retention of desired properties of the protein.

The basic properties of proteins from various sources require study in order to relate their molecular properties to their physical properties, and their physical properties to their functional (or performance) properties, through theoretical or correlative techniques. The critical molecular properties needing identification include molecular weights and distribution, ionization properties, reactive side chains, and primary, secondary, tertiary, and quaternary structure and morphology. Physical aspects to be characterized include hydration properties such as solubility in various media, suspendability, swelling, gelling, and rheological properties such as viscosity or apparent viscosity, yield stress, time dependency, shear dependency, and creep and relaxation. Thermal aspects include gelation and coagulation, while surface properties include hydrophilic and lipophilic properties, and surface absorption and adsorption.

For data on performance characteristics, studies are required on reactivity between starch, fat, flavoring, and other food ingredients, and on relationships between performance properties and chemical and physical properties.

Examples of process research would be concentration and isolation of protein materials, and methodologies for restructuring protein materials, or combining proteins with other materials. The effect of processing conditions on physical properties, and the influence of changes in the latter on organoleptic (taste, smell) characteristics of the final product both need to be studied.

Potentials for Improving Protein Quality in Plants by Genetic Means

Geneticists and plant breeders have, in recent years, succeeded in developing or identifying mutations in corn, barley, and sorghum that have significantly higher relative levels of lysine, as well as favorable alterations in levels of other amino acids, in their seed proteins. This achievement raises questions of the extent to which similar mutations are possible in other grains or crop plants, and also brings up the question of this kind of genetic manipulation's ultimate limits.

The single gene mutations that substantially increase lysine content in corn, barley, and sorghum involve changes in the proportions of the few protein species that normally constitute the storage protein complement of seeds, but apparently without affecting their amino acid composition.

Apparently, the situation is different in the case of rice and wheat. Rice has a low proportion of prolamine to begin with, and no prolamine-depressing mutation would have much effect in altering amino composition. Wheat does contain a sizable proportion of its total seed protein as prolamine, but mutants that cause its repression are recessive. The hexaploid nature of the wheat species combines genomes of three closely related diploid species. The probability that a similar mutation would occur in all the others at the same time is obviously extremely small.

The suppression of the synthesis of less desirable protein fractions, and the secondary increase in synthesis of fractions with greater biological value, may also be effective in legumes which, in the case of *Phaseolus,* show similar storage protein heterogeneity.

Biological Nitrogen Fixation

Enhancement of biological nitrogen fixation, whether symbiotic or nonsymbiotic, requires greater understanding of the processes themselves, and of the organisms that effect the processes. The protein nature of the nitrogenase complex that catalyzes nitrogen fixation in organisms is fairly well understood. Research is needed to determine the crystalline enzyme components, the role of ATP in the system, the mechanism whereby iron and molybdenum are incorporated into the enzyme, and the energetics and kinetics of the overall reaction.

The genes coding for nitrogenase in bacteria have been successfully transferred from one species to another. Thus, the genetic potential exists for extending nitrogen-fixing capability to a variety of economically important organisms.

In nitrogen-fixing legumes, a better understanding is needed of the genetics of both the host species and the bacterial endophytes. In the breeding of improved legume cultivars, insufficient attention has been given to these host/ endophyte relationships. Useful application of biological nitrogen fixation to grasses requires better understanding of the genetic and biochemical compatibility of host and endophytes.

Limitations to increased yield in legumes seem to be related not only to conditions affecting the availability of useful *Rhizobium* strains and the adequacy of present inoculation techniques, but also, in the case of soybeans at least, to an insufficiency in photosynthate energy required to maintain optimum nitrogen inputs. A broad attack is needed on the many physiological and agronomic aspects of nitrogen-fixing systems of known or potential agronomic significance.

POTENTIALS AND RESEARCH NEEDS IN SPECIFIC PROTEIN RESOURCES

Grain Crops for Food and Feed

The tremendous and relatively unexplored genetic diversity of cereal grains provides great promise for expanded food and protein production. An accelerated genetic search for increased protein quantity and quality in the major cereals requires medium- and long-term funding. These genetic questions also call for considerable research in fundamental scientific areas relating to genetics, and in this respect represent an appropriate area of NSF concern. For example, comprehensive biochemical research on the uptake and translocation of nitrogen in crop plants, as well as related seed protein metabolism in the cereal grains especially, can lead to the development of genetic or other means for increasing seed protein quantity and quality. There is a need for expanded basic studies on the biochemical aspects of plant physiology and metabolism.

Rapid, accurate procedures for screening a variety of crops for protein nutritional quality need to be developed, for use by plant breeders, to select superior lines. Such research requires reevaluation or review of bioassay procedures and their pertinence to human and livestock animal requirements.

Increasing soybean yields by breeding requires use of germ plasm from mainland Asia. Another approach to the soybean yield problem is to determine the cause or mechanism of oxidative photorespiration in vegetative soybeans and other legumes. This mechanism limits carbon fixation and, therefore, grain yield.

Symbiotic association of nitrogen-fixing bacteria with roots of certain grasses and corn suggests that similar associations with cereals can be identified or developed, so as to allow large savings in energy because of reduced need for nitrogen fertilizer.

Cereal Protein Technology

The normal abundance in the U.S. of low-cost grains and their underutilized byproducts suggests the desirability of initiating greater scientific and technological efforts to upgrade their food use and nutritional value.

New technologies and processes need to be perfected for separating upgraded protein products from grains and their industrial byproducts. These methods would include improved techniques for producing stable edible protein concentrates from wheat milling byproducts, better methods for separation of wheat gluten by aqueous processes, and separation of edible protein isolates from other cereals and their byproducts. Along with an improved technology for preparing protein concentrates, new food-processing applications for proteins in formulated food products should also be developed.

Research is under way in these areas, but with low-priority status, in the U.S. Department of Agriculture (USDA), the state institutions, and some food industry laboratories. To stimulate this important application of technology, an economic and marketing feasibility survey is needed.

Oilseed Proteins

Soybeans represent the single largest source of oilseed protein for both animal and human consumption, and most technology for the food use of oilseed proteins relates to soybeans and a spectrum of products derived from them. A number of other oilseeds, e.g., cottonseed, peanuts, sunflowers, rapeseed, and sesame, have potential for similar utilization; however, the necessary technology for production of food-grade products from these materials is not fully developed. Additional research is needed on all these oilseeds, including soybeans, to solve problems involving flavor, functionality, color, antinutritional factors, processing technology, and many other factors.

Research and development in six food-processing and utilization areas will be essential if oilseed proteins are to achieve maximum acceptance in human foods. Specifically,

1. Protein and nonprotein component interactions during processing must be identified.
2. Fundamental physical and chemical characteristics of the proteins of oilseeds, as related to their functional properties, need to be studied.
3. Screening methods must be developed for determining functional properties of oilseed proteins with respect to their utilization in food systems.
4. Identification of components responsible for undesirable flavors and development of processing technology to eliminate these from food products are essential.
5. Investigation should be undertaken of modification of the functionality of oilseed proteins by physical, chemical, or enzymatic means.
6. Assessment is needed of the level at which the presence of flatus-producing oligosaccharides in oilseed products assumes practical significance, and technology to minimize this problem needs to be developed.

The efforts being devoted to these problems in USDA, the state institutions, and the food industry require stimulation, and the desirability of a selective role on the part of NSF is clearly evident.

Food Legumes

Taking into account the major problems that need to be overcome in production, utilization, and marketing of food legumes, the following recommendations are offered:

In food legume *production,* research is needed to:

1. overcome genetic-physiological barriers to higher seed and protein yield;
2. improve control of and resistance to disease and insect pests;
3. promote greater efficiency in cultural systems; and
4. reduce the deleterious effects of adverse environmental factors.

In *utilization* research, the most urgent priorities are to:

1. develop convenient and rapid quantitative methods to be used, by breeders, for the estimation, identification, and removal of undesirable or toxic constituents in legume seeds;
2. develop more rapid and valid methods for estimating the nutritive value of legume proteins, and apply this new technology to the improvement of protein quality in commercial seed types;
3. study combinations of legumes with cereal products and other staple foods, with the objective of improving the nutritional properties and digestibility of both; and
4. develop improved, stable, processed dry legume products that may be prepared for eating quickly, i.e., with a minimum of energy (fuel) input.

Livestock Animal Production

U.S. animal industries are capable of producing most of the fresh meat consumed in the U.S., plus some for export, until the year 2000. However, in order to do so, great advances will be necessary in the productivity and efficiency of animal production enterprises. These advances can be achieved through increased research in (1) recycling of animal wastes, (2) further use of byproducts, wastes, and other alternative feed sources, (3) improvement of animal reproduction and growth efficiency, (4) greater use of forages in animal rations, (5) increased efficiency of nonprotein nitrogen utilization by animals, and (6) development, through breeding programs, of high-efficiency animals that can effectively utilize more forage rations.

In regard to these problems, research sponsored by USDA and the state universities and experiment stations is inadequate in relation to the urgency of the problems. These agencies must expand and intensify their activities accordingly, and NSF can contribute to progress by selective funding of research in animal reproduction and growth efficiency, and by supporting innovative approaches in the recycling of animal wastes.

Animal Protein from Dairy Products

The supply and utilization of milk in the U.S. dropped from 56,700 million kg in the early 1960s (296 kg per capita in 1960) to about 53,500 million kg the early 1970s (253 kg per capita in 1973). It is estimated that by 1980, per capita dairy food consumption in the U.S. will be down to 237 kg.

It is not likely, that is, that U.S. per capita milk consumption will increase. At present the American consumer perceives no nutritional need for increased dairy consumption, although this conception overlooks the importance of milk as a calcium source. It would take increased government-financed subsidies to produce more, but it is unlikely that the government will take steps to increase production capacity as long as other countries can produce surplus milk more cheaply than the U.S. can. Demands, therefore, will probably be met increasingly by imports.

This situation requires that in the next 10 years, government-sponsored research on dairy products be strengthened by 30%, and industry research by 50%, over present levels. For primary dairy products and for dairy analogs, research and related efforts are needed to:

1. improve quality and convenience of the established products, on the basis of market research guidance;
2. develop new dairy products and concepts that are marketable and competitive with fruit juices and soft drinks;
3. perfect a rapid, automated cheese production and ripening process that that would increase the competitiveness of cheese in both domestic and export markets;
4. develop new processing and preservation methods for milk, so as to increase its useful storage life, reduce bulk, and make milk a significant protein resource suitable for worldwide shipment and trade;
5. develop dairy analogs based on vegetable proteins;
6. conduct nutritional studies to clarify the role of nonlipid dietary com-

ponents, as well as milk-fat and dietary cholesterol, with respect to coronary heart disease;

7. optimize the food technological utility and functionality of dairy proteins as replacement proteins in fabricated foods, taking into account safety as well as nutritional factors; and

8. undertake economic and marketing studies to determine both the feasibility of increasing U.S. dairy exports, and the most favorable product mix of natural and analog dairy products.

Areas suggested for research into secondary dairy products include (1) chemical modification and upgrading of whey proteins into useful new products, (2) whey protein fractionation and characterization; (3) fundamental investigation into improving sensory and organoleptic properties of whey for applications in foods, (4) clarification of galactose metabolism in humans as a first step to wider utilization of lactose, and (5) development of whey products for the world market as protein supplements to upgrade protein-deficient diets.

All the agencies concerned with dairy research, i.e., industry, USDA, and the state universities and experiment stations, have roles and responsibilities in attacking these problems more vigorously. The call for innovations in food science also suggests that NSF could usefully support selected projects in the areas indicated.

Animal Protein from Meat, Poultry, and Eggs

There is great potential for expanded development, production, and utilization in the meat and egg industries. The utilization of this potential will depend on research and development inputs, and on the realism of regulatory constraints in terms of risk-cost-benefit considerations. It is also apparent that energy availability and cost, environmental issues, and governmental policy decisions will have far-reaching effects on the future availability of meat and eggs.

A significant expansion of the supply of animal protein for human consumption could be brought about as a result of research into use of animal tissues that are at present diverted from the market by health or palatability considerations, or by government restrictions on otherwise safe and nutritious products.

Many packinghouse raw materials, such as visceral organs, are currently processed into livestock and pet feeds. Processes similar to those used to produce fish protein concentrates have been developed for the production of edible meat protein concentrates from the various offal tissues. However, further studies are needed in this area, as well as review of regulations to permit their use in the food supply.

Technical knowledge now available to the meat industry could result in increasing the output of processed meat products by over 50%, through appropriate extension or supplementation with plant proteins.

Consumers are concerned with the possible relationship of diet and coronary heart disease. Attention centers on cholesterol and animal fats. Because the consumption of nutritious foods may be inhibited by adverse publicity based on inadequate scientific evidence, it is imperative that well-planned, long-range studies be implemented to clarify these questions.

Rigid and frequently outdated standards of identity discourage the development of new or improved products, which could extend the quality and variety of the national protein supply. Other standards, e.g., microbiological standards, increase cost to the consumer without demonstrating improvements in product quality or safety as a result of their enforcement. Overregulation, in short, adds to product cost, channeling much industry research funding into matters concerned primarily with regulatory compliance.

Broad areas of research have been receiving attention from industry, the USDA, and the state universities and experiment stations, but such activity requires far greater support from funding sources than has been the case heretofore. As regards relatively basic research, there are a number of areas where NSF support would help stimulate the solution of serious and long-standing problems.

Aquatic Proteins

Most of the U.S. fishery stocks traditionally used by Americans for food are either fully exploited or depleted. There are, however, species even within the present, limited economic control zone—not to mention the larger resources within the proposed 200-mile zone—that have remained largely un- or under-exploited. It is estimated, for example, that between 100,000 and 500,000 MT of capelin could be landed yearly on the northwestern Atlantic coast. This fish could be offered in the form of engineered or fabricated foods that would be more familiar to the public. Squid, likewise, is most suitably utilized in textured and engineered food products.

Much more needs to be known about the biology and behavior patterns of aquatic animals, and techniques need to be developed for locating, harvesting, preserving, and processing this resource. Polyculture, which relies on the growing-together of a number of fish species of varying feeding types, presents opportunities for attaining very high yields per hectare by taking advantage of symbiotic relationships among the different species. The high yields in such systems can be maintained without competing with nonruminant farm animals for feed. Species with maximum productivity potential in warm freshwater pond polyculture systems include carp, buffalofish, tilapia, white amur, mullet, milkfish, and catfish.

Capture fisheries represent the major focus of aquatic protein resource development. Antarctic krill, for example, is the single largest natural source of animal protein on this globe, and probably 45 million MT of it could be harvested yearly without compromising the availability of the resource. In view of the lead taken principally by Russia, and, to a lesser extent, by Japan, in krill harvesting and utilization, the U.S. must now decide what commitments it should undertake in the management and utilization of this resource. It seems prudent to advise allocation of funds at levels sufficient at least to undertake a technical and economic feasibility study of U.S. participation in and utilization of the krill harvest.

As regards support for research and development, the financial and political decisions will have to be made by government, since industry will not initially invest the hundreds of millions of dollars required to perfect the tools needed to produce and utilize increased tonnage of raw aquatic material. New types of suitably equipped fishing vessels will have to be designed and constructed.

New methods of locating, harvesting, preserving, and processing must be developed. New toxicological and nutritional information will be necessary to develop regulations for monitoring the quality and safety of the new aquatic food products. Investigations will be needed in biology, genetics, animal nutrition, and ecology of aquatic organisms. The National Science Foundation could most appropriately provide funding for studies in oceanography, ecology, physiology, basic biology, and other background areas.

Potatoes

The potato has protein levels comparable to those of cereal grains; indeed, cultivars containing 17–18% protein (dry weight basis) have been identified. The crop, clearly, does not merit the status of a "poor man's" energy food.

With the introduction of new potato varieties, this crop's yields per hectare have increased nearly 300% in the past 20 years. Through intensified breeding studies, exploration of hybridization should be continued, in order to expand adaptation, and improve disease and insect resistance, nutritive value, and yield; the ideal polyploid level for optimum productivity needs to be determined.

Systematic study is needed on factors affecting productivity and nutritional quality. These factors include optimum stage of maturity, effects of fertilization and irrigation, and possible benefits of multiple cropping with early and late maturing varieties, and with other crops. (This last factor is relevant especially to potato culture in warmer environments.)

Researchers need to analyze potatoes for quantity and quality of various proteins, evaluate their amino acid composition, and determine whether or not breeding can alter protein ratios, so as to improve the overall protein nutritive quality. Simple screening methods for protein quality and quantity are needed to assist breeders in analyzing large potato populations.

Much work also needs to be done on the reclaiming and upgrading of potato-processing wastes, with emphasis on recovery of proteins and amino acids.

Nonphotosynthetic Single-Cell Protein

The role of single-cell protein as a supplement to the world protein supply is now well established. Research and development on SCP production have been intense for over a decade, and as a consequence there exist a number of large SCP plants in operation for animal feed production; several more are under construction. The problems being addressed today relate to second- and third-generation processes for SCP production for both animal feed and human food.

No single raw material or organism will provide *the* ultimate SCP process. Consequently, it is essential to evaluate, in parallel, several process alternatives, to appreciate fully the flexibility available in the use of SCP. There is no specific recommendation of substrates, but it is clearly the overall view of the experts that alcohols and cellulose hold the greatest potential for the U.S., and therefore should receive priority consideration.

It is believed that cell yield is the single most important economic factor in the fermentation process, and that great stress should be placed, in practice, on approaching the theoretical fermentation yield. Improved processes for RNA removal would involve study of RNA levels in cells, the role and activation of endogenous ribonucleases, and their control by means of genetic and cell physiology factors.

More efficient use could be made of the proteins within the cell if economical means for their recovery were available. Selective isolation of proteins would also be a method of avoiding the RNA problem. Studies are needed of SCP engineering properties, interactions with food constituents, and use in structure-forming operations. Dewatering and drying comprise one of the most significant cost factors in the overall process. Study is needed on membrane processes, improved methods of mass transfer, and the effect of drying on functional properties.

Research on nonphotosynthetic SCP clearly needs much wider support in the U.S., in order to increase production of protein and other useful products, especially from waste. At present in the U.S., such research and development activities are confined to industry and a few universities. The growing urgency in the U.S. for waste recovery and recycling—the need to reprocess livestock animal waste and manure for refeeding is only one example—suggests a priority area for NSF funding.

Photosynthetic Single-Cell Protein

Photosynthetic single-cell protein is produced in the cells of microscopic plants (algae) that grow in suspension in the waters of shallow, illuminated ponds. These ponds contain culture medium that consists of simple salts—such as carbonates, nitrates, and phosphates—dissolved in water. Depending on the genus, the cells may be separated from the growth medium by screening, filtration, coagulation either by flotation or sedimentation, and centrifugation.

During the next decade, steps should be taken to:

1. study the relationship of algal species to algal nutritional characteristics, including protein quality, and the influence of ratios of critical substrate nutrients, including consideration of water-quality factors;
2. study productivity as a function of species, predators and pathogens, nutrient mix, physical parameters such as detention period, mixing, recirculation, and waste as a source of nutrients; and
3. study processing of algae to produce various products, including decolorized and bleached algae, algal pigments, and spun algal protein; and study algal preservation by dehydration, canning, drying, freezing and freeze-drying.

Leaf Protein

Green leaves are the largest producers of protein in the world, supplying protein to other plant tissues including the crop seeds that nourish humans and animals. Indeed, the protein in the 1973–74 U.S. alfalfa crop was almost twice as much as that in the 12.5 million MT of soybean meal utilized in the U.S. that same year.

Process research is well developed for a commercial system that would be added to a conventional dehydration plant to recover whole-leaf protein. When economic feasibility studies are completed by the USDA, a full-scale demonstration plant will be recommended for construction at the site of a commercial dehydration plant.

Process research for an on-the-farm-type leaf protein recovery system (in connection with silage or hay production from the press cake) has been undertaken by workers at the University of Wisconsin and elsewhere. This work involves low-cost equipment development and further research on production and quality of the silage and/or hay produced.

Research applicable to both types of systems is needed for optimization of unit operations, for higher-value utilization of the residual juice solubles fraction, and on economic analysis of the several possible variants in the systems.

Denatured white (insoluble) products are made by heat coagulation of chlorophyll-free alfalfa juice after prior removal of the green protein fraction. A great deal of further research is needed to increase yields of this white protein, to increase its purity, and to explore its utilization possibilities in various types of food.

When *Nicotiana* (tobacco) species are used as raw leaf materials, a white protein (Fraction I protein) can be obtained readily in pure crystalline form. This tasteless, pure-white product should have special value where high purity is needed. Research is needed on growing these plants on an intensive scale, on determination of the economic value of the crystalline protein, and on the economics of its production.

It may be concluded that leafy plants have tremendous potential for supplying an important proportion of the protein requirements of both monogastric animals and man by the years 1985-2000. What is needed is a coherent, well-financed, multidisciplinary research effort in the agronomic, genetic, chemical, engineering, nutritional, toxicological, microbiological, and food technological aspects of leaf protein production.

Chemical Synthesis of Nutrients

The possibility exists of filling some of humankind's protein needs by non-traditional means, particularly by chemical synthesis. Synthetic vitamins and amino acids are, of course, already in common use. While the cost of their chemical synthesis is relatively high compared to the cost of products made by fermentation, the use of mixtures made from a common intermediate might considerably reduce the cost.

Synthesis of industrial fatty acid from carbon monoxide was conducted in wartime Germany, and increased efficiency is possible. The synthesis of glycerol for human food has also been investigated, particularly by the National Aeronautics and Space Administration, as a potential energy source for a planetary base. A more advanced approach involves 1, 3-butane diol, which is metabolized with 50% greater energy output than are sugars or glycerol.

Recent studies have shown that normal paraffins can provide some metabolic energy to chickens. There is a strong possibility that an efficient and relatively high-yielding synthesis of ATP can be developed using HCN as a starting material for adenine. All such developments, however, are clearly in the area of long-range prospects.

RESEARCH RECOMMENDATIONS

The reports of the working groups identify a large number of important research areas and projects, from which only a limited number have been selected for the recommendations that follow here. Most research that is already of major ongoing concern to USDA and the state agricultural institutions in the U.S. has been excluded only because of the special purpose of this report, and not because of any judgment as to its relative importance. The principal criterion for selection was the research's applicability to (1) an area of importance that complements or underlies traditional agricultural research and is at present inadequately supported by the USDA, the state agricultural institutions, or any other source; or (2) an unconventional area not now receiving an emphasis commensurate with its potential. No meaningful further subdivision of priority rankings can be assigned to the basic and long-term research recommended because too many uncontrollable and unpredictable factors are involved.

Fundamental Mission-Oriented Research

Nutrition

1. Protein requirements of human subjects of various ages and physiological states should be evaluated by means of improved metabolic balance techniques.

2. Existing biochemical and biological methods for the evaluation of protein quality need to be improved to reflect more closely the nutritional requirements of humans and livestock, and these methods need to be applied to new or novel protein sources as well as processed protein foods of all types. The urgent needs of plant breeders and regulatory agencies for rapid methods of protein quality evaluation should be taken into account in this research.

Toxicology

Basic research should be undertaken on the toxicological hazards associated with new protein sources, and with conventional proteins processed in new ways. This research should be followed, when appropriate, by clinical trials, and by efforts to remove, through processing or other means, toxic factors identified in the animal or clinical trials.

Biological Nitrogen Fixation

The subject of nitrogen fixation in crops requires comprehensive study. This study should consist of basic biochemical and genetic research on the nitrogen and carbon metabolism of plants and microorganisms, with the objective of reducing the need for synthetic nitrogen fertilizer.

Mission-Oriented Research
in Specific Resource Areas

Grain Crops for Food and Feed

1. The metabolic process of oxidative photorespiration in cereals, legumes, and leguminous oilseeds should be investigated. This process seriously limits fixed carbon accumulation and thus reduces potential crop yields. The objective should be to identify genetic or other means to control this undesirable metabolic process.

2. Research on symbiotic and nonsymbiotic nitrogen fixation in cereals should be expanded, with emphasis on development of nitrogen-fixing microorganisms compatible with host cereal species.

3. Basic research to provide new sexual and asexual methods for breeding more productive crops with higher protein potentials should be intensified. Such studies would involve identification of specific genes and gene groups, use of cell culture, somatic hybridization and chemical stimulation of gene compatibility for broad sexual crosses, as well as other innovative techniques.

4. The uptake of nitrogen in crop plants, and the related protein metabolism of seeds, particularly in the cereal grains, should be studied more extensively in order to identify genetic and other means for increasing protein quantity and quality without seriously compromising crop productivity and other important qualities. This will require improved screening methods to assist plant breeders in the rapid identification of desirable cultivars in protein improvement breeding programs.

Cereal Protein Technology

New technologies need to be developed for separating, recovering, and concentrating the protein fractions of cereal grains (wheat, corn, sorghum, barley, oats, rice, triticale, rye), and processed cereal byproducts. Attention should also be given to development of new processes for reconstituting or combining cereal protein fractions with other constituents to produce attractive new protein foods such as meat analogs, meat extenders, and beverages.

Oilseed and Legume Proteins

1. Physical, chemical, and enzymatic methods of modifying the functionality of oilseed and legume proteins need to be studied to facilitate development of protein materials with wide versatility and acceptability in formulated foods.

2. Studies of the basic cellular and subcellular structure of oilseeds and legumes should be intensified, with attention to the location and form of primary constituents (proteins, oils, carbohydrates, etc.), in order to permit development of more efficient technologies for protein and oil recovery with retention of optimal functional and nutritional characteristics.

Livestock Animal Production

1. Research on the feeding value of various fractions of animal and vegetable wastes for different livestock species (beef, swine, and poultry)

should be expanded, and technologies, such as fermentation with appropriate microorganisms, or silage treatment, need to be developed to minimize toxicity and unpalatability, and to upgrade the nutritive value of waste materials.

2. Studies should be conducted of the carry-over, into animal tissues used for human food, of possible toxic or pathogenic factors related to feeding recycled wastes of various kinds to livestock.

Dairy Products, Meat, Poultry, and Eggs

Sanitary and microbiologically safe technologies need to be developed for reclaiming food products from dairy byproducts, defective livestock animals, muscle and organ tissues, and poultry and eggs rejected for food use and used only partially (for livestock and pet feeding) under present food laws and grading standards.

Aquatic Proteins

1. The basic problems affecting the development and economic efficiency of aquaculture require more thorough investigation. Studies should include further identification of optimum species for monoculture and polyculture systems, and examination of the problems in breeding and culturing these species, including their metabolic and nutritional requirements and diseases to which they may be susceptible. Polyculture, which can take advantage of symbiotic relationships among several different species, should be further developed to increase efficiency of feed utilization and thus reduce competition with nonruminant farm animals for feed.

2. There should be a comprehensive feasibility study on the harvesting and utilization, for human consumption, of Antarctic krill. The study should assess integrated harvesting technology, acceptability of possible food products, use of byproducts such as chitin, and potential profitability. Since most krill resources occur primarily in international waters, apparently beyond most countries' present or future jurisdictional limits, and because the U.S.S.R. now leads in the development and application of the relevant technology, NSF should develop a collaborative effort with the Soviet Union, if an appropriate agreement can be negotiated.

Nonphotosynthetic Single-Cell Protein (SCP)

1. Studies should be done to clarify the nature, occurrence, and mode of action of substances giving adverse reactions in human feeding, either occurring naturally in, or produced during the processing of, bacteria, yeasts, or fungi. In addition, more economical methods are needed to reduce nucleic acid content of SCP.

2. Efficient methods should be developed for the selective isolation of proteins free from nucleic acids and other undesirable constituents, and for producing such proteins with desirable functional and organoleptic properties.

3. SCP technology should be expanded to waste processing, and recovery for animal feeding, utilizing materials such as cellulosic and other crop and animal wastes, sewage, and industrial food wastes.

4. Ways should be found for improving cell yields and increasing the efficiency of heat and oxygen transfer in fermentors, taking into account cooling difficulties in tropical environments, and cell-yield limitations due to inadequate oxygen supply. Ways of improving efficiency of cell harvesting or collection, and of dewatering and drying should be studied, taking into consideration effects on protein functionality and nutritional properties.

Photosynthetic Single-Cell Protein

1. Information should be gathered on the toxicology, food/feed safety, nutritional value, and acceptability as food of algal sources.
2. Economically feasible techniques need to be developed for processing algae as human food, including means for decolorizing or bleaching, recovery of algal pigments, isolation or concentration of protein constituents, and application of algae to food uses; also means for preservation by common technologies need to be developed.

Leaf Proteins

1. There is a need for comprehensive research, technological development, and testing of an integrated on-the-farm-type system for recovery and direct feeding, to nonruminants, of leaf protein products, including evaluation of the nutritional and toxicological implications of such feed use.
2. Development of technology for recovery of leaf protein concentrates and isolates for food use should be intensified. Attention should be directed toward evaluation of nutritional and food safety aspects, as well as functionality and organoleptic qualities, of concentrates and isolates used as ingredients in formulated or fabricated foods. This work should include comprehensive study of the unique properties of *Nicotiana* (tobacco) leaves, which permit easy separation and recovery of relatively pure protein, and exploration of agronomic and other factors that relate to the optimal production of tobacco for such use.

Advanced Science and Technology

Innovative Technology for Protein Utilization

Research should be conducted to gain a basic understanding of physical and chemical properties of protein molecules. The separation and restructuring of plant proteins should be studied, and the application of chemical engineering technology to the development of edible protein.

Targets of Opportunity

Funds should be made available for innovative exploratory research yet to be identified.

CONCLUSION

In closing, may we indicate that, notwithstanding current expenditures of over $1,000 million a year in the U.S. on relevant agricultural research, it is our conviction that many useful and important opportunities still exist for productive complementary support, by NSF, of research in the basic biological and biochemical sciences that are the foundations for all agricultural technology, and for innovative food science applications. In addition, it would certainly reflect the national interest to explore, through a modest long-term investment on the part of NSF, the contributions that various unconventional food sources might make to U.S. and world food supplies late in this century by supplementing agricultural food production.

THE ROLE OF ANIMAL PROTEIN

Charles N. Dobbins, Jr.

College of Veterinary Medicine and
Cooperative Extension Veterinary Department
University of Georgia
Athens, Georgia 30602

Some people have voiced the opinion that animal agriculture is wasteful and should be on its way out in favor of grain production. It has been predicted that if we continue our present feeding practices, the world population will use all of the grain supplies it can produce by 1985.

We hear such statements as: "For the first time in history, we can see a connection between the eating habits of the U. S. citizen and the hunger for millions of others. Hungry people see our heavy meat diet taking a disproportionate share of the world's food supply." They would have us feel guilty for the abundance we produce.

The statistics these people use are quite misleading and would have you believe animal agriculture should be discontinued. To be sure, we may change some of our feeding techniques, sources of animal feeds, and even types of animals.

In the long run, there must be a balance between animal and plant agriculture if this world is to be fed. Each has its place and must be properly utilized.

Contrary to the opinions of many, livestock and poultry will play a key role to provide food for the world because of their ability to use forages, roughages, and byproducts. This point has been grossly overlooked in the attempt to show grain requirements to produce meat, milk, and eggs.

Even the comparison of grain/soybean protein versus milk/meat/egg protein is not entirely accurate. Plant protein is generally inferior to animal protein. For example, animal protein is more available than vegetable protein to humans for body maintenance and growth as expressed in NPU's (Net Protein Utilization Value). This value may be expressed as follows: eggs—100%; fish—84%; red meat and poultry—80%; milk—75%; defatted soybean flour—72%; rice—67%; corn—56%; wheat—62%. This means that almost all egg protein is available for use when consumed by humans, whereas only 56% of corn protein is available. Instead of 1.14 pounds of vegetable protein needed to produce a pound of animal protein in dairy cows, the figure should be .95 pounds in terms of protein available to humans.

Do you realize that only 6% of the world's ruminants are located in the United States but produce about 19% of the total animal food output? In developing countries, where over 60% of the world's ruminants reside, they account for only 22% of the output. Animals of low genetic quality, poor disease control and husbandry practices, coupled with cultural/religious prejudices, severely limit animal production.

What do animals actually eat in the United States? The components of their ration are as follows: pastures—32%; hay—32%; processed feed—8%; feed grains—27%; wheat and rye—1%. By being able to convert roughages, forages, and by products into human food, animal agriculture will play a key role in the race against the world food shortages.

It has been estimated that animal production needs to be expanded at the annual rate of 3 percent. With more pressure being placed on grain by the consumption by humans, we need to be in a better position to evaluate byproducts and new feedstuffs for animals. This is especially important when you consider that from birth to market perhaps 80% of the beef animals' lifetime diet is forages, and that 75% of the beef protein is produced before animals go on a concentrate diet.

For example, consider a recent development by the Extension Veterinary Department at the University of Georgia. We have developed a process to convert food waste into a nutritious, palatable animal feed ingredient. Not only does this process reduce pollution by keeping this valuable product from sanitary landfills, it provides a method of producing a new animal feed ingredient that analyzes approximately 22% protein containing all essential amino acids plus 20% fat. The end product is in the form of a dry meal that can be readily utilized by all classes of livestock and poultry. Special collection techniques make this process commercially feasible in towns or cities in which a minimum of 15 tons of raw food waste is available on a daily basis. Based on today's prices, the final product is nutritionally worth approximately $170 per ton when compared to soybean meal and No. 2 yellow corn. It costs approximately $85 per finished ton to collect the raw material and process it.

A special stabilization process has been developed that makes it possible to hold both animal and vegetable materials for long periods of time without refrigeration and without decomposition. Recent tests have proven that waste ranging from trash fish on fishing boats, waste from vegetable-packing plants to forages and even animal manure can be stabilized and held for long periods of time without decomposition. These products may form the basis of an animal ration for the production of meat, milk, and eggs for human consumption. Literally dozens of protein and energy sources are available for animals that humans either can't consume or would find very unappetizing.

Non-ruminants are perhaps the biggest competitors with man in terms of their use of grains and oil seeds. On the other hand, broilers can convert about 2 pounds of grain into 1 pound of meat.

The dairy cow, on the other hand, is probably the most efficient recycling animal available. It has been shown that dairy cows could produce milk, although not quite as much, on a 100% forage diet. If some urea, as a protein concentrate replacement, were used it would make the dairy cow totally noncompetitive with man for grain supplies.

In addition to being a source of human food, animals serve other useful purposes such as power, revenue, fuel, and byproducts. In many parts of the world, animals will provide power for the intensive cropping necessary to help feed the population.

Have you thought about the value of health aids from animals such as heparin and insulin or commercial items such as leather, glue, adhesives, fatty acids, lubricants, cosmetics, paint driers, liquid detergents, fertilizer, and a thousand other products?

We need to use our imagination, using both traditional and nontraditional products for animal feeds as well as domesticated and wild animals as sources of animal protein. The natural balance of game animals in a system frequently uses the available natural forage more efficiently since grazers, browsers, and tree-leaf-eating mammals do not demand one particular forage type. Resource management also includes proper utilization of forage plants by not permitting overgrazing and other practices that are detrimental for future production.

With vast semiarid areas, animal protein could be derived by a wide variety of herbivores without competing with man's food.

It is clear that animals, especially ruminants, will be a source of human food in years to come. In the long run, meat, milk, and eggs would give the world a few extra years in which to solve its population problems.

FORTIFICATION OF FOODS WITH VITAMINS AND MINERALS

Walter Mertz

U.S. Department of Agriculture
Agricultural Research Service
Nutrition Institute
Beltsville, Maryland 20705

Fortification of foods with essential micronutrients is one of the great accomplishments of nutritional science, and its benefits to mankind rank with those of the greatest medical discoveries of this century.[1] The virtual disappearance of pellagra and rickets and the substantial reduction of iodine deficiency goiter in the United States are the most outstanding examples of success. Those benefits outweigh by far other aspects that were not nearly as successful—for example, attempts to eliminate iron deficiency anemia by iron fortification. Yet, from the point of view of the nutritionist, even the most successful fortification programs are compromise solutions. The ideal solution, and the ultimate goal of national and international nutrition policies, must be to make available to all people diets that meet all nutrient requirements. When this goal is met, fortification will be unnecessary, and a great amount of scientific effort now being spent on problems of fortification can be used elsewhere.

Unfortunately, this ideal situation is unlikely to be achieved in the foreseeable future, either in the United States or abroad. Therefore, programs of enrichment and fortification will not only maintain but increase their scope to reach more people and include more micronutrients, as our knowledge of human requirements and of the existence of deficiencies increases. The potential benefits to human health of an enrichment program on a global scale are enormous if the program is based on sound scientific and technological knowledge and if experience gained from past errors can be applied. The cost-to-benefit ratio of enrichment with micronutrients is among the most favorable of any nutritional or other intervention. The following discussion will examine the various conditions necessitating fortification policies, evaluate the state of scientific knowledge pertinent to such policies, and point out problem areas where our knowledge must be increased if future fortification efforts are to be effective. The fact that problems of mineral nutrition are treated preferentially is not meant to detract from the importance of the vitamins; it merely reflects the greater gaps in our knowledge of the inorganic micronutrients.

SITUATIONS CALLING FOR FORTIFICATION PROGRAMS

Fortification should be considered as one solution—but not necessarily the only one—whenever the food intake of a substantial part of a population falls significantly short of the human requirement for one or more micronutrients. Alternative measures, such as supplementation of high-risk groups with vitamin and mineral pills or qualitative changes in dietary practices, have

151

been considered in the past and, under certain conditions, are of considerable merit.

1. *Influences of the geochemical environment.* There are wide areas in the world with absolute or conditioned deficiencies of soil minerals. These deficiencies can be reflected in low concentrations of minerals and trace elements in drinking water, agricultural crops, and in the tissue of farm animals, and result in marginal or deficient intakes from food.[2] Man's dependence on the geochemical environment is greatest for mineral elements occurring in anionic form—for example, fluorine, iodine, selenium, and molybdenum; for all these elements pronounced excesses or deficiencies in human populations are known. Many areas in the world are iodine deficient, and although iodization of salt has alleviated deficiency in many regions, it is not yet practiced universally in an effective manner. Equally large areas are so low in fluorine that fluoride enrichment of drinking water can produce substantial benefits for dental health of children and, perhaps, for the bone health of the middle aged and elderly as well. Our knowledge of the regional distribution of selenium is incomplete, but some areas in the United States and a large part of New Zealand are known to be selenium deficient to such a degree that blood levels of this element in human subjects are significantly reduced.[3] Molydbenum deficiency is not known to exist in man, but it does occur in farm animals in some areas of Australia. The main problem with this element is that an excessive concentration in the environment can result in conditioned copper deficiency. Such situations have been described in detail for certain provinces in the U.S.S.R.[4] Selenium deficiency and its consequences are now being investigated in New Zealand; the beneficial effect of a high copper intake in the subjects suffering from excessive molydbenum exposure in the U.S.S.R. has already been demonstrated. Fortification of certain foods is one alternative that needs careful consideration in these countries. Systematic efforts to define trace-element imbalances in man caused by the geochemical environment are just beginning on a world-wide basis.[5] A reasonable amount of information exists for iodine, but for man the potential problems with other important elements can only be inferred from experiences in farm animals.[6]

2. *Influences of the food supply.* In all situations where substantial segments of a population do not have access to sufficient foods to prevent undernutrition and malnutrition, the only real solution lies in measures to improve food production, distribution, and protection. Such measures require much effort and time before they have a measurable impact on the nutritional status of those affected. In the interim, programs providing dietary supplements to increase the nutrient intake can have immediate health benefits. Diets resulting in undernutrition and malnutrition are not only quantitatively deficient, but in most instances are unbalanced with regard to high-quality protein, vitamins, and essential trace elements. The supplements, therefore, must not only furnish protein and the essential micronutrients, in proportion with their energy content, but must carry these latter substances in such concentrations that they complement the total food intake of the recipient population. Programs abroad that supply energy and protein to improve a deficient intake of population groups have done much good, but unless the supplements also contain essential micronutrients, either naturally or by fortification, they produce less than optimal results. It is increasingly recognized that pure forms of malnutrition are extremely rare or nonexistent under field conditions; malnutrition is almost always complicated by deficiencies of essential micronutrients.

The predictable trend toward greatly increased production of concentrated vegetable protein products, which are of good protein quality but lack several essential micronutrients in available form, must alert the planners of nutrition policies to pay increased attention to this latter group. These substances are required in trace amounts only, so the added cost of fortification is small in relation to the expected benefits. A zinc-deficient organism does not grow, even when all other nutrients are present in the diet in luxury amounts, and in marginal zinc deficiency the amount of food required to produce a certain growth rate is substantially greater than that required when the zinc intake is adequate. These considerations are valid for all essential micronutrients.

3. *Trends and preferences influencing food intake.* Even when an abundance of foods is available to a population at reasonable prices, the micronutrient intake can be compromised by certain trends in the style of living and eating. The increasing use of fossil energy during this century has led to the mechanization of many chores of life and to the reduction of energy expenditure of large population segments in the developed countries. This reduction of food intake necessary to avoid overweight is believed to be one of the causes of the substantial incidence of iron deficiency in the United States. With the average concentration in American diets of 6 mg iron/1000 kcal, a physically very active woman of child-bearing age would have no difficulty obtaining her Recommended Dietary Allowance of 18 mg from a 3000 kcal diet without becoming overweight. With the now customary lifestyle, however, it would be unrealistic to assume that a substantial number of women in the United States have that caloric intake. A second trend is the dilution of our food supply with products furnishing substantial amounts of energy but not of essential micronutrients. The high consumption of sugar in the United States is of concern to many nutritionists. The average sugar intake adds 400–500 kcal to the daily intake of each individual, but no micronutrients. Cereal products constitute approximately 25 percent of the average energy intake of the U.S. population.[7] Those produced from low extraction grade white flour carry few of the essential micronutrients originally present in the grain, and even enriched products are not equivalent to the grain in respect to all essential micronutrients. Thus, a substantial part of our food intake does not furnish its share of vitamins and mineral elements, placing an increased demand on the rest of the diet to furnish the daily requirements of these substances. The assessment of this situation varies among nutritionists, but there is reasonable agreement that any substantial increase in the consumption of foods, not carrying their share of essential nutrients, at the expense of conventional foods must be regarded with concern, unless such products can be enriched with vitamins and mineral elements in an available form.

4. *Exclusive formulae.* The best example of exclusive formula nutrition, total parenteral alimentation, is a clinical problem, of importance only to a very small segment of the 'population. However, the developments in this field have important consequences for enrichment policies and philosophies pertaining to other exclusive formulae of wide use and great public health importance.

With increasing purity of the ingredients and the reduction of the levels of contaminating heavy metals, essential elements are also reduced to concentrations that do not meet human requirements. Enrichment with essential trace elements is as important as the long-standing practice of enrichment with vitamins. Deficiencies of zinc,[8] copper,[9] and chromium [10] have been described in patients receiving total parenteral alimentation, emphasizing the need to consider a much larger number of elements than has been considered in the past, perhaps even those trace elements that have been shown to be essential only in animal experimental models. The same demands must be met by infant formulae and dietary formulations administered to patients over long periods of time at the exclusion of conventional foods.

FORTIFICATION IN THE FUTURE: NEEDS AND CONSTRAINTS

Fortification policy, in order to be effective, must be dynamic and must utilize as completely as possible and as soon as possible new knowledge of the nutritional status and of human requirements produced by nutrition research. Our knowledge of essential micronutrients should never be considered complete; therefore, the list of vitamins and trace elements used in fortification must be always open to revision. This attitude is reflected in a recent statement of a subcommittee of the Food and Nutrition Board proposing considerable changes of fortification guidelines.[7] The inclusion of zinc among the nutrients proposed for fortification is a significant step based on the growing awareness of marginal zinc intakes in parts of the U.S. population. This step can be expected to be followed by others in the future. Additional trace elements are now of substantial interest in human nutrition, and many mineral interactions are known that may increase or decrease the human requirement.[11] Finally, a number of trace elements have been identified as essential in one or two animal species and, while there is no knowledge as yet of human requirements and nutritional status, there is a possibility that the supply may be suboptimal. A discussion of five major problem areas related to fortification programs follows. In some of these areas, newly acquired knowledge can be applied immediately to improve existing programs, but in others, many important questions must be answered through research, before the solutions can be put into practice.

1. *Human requirements and nutritional status.* In those cases where the human requirement for a micronutrient is reasonably well known and sufficient data on the nutrient content of foods are available, an approximate evaluation can be made of whether the national food supply furnishes abundant, sufficient, or marginal amounts of the nutrient in question. In the first case, no intervention is necessary. In the second, a detailed assessment of the intake of different population groups is needed, whereas the third case, a marginal or insufficient supply, calls for intervention to remedy potential deficiencies, particularly if the biochemical or medical assessment of the population indicates a marginal nutritional status.

The essential trace element copper was believed to belong to the first category and has not been considered for fortification of foods.[7] Copper deficiency in free-living adult human subjects was not known, and analytical data indicated that copper intakes ranged between 2 and 5 mg/day, readily meeting the requirement of 2 mg/day. Recent developments, however, suggest that the state of copper nutrition in the U.S.A. must be reevaluated. Mild copper deficiency in experimental animals results in hypercholesterolemia, particularly in the presence of high levels of zinc.[12] Although no data do as yet indicate marginal copper deficiency as a cause for elevated cholesterol levels in humans, the association in animals is strong. Furthermore, reexamination, with modern methods, of the copper concentration in foods has consistently shown that the daily intake is much lower than the 2 to 5 mg reported previously: the average daily copper intake from a mixed diet is probably close to 1 mg, about one-half of the estimated human requirement.[13] Reexamination, with modern analytical methods, of human balance studies should provide the basis for decisions concerning copper fortification programs.

Zinc is an example of an element of the second category: the daily intake may furnish or be slightly below the human requirement.[14] Recent research already has identified population groups that are at risk of marginal or deficient intake. Although the available data are still limited, they alert us to the possibility that marginal zinc deficiency may not be uncommon in the United States. This recognition led to the recommendations for zinc fortification by the Food and Nutrition Board Subcommittee; it is already implemented by most of the infant food manufacturers.

Iron is the best example for an element in insufficient supply. The Recommended Dietary Allowance of 18 mg for women of child-bearing age is based on solid scientific evidence but is practically unattainable for most women living in the United States. Although the iron fortification program increased the average intake of this element by approximately 25 percent, the program was not fully successful: the incidence of iron deficiency is still substantial. Some potential reasons will be discussed later.

Two elements, selenium and chromium, have been known as essential for almost 20 years. Large areas with selenium deficiency in soils are known, and selenium supplementation of animal feeds is practiced widely. Marginal intakes by the human population are known to occur in New Zealand,[3] and perhaps other areas, but many more data of the selenium intake in the United States are needed before the nutritional status of the U.S. population can be assessed. Chromium deficiency is known to occur in human subjects suffering from protein-calorie malnutrition [15] and is suspected to occur in a marginal form in elderly people in the United States. Although the minimum human requirement for absorbable chromium is defined at around 10 μg/day, problems of analysis and our incomplete understanding of the availability of chromium compounds do not yet allow an assessment of the nutritional status.

Deficiencies of the "newer trace elements" can be consistently produced in experimental animals (Si, V, Ni, As, Sn), but human requirements [16] are not known. Such knowledge may well come from research in total parenteral nutrition and may stimulate efforts to include some or all of these elements in fortification, at least of highly purified, exclusive formulae.

2. *Availability.* The Food and Nutrition Board has stated that micronutrients used for fortification must be "physiologically available." [7] The knowledge of biological availability of trace elements has substantially increased in this decade. The major example of progress is the agreement on the relative biological value of iron compounds for animal species. Although the now accepted concept of the non-heme iron pool has deemphasized the importance of small differences in biological value of iron compounds, it can be stated that some iron preparations still used for fortification do not enter into the non-heme iron pool, and are nutritionally of little or no value. The use of iron compounds of good biological availability is increasing, so that the share of these in the fortification program may now be greater than it was in 1970 (TABLE 1). There still remain a number of important questions: for example, whether the avail-

TABLE 1

USE OF FORTIFICATION IRON IN CEREAL PRODUCTS

Total Amount	1966	1968	1970
(kg)	73,950	99,809	120,657

Compounds Used in 1970

	% of Total
Reduced	31
Ferric orthophosphate	18
Sodium-iron pyrophosphate	16
Ferrous sulfate	20
Ferric ammonium citrate	0–5
Other	10–15

ability data obtained from animal experiments are valid for human subjects, how processing (e.g., baking, heating) influences biological availability and whether enough food-grade iron compounds of high availability (for example, ferrous sulfate or reduced iron of a favorable surface:mass ratio) can be produced to improve the overall value of the iron fortification program.[17] The possibility of using heme iron for fortification is of great (albeit only academic) interest, but the study of ascorbic acid chelates or fructose complexes offers additional promising approaches.

Much less is known about the biological availability of zinc compounds to man. A variety of zinc salts and complexes appears to be readily available to the experimental animal, but the experience in human subjects is almost completely restricted to zinc sulfate. In view of the active interest in zinc fortification, the biological availability of potential fortification compounds should be measured in carefully controlled human studies.

The biological availability of selenium also appears to depend on the chemical form. The most effective compound, designated Factor 3, has not yet been identified, but its biological activity and availability are approached by certain monoselenodicarboxylic acids.[18] Seleno methionine appears to be better utilized by human subjects than selenite.[19] Naturally occurring copper compounds concentrated from plant material appear to be better utilized by experimental animals than simple copper salts,[20] and certain silicon compounds are believed to be completely nonavailable to animals.[21] Chromium is biologically most effective in form of a "glucose tolerance factor" occurring in yeast and other foods; this compound has been tentatively identified as a dinicotinic acid chromium complex; its complete structure is not yet known. Absorption of simple chromium salts, such as chromic chloride in the human subject, is generally less than 1 percent of a given dose—that of chromium naturally occurring in food is probably much higher.[22]

These differences in biological availability of various trace elements emphasize the need for careful study of biological availability of trace elements to man, if new fortification programs are to be effective.

3. *Interactions.* Interactions among fortification nutrients must be considered in any decision to add to the number or increase the level of nutrients in fortification practices. The main question must be: Does an increase of

fortification levels or the addition of a new nutrient lead to imbalances in the diet? Innumerable examples of nutrient interactions are known from animal experiments. Interactions exist between macronutrients on one hand and vitamins and mineral elements on the other, between vitamins and mineral elements, and among mineral elements. It is possible that disturbed balances among interacting nutrients are as important as the absolute levels of the individual components in the diet. For example, the ratio calcium:phosphorus is believed to be an important determinant of bone health. A decision to increase the calcium intake of the population through fortification must take into account the consequences for the calcium:phosphorus balance. The dietary intake of phosphorus in the United States far exceeds that of calcium; therefore, any increase in calcium fortification would improve the ratio and should be beneficial. On the other hand, excessive calcium can, under certain conditions, reduce the biological availability of zinc and iron. Of great immediate importance, in the light of recent recommendations for zinc fortification, is the postulated antagonism between zinc and copper.[12] Marginal copper deficiency results in elevated serum cholesterol levels of experimental animals, and this effect is aggravated by high levels of zinc. Thus, the copper intake and status must be carefully examined before a zinc fortification program can be considered safe. While these examples emphasize the need for caution, other examples of interactions may stimulate a more aggressive fortification policy. One such example is the interaction of selenium with heavy metals, such as mercury and cadmium.[23] Selenium has been shown to protect against the effects of excessive exposure to these metals; thus, it is possible that a selenium supply that is adequate under ordinary conditions might be marginal in a heavily contaminated environment. In this situation a health benefit could be expected from selenium fortification, even though there might be no overt indications of a deficient intake.

Iron fortification has already created marked changes in the balance of trace elements naturally present in cereals (TABLE 2). It is not known whether these imbalances are of significance when evaluated as part of the total intake from a mixed diet.

4. *Interactions of fortification nutrients with the carrier food.* As has been discussed above, iron compounds of reasonable bioavailability enter into equilibrium with the non-heme iron pool of the gastrointestinal tract. It is now well known that the biological availability of this pool is dependent on the ingredients of the diet; some enhance, others degress availability. The two

TABLE 2

RATIO OF ESSENTIAL TRACE ELEMENTS TO IRON *

Ratio	Whole Wheat	Patent Flour	Enriched Flour (40 mg/lb; ≃88 ppm)
Zn/Fe	0.84	0.86	0.067
Cu/Fe	0.1	0.2	0.015
Mn/Fe	1.32	0.81	0.063
Mo/Fe	0.003	0.026	0.002
Co/Fe	0.0006	0.0005	0.00004

* Calculated from Czerniejewski *et al.*, 1963, *Cereal Science.*

known dietary factors that greatly increase the absorption of non-heme iron, when present with iron in the same meal, are ascorbic acid and an as yet unidentified factor in meat. Depending on the quantity of these enhancing factors present, the absorption of non-heme iron can be increased as much as four- or five-fold. On the other hand, several nutrients and nonnutrients, potentially present in meals, have been found to depress non-heme iron absorption significantly. Among those are phytates, phosvitin of egg yolk, calcium and phosphate salts, tannic acid of tea, EDTA, and antacids. The potential influence of dietary fiber on the availability of non-heme iron is still under investigation.[24] These well-known enhancing and depressing effects should be taken into consideration when a carrier food for iron enrichment is selected. Iron enrichment of a food containing meat, ascorbic acid, or both, would obviously be much more beneficial than enrichment of a food containing high levels of phytate. Similar interactions of other trace elements are poorly understood, although it is known that the zinc present in animal products is more readily available than zinc in products of vegetable origin.

Interactions of the fortification micronutrient with the carrier food also can affect consumer acceptability of the enriched product. Trace elements are powerful catalysts that can accelerate undesirable reactions, leading to off-color, off-flavor, or off-taste qualities in the products. Biologically available forms of trace elements are generally also reactive in the carrier food before it is consumed, and inert forms of trace elements that do not react with the carrier are unlikely to be readily available for absorption. Thus, the choice of a particular form of an element for fortification must take into account nutritional, as well as technological, considerations, if the enriched product is to be acceptable and at the same time is to contain the enrichment agent in an available form.

5. *Selection of a suitable carrier food for fortification.* The most important consideration in the selection of a carrier food must be its availability to the target population. Target populations can usually be broadly defined as certain age or sex groups particularly at risk from deficiency; groups may be narrow segments of the population in one case or represent a large proportion in another. The vitamin D requirement of adults in the United States appears to be met by endogenous synthesis; thus, the main target groups of vitamin D fortification are infants, children, and adolescents. The groups at greatest risk of marginal chromium deficiency in the United States may be pregnant women and middle aged and elderly subjects. Fortification with vitamin B_6, if it is to be considered, would have to address pregnant women and, perhaps, users of oral contraceptive steroids, whereas the existing fortification with the other B vitamins is directed to the total population.

In view of the potential risks of any fortification program discussed above, the ideal carrier should be a food that is consumed preferentially by the intended target group and that is of minor importance for those population groups not in need of the fortification nutrient. Infant formulae are an ideal example; they are used exclusively by the target population. Milk is preferentially consumed by growing subjects, although not restricted entirely to this group. Flour and baked products are widely consumed by all but the youngest age groups and are therefore good carriers for fortification nutrients that are directed to the population as a whole. The results of fortification of flour with vitamins of the B group have been excellent. On the other hand, the suitability of this carrier might be questioned for iron fortification, mainly directed to children and women of child-bearing age. Salt and drinking water reach all of the population in predictable amounts. They are inexpensive and can be considered ideal carriers for fortification programs directed to all age groups.

The requirement for some vitamins and trace elements depends on the intake of certain macronutrients. This allows the design of almost ideal fortification programs, by adding the required micronutrient to those foods that determine the requirement. The best known example is the dependence of the vitamin E requirement on the dietary intake of polyunsaturated fatty acids. Oils with a high content of polyunsaturated fatty acids naturally carry vitamin E, so that any increased requirement is automatically met. The chromium requirement is believed to be increased by a high intake of refined sugars. If chromium fortification should ever become necessary, sugar might be considered as a promising carrier.

Soft drinks and snack foods, very popular with adolescents, are potentially good carriers of micronutrients to make these products nutritionally more complete or to counterbalance the effects of nutritionally undesirable additives, such as phosphates or EDTA in soft drinks.

CONCLUSION

Knowledge of human nutrient requirements and of individual essential nutrients is increasing and can be expected to increase further in the future. As methods for assessing the nutritional status of population groups are improved, nutrition surveys will be increasingly effective in defining nutrients for which a risk of marginal intake exists. As nutritional practices and the exposure to certain nutrients change, needs for fortification measures also change. These changes are not necessarily in the direction of increasing the number and concentration of nutrients in fortification; there may also be a reduction or elimination of nutrients, if the need for fortification no longer exists. Fortification programs are not substitutes for measures to insure an ample supply of nutritious food to all people to meet their nutrient requirements for optimal health; these programs should not be considered more than interim measures. In order to be effective, fortification programs must incorporate the latest scientific knowledge of human requirements, nutrient interactions, and of biological availability. This knowledge has substantially increased, but many problems are still to be resolved by nutrition research.

REFERENCES

1. AYKROYD, W. R. 1970. Conquest of deficiency diseases. Achievements and prospects. World Health Organization, Basic Study No. 24. Geneva, Switzerland.
2. SUBCOMMITTEE ON THE GEOCHEMICAL ENVIRONMENT IN RELATION TO HEALTH AND DISEASE. 1974. Geochemistry and the Environment. National Acad. Sci. Washington, D.C.
3. ROBINSON, M. F. 1975. The moonstone: More about selenium. The Nutrition Society of New Zealand : 13–30. Palmerston North, New Zealand.
4. KOVAL'SKIY, V. V. & G. A. YAROVAYA. 1966. Molybdenum-infiltrated biogeochemical provinces. Agrokhimiya 8: 68–91.
5. WHO EXPERT COMMITTEE. 1973. Trace elements in human nutrition. Annex 1. World Health Org. Tech. Rep. Ser. No. 532. Geneva, Switzerland.

6. MERTZ, W. 1976. Trace elements in animal nutrition. Can a great potential be realized? *In* Nuclear Techniques in Animal Production and Health. Intern. Atomic Energy Agency : 3–15. Vienna, Austria.

7. FOOD AND NUTRITION BOARD. 1974. Proposed fortification policy for cereal-grain products. Nat. Acad. Sci. Washington, D.C.

8. SANDSTEAD, H. H., K. P. VO-KHACTU & N. SOLOMONS. 1976. Conditioned zinc deficiencies. *In* Trace Elements in Human Health and Disease. Vol. I, Zinc and Copper. A. S. Prasad, Ed. : 33–49. Academic Press. New York.

9. KARPEL, J. T. & V. H. PEDEN. 1972. Copper deficiency in long-term parenteral nutrition. J. Pediat. **49:** 246–258.

10. JEEJEEBHOY, K. N., R. CHU, E. B. MARLISS, G. R. GREENBERG & A. BRUCE-ROBERTSON. 1975. Chromium deficiency, diabetes and neuropathy, reversed by chromium infusion in a patient on total parenteral nutrition (TPN) for 3½ years. Clin. Res. **23:** 636A.

11. UNDERWOOD, E. J. 1977. Trace elements in human and animal nutrition. 4th Edit. Academic Press. New York.

12. KLEVAY, L. M. 1973. Hypercholesterolemia in rats produced by an increase of the ratio of zinc to copper ingested. Am. J. Clin. Nutr. **26:** 1060–1068.

13. KLEVAY, L. M. 1975. The ratio of zinc to copper of diets in the United States. Nutr. Rep. Intern. **11:** 237–242.

14. FOOD AND NUTRITION BOARD. 1974. Recommended dietary allowances. National Acad. Sci. Washingon, D.C.

15. GURSON, C. T. & G. SANER. 1973. Effects of chromium supplementation on growth in marasmic protein-calorie malnutrition. Am. J. Clin. Nutr. **26:** 988–991.

16. MERTZ, W. 1974. The newer essential trace elements, chromium, tin, vanadium, nickel and silicon. Proc. Nutr. Soc. **33:** 307–313.

17. FOOD AND NUTRITION BOARD. 1971. Extent and meanings of iron deficiency in the U.S. Summary Proceedings of a Workshop. National Acad. Sci. Washington, D.C.

18. SCHWARZ, K. & A. FREDGA. 1969. Biological potency of organic selenium compounds. J. Biol. Chem. **244(8):** 2103–2110.

19. GRIFFITHS, N. M., R. D. H. STEWART & M. F. ROBINSON. 1976. The metabolism of [^{75}Se] selenomethionine in four women. Brit. J. Nutr. **35:** 373–382.

20. MILLS, C. F. 1955. Availability of copper in freeze-dried herbage and herbage extracts to copper deficient rats. Brit. J. Nutr. **9:** 398–409.

21. SCHWARZ, K. 1974. New essential trace elements (Sn, V, F, Si): Progress report and outlook. *In* Trace Element Metabolism in Animals. II. W. G. Hoekstra, J. W. Suttie, H. E. Ganther & W. Mertz, Eds. : 355–380. University Park Press. Baltimore, Md.

22. MERTZ, W. 1969. Chromium: Occurrence and function in biological systems. Physiol. Rev. **49:** 163–239.

23. PARIZEK, J., J. KALOUSKAVA, A. BABICKY, J. BENES & L. PAVLIK. 1974. Interactions of selenium with mercury, cadmium, and other toxic metals. *In* Trace Element Metabolism in Animals. II. W. G. Hoekstra, J. W. Suttie, H. E. Ganther & W. Mertz, Eds. : 119–131. University Park Press. Baltimore, Md.

24. MONSEN, E. R., L. HALLBERG, M. LARYSSE, D. M. HEGSTED, J. D. COOK, W. MERTZ & C. A. FINCH. 1977. Estimation of available dietary iron. Am. J. Clin. Nutr. In press.

THE USE AND ABUSE OF FOOD TECHNOLOGY IN THE QUALITY OF OUR FOOD SUPPLY

Samuel A. Goldblith

Department of Nutrition and Food Science
Massachusetts Institute of Technology
Cambridge, Massachusetts 02139

INTRODUCTION

The late Mr. Justice Holmes stated that, "Man must share the actions and passions of his time at the peril of being judged not to have lived." Thus I agreed to talk on the subject that was assigned to me—a difficult one. It can be approached from a number of different viewpoints:

1. The consumerist movement point of view.
2. The historical point of view.
3. The futuristic point of view of world needs.
4. The nationalistic point of view.
5. The development of science and technology and its influence.
6. Man's desires *vs.* man's nutritional needs.
7. The pragmatic point of view.

I have chosen to attempt to discuss this subject using all points of view.

It is obvious that this is a controversial subject evoking deep-rooted feelings and has often resulted in legislation in the U.S.A. based on the emotional passions of the time rather than on scientific facts. I believe we should recognize that while the statement by Chancellor-Emeritus of the University of California, Professor Emil M. Mrak, may be an oversimplification, it is, by and large, correct. This statement, as I recall it, is: "There are no bad chemicals; only bad ways of using these chemicals insofar as food is concerned."

THE DELANEY AMENDMENT AND THE DEVELOPMENT OF ANALYTICAL CHEMISTRY

Perhaps no single piece of legislation has caused as much controversy as has this amendment to the Food and Drug Laws, which in effect declares illegal any compound or chemical that causes cancer. This amendment gives no consideration to:

1. The amount needed to cause cancer in laboratory animals.
2. Laboratory animals being different from humans in their response.
3. The spectacular developments in analytical chemistry that led to what is known as the "vanishing zero."

The Delaney Amendment does not take into account the fact that in the biological sciences, there is no "zero" nor is there "100 percent." One forever lives in the area between black and white, and one must consider risk and benefit, cost and effect.

One spectacular illustration of the abuse of the Delaney Amendment is the

161

aminotriazole incident of 1961. Here, you may recall, is a real example of the abuse of a chemical by a farmer who used aminotriazole in a cranberry bog just prior to harvest, contrary to written directions. Minute amounts of amino-triazole were found in a few cranberry samples, and a national alarm was sent out—far beyond any justification for the few parts per million of aminotriazole found in a few samples representing but a very small part of the production of the cranberries. The result was simply a disaster for the cranberry industry for several years.

Another example lingers with us today—the cyclamate story. Canada, The Netherlands, Belgium, Switzerland, West Germany, and Spain permit the use of cyclamates up to a maximum recommended intake of 3.5 grams per day. The United States banned cyclamate, almost ruining several canning companies who had just canned their annual pack of dietetic fruit when the ban was announced. The ban was based on flimsy evidence of a feeding study of a *mixture* of cycla-mate and saccharin only. In the United States, this ban exists to this very day.

To me, this is an administrative ban based on the passions and emotions of a few people rather than on scientific evidence. This ban is as emotionally rooted as was the approval of saccharin by President Theodore Roosevelt in 1906, which was based on Wiley's wish to get the Pure Food and Drug Act passed. Wiley acceded to Roosevelt's demand to permit the use of saccharin (and to not have it included as a "poison"). Again, human emotions overruled the scientific wisdom *of that time*—Roosevelt was a diabetic. This does not mean that I believe saccharin to be unsafe or to be carcinogenic. I cite this story to indicate the emotionalism involved, as well as to remind us that cycla-mate was banned on a study based on a mixture of cyclamate plus saccharin.

As analytical chemistry has developed, the erroneous and fallacious basis of the Delaney Amendment becomes more and more obvious.

Legislation and regulation must be based on the science of the time and be designed to react to changes in science and in world affairs. We and the poli-ticians must learn that there is no such thing as "zero molecules" and that cause and effect, risk and benefit must be considered. There is some risk in every-thing; every benefit has a cost; and wiser behavior means not escape but our informed choice.[2] Moreover, we must learn that food is a complex conglom-erate of chemicals, all of which, in all probability, if fed in sufficiently high amounts (e.g., salt and/or methionine—both needed by man) can cause cancer —*if fed in sufficient quantities or if embedded in an organ.*

Monsodium glutamate is always consumed by mouth, yet the hue and cry of the anti-glutamate movement is based primarily on injection of the com-pound into the brain!

EXAMPLES OF CURRENT CONTROVERSIES—THE TWO POINTS OF VIEW

Butylated hydroxy toluene (BHT) is decried as a "bad chemical" by the consumerist movement. Yet scientifically we know that peroxidation of fats may very easily lead to cancer in some cases. Moreover, the use of antioxidants has permitted long-term storage and utilization of cold breakfast cereals. If Burkitt's hypothesis is correct relative to lower bowel cancer being due to inade-quate fiber in the diet, then surely BHT, BHA, and other antioxidants are important and needed in our Western civilization today, both to prevent peroxi-dation of fats and at the same time to permit more fiber in the diet in an acceptable form—"Food is not food until it is eaten," to quote the eminent nutritionist Professor Samuel Lepkovsky.

Will we go back to the diet of one hundred years ago? Who will farm the farms? How will the world be fed? Let us look at the matter of nitrites, nitrosamines, and botulism. Without going into the massive literature on the subject of nitrosamines and cancer which still is, in my judgment, based on supposition and unproven theory of formation in the stomach, let us recall the following:

1. Nitrites and nitrates have been in use (as an impurity in salts) since 3000 B.C. in Mesopotamia as well as in China and India. Thus we have history of extended usage.

2. Nitrites are effective agents against botulinum organisms, and together with salt, have made the canned ham industry possible as well as other cured meats which have permitted the feeding of people over long voyages on sea and on land. Nitrite/nitrate made possible the exploration of the New World in the Middle Ages as well as the thriving trade in the Mediterranean countries before the Common Era.

The nitrosamine issue has brought to the fore three important matters:

1. The developments in science and technology that have reduced the amount of nitrite from the 200 ppm authorized by the U.S. Department of Agriculture in 1925, and, later, the deletion of the addition of sodium nitrate. At that point in time, the greatest worry of nitrite/nitrate was its effect on hemoglobin. Yet surveys in 1936 and 1970 showed less than 75 ppm nitrite in cured meats and less than 130 ppm in shelf-stable and pasteurized meat products.

2. The theory of nitrosamine formation and its possible effect have led to extensive studies by the meat industry which have eliminated the use of nitrate entirely and reduced the use of nitrite. They equally well have demonstrated the need of nitrite to prevent botulism in cured meats.

3. A third significant point is that nitrates are normally found in saliva *without eating cured meats*. Moreover, nitrates are found in fairly substantial quantity in untreated vegetables.

We do not have all answers either con or pro nitrites, and epidemiological studies show that stomach cancer has been reduced in America over the past decade.

One can look at this matter of nitrites in foods from two points of view. On the one hand, the use of 200 ppm in 1906 could have been considered an abuse of additives (*in hindsight*). Nevertheless, the other side of the story is that industry began in 1970 a series of extensive and expensive studies which have led to the reduction of nitrites in meats and shown the minimum needed for protection of man from botulism. But the story on nitrites in cured meats is not finished. Much more research is needed to objectively assess the nitrosamine problem.

Yet of this one can be certain: Cured meats and fish have played an important role in the feeding of man over the ages. Again accepting the proposition that "Food is not food until it is eaten," mankind will not accept insipidity in its food supply any more than it will in that other great urge that governs man! Secondly, nitrites have contributed to the safety of man's food supply.

CHEMICALS IN FOODS: BOON OR DISASTER—NEED FOR MANKIND

One of the abuses of a simple chemical may be common table salt in baby foods. This has been to please mothers, however, rather than to satisfy the baby's nutritional needs. Yet one can hardly blame industry for attempting to satisfy customers' needs and desires. At the other end of the spectrum is the tremendous growth in population in the world—far greater in the lesser developed countries than in the developed countries. Yet, North America has continued to provide food for these less developed countries to help them keep pace with their burgeoning population. India, the U.S.S.R., France, etc., have many more workers on the farm than the U.S., but our productivity is far greater, where only 4 percent of our population is, and has been made possible through inputs of pesticides, herbicides, fertilizers, water, agricultural machinery, and petroleum, not to mention tremendous increases in knowledge about agricultural science and technology, agricultural genetics, soil husbandry, etc. Without these agricultural inputs, it would be virtually impossible for North America to feed the world.

Thus, we end up balancing on the edge of a sharp knife—the risk *vs.* the benefit of a bounteous food supply with these agricultural inputs or triage on the other hand. What is your preference?

FOOD TECHNOLOGY

Food technology began as an art and has resulted in a scientifically based technology expressed by engineering operations. The eminent Brillat-Savarin stated that "The destiny of nations is determined by the manner in which they feed themselves."

The need to preserve food dates back to ancient Egyptian and Sumerian civilizations. It has been the cornerstone that made urbanization possible, that has made possible the carryover of foods from one harvest season to the other, that has been the difference between success and failure in battles, and that helped to make Jules Verne's dream of man on the moon a reality.

Yet, we hear so much negativism about our technology. Again if we accept Professor Lepkovsky's basic premise that "Food is not food until it is eaten," I would also add to it his proposition that food must be consumed with gustatory delight, and the latter adds to the nutritive value of foods beyond mere calories, protein, fat, carbohydrates, minerals, and vitamins.

Processing has negative aspects. It produces white bread from wheat flour which has had many vitamins and minerals removed. So we add them back. While I decry and dislike the bread we call "wind pudding," you and I do have *freedom of choice,* so I eat oatmeal bread, whole wheat bread, etc. This is possible because we live in a free society under the free enterprise system where science and technology can flourish. To accommodate the bulk of Americans who prefer white bread, technology adds back the missing nutrients. Moreover, for those who need it, higher protein breads are available at reasonable prices.

We have developed convenience foods—be it soluble or freeze-dried coffee or potato crisps made from dehydrated potatoes. We have developed complex engineered foods from soya—extenders, frozen, canned, cured, etc.—all to respond to needs expressed by the consumers. Is it an abuse to make the "golden nugget" of the Orient a cheaper source of vegetable protein for Westernized society? I think not.

While we may decry the use of technology to make vegetable oil-based creams, and vegetable-based protein products, the fact of the matter is that the public wants them for convenience and for health and/or religious reasons. Is it wrong to use science and technology to make whey protein (from the throwaway by-product of cheese manufacture) a utilizable nutritional source of protein with functionality, as well as thereby improving our ecology and environment?

Food science and technology have cut down peeling and trimming losses, satisfied consumer needs, improved the microbial quality of our food supply, and prevented favism, mycotoxin formation, anti-tryptic activity, haemagglutinins in soybeans, etc.; and food additives can reduce and improve acceptability. Food science and technology's stature today, in this bicentennial year, from a nutritional point of view, is better than that 200 or 100 or even 50 years ago. Try a visit below decks to the frigate U.S.S. Constitution in Boston, or look at the almost doubling of our life span since 1775.

True, we have much to do. "The development of knowledge," as Pascal said, "is like a growing sphere." As the sphere of knowledge grows, "it exposes a greater surface to the unknown." I believe our food science and food technology have benefitted mankind far more than it has hurt man:

1. We are better fed and better nourished than ever before.
2. Urbanization, whether we like it or not, has been made feasible.
3. We now have recognized the immortality of nature and are doing something about it.
4. We have improved our ecology and environment.
5. We are learning more about the chemicals in our food supply but need to learn more about their interaction. Without food science, this is impossible, and without the free enterprise system in a democratic society, the development of new knowledge is impossible.
6. We are helping to maintain free societies, and we are providing humanitarian relief with food.

SUMMARY AND CONCLUSIONS

I have attempted to present some of the facets of a difficult topic. In my judgment, they lead to four conclusions that are undebatable:

1. Food additives, processing, and technology can benefit from an analysis of risk *vs.* benefit.
2. Legislation and regulations based on scientific data are far better for mankind than regulations governed by emotions.
3. To achieve proper regulations at minimum risk and maximum benefit to mankind, research is a *sine qua non* upon which to develop sound regulations.
4. While we have taught people how to make a living, we need to teach them how to live; people succeed but know not how to cope. People buy and pay more for an "organic" tomato they do *not* need, yet refuse to buy iodized salt that they *do* need. Thus we need educational reform in food science and nutrition—teaching people at the elementary school

level where childrens' minds are like sponges. We have two kinds of capital—green capital ($) and grey capital. We reserve education in food science, nutrition, and medicine for university specialization. Yet, we all need to know and to understand our food and medical needs throughout life. Why not fill the grey capital of *young* brain cells with knowledge of their fundamental needs?

The pathway to wholesome food optimized will always be grey, tortuous, and narrow, veering between black and white, and only educated judgments based on scientific facts are our hope in feeding the world on the one hand and not abusing the use of chemicals in our food supply and in our environment and thus renewing our natural resources. We must move to a more informed and more rational society. "We need a better process than the adversary process to solve the complex scientific problems we now face—the 'trans-scientific' issues, such as moral values, aesthetics or personal preferences." [2]

Scientific questions which require specialized knowledge remain blended with value questions in which all citizens should have a voice. But it must be an *informed, educated citizenry*.

In 1579, John Lyly recommended for the 1570's, "A diet wholesome, but not excessive." The food industry provides us, in the 1970's, with a wholesome diet. As to excessiveness—well, that is a personal matter to each of us.

REFERENCES

1. BINKERD, E. F. & KOLARI, O. E. 1975. The history and use of nitrate and nitrite in the curing of meat. Food Cosmet. Toxicol. **13:** 655–661.
2. HALL, R. L. 1973. A diet wholesome, but not excessive. Food Technol. (Chicago) **27**(7): 61, 63–66.

GENERAL DISCUSSION

Samuel A. Goldblith, *Moderator*

Department of Food Science
Massachusetts Institute of Technology
Cambridge, Massachusetts 02139

DR. DONALD WATKIN (*HEW, Washington, D.C.*): Dr. Greenland, do you have any information based on your Nigerian experience on how much capital is required to bring about the results that you've already produced and any projections as to what would be needed to bring the quality of nutrition up to what you would regard as adequate for Nigeria?

DR. GREENLAND: I don't think there is any single answer to that. It depends entirely on the way in which you want to adjust the diet, and who's going to do the paying.

I mentioned at the start that the humid tropics, in Africa in particular, are dependent on small farmers. The average cultivated farm holding in Nigeria at present is 1.1 acre, half a hectare. What it costs in terms of bringing that nutrition level to that farmer up to a desirable scale is really impossible to estimate because the nutrition depends on not only what's grown, an awful lot is still gathered from the bush that's around and has particularly important influences on nutrition in the diet.

You can't divorce, I think, the question of just increasing the cost to the individual farmer of doing something for his own diet, from the cost of changing the whole economy of the country from an entirely subsistence level to a level wherein there is a large additional income that is going to produce the other aids to life that are needed.

A lot of people at the moment dismiss Nigeria, and I think Nigeria is mostly on the U.S. aid list at the moment because of the oil money there, which is large in amount. But it's doubled per capita income in the country from $120 a head to about $250. There is still such an enormous amount to be done in terms of making any increases in gains in the country really work. The problems I mentioned of communications and of roads, those are terribly real and most of where the money is going at present. The costs of improving port facilities to get the things that are so badly needed into the country are enormous. The problems of government are so tremendous that I don't think that one at present can divorce the costs for an actual increase in nutrition from the other costs of development.

DR. BARTON H. MARSHALL (*Silver Spring, Md.*): Did I understand you correctly, Dr. Greenland, that you had success with no till agriculture without herbicides?

DR. GREENLAND: Yes, in fact roughly what the people still use in the forest areas of West Africa is simply essentially a divil stick, and they will poke a little hole and drop the May seed in. And that's it.

The weed control, of course, is really the major problem for them. And when I said that labor was both too little and too much, shortly after planting if you're not using herbicides then certainly labor is not enough to give you real control of the weed problem and they lose an awful lot of crop from weeds.

In that slide I showed of yields falling to zero in three or four years, there

167

was a curve showing what happened even if you put fertilizers on and left the weeds or if you didn't put fertilizers on but weeded. The weeds are almost as much a problem as the fertility change.

But if you're practicing, as most of the farmers do, shifting cultivation, you don't let your land go back into bush after two years. And this is just when the weeds beat you. But the redevelopment of the cover, of course, is one of the reasons why they have managed to keep a stable productive system going for several hundreds of years; whereas if we try and mechanize it no one yet on the non-valley bottom land has produced a mechanized system which will produce continuously on the upper slope soils. Because when you mechanize you have no choice but to grow a bumper crop. You've got no choice but to leave the soil exposed for a period. You lose your top soil and you lose your nutrients and you're yields decline. Management is blamed, but nine times out of ten the trouble is lack of proper care of the soil. Unless you use perennial crops, tree crops, all the successful development schemes in South America as well as Africa have depended upon perennials, in some form or other. If you try and mechanize in other ways you don't get that.

The divil stick and the no till without herbicides does work—but at a fairly low productive level.

DR. JOHN R. OPPENHEIMER (*Johns Hopkins University, Baltimore, Md.*): Dr. Rawlins, you mentioned in the beginning of your talk that salt deposition was a problem, and I don't know whether you actually came up with a solution or not.

DR. RAWLINS: Well, the solution to the problem of salt in most cases is to prevent the depercolation that causes the water table to rise. I don't think I brought that out. By controlling water and preventing this tremendous depercolation, then the naural drainage capacity of many salts will be sufficient and the water table won't rise. That's the answer: preventing depercolation. Certainly that's the answer to Egypt's problem, at the present time.

DR. BARTON H. MARSHALL: What about the use of highly saline water, such as we have in the Colorado River?

DR. RAWLINS: Contrary to what most people believe, the Colorado River is not highly saline. It has about 860 parts per million of total dissolved salts at Imperial Dam, which is a very good water. Many places in Israel are using 3,000 parts per million in water.

High frequency irrigation, drip irrigation particularly, makes it possible to use more highly saline water, primarily because the water content of the soils remains high and you dilute the salts more and it makes it possible to use more saline water. I go into this in considerably more detail in that *Science* article in the food issue a year ago in May.

DR. R. W. F. HARDY (*E. I. du Pont de Nemours & Co., Wilmington, Del.*): I'm wondering if there is any information on how much you can improve the efficiency of water use in the plant itself. Can a plant use half as much water and come up with the same amount of yield? Is there any work going on there?

DR. RAWLINS: A lot of work has been done in that area, kinetic value cultural station and others have used stomatal control compounds and other things to try to stop wasteful transpiration use. I don't think there is any hope. The basic problem is that the stomates must be open for carbon dioxide to diffuse in, carbon dioxide is absorbed on a wet surface, and water diffuses out the same pathway.

Now, there are some crops—pineapple and others—whose metabolism fixes carbon dioxide at night. The stomates are open at night and absorb the CO_2. It's stored, and then the stomates can be closed during the day when transpiration would be high.

There are some long-range possibilities that these kinds of things could be adapted to plants. But in the near future I think there is very little hope that we can really stop transpiration. Transpiration seems to be almost dependent upon the number of acres, on the crop area, that you have. By increasing the production per unit crop area you therefore increase the production per unit water considerably. And so I think by putting the necessary inputs in to raise productivity per unit area we can save water in that sense. I think that's the main thrust that we can use.

DR. D. J. GREENLAND: I'd like to correct one comment you made on behalf of my colleagues at some of the other international institutes, when you commented that high-yielding varieties won't perform as well as some of the traditional varieties under irrigation, particularly rice, I think. The International Rice Institute has shown pretty unequivocally that within the very wide spectrum now of the high-yielding varieties many of these perform much better both under very good conditions and under very poor input conditions. At the International Institute for Tropical Agriculture in Nigeria, we have been looking very deliberately at the development of materials for low input conditions as well as high input conditions. Simet in Mexico is doing the same for maize and wheat. Again, broad performance across a very wide range of high and low fertility conditions is a characteristic of most of the new materials coming from the institutes. And I think it's propagating a myth to talk about the high yielding varieties only performing well under high input conditions. They are well adapted to both very low input as well as high input conditions. I think it's important that that is recognized.

DR. RAWLINS: I appreciate that very much. You certainly know far more about that than I. I'm only quoting the literature. I appreciate that correction.

MS. SUSAN GREENBERG (*Simon Fraser University, Vancouver, British Columbia*): Dr. Milner, could you elaborate on any large-scale methods for reclaiming of organic wastes and what methods are in practical use in the United States today?

DR. MILNER: Actually there is a lot going on in research and even in the engineering phases here. I indicated, for example, that one of the major areas for more extensive research is the reclaiming of wastes from livestock feeding operations and so forth. There is a great deal of activity going on by the producers themselves, and the Food & Drug Administration is now working on protocols for this research. There are all kinds of proposals for the recovery of bagas and other cellulosic wastes. These things seem to have hit an impasse at the moment. We know a great deal of research and development has been done, but it all boils down to the question of economics, as to whether this will move very quickly from the laboratory into the practical area. Clearly the economics have not yet been established.

I didn't mention that one of the recommendations was to intensify the use of the fermentation approach to upgrade organic wastes.

DR. MOSSEF EL MAN (*Weizmann Institute, Israel*): I would like to suggest another approach that was not mentioned by the speaker: utilization of the wild relatives. In our department in the Weizmann Institute we analyze the wild relatives of wheat that grow in Israel. In some lines we found more than 30% protein in grain collected in the field and without fertilization. This is an excellent source of genetic material for the improvement of protein content in wheat grain. This source of wild material, wild relatives, was not studied and was not utilized in this direction.

DR. MILNER: I would have to differ with you in this regard. When you read the complete reports you'll see that high protein cultivars selected from wild strains, and initially as a matter of fact in North Africa, have already been cranked into research. There are now commercial varieties being furnished around the world—particularly through the University of Nebraska where in connection with A.I.D.—in which there is at least 5% increase in protein.

DR. EL MAN: This is not wild material, this is cultivated. They found two cultivated materials, and they were able to increase the protein content only to 18% in wheat. Now, in this wild material there is 35% protein in the grain. It's a completely different level.

DR. MILNER: Thank you. I hope you bring this to the attention of the American scientists. Perhaps they haven't heard of it.

DR. ARTHUR MILLER (*Philadelphia*): I had the opportunity to work on a National Science Foundation project involving studies concerning ground beef production in the United States. We were looking at the cost of regulations. It seemed to be a simple task at first. But in looking at the details, no one really had the information, and we had to do quite a lot of legwork. How can we possibly avoid this sort of situation, with new and different proteins, when we can't even do this with the almighty hamburger?

DR. MILNER: You are referring to restrictions as far as food and drug laws in this country?

DR. MILLER: Well, the cost involved with regulations. Now, when we're talking about new products, as it turns out, talking about quite a lot of regulations.

DR. MILNER: You realize you've opened a hornet's nest here which is another subject, and we do have authorities in this room like Dr. Oser over here who I am sure would be glad to propound on this subject for any infinite amount of time.

As a matter of fact you'll find in the final documentation a chapter written by Dr. Oser in which he deals specifically with this problem. What to do about it, I don't know. This is the area of public policy in the United States.

By the way, one thing I went over very quickly. We are proposing research on the reclaiming of animal products which are now rejected under our terribly overstrict marketing and grading systems.

DR. ANDRE BOLAFFI (*Dunkin Donuts of America, Randolph, Mass.*): Max, in your opinion, in reference to all sources of nonconventional proteins and technologies that you listed, which one or two priorities do you see as having the best chance of success from an economic point of view, from a practical point of view, from an availability point of view?

DR. MILNER: Well, as I indicated, perhaps the greatest excitement of all end research on increased food production at the present time is in the cereals. The plant breeders, particularly the cereal breeders, are just beginning to realize the diversity of possible ways to go in terms of cereal breeding. There is still tremendous potential unexplored. Without any question, this is one of the very major priorities, and that's why we listed it very close to the top.

With reference to other innovative sources of protein, in Chicago yesterday soy beans were $6 per bushel. Now, that's up quite a bit from what they were six or eight months ago. The forecast is that notwithstanding our soy bean crop being down some 18% this past year, soy bean prices will, as a matter of fact, drop this next year probably to $5.50 a bushel. The point is that this is the major world protein resource for animal feeding. And that is the benchmark. And as long as those prices prevail, these new innovative approaches are not going to come in very fast. And that opens another story as well, because as you heard at this meeting more people are hungry than ever before, yet at the international marketing level cereals and grains are cheaper than they have been and we wonder how farmers are making a living.

Dr. MICHAEL RABIN: Dr. Dobbins, what preservative is there in the material that enables you to keep it for 7 weeks· And has it been dehydrated or cooked?

Dr. DOBBINS: How many of you know, raise your hands, what I'm talking about if I say corn silage? About half, I guess. We're taking a simple takeoff on ensiling to do this, and it's in a wet state at that particular point. We have selected different lactobacilli that we add the culture to a 500 gallon tank one time, and as food waste is put in each day it's stirred up enough, apparently there are enough growth and enough nutrients there to make it work. And we do dehydrate at the end, but we don't have to. We can feed it wet, if we have the facilities. But for flexibility and use by all species we do dehydrate it.

Dr. RABIN: You don't put in any preservatives?

Dr. DOBBINS: Not at the beginning. The sample that you saw pass by had no preservatives. We didn't need to add an anti-oxidant because our fat level was about 12%. But we have now improved both the protein from 18 to 22% and the fat level from 12 to 20%. So now we would need to add an anti-oxidant.

Dr. RABIN: You're a veterinarian. What is the state of the health of these animals on this feed? Cows today drop dead from heart disease, they get diabetes, Bangs disease, and all the rest of these things that humans do. I'm wondering, as far as the nutritional value of this material is concerned, what is the health of the animals?

Dr. DOBBINS: I think you would recognize right off the bat that this is an animal feed ingredient, not a total ration. On bovine-type diets we can't go as high as 25% because of the high fat level. In fact it works better in swine and in chickens. And there we're going with 15–25%. We've been doing studies on both of them; no problems health-wise, pathogen-wise or this sort of thing. In fact we've used salmonellas and we haven't used tuberculosis, obviously, in our work. We use salmonellas as our guide organism to make sure that the process does remove the pathogens from the problem.

Essentially it's a combination of a drop of pH. We can get a drop in pH in these holding tanks down to 3.8 in roughly 96 hours. If the weather is warm we can do it quicker than that. In addition to that we do have the dehydration phase, which is a temperature time exposure.

Dr. RABIN: Do you find that pigs get diarrhea on cooked garbage?

Dr. DOBBINS: Let me make sure that I understand you. Cooked garbage— are you talking about bio meal or the traditional?

Dr. RABIN: No, the usual stuff.

Dr. DOBBINS: Yes. There's no way to regulate fat content primarily, and of all the other problems associated with garbage feeding, not to mention pollution problems.

Dr. R. D. SEELEY (*Anheuser-Busch, Inc., St. Louis, Mo.*): What kind of a drying system do you use?

DR. DOBBINS: We have used three or four. The one that we find the most economical is an adaptation—in fact, we have not been able to find commercially available equipment that will do the job. We have had to modify everything that we've tried. One of the problems is in getting people, engineers and such, interested in a process that is marginal from a commercial standpoint and in working with people on developing these side feed ingredients. We are using a steam-jacketed pressure rise cooker with an agitator on the inside but have had to modify many parts so it would handle this particular product.

This product handles differently apparently from anything anybody has tried. We've had several engineering groups just give up on it. And it becomes plastic at one stage of the drying. It will just tear the agitator completely out if it's not designed correctly.

DR. GOLDBLITH: Have you found any concentration of pesticides in the animals due to the recycling and so on? Or do you destroy these in the processing?

DR. DOBBINS: We have purposely added pesticides because we figured someone (if we're doing this on a commercial basis and a restaurant is involved) is going to drop some roach or ant pellets or something somewhere in the line, and we want to see what happens. We were concerned about glass too. We found that there is such a dilution factor involved in this, as well as perhaps breaking some of these products down, that we have not had a problem. Even glass winds up as sand as it completes the whole process. So our big problem, frankly, is how to get polished aluminum out of the thing. We have almost a side industry on the side of tableware, of silverware. It almost pays for the process.

DR. HERBERT P. SARETT (*Mead Johnson Research Center, Evansville, Ind.*): Dr. Mertz, I wonder about your statement that fortification programs are compromises until there is enough food for everyone—I think this could be misleading. I think fortification programs have to continue with conventional foods as they have for the past 35 years to get the thiamine and niacin and some of the other nutrients that you pointed out have done some good. I think that there has to be a type of fortification program, which may not be called fortification, but the addition of the proper nutrients with the new protein sources that Dr. Nolan was talking about. You can't feed these isolated single-cell proteins or soy protein isolates to the world without putting in the nutrients that animal protein or the other proteins that they are substituting for in the diet had provided.

You have to build many new foods from these new sources to increase and improve the world's supply with judicious fortification at the proper level, the proper blanket of nutrients that will make these nutritious based on the new knowledge. And also I would like to comment at the same time in relation to your discussion of the need for flexibility of fortification programs. You pointed out the recommendations made several years ago by the National Academy for adding to this list. We still have the same thiamine, riboflavin, niacin, and iron that we had in 1941, and here it's 35 years later when we know that other nutrients are needed.

Now, there is one further aspect of that, and that is that you didn't include to use iron properly; it not only has to be available but you need copper and you need folic acid. These haven't been in the flour in which the iron has been put and increased and the form changed and everything else. And until we look at all these things and do all these things to improve the world food supply, I think we're going to have problems.

DR. MERTZ: Dr. Sarett expressed what I could have expressed had I had more time. When it comes to the flexibility of regulations that we must have, I agree with you on that, Herb. I do not necessarily agree with you on the first point. I am perhaps a little bit idealistic. What I see as the ideal solution, perhaps not to be achieved in the next 200 or 500 years, is the availability of a complete diet to everyone from which those persons get all their nutrients. I am fully aware that for all those years until we get there, if we ever get there, fortification is absolutely necessary. I should have pointed out very strongly, but I didn't, that a particular need exists for the understanding of fortification principles and of principles that guide the availability of nutrients for the new unconventional food, such as meat analogs.

DR. E. M. WIDDOWSON (*Addenbrooke's Hospital, Cambridge, England*): I was very interested in your last comment Dr. Mertz, that what we need is more information about the requirements. We are facing this too in Britain because we are trying to draw up a new edition of our recommended food intakes. We just have to grub around the old literature; nothing much seems to have been done since we last prepared these tables. I would very much like to know if anyone is doing any work on this subject in this country? There certainly isn't anyone in Britain.

DR. MERTZ: Dr. Widdowson, I agree with you. Everyone who has to look at the existing recommendations and has to address the question of how they can be revised, finds himself confronted with the fact that very little is being done. In the past few years, however, some new knowledge has come out.

An important new insight is the concept of a non-heme iron that can produce a tremendous noticeable, measurable benefit in iron nutrition. Another is the demonstration of marginal zinc deficiency in this country, which has led already to an approximation of the human requirement in a very few years. If this work continues, we will have much better knowledge of requirements of different age groups.

Thirdly, we have some information now, as yet unpublished, on the human requirement for chromium, as one example of the new trace elements. And we have accumulated out of the New Zealand group in Dunedin a very considerable amount on knowledge of selenium intakes that lead to slight metabolic imbalances. In other words, we can now make an educated guess as to selenium requirement.

And finally, I'm happy to report that work is now going on in several outfits here in this country that finally starts measuring the effect of dietary fiber on the availability and requirement of essential trace elements. And I think this will also be a very important point.

But we all wish there would be ten times as much work.

DR. MICHAEL RABIN: Dr. Mertz, I was glad to hear you begin to talk about the quality of our food. Now, you spoke of the minimum daily requirements. With such human variability—I'm looking at this from the clinical standpoint because I treat patients—how can we ever discover what the human requirements are? There must be an approximation.

Now, when you talk about the different elements in foods, are they the only things that are in a whole food? That we only restore part of them? Most of our deficiencies in food are the result of processing. Where you take the whole food and you don't have any problem, when you take away the processed foods you eliminate the problem. So what I'm saying is that this just doesn't gel with the current opinion of various authorities in the field, those who work with patients.

DR. MERTZ: Dr. Rabin, the human nutritionist, in contrast to the clinical nutritionist, addresses himself to a healthy population. And in the recommended dietary allowances this is very clearly stated. The range of requirements in healthy people is probably less than what you find in your own practice. I would say that with all the doubts that every scientist has and should have, that the recommendations which the Food & Nutrition Board has come up with are the closest estimates we can make.

Some of these estimates are based on rather flimsy or incomplete data, but it is the best estimate that can be made. And we are reasonably sure that if this requirement is met, that let's say of 15 milligrams of zinc or let's take the iron or vitamins, that the risk of deficiency in healthy people is minimal.

Ms. ELLEN BAUM (*Yale University, New Haven, Conn.*): Dr. Goldblith, I agree with a couple of things you were saying. Clearly additives in the food have really cut down on some of the food diseases. But a couple of things you said I just don't agree with at all.

First of all, you say we have white bread because the consumer really wants it. But at the same time you talk about education and how we have to really work on nutrition education. Do you really think that it is entirely a consumer's choice that they're having white bread?

DR. GOLDBLITH: Absolutely. You can go to any supermarket today and buy all the whole wheat bread, all the oatmeal bread that you want. It's your choice in this free society. And if you have good education, you'll eat oatmeal bread like me.

Ms. BAUM: Okay, what about Saturday morning TV shows where the kids see for 15 minutes in a half an hour program or 15 minutes in an hour program, how they should want sugar-coated cereals, how they should want Twinkies. That's a kind of education. How do you respond to that kind of problem?

DR. GOLDBLITH: I respond to that very simply and based on Burkett's Syndrome. If that's true, give them sugar but give them the cereal to go with it. You may not like my answer, you may not agree, but there it is.

Ms. BAUM: Okay. Then one more question. Do you really think that food is cheaper? You talked about it being actually cheaper than when you had added processing, probably because of the lack of waste that you would have. But I don't understand how that could be. Soy products are actually much more expensive.

DR. GOLDBLITH: Not all the soy products are expensive. You go out and buy soy flour and you can enrich your own bread and you can make it much cheaper. But if you want fancy convenience foods, you'll pay the price. You don't have to buy convenience foods. You can cook at home and spend 7 hours a day, as they did in 1776, doing the cooking.

Ms. BAUM: I don't think that's the option. I mean you don't have to cook for hours.

Ms. DEBRA HAMILTON (*National Public Radio*): We have been talking about cereals this morning, and it's known that nitrates are used to prolong their shelf life. But on the subject of sodium nitrates—

DR. GOLDBLITH: Cereals?

Ms. HAMILTON: Your abstract mentions that antioxidants have made possible the longer shelf life of cereals. But then you refer to nitrates as reducing botulism in meats. That's what I want to address—sodium nitrates in meats. It wasn't brought up that this is a possible cause of cancer, that it is an acknowledged enzyme destroyer, that it is highly dangerous to children and can cause serious damage to anemic persons. My question is can you assure the public that the amounts of sodium nitrates in their daily diets will not destroy their enzymes to a harmful extent?

DR. GOLDBLITH: I did say that the cancer story on nitrosamines was brought out. I did say that, together with nitrites, nitrosamine and botulism all in the same paragraph. And I have the statement as I read it right here. And *that* cancer theory is based on supposition as yet not proven. The incidence of cancer of the stomach in the United States, I also said, has gone down tremendously.

MS. HAMILTON: Can you assure the public—

DR. GOLDBLITH: I cannot assure the public of anything unless I have hard scientific data. And those hard data, being a scientist, I recognize can change as science advances and just gives us more unknowns.

MS. HAMILTON: Can you tell us what's holding back that scientific data?

DR. GOLDBLITH: Certainly. Money to do it with. Now, let me just also add another point or two along that line. No reputable scientist, as I said before, will give a definite yes or a definite no, but I think the benefit to mankind of using nitrites far outweighs the risk of stomach cancer.

MS. HAMILTON: One last question and then we'll go to lunch and eat our chemicals, additives and whatnot—

DR. GOLDBLITH: No, we're going to eat *food*, in case you're interested. Food is composed of chemicals.

MS. HAMILTON: On sodium sulfite, this is a chemical used to restore the color to rancid meat that has turned black, and also to eliminate the—

DR. GOLDBLITH: Sorry M'am, but Dr. Harvey Wiley in 1906 prohibited the use of sodium sulfite in meat products, and it is illegal to use it to this day for the reason you pointed out and is *not* used.

PROTEIN-CALORIE DEFICITS IN DEVELOPING COUNTRIES

M. Béhar

Nutrition Unit
World Health Organization
Geneva, Switzerland

Twenty years ago, we were invited to present a paper on severe protein-malnutrition in children [1] in a meeting organized by this same Academy. In reviewing that paper for this presentation, it was very frustrating to find that the basic principles we stated there in regard to the nature of the problem and its epidemiology are as valid today as they were 20 years ago. As most other workers in the field, we were then particularly concerned with the severe forms of protein-calorie malnutrition (PCM): kwashiorkor and marasmus. These individual cases occupied a large proportion of pediatric beds in hospitals of most developing countries, and we were interested in finding better ways to treat them. But also we were studying these cases as a basis for understanding the responsible factors better and for designing possible preventive measures. The interrelations of kwashiorkor and marasmus were recognized then, as well as the fact that both protein and calories should be considered together in the epidemiology of the problem. We were also beginning to understand that the severe clinical cases that we were seeing in the hospitals were only the visible part of a much greater problem affecting the communities from which these children came. With the knowledge then available on the epidemiology of PCM, we were also starting to explore some specific measures for its prevention. I would like now to review what progress we have made, if any, in the understanding of the nature and magnitude of the problem, its epidemiology, and in designing preventive measures.

NATURE AND MAGNITUDE

In regard to the nature of the problem, it is now clear that our main concern should not be the extreme clinical conditions of PCM (marasmus and kwashiorkor), but the subclinical chronic states of PCM affecting primarily children but also to some extent adults of large population groups in most developing countries. This includes areas where the extreme clinical conditions are now seldom seen.

The condition is frequently present from birth. It is manifested as low birth weight even in babies born at term (small-for-date babies), which in some countries may represent up to 30% of all live births.[2] Chronic subclinical malnutrition of the mother, during her early childhood and during pregnancy, seems to be the main factor responsible for this condition,[3] which contributes to the very high rates of infant mortality in developing countries.[4] PCM becomes more serious during the weaning and postweaning period where most of the severe clinical cases are seen, but persists in older children and even in adults. Still the only practical way that we have to assess subclinical PCM is the rate of growth in children. The method, of course, is not specific and is of no value in adults. Work is still needed for a better understanding of the functional alterations resulting from chronic PCM and their consequences for the individuals and their communities.

The efforts that have been made in the last years for understanding the possible role of PCM in mental development,[5] physical work output,[6] or resistance to infections [7] are still, in my view, not conclusive. Their real causative relationship with malnutrition *per se* is not clear. Nor is their public health and social significance in the context of the situation in which these people live. It is becoming clearer, for instance, that the mental retardation and other behavioral changes observed in children who have suffered from malnutrition are more related to the accompanying deficiencies of psycho-social stimulation [8] and could be overcome by proper environmental stimulation.[9] The work demonstrating limitations in work output of malnourished adults needs to be interpreted in terms of its significance for these individuals, their families, and society in relation to their actual needs and opportunities for work under the socioeconomic structure in which they live. We still need to know more about the magnitude of alterations in different defense mechanisms to infections related to malnutrition and the relative importance for individuals suffering not of severe advance malnutrition but of subclinical chronical forms. I am not denying the importance of these functional alterations resulting from malnutrition; to the contrary, I want to emphasize that it is in the area of assessing the effects of malnutrition as it commonly occurs, in individuals, families, and societies that more precise and pertinent information is needed. This is not, I recognize an easy field. It is not always easy to separate the causes from the effects, as well as from other interrelated variables. In any case, although I recognize that more information in this field of knowledge would be useful, I also believe that if to the best of our knowledge we consider that a population is suboptimally nourished, we must be concerned about it and we must do whatever we can to remedy the situation. Adequate nutrition for the whole population should be seen primarily as a human right and not only in terms of its economic or other implications for society.

In the last few years, particular and urgent attention has been paid to the critical situations of famines, from which whole population groups have been suffering. This is understandable because famines are unacceptable at this stage of our scientific and technological development. It can be considered, however, that individual cases of severe PCM in a community and famine in whole population groups both result from additional stresses at the individual or community level, which break the very delicate equilibrium in which these populations manage to survive. Viewing the problem in this way, one can see that it is as unsatisfactory to take care only of the emergency situation of a famine as it is to treat only the individual cases appearing in a community without concern for the fundamental causes responsible for these populations being at such risk. Our efforts must therefore focus on preventing chronic subclinical malnutrition; and this is still very much neglected. In regard to the magnitude of the problem of PCM, we must recognize that our estimates are not adequate. Various attempts have been made recently to determine the prevalence of PCM on a worldwide basis,[10, 11] and I do not believe that we can learn more from further analysis of this type. We know that protein-calorie malnutrition occurs in various degrees of severity wherever there are people living in poverty, with low educational level, poor sanitary conditions, in a disorganized society and without adequate public services or with no services at all; this of course occurs mainly in the developing countries. But again unless there is a clear definition of the particular categories of people

TABLE 1

AVERAGE PER CAPITA DAILY SUPPLY OF ENERGY AND PROTEIN (1970)

Country	Energy (Kilocalories)	Proteins (Grams)	Energy as % of Requirements	Protein/ Energy Ratio
Japan	2,470	76.2	106	12.3
Sweden	2,800	83.8	104	11.9
Brazil	2,600	63.8	109	9.8
Chile	2,460	70.9	101	11.5
Costa Rica	2,470	63.0	110	10.2
Mexico	2,560	65.1	110	10.1
Nicaragua	2,380	70.1	106	11.7

* Data from: "The State of Food and Agriculture, 1974." FAO, Rome, 1975.

affected and the reasons why they are affected, a presentation of the countries with problems of PCM has no useful purpose. In most cases adequate data on this breakdown are not available.

The problem of PCM is not one that can be analyzed on a national basis, taking the countries as units. This is as true for prevalence of the conditions as it is for dietary intake as one of its determining factors. Unfortunately, however, we still see analysis of PCM in terms of per capita intake of calories and proteins on a national basis. Just to illustrate the fallacy of such analysis, I have taken from a recent publication of FAO [12] data on average daily per capita availability of food energy and protein for a few selected countries (TABLE 1). We know that protein-calorie malnutrition is not a problem in two of them: Japan and Sweden. In the five Latin American countries selected (Brazil, Chile, Costa Rica, Mexico, and Nicaragua), the nutritional problem exists in varying degrees of public health significance. In some of them, it is a serious one. You will notice that no significant differences are observed in the availability of energy. When it is expressed as percent of requirement, the energy availability in all the countries is slightly more than adequate. I think that the same can be said for protein availability, expressed in grams per capita. No attempt was made to express it in percent of requirements since, due to the variability in protein sources, this average value has even less meaning than for energy. Nevertheless, we see again that the protein/calorie ratios are within an acceptable range. Although the figures for the Latin American countries are slightly below those for Japan and Sweden, this difference should not be of importance if we accept the present idea that calories rather than proteins are the limiting factor in the diet of populations suffering from protein-calorie malnutrition. But we will come later to this point. It could be argued that the figures of average per capita availability have some meaning only when they fall below the recommended requirements because they will then clearly indicate that the needs of at least part of the population will not be satisfied. Most of the developing countries do in fact have figures below the average requirements for energy and protein. Differences between the total developed countries and the total developing ones are shown in TABLE 2. I would question, however, if this difference is *the cause* of the problem or if it is not rather *a manifestation* of more fundamental causative factors. We might be confusing a symptom with the cause of the disease. This is, I think, a fundamental question because the belief is still too common that *the* solution to malnutrition is increased food availability. I do not believe that this is even possible on a continuous basis without correcting other factors determining low effective demand. Even if increased food availability (supplies) were possible at the national or even community level, I do not believe this would eliminate malnutrition in most of the people suffering from it.

CAUSES OF PROTEIN-CALORIE MALNUTRITION

I would like to start this part of my presentation with some considerations about the present controversy between those who still consider that proteins are the main limiting factor in the diets of populations suffering from malnutrition and those who believe that calories are rather to be blamed.

Since I might be considered among those who are being accused of overemphasizing the importance of proteins and neglecting calories, I would like to quote from the paper presented 20 years ago to which I referred earlier. In that paper, we said: "In the majority of the regions of the world in which kwashiorkor is found, children after weaning receive diets that are deficient not only in proteins but also in calories." It is, however, pretentious to try and justify our previous position; knowledge progresses, fortunately, and what is important is to analyze what we know now.

It was demonstrated in a recent INCAP study,[13] among others, that the addition of proteins to the usual diet cannot completely correct the problem of protein-calorie malnutrition in preschool children. For more than two years, a soy protein concentrate plus lysine with vitamins and minerals was added to corn "tortillas," the main item in the diet of the population studied. It was not possible to demonstrate a significant effect of this addition in correcting the low birth weight of babies, the insufficient weight gain in preschool-age children, nor in improving other parameters used to assess nutritional status. Nevertheless, it is very interesting that a reduction in the severity and duration of common infectious diseases was observed in the groups regularly eating the enriched tortillas. The mortality in the 1–5-year-old children was also significantly reduced. This is an important observation, but if insufficient protein in their diet had been the main factor responsible for poor nutritional status of this population, one would have expected better

TABLE 2

AVERAGE PER CAPITA DAILY SUPPLY OF ENERGY AND PROTEIN (1969–71)*

	Energy as % of Requirement	Proteins (Grams)
Total developed countries	123	96.4
Total developing countries	95	57.4
World	104	69.0

* Data from: "The State of Food and Agriculture, 1974." FAO, Rome, 1975.

results. Would the situation have been different if calories instead of proteins had been added to the diet? I do not believe that we have as yet convincing experimental data to answer this question as applied to small preschool children having the type of diets common in most areas where protein-calorie malnutrition occurs. Some preliminary observations [14] suggest that preschool children fed *ad libitum* with a corn and beans based diet can more easily satisfy their caloric needs and grow adequately if fat is added to increase the calorie density of the diet. But these were clinical observations by necessity of very short duration (3 weeks) and with a small number of children (only four). More evidence is needed therefore on the possible effects of adding calories to the diets.

In this protein-calorie controversy, some workers, probably more realistic, say that neither proteins nor calories but total food intake is the main limiting factor responsible for PCM in preschool children in most parts of the world. However, direct personal observations in poor rural communities of Guatemala living on a diet based on corn and beans tend to show that even where preschool age children have access to sufficient amounts of the family foods, the amount they actually consume is below their requirement, and protein-calorie malnutrition occurs. Analysis showing that there is no correlation between the total calories consumed by the family and those consumed by the preschool child [15] substantiate, I believe, these observations. Why is it that they are not able to eat more? I can only offer as hypothesis the following possible explanations:

1. The diet may be somehow inadequate for them in terms of bulk (calorie density), other physical or organoleptic characteristics, or in nutrient balance. It is in fact known that animals consume less than will be required to satisfy their caloric needs when put on an imbalanced diet. We have also observed in clinical-metabolic studies that children do the same when offered an imbalanced or otherwise inadequate diet. This is probably a defence mechanism against more serious metabolic disturbances.
2. Their appetite is reduced by the frequently occurring infections, even if they are mild and not recognized as diseases, or by other environmental factors.
3. Their actual requirements are reduced as a consequence of previous malnutrition during their earlier life, and they are "adapted" to a lower level of metabolic needs with slower growth rate and lower activity than normal children of the same age.

I do not believe that we have enough evidence from field conditions to substantiate any of the hypothesis, despite some observations suggesting that all three may be operating. Whatever the explanation, the fact is that the solution for these children could not simply be to eat more of what they are eating. They cannot. These observations and comments are made primarily on the basis of our own observations in Central America, particularly of Indian populations living in the highlands of Guatemala. I am conscious of the danger of generalizations; the situation, of course, would be different in other areas where small children are actually starving. In any case, a more critical analysis of the situation is needed before jumping to conclusions that might orient actions in the wrong direction.

A conclusion that can be drawn from the above discussion is that neither protein alone, nor calories alone, nor even food alone can be incriminated as the only factor responsible for the occurrence of protein-calorie malnutrition in small children in developing countries. What other factors should then be considered?

In the first place, we would like to insist once more on the importance of the common infectious diseases of childhood and other infections and infestations. Even if they are mild or not even noticeable, these children are almost continuously suffering from them, the infections reduce their appetites, their reaction to external stimula and may have significant effects on the absorption and metabolism of nutrients. This has been well documented [16] but is still frequently ignored when designing so called "nutrition programs."

Where children are consuming a diet that seems to be just sufficient to satisfy their nutritional requirements if they eat enough, the effect of these infections seems to be the main factor responsible for maintaining them in a state of chronic deficiency and for precipitating the appearance of severe clinical malnutrition in some of them. Observations made by Arroyave [17] in Guatemalan preschool children fed under controlled conditions with their usual diet based on corn and beans plus a few vegetables, showed that those who did not suffer from frequent infections during the observation period maintained an acceptable nutritional level and progressed adequately in weight and height. Those suffering from frequent infections did not. These observations strongly suggested that the main mechanism by which infections interfere with adequate nutrition was a voluntary reduction in food intake (anorexia). We recognize that efforts should be made to insure that children living in these conditions should not be deprived of the available foods during infections and particularly during the period of convalescence. In convalescence, if possible, they should be offered even more to allow for recuperation of what they have lost during the period of disease. But it is difficult to accept the suggestion that has been made that the recommended allowances of these children be increased as a means of counterbalancing the effects of infections because, as indicated, anorexia is the main mechanism by which they operate. It is still to be proved that a significant improvement in the quality of the diet could correct this situation. So far all we can conclude is that the control of diarrhoeas and other common infections must be considered necessary to correct malnutrition as it occurs in small children in most developing countries.

In addition to infections, other environmental factors also seem to be operating as determinant or contributing factors to malnutrition in small children. In a small Mexican community, Cravioto compared the past and present characteristics and family circumstances of children who developed severe PCM and of controls matched at birth for gestational age, body weight, and height.[18] The variable most significantly associated with malnutrition was found to be the amount of stimulation in the home and mother's behavior toward her child. Cravioto concluded that the type of child care, as influenced by the general culture of the mother and her contacts with the outside world, could explain the development of severe malnutrition in some families that could otherwise not be differentiated. Cravioto's report provides no direct information on the usual diets of these children. However, he reports that there were no differences in family size, per capita income, and source of income between the families of the children who developed severe PCM and those who did not. It could, therefore, be assumed that the same types of food were available to the two groups of children, as has been frequently observed. The question remains, however, whether or not the inadequate mother-child interaction of the children who developed malnutrition was influenced by their early manifestations of malnutrition as Cravioto himself has previously found. Also, we do not know how valid these observations could be in other sociocultural settings, or to what extent they would apply to the chronic state of subclinical malnutrition affecting the majority of children in poor communities. It may only affect the development of the severe clinical forms. Regardless, Cravioto's observations are important and point to the need for considering in the epidemiology of malnutrition other environmental factors in addition to diet and infections. For instance, recent studies by Viteri [19] have shown that experimental animals (rats) fed a balanced diet in sufficient or restricted amounts and submitted to a program of increased physical activity, grow better than animals restricted in their movements in spite of identical intakes. Observations of children recovering from PCM [20] indicate that they behave in a similar way. Increased physical activity enhances their growth and the repletion of lean body mass. We can assume, therefore, that the physical activity represented by playing and other movement might have a direct effect on the efficiency of nutrient utilization, in addition to offering more opportunities for psychosocial stimuli. It is a common observation that in developing countries small children in poor families usually have less physical activity than children of families with higher income. This is probably because the poorer children are frequently sick or, for cultural or other reasons including space available, opportunities for playing and time devoted to them by other family members are less.

What I am trying to bring out of this discussion is that nutrition is not only a matter of food as is commonly thought. We began by discussing why per capita food availability has no meaning for assessing the existence of malnutrition in preschool age children on a national or community basis, or even on a family basis. We then presented arguments suggesting that for small children, at least, even food availability on an individual basis, and even food intake in certain circumstances, cannot be claimed to be the only factor explaining the existence of malnutrition. This of course has an important bearing on the consideration of measures to control malnutrition. It may explain why efforts to prevent PCM that have been addressed specifically to different aspects of the food problem (i.e., supplementation, enrichment, nutrition education) have so far given very disappointing results.

PREVENTION OF PCM

We recognize that actions carried out directly by the health sector cannot eliminate the problem of PCM. Nevertheless, and even if no other, more fundamental measures are taken, health service actions could significantly improve the situation and at least prevent the appearance of the severe clinical forms and reduce the risk of permanent damage or mortality from associated diseases. At present, the main limitation for the health sector to fulfill this function in most countries is its low coverage. Populations at greatest risk of malnutrition are those with the least access to health services. Even when some types of health services are available to these populations, their functions are often limited to curative services with little or no efforts for prevention. Malnutrition is usually not even recognized unless it is clinically manifested in an advanced form. The provision of basic health services to the entire population could by itself result in a significant improvement in the nutritional situation and could offer the opportunity, not now available, for implementing more direct nutrition-oriented interventions. Provision of such basic health services will require a complete reorganization of the structure and functions of the health delivery system as it now exists in most countries. It requires a shift from a highly specialized, expensive and mainly curative type of system available only to a privileged minority, to generalized services providing basic preventive and curative services to everyone. In order to achieve this, a greater direct community involvement is needed as well as the rational utilization of available resources including adequately trained non-professional workers. Even more fundamentally, it will require a significant reorientation in the socioeconomic developmental policies and therefore the will and capacity of governments to produce these changes.

In reviewing the measures that the health sector could do for the prevention of PCM, I would like to analyze, in the light of what we have learned in the meantime, the measures that we discussed in the paper mentioned earlier, presented to the Academy 20 years ago.[1]

We discussed among the dietary measures to be recommended, particularly for the weaning process, the need for replacing the starchy foods commonly consumed during weaning with other foods that could improve the protein/ energy ratio of the children's usual diet. Primarily for economic reasons, we discarded for most populations in need the possibility of using milk or other foods of animal origin. We were therefore suggesting the possibility of developing nutritionally adequate and less expensive foods based on vegetable sources. Studies to produce what was going to be known later as INCAPARINA were then starting. Formulae to fit different local conditions were afterwards developed and tested. One of them has been in commercial production in Guatemala since 1961.[21] Many other products based on the same principles have since been developed and widely used in different parts of the world.[22] Still new products are being developed and tested.

It has been frequently said that INCAPARINA has been a failure and that the whole approach is wrong. I would like to challenge that statement and to analyze what we have learned from the experience of making such a product commercially available in Guatemala. One judgment of failure is based on the fact that PCM is still prevalent in the country more than 10 years after the product has been available. To this we would argue that INCAPARINA was never developed with the idea that it was going to be *the* solution to the complex socioeconomic problem of malnutrition. The only intention was to make available, using the new scientific and technological knowledge, a food for small children, during and after weaning—a food that would be nutritionally adequate, culturally acceptable, less expensive than other available foods of similar value, and produced locally and with locally available materials. We believe that all these objectives have been achieved. The product is available in stores selling these foods even in the small cities and most villages. It has been well accepted by the population as well as by the physicians and public health personnel who recommend its use. The government and other public and private agencies use it in supplementary feeding programs. The majority, however, is bought directly by the consumers. The sales have been steadily increasing and for many years have reached a level that makes the product, which has never been subsidized, a commercial success in spite of its very low selling price. It may still be asked, as we have done ourselves, who is using it? What has been its impact in nutritional terms for the population of the country? To the first question we can answer that the main users of the product have been low- and middle-income people mainly in the cities. It is bought primarily, though not exclusively, for children. It is not consumed regularly by poor people in the rural areas who could benefit from it, because they are not in the cash economy, but rather on an agricultural subsistence one. This is, of course, an important limitation which, we now understand better, any industrialized product distributed through the regular commercial channels will have. But the product is still helping a significant and important proportion of the population that would otherwise be in a much more difficult situation to feed their children properly, particularly in light of the recent rapid and drastic increase in the price of foods.

It is now thought that particularly for people living on subsistence agriculture, nutritionally adequate food mixtures, prepared at home, with locally available foods (home weaning foods) would be a more practical solution for the weaning of children than industrially prepared foods. This idea, however, has still to be tested under actual field conditions. Even if it is nutritionally and economically feasible, as is probably the case for many population groups, important changes, not easy to achieve, may still be needed in the beliefs and practices of feeding small children.

The answer to the second question of what nutritional impact the availability of the product has had in Guatemala is of course much more difficult. The nutritional situation of the general population has improved in the last 20 years, at least in terms of the incidence of severe forms of PCM, which is now much less frequent than 20 years ago, and in terms of reduction of the rates of mortality of infants and preschool children, which are influenced by malnutrition. We cannot, however, assess how much the availability of INCAPARINA, nor any other single measure, could have contributed to this change. It seems to be more directly related to an increased availability of health and other public services and to improvements in the overall socioeconomic conditions of large sectors of the population.

The second possible preventive measure we considered in our 1957 presentation was that of amino-acid supplementation of staple foods. This was considered as a possibility if the biological value of the dietary proteins was found to be more of a limiting factor than their concentration. A great deal of new knowledge and experience has since been gained on this subject. It has been clearly demonstrated that the utilization of cereal proteins, when tested as the only or main source of proteins in the diets of small childien, can be significantly improved by adding the amino-acids in which they are deficient.[23] However, it has not been possible to demonstrate this beneficial effect when dealing with mixed diets as commonly used. The amino-acid deficits of the staple may be in this case corrected by the other foods; or other amino-acids or total protein concentration may become more limiting.

In fact two recent large field trials of lysine supplementation of rice and wheat have to our knowledge failed to show any improvement in the nutritional situation of the populations living with these cereals as the staple.[24] In our opinion, however, these results should not be interpreted as indicating that the protein quality and concentration of these diets are adequate or that they could not be improved. As we have discussed earlier, there are other factors of cultural or environmental nature or related to the foods themselves that limit the total food consumption of the children. Under these circumstances, we cannot expect benefits from improving protein quality or even concentration if the total energy intake is below the requirements for these children.

Another possible action that we discussed for the prevention of PCM in our previous presentation was nutrition education. I believe that in spite of large and sometimes costly efforts in this direction, we have indeed advanced very little. We do not understand the real need and value of this measure, and if so how it could best be implemented. We also do not have clear objective evidence of its possible role in preventing PCM as it occurs in developing countries. Most probably, if properly oriented and conducted, nutrition education can contribute. But I believe that here again its role as *the* required solution of the problem has been overemphasized. A better knowledge of nutrition would not overcome the scarcity of foods in amount and in variety for the family as a whole if this scarcity is primarily related to economical limitations. Nor could it overcome the reduced intake of small children due to infections and other factors that we have discussed. In fact, we believe that in most instances mothers know enough to feed their children better than they do. If they do not apply this knowledge, it is frequently because they do not have the resources and other facilities to do so. Under these circumstances, nutrition education could therefore be useful only as a supportive measure to more fundamental actions oriented to correct the basic responsible factors, which have been indicated in the previous sections.

Finally, in our 1957 presentation we said that "efforts directed towards improving environmental sanitation and controlling communicable diseases should considerably reduce the number of children developing kwashiorkor, even though they will not eliminate the chronic malnutrition present in most children in rural and poor urban groups in the so-called underdeveloped areas." This statement is as valid today as it was 20 years ago. As we have indicated earlier, we believe now that if the diarrhoea and other infections these children are so frequently suffering from were controlled, not only would the severe forms of PCM be less frequent, but also their overall nutritional situation would be improved.

Another measure that has been widely implemented for the past 20 years is direct supplementary feeding for children and other persons at risk. This measure is not being discussed here because we do not think that it can be included among the measures for the control of PCM; that is, it cannot help to eliminate its responsible factors. It is at most a palliative need, which indicates our failure in implementing effective preventive measures.

We can then conclude that we have not really advanced much in terms of designing effective actions for the control of PCM. We are, in regard to this problem, almost where we were 20 years ago. We have learned that some actions based on the present scientific knowledge and technological developments could help; but what has only been clarified and strengthened with the experience gained is our conviction that the fundamental causes of the problem are of social and economic nature and that these factors are the ones limiting the possibility of effectively applying available knowledge. Let us hope that 20 years from now other people discussing this subject will have more positive experiences to analyze.

186 Annals New York Academy of Sciences

REFERENCES

1. BÉHAR, M., *et al.* 1958. Principles of treatment and prevention of severe protein malnutrition in children (kwashiorkor). Ann. N.Y. Acad. Sci. **69:** 954–968.
2. MATA, L. J., *et al.* 1974. Antenatal events and post-natal growth of children. Western Hemisphere Nutrition Congress IV. Bal Harbour, Florida. August 1974.
3. LECHTIG, A., *et al.* 1975. Effect of food supplementation during pregnancy on birthweight. Pediatrics **56**(4): 508–520.
4. HABICHT, J. P., *et al.* 1974. Maternal nutrition, birthweight and infant mortality. *In* Size at Birth. K. Elliot & J. Knight, Eds. : 353–377. Associated Scientific Publishers. Amsterdam.
5. CRAVIOTO, J., L. HAMBRAEUS & B. VAHLQUIST, Eds. 1974. Early Malnutrition and Mental Development. The Swedish Nutrition Foundation. Almqvist & Viksell. Uppsala, Sweden.
6. VITERI, F. E. 1976. Definition of the nutrition problem in the labour force. *In* Nutrition and Agricultural Development. N. Scrimshaw & M. Béhar, Eds. : 87–98. Plenum Press. New York.
7. FAULK, W. P., L. J. MATA & G. EDSALL. 1975. Effects of malnutrition on the immune response in humans: a review. Trop. Dis. Bull. **72:** 89–103.
8. CRAVIOTO, J. & E. DELICARDIE. 1972. Environmental correlates of severe clinical malnutrition and language development in survivors from kwashiorkor or marasmus. *In* Nutrition, the Nervous System and Behaviour : 73. PanAmerican Health Organization. Washington, D.C.
9. MCKAY, H., A. MCKAY, & L. SINISTERRA. 1974. Intellectual development of malnourished preschool children in programmes of stimulation and nutritional supplementation. *In* Early Malnutrition and Mental Development. **5:** 226–232.
10. BENGOA, J. M. 1970. Recent trends in public health aspects of protein-calorie malnutrition. WHO Chronicle **24:** 552–561.
11. MAYER, J. 1976. The dimensions of human hunger. Sci. Am. **235**(3): 40–49.
12. FAO. 1975. The State of Food and Agriculture, 1974. Rome.
13. URRUTIA, J. J., *et al.* 1975. Reporte preliminar del Efecto biológico de la Fortificación del Maiz con Harina de Soya y Lisina. Primera Conferencia Latinoamericana sobre la Proteina de Soya. Noviembre 1975, Mexico, D.F.
14. Instituto de Nutrición de Centro America y Panama. Unpublished data.
15. FLORES, M. 1976. Food attitudes to actualize community nutrition education. *In* Nutrition and Agricultural Development. N. S. Scrimshaw & M. Béhar, Eds. : 275–287. Plenum Press. New York.
16. MATAL, L. J. 1977. The Children of Santa Maria Cauqué. MIT Press. Cambridge, Mass. In press.
17. ARROYAV, G. & O. PINEDA. 1974. Experiences with meeting protein requirements of preschool children with diets of corn and beans. Effect of morbidity. *In* Influence of Environmental and Host Factors on Nutritional Requirements. N. Shimazono, Ed. : 121–134. Japanese Panel of Malnutrition. US Japan Cooperative Medical Sciences Programme. Tokyo.
18. CRAVIOTO, J. & E. R. DELICARDIE. 1976. Microenvironmental factors in severe protein-calorie malnutrition. *In* Nutrition and Agricultural Development. N. Scrimshaw & M. Béhar, Eds. : 25–35. Plenum Press. New York.
19. VITERI, F. 1973. Efecto de la Inactividad sobre el Crecimiento de Ratas alimentadas con una dieta adecuada, a niveles de Ingestión calórica normal y restringida. *In* Nuevos Conceptos Sobre Viejos Aspectos de la Desnutrición : 207–229. Academia Mexicana de Pediatria. Mexico.
20. TORUN, B., *et al.* 1975. Effect of physical activity upon growth of children recovering from protein-calorie malnutrition (PCM). Presented at the Xth International Congress of Nutrition, Kyoto, Japan. August 1975.
21. SHAW, R. L. 1973. Incaparina: The market development of a protein food. Tropical Sci. **14**(4): 347–371.

22. DeMaeyer, F. M. 1976. Processed weaning foods. *In* Nutrition in Preventive Medicine. World Health Organization. : 389–405. Monogr. Ser. No. 62. Geneva.
23. Bressani, R., L. G. Elias & R. A. Gomez Brenes. 1971. Improvement of protein quality by amino-acid and protein supplementation. *In* International Encyclopaedia of Food and Nutrition. Nutritional Role of Proteins and Amino Acids. Vol. II, Chapter 10. E. J. Bigwood, Ed. : 475–540. Oxford, England.
24. USAID. Unpublished data.

PRENATAL NUTRITION

E.M. Widdowson

Department of Medicine
Addenbrooke's Hospital
Cambridge, England

The title of my paper, "Prenatal Nutrition," in the context of the subject of this session, "Problems and Solutions in Developing Countries," suggests that my remit is to discuss the effects of deficiencies in the mother's diet on the nutrition of her fetus. In some countries, mothers suffer from a chronic shortage of food during pregnancy as they do during the rest of their lives, but in others, even where protein-energy malnutrition is common in young children, the women are not necessarily malnourished. In southern Uganda, for example, women show no signs of dietary deficiency, although their young children may well be suffering from kwashiorkor.

Undernutrition during pregnancy, whether chronic or acute, is no new problem. There were food shortages in Europe during and after W.W. I, and many papers were published describing the effects of these on the size of the babies at birth. Many of them were inconclusive and contradictory, probably because the conditions were not sufficiently carefully defined. Krogman [1] refers to 29 authors who reported a decrease in birth weight and to another 26 who found no change.

In the period between the two wars many surveys were made to find out the effects of inadequate diets eaten by poor women in various parts of the world on the birth weights of their babies. Some of this work was summarized by Barcroft [2] and Garry & Wood.[3] The conclusion was that children born to women at the lower end of the socioeconomic scale were generally a little lighter at birth than those of women living in more affluent circumstances, and that nutrition was probably one of the responsible factors.

W.W. II again brought food shortages to Europe and other parts of the world. These were sometimes brief and acute and in other instances prolonged but less severe. Into the first class falls the period of hunger in Holland lasting from September 1944 to May 1945, when the transport system was paralyzed by a strike. The well-known papers by Smith [4, 5] showed that there was a sharp decline in birth weight in Rotterdam and The Hague during this time, being at its lowest between December and May. The estimated energy available in the rations for pregnant women during this time was less than 1000 kcal/day. The birth weights rose again as soon as Holland was liberated and food became available. Holmer [6] reached the same conclusions in a different way. He analyzed records of birth weights at another Dutch hospital in The Hague. In the first half of 1945 the number of children under 3000 g at birth was 41% of the total, in 1942 it had been 24%.

Another wartime study was conducted by Antonov,[7] who described the weights of babies born in Leningrad from August 1941 until January 1943. The period of acute food shortage lasted from September 1941 to February 1942. The average birth weight of babies born at the State Pediatric Institute fell by 500 to 600 g during the period of famine, but the decline in birth weight may not have been entirely due to lack of food for, as in other similar studies, the women had many other problems.

Dean [8] took the opportunity while we were working in Germany in 1946–49 to analyze the records of 22,000 births at the maternity hospital in Wuppertal during the years 1937–48. The average birth weight was lowest in 1945, the time of greatest food shortage, when it was 185 g less than it was in 1937. There was also a small reduction in body length. This was in spite of the fact that the rations for pregnant women provided 1000 kcal a day more than those for other adults. However, we know from experience that the mothers in Germany did not eat their extra rations themselves but shared them with the rest of the family.

Smith [4, 5] and Dean [8] realized that average birth weights might be misleading, and they also gave their results in terms of percentiles. Their results are summarized in TABLE 1. At each percentile the weight was lower during the time of greatest food shortage than it had been before the war, and the differences was greater in Holland, where the deprivation was more severe. Following the lead of Lubchenco et al.[9] in Denver, many investigators have constructed fetal growth curves from cross sectional data on birth weights at

TABLE 1

WEIGHTS (IN GRAMS) OF CHILDREN BORN IN THE HAGUE AND WUPPERTAL BEFORE AND DURING THE TIMES OF FOOD SHORTAGE

Percentile	The Hague			Wuppertal		
	1938–39	January-April 1945	Decrease	1937–38	1945	Decrease
10	2920	2680	240	2800	2630	170
25	3130	2910	220	3100	2950	150
50	3440	3200	240	3400	3250	150
75	3760	3440	320	3710	3550	160
90	4000	3640	360	4000	3850	150

various gestational ages in different countries, either using average weights or percentiles. The places and countries from which these originate include Baltimore [10] and Portland [11] in the United States, Canada,[12] Britain,[13] Holland,[14] Japan,[15] Israel,[16] South Africa,[17] India,[18] Brazil,[19] Ceylon,[20] Yugoslavia,[21] and Nigeria,[22] and there are many others. Some of them are summarized by Gruenwald.[23, 24] Of particular interest is the information given by Gruenwald et al.[15] about birth weights in Japan in 1945/46, 1957/58, and 1963/64. Over the first 12 years the mean birth weight at each gestational age from 33 to 43 weeks increased by 100 to 200 g, and this was followed by a smaller increase over the next 6 years. The earlier increase was believed to be indicative of a recovery from wartime deprivation, but there is evidence that the further increase resulted in birth weights that were higher than those before the war.

Investigators in Guatemala have approached the problem experimentally. They gave food supplements to undernourished mothers during pregnancy and found that their babies were heavier than babies born to mothers who had had no supplement. Further the effect on the birth weight was greater with a larger supplement than with a smaller one.[25]

Taking all these investigations together we must conclude that a shortage of food and of total energy in a previously well-nourished population, which includes pregnant women, has led in the past to a reduction in the average weight of the baby at birth, and the greater the deficiency the greater the effect. This has been so even if special rations were provided for pregnant women for, as I have said, in times of food shortage any extra food acquired by one member of the family tends to be shared by all. With the return to plenty there is a recovery of the birth weight to its original average or even above. Similarly, the provision of a dietary supplement to poorly nourished women during pregnancy has resulted in higher birth weights as compared with the birth weights of infants of women whose diets were not supplemented. The changes are not large, but they have been significant, and during the remainder of my talk I am going to discuss the reasons why the nutrition of the mother should affect the birth weight of her baby, and what the consequences of being born small may be.

All the nutrients the fetus needs come ultimately from the mother's blood, and one might suppose that its composition would be important in determining the rate of fetal growth. This is not so, for the composition of the plasma is

TABLE 2

SOME CAUSES OF AN INADEQUATE BLOOD SUPPLY TO THE FETUS
AND CONSEQUENT INTRAUTERINE UNDERNUTRITION

Undernutrition of the mother
A small mother
An inadequate placenta
More than one fetus in the uterus
Implantation at a site where blood supply is poor
Disease of the mother

much the same, not only in women all over the world, but also from one species to another throughout the mammalian kingdom. There are a few instances where the composition of the mother's blood can affect the development of the fetus but, generally speaking, it is the quantity of blood reaching the fetus that determines its rate of growth. This is true within the human species, and it is true when we compare one species with another. Anything that reduces the blood supply to the fetus, therefore, will interfere with its nutrition and hence its growth. Undernutrition does this by causing a fall in cardiac output and blood pressure,[26-28] and this explains at once why the blood supply to the fetus may be low.

Undernutrition of the mother is not the only reason for too small a blood supply. TABLE 2 lists some others, and each may be modified by the mother's state of nutrition. First, the size of the mother. We have to turn to other species for the best demonstration of this. Walton & Hammond[29] crossed very large and small breeds of horses in both directions. The size of the foal at birth hinged on the size of the mother. The Shetland mare, with her small circulatory system and uterine blood supply, produced a much smaller foal than the Shire mare. The former weighed 17 kg, the latter 53 kg. The Shetland mare was able to nourish her fetus as well as she would a pure-bred Shetland fetus, but she could do no more. Her foal was small for nutritional, not genetic reasons, even though the mother herself was well-nourished and genetically small. After birth the genetic influence of the large father became apparent, and the small crossbred foal grew more rapidly than a pure-bred Shetland one. Similar studies have been made on cattle, sheep, and mice.[30-32]

Small women tend to have smaller babies than large ones, whatever the size of the father has been. This has been shown to be true within one country,[19, 33, 34] and also if a small race is compared with a large one.

The placenta is a vital organ so far as nutrition of the fetus is concerned, and one must always remember that the fetus grows its own placenta and probably makes it as large as its nutritional and other possibilities allow. Winick et al.[35] have shown that the weight of the placenta and of its protein and RNA increase linearly to term, but cell division stops about one month before. Some substances, such as oxygen, carbon dioxide, and water diffuse across the placenta in both directions where the fetal and maternal blood streams are in most intimate association; at first sight others such as glucose may appear not to do so because the concentration in the plasma of the human fetus is lower than in maternal plasma. There may be another explanation, however, for the rate of removal of the glucose on the fetal and maternal sides of the placenta may not be the same, and this might explain why in ungulates there is more sugar in maternal than in fetal blood. For other substances there appears to be an active transport mechanism, because they are at a higher concentration in fetal than in maternal plasma. This is true, for example, of amino acids, calcium, phosphorus, and potassium. The placenta itself, moreover, has a high rate of growth and metabolism, particularly in early pregnancy, and it may alter organic substances during their passage through it. Synthesis of proteins, enzymes, nucleic acids, high-energy phosphates, and hormones are all part of the life of the placenta. Anything, therefore, that interferes with the normal development of the placenta is likely to affect the fetus. Generally speaking, a fetus that is small for whatever reason has a small placenta,[36-38] with a smaller vascular bed and less protein and fewer cells in it than a large one.[39] Pathological changes in the placenta such as infarcts, haemangiomas, and areas of premature separation or thrombosis of large fetal blood vessels are likely to lead to fetal undernutrition.[40]

The placenta is a transient organ. It grows, lives its life, and ages like other tissues of the body. One of the signs of aging is the calcification of its blood vessels, which must interfere with the circulation of blood through it. Sometimes the placenta begins to age prematurely, just when the fetal requirements for nutrients are approaching their highest. Even in normal, full-term human births there are signs that the placenta is not able to provide the fetus with enough nutrients to maintain its previous rate of growth, which begins to fall off after about the 36th week.[9, 10, 41] This is even more likely to occur if the baby is not delivered till it is post-mature, and such babies may even lose weight or die of intrauterine anoxia.[42]

The early stages of gestation present the fetus with no nutritional problems, however many there are inside the uterus. Later, however, the number of fetuses sharing the blood supply to the uterus affects the growth of each individual. The weight of the fetus is independent of numbers in the uterus until about the 26th week of gestation, but thereafter twins grow more slowly than singletons, triplets still more slowly, and quadruplets more slowly still.[41] Twins have smaller placentae than singletons, and triplets and quadruplets smaller placentae still.[36, 41] The length of gestation tends to be reduced in multiple pregnancies, and this further limits the weight at birth.

Multiple births do not always produce babies of uniform size. One twin is often larger than the other, and this occurs in animals, too. If, for example, there is one small mouse or piglet in a large litter we know that the embryo is likely to have been implanted at a site in the uterus where the blood supply is not as good as elsewhere. In the pig, placental blood flow has been shown to be positively correlated with the weight of the fetus and the weight of the placenta.[43] Disease of the mother can also hinder the growth of the fetus by reducing the supply of blood to it. Chronic hypertensive cardiovascular disease acts in this way, as does toxaemia if it is prolonged and severe.[44]

There seems no doubt, therefore, that a small blood flow to the placenta and fetus prevents the fetus from attaining its potential size. Why does a reduced blood flow have such a profound influence on fetal growth? Many of the nutrients probably reach the fetus in ample amounts even if the blood supply is small. There must be a limiting nutrient in every case, perhaps a specific amino acid, or all amino acids, or a mineral, or a vitamin, or total energy. Barcroft[45] believed that oxygen was the substance most likely to limit the growth of the fetus, particularly towards the end of gestation; in some species the possibilities for the fetus to get oxygen are almost exhausted by term. The human fetus is protected from hypoxia to some extent by having a special fetal haemoglobin which has a greater affinity for oxygen than adult haemoglobin. Women who live at high altitudes have smaller babies than those who live at sea level,[9] and those who smoke a great deal tend to have smaller babies than those who do not.[46-48] Since a major function of the placenta is to transfer oxygen to the fetus, the effects of very high altitudes are perhaps obvious, but here it is the composition of the mother's blood and the oxygen carried by the haemoglobin that is the trouble. Much work has been done on placental gas exchange in sheep, but here there is a genetic adaptation in some breeds in that they produce a different haemoglobin as the altitude goes up. Hypoxia probably affects the transfer of most nutrients by limiting the provision of energy, for the sodium pump for example. All in all it is not surprising that babies born at high altitudes are a little light in weight. Carbon monoxide, produced by tobacco smoke, has a very high affinity for haemoglobin. It diffuses readily across the placenta, and the concentration of carbon monoxide in fetal blood is generally greater than in the maternal. Carbon monoxide, like high altitudes, may produce relative hypoxia in the fetal tissues and so hinder their growth,[49] but the nicotine from the inhaled cigarette smoke may make matters worse by constricting the blood vessels and so reducing the supply of blood.

In conclusion, I want to say something about the consequences of being born small. All the evidence goes to show that babies born small for their gestational age, for whatever cause, do not grow particularly rapidly after birth. They show no signs of the catch-up growth that is so characteristic of rehabilitation after undernutrition at older ages, and they remain small for a very long time.[50-53] If the father has been tall, his genes may influence the rate of growth after birth, and a small baby may become a tall adult, though perhaps not quite as tall as he might have been had his father married a taller, better nourished, or more healthy wife.

The reason the small baby does not grow very rapidly is because it is not hungry enough to take enough food to enable it to do so. This is more clearly shown by animal experiments.[54] Pigs and guinea pigs that are small at birth remain behind their larger littermates during the whole of the growth period and become smaller adults. On the other hand, children and animals that are deprived of energy when they are older become extremely hungry, and as soon as food is made available they take a great deal of it and consequently gain weight fast.[55, 56] We have suggested that if the individual has been retarded in growth and is therefore small at the age when the appetite centers are developing in the hypothalamus then the appetite will be "set" at a level appropriate to the size and rate of growth at that time.[57] Dörner & Staudt[58] have demonstrated that in man the organization of the nuclei and tracts takes place between the 4th and 7th months of fetal life. Appetite control comes into play immediately after birth. A small size at this time is inevitably associated with an appetite geared to this small size, and hence the baby grows slowly and remains small.

Does this matter? How much of a disadvantage is it to the individual to be undernourished *in utero* and therefore small at birth and small in later life? A small newborn baby or animal has greater problems over thermal regulation and maintenance of blood sugar than a large one but, once the immediate postnatal period is past and so long as nutrition and the environment become satisfactory, there seems no particular disadvantage in growing along the 40th rather than the 60th percentile. It is true that the organs of a small individual are small, and if taken out of the body and analyzed they might be condemned as having fewer cells in them than in those of larger ones, but as far as we know these small organs are quite capable of performing their proper physiological functions in the small individual to which they belong.

What happens to the child after birth is far more important for its physical and mental well-being than what happens to it before. In the uterus it is protected to a large extent, however poor the environment into which it will be born. Nutrition may be a little inadequate, but never as inadequate as it can be after birth. Moreover, mental stimulation, which is so important in development after birth, plays little or no part before birth, and if it plays any part it is the same for all. A big newborn baby may be desirable and beautiful, but the small one is beautiful also, in babies as in businesses, and both large and small need the same good nourishment and mental stimulation if they are to fulfill the potential with which they have been endowed.

REFERENCES

1. KROGMAN, W. M. 1941. Growth of Man. Vol. 20 of Tabulae Biologicae. Junk. Den Haag, The Netherlands.
2. BARCROFT, J. 1946. Researches in Pre-natal Life. Blackwell Scientific Publications. Oxford.
3. GARRY, R. C. & H. O. WOOD. 1946. Dietary requirements in human pregnancy and lactation. A review of recent work. Nutr. Abstr. Rev. **15**: 591–621.
4. SMITH, C. A. 1947a. Effects of maternal undernutrition upon the newborn infant in Holland (1944–45). J. Pediatr. **30**: 229–243.
5. SMITH, C. A. 1947b. The effect of wartime starvation in Holland upon pregnancy and its product. Am. J. Obstet. Gynecol. **53**: 599–606.
6. HOLMER, A. J. M. 1949. De voeding in de Zwangerschap. Voeding **10**: 134–139.
7. ANTONOV, A. N. 1947. Children born during the siege of Leningrad in 1942. J. Pediatr. **30**: 250–259.

8. DEAN, R. F. A. 1951. The size of the baby at birth and the yield of breast milk. *In* Studies of Undernutrition, Wuppertal 1946–9. Spec. Rep. Ser. Med. Res. Coun. No. 275: 346–378. HMSO. London.
9. LUBCHENCO, L. O., C. HANSMAN, M. DRESSLER & E. BOYD. 1963. Intrauterine growth as estimated from live-born birth weight data at 24 to 42 weeks of gestation. Pediatrics (N.Y.) 32: 793–800.
10. GRUENWALD, P. 1966. Growth of the human fetus. I. Normal growth and its variation. Am. J. Obstet. Gynecol. 94: 1112–1119.
11. BABSON, S. G., R. E. BEHRMAN & R. LESSEL. 1970. Fetal growth: liveborn birth weights for gestational age of white middle class infants. Pediatrics (N.Y.) 45: 937–944.
12. USHER, R. & F. McLEAN. 1969. Intrauterine growth of liveborn Caucasian infants at sea level: standards obtained from measurements in 7 dimensions of infants born between 25 and 44 weeks of gestation. J. Pediatr. 74: 901–910.
13. THOMSON, A. M., W. Z. BILLEWICZ & F. E. HYTTEN. 1968. The assessment of fetal growth. J. Obstet. Gynaecol. Br. Commonw. 75: 903–916.
14. KLOOSTERMAN, G. J. 1966. Prevention of prematurity. Ned. Tijdschr. Verloskd. Gynaecol. 66: 361–379.
15. GRUENWALD, P., H. FUNAKAWA, S. MITANI, T. NISHIMURA & S. TAKEUCHI. 1967. Influences of environmental factors of foetal growth in man. Lancet 1: 1026–1029.
16. TSAFRIR, J. & I. HALBRECHT. 1973. Birth weight in various populations in Israel. Soc. Biol. 20: 71–81.
17. JAROSZEWICZ, A. M., D. E. W. SCHUMANN & M. P. KEET. 1975. Intrauteriene grocistandaarde van Kaapse Kleurling babas. S. Afr. Med. J. 49: 568–572.
18. LAKSHMINARAYANA, P., S. NAGASAMY & V. B. RAJU. 1974. Foetal growth as assessed by anthropometric measurements. Indian Pediatr. 11: 803–810.
19. ARAUJO, A. M. DE & F. M. SALZANO. 1975. Parental characteristics and birthweight in a Brazilian population. Hum. Biol. 47: 37–43.
20. SOYSA, P. E. & D. S. JAYASURIYA. 1975. Birth weight in Ceylonese. Hum. Biol. 47: 1–15.
21. NIKOLÍC, L. 1973. Intrauterini rast zivorodene dece. Jugosl. Pedijatriya 16: 131–139.
22. BRUETON, M. J. 1975. The use of clinical gestational age assessment in the construction of standards for birthweight in a rural Nigerian community. Acta Paediatr. (Stockholm) 64: 537–540.
23. GRUENWALD, P. 1968a. Growth Pattern of the Normal and Deprived Fetus. *In* Aspects of Prematurity and Dysmaturity. J. H. P. Jonxis, H. K. A. Visser & J. A. Troelstra, Eds. : 37–45. H E. Stenfert Kroese. Leiden, The Netherlands.
24. GRUENWALD, P. 1974. Pathology of the deprived fetus and its supply line. *In* Size at Birth : 3–19. Ciba Foundation Symposium 27. Associated Scientific Publishers. Amsterdam, The Netherlands.
25. HABICHT, J. P., A. LECHTIG, C. YARBROUGH & R. E. KLEIN. 1974. Maternal Nutrition, Birth Weight and Infant Mortality. *In* Size at Birth : 353–377. Ciba Foundation Symposium 27. Associated Scientific Publishers. Amsterdam, The Netherlands.
26. LANDES, G. & R. ARNOLD. 1946–47. Weitere Untersuchungen über den Kreislauf bei Ödemkrankheit. Klin. Wochenschr. 24/25: 654–657.
27. KEYS, A., A. HENSCHEL & H. L. TAYLOR. 1947. The size and function of the human heart at rest in semi-starvation and in subsequent rehabilitation. Am. J. Physiol. 150: 153–169.
28. HOWARTH, S. 1951. Cardiac output and the peripheral circulation. *In* Studies of Undernutrition, Wuppertal 1946–9. Spec. Rep. Ser. Med. Res. Coun. No. 275: 238–258. HMSO. London.
29. WALTON, A. & J. HAMMOND. 1938. The maternal effect on growth and conformation in Shire horse-Shetland pony crosses. Proc. R. Soc. London Ser. B. 125: 311–334.

30. JOUBERT, D. M. & J. HAMMOND. 1958. A cross breeding experiment with cattle with special reference to the maternal effect in South Devon—Dexter crosses. J. Agric. Sci. (Camb.) **51:** 325–341.

31. HUNTER, G. L. 1957. The maternal influence on size in sheep. J. Agric. Sci. (Camb.) **48:** 36–60.

32. DICKINSON, A. G. 1960. Some genetic implications of maternal effects. An hypothesis of mammalian growth. J. Agric. Sci. (Camb.) **54:** 378–390.

33. McKEOWN, T. & R. G. RECORD. 1954. Influence of pre-natal environment on correlation between birth weight and parental height. Am. J. Hum. Genet. **6:** 457–463.

34. CAWLEY, R. H., T. McKEOWN & R. G. RECORD. 1954. Parental stature and birth weight. Am. J. Hum. Genet. **6:** 448–456.

35. WINICK, M., A. COSCIA & A. NOBLE. 1967. Cellular growth in human placenta. 1. Normal placental growth. Pediatrics **39:** 248–251.

36. McKEOWN, T. & R. G. RECORD. 1953a. The influence of placental size on foetal growth in man with special reference to multiple pregnancy. J. Endocrinol. **9:** 418–426.

37. McKEOWN, T. & R. G. RECORD. 1953b. The influence of placental size on foetal growth according to sex and order of birth. J. Endocrinol. **10:** 73–81.

38. IYENGAR, L. 1973. Chemical composition of placenta in pregnancies with small-for-date infants. Am. J. Obstet. Gynecol. **116:** 66–70.

39. WINICK, M. 1967. Cellular growth of human placenta. III. Intrauterine growth failure. J. Pediatr. **71:** 390–395.

40. GRUENWALD, P. 1968b. Problems in the pathologic study of the placenta. *In* Aspects of Prematurity and Dysmaturity. J. H. P. Jonxis, H. K. A. Visser & J. A. Troelstra, Eds. : 21–23. H. E. Stenfert Kroese. Leiden, The Netherlands.

41. McKEOWN, T. & R. G. RECORD. 1952. Observations on foetal growth in multiple pregnancy in man. J. Endocrinol. **8:** 386–401.

42. CLIFFORD, S. H. 1954. Postmaturity—with placental dysfunction. J. Pediatr. **44:** 1–13.

43. COOPER, J. E., I. R. McFADYEN & R. WOOTTON. 1976. Measurement of placental blood flow in the pig and its relation to foetal development. Communication given to the Neonatal Society, London. November 4th.

44. LUBCHENCO, L. O., C. HANSMAN & L. BÄCKSTRÖM. 1968. Factors influencing fetal growth. *In* Aspects of Prematurity and Dysmaturity. J. H. P. Jonxis, H. K. A. Visser & J. A. Troelstra, Eds. : 149–166 H. E. Stenfert Kroese. Leiden, The Netherlands.

45. BARCROFT, J. 1944. Nutritional functions of the placenta. Proc. Nutr. Soc. **2:** 14–18.

46. LOWE, C. R. 1959. Effect of mother's smoking habits on birth weight of their children. Br. Med. J. **ii:** 673–676.

47. HERRIOT, A., W. Z. BILLEWICZ & F. E. HYTTEN. 1962. Cigarette smoking in pregnancy. Lancet **i:** 771–773.

48. LONGO, L. D. 1970. Carbon monoxide in the pregnant mother and fetus and its exchange across the placenta. Ann. N.Y. Acad. Sci. **174:** 313–341.

49. FORSTER, R. E. 1973. Some principles governing maternal—foetal transfer in the placenta. *In* Proc. Sir Joseph Barcroft Centenary Symposium. R. S. Comline, K. W. Cross, G. S. Dawes & P. W. Nathanielsz, Eds. : 223–237. Cambridge University Press. Cambridge.

50. DRILLIEN, C. M. 1970. The small-for-date infant: etiology and prognosis. Pediatr. Clin. North Am. **17:** 9–24.

51. BABSON, S. G. & D. S. PHILLIPS. 1973. Growth and development of twins dissimilar in size at birth. New Engl. J. Med. **289:** 937–940.

52. BECK, G. J. & B. J. VAN DEN BERG. 1975. The relationship of the rate of intrauterine growth of low-birth-weight infants to later growth. J. Pediatr. **86:** 504–511.

53. BJERRE, I. 1975. Physical growth of 5-year-old children with a low birth weight. Stature, weight, circumference of head and osseous development. Acta Paediatr. (Stockholm) **64:** 33–43.
54. WIDDOWSON, E. M. 1974. Immediate and long-term consequences of being large or small at birth. A comparative approach. *In* Size at Birth. Ciba Foundation Symposium 27 (New Series). K. Elliott & J. Knight, Eds. : 65–82. Elsevier. The Netherlands.
55. RUTISHAUSER, I. H. E. & R. A. McCANCE. 1968. Calorie requirements for growth after severe undernutrition. Arch. Dis. Child. **43:** 252–256.
56. ASHWORTH, A. 1919. Growth rates in children recovering from protein-calorie malnutrition. Br. J. Nutr. **23:** 835–845.
57. WIDDOWSON, E. M. & R. A. McCANCE. 1975. A review: New thoughts on growth. Pediatr. Res. **9:** 154–156.
58. DÖRNER, G. & J. STAUDT. 1972. Vergleichende morphologische Untersuchungen der Hypothalamus differenzierung bei Ratte und Mensch. Endokrinologie **59:** 152–155.

INFANT FEEDING IN NATIONAL AND INTERNATIONAL PERSPECTIVE: AN EXAMINATION OF THE DECLINE IN HUMAN LACTATION, AND THE MODERN CRISIS IN INFANT AND YOUNG CHILD FEEDING PRACTICES

Michael C. Latham

Division of Nutritional Sciences
Cornell University
Ithaca, New York 14853

Indications are that world yields of cereal grains, and that of many other major food crops, will be gratifyingly high in 1976. However, this has been a disastrously bad year in the world as far as human breast milk production is concerned. Our estimates indicate that total world production of human breast milk may be 12 billion liters short of production potential. This "loss" in monetary terms is in the order of $6 billion. Whereas total grain production has steadily increased over the last four decades, total production of breast milk has declined quite dramatically.

At this moment in 1976 there are probably over 120 million infants alive in the world. If all their mothers were in full lactation, providing appropriate quantities of milk for them, they would during the year produce over 30 billion liters of milk. This would provide 22,500 billion kilocalories and 400 billion grams of protein. The value of this milk at U.S. supermarket prices for whole fluid cow's milk would be about $15 billion, and yet the cow's milk would provide less energy than the human milk.

Since W.W. II a network of some 10 excellent international research centers has been established around the world with the objective of conducting research designed to improve food production, and to increase yields of specific food crops. IRRI in the Philippines and CIMMYT in Mexico are perhaps the best known. These 10 centers together are working on rice, maize, wheat, millet, sorghum, legumes, potatoes, vegetables, and animal production. The total budget of these centers in 1975 was about $50 million.[1] Where is there a comparable institute conducting research to help ensure an adequate supply of breast milk? There is no such institute, yet breast milk is the only natural food product that is complete in its content of nutrients, that can serve as the only food of a human during his period of most rapid growth, and that is produced on every continent.

We have on our hands a crisis in infant feeding practices and yet one that has neither caught the headllines nor interested the economists, despite its huge economic implications, and it is an issue that most nutritionists have ignored.

THE PRESENT WORLD SITUATION

What is the present global situation with regard to breast milk production? We can only make educated guesses because food production figures, be they Food Balance Sheets or other reports, seldom include breast milk.

The world can be divided into three perhaps unequal groups. There are those areas first where the majority now bottle-feed their infants, second those where breast-feeding remains the principal means of infant feeding, and a third intermediate group that are mainly in transition from breast to bottle.

It is clear that almost all of North America, Western Europe, and Australasia have become arid zones and fall into the first group. Their yield of breast milk in relation to their populations is extremely low. Only a few oases remain in these continents. In several Caribbean nations, in certain parts of Latin America, in some Asian countries such as Hong Kong and Singapore, and in a number of urban centers elsewhere only a minority of mothers are still breast-feeding their 3-month-old infants. These nations and communities also fit into the first group.

The second group where breast-feeding still predominates includes a large part of Asia including China and India, the world's most populous nations, and nearly all of black and brown Africa.

The third group where bottle-feeding is to a greater or lesser extent replacing breast-feeding includes many urban populations in Asia and Africa, much of Central and South America, and some of Eastern Europe.

In very few countries are there any regular collection and publication of figures on rates and duration of breast-feeding. The World Health Organization is now sponsoring a study on breast-feeding in several countries. To illustrate the situation in a few countries figures are presented from studies undertaken by our group at Cornell. These are based often on small samples, and in all cases the data were collected as part of a nutrition study not related to the prevalence of breast-feeding (TABLE 1).

TABLE 1

LENGTH OF BREAST-FEEDING IN DIFFERENT COUNTRIES *

Country, Author, Year and Number	Never Breast-Fed (%)	Age Breast-Feeding Stopped		
		0–5 Months (%)	6–12 Months (%)	Over 12 Months
Colombia (Englberger) 1972 (N=135)	9	26	51	14
Hong Kong (Woo) 1974 (N=113)	50	32	18	0
N.E. Brazil (Drummond) 1974 (N=82)	—	13	79	8
India-Punjab (Levinson) 1971 (N=496)	—	near zero	8	92
Jamaica (Evans) 1972 (N=91)	—	24	64	12
Jamaica (Almroth) 1976 (N=138)	—	26	52	20
Philippines (Popkin) 1975 (N=314)	—	12	11	77

* Data are taken from unpublished studies (Masters degree or Ph.D. theses) done at Cornell.

TABLE 2

LENGTH OF BREAST-FEEDING IN ST. VINCENT *

	Age Breast-Feeding Stopped		
	0–4 Months (%)	5–12 Months (%)	Over 12 Months (%)
1967 (Beaudry) N=163	15	69	16
1974 (Greiner) N=193	31	54	15

* From T. Greiner, "Commercial infant foods and malnutrition in St. Vincent." Presented at Am. Anthropol. Assoc. Mtg. Washington, D.C., Nov. 18, 1976.

In St. Vincent, where we have had surveys in 1968 and 1974, an apparent decline in the duration of breast feeding is seen (TABLE 2).[4]

TRANSITION IN INDUSTRIALIZED COUNTRIES

The change from breast to bottle in the industrialized countries of North America and Western Europe was not without its serious problems, ones that are similar to those encountered now in the developing countries or poor communities where today the bottle has replaced the breast.

In Chicago in 1934 mortality per 1000 infants in the first 9 months of life was 10 times as high in artificially fed than in partially breast-fed infants, and 50 times higher than in totally breast-fed children.[2] In a study of feeding in relation to morbidity and mortality of infants from birth to 7 months in Liverpool from 1936 to 1942, morbidity per 1000 was twice as high and mortality more than five times as high in bottle fed as in breast-fed infants.[3]

TRANSITION IN DEVELOPING COUNTRIES

Among countries that have moved rapidly from breast- to bottle-feeding, the situation has been well documented in Chile. The very rapid decline in rates of breast-feeding there should prevent complacency in any nation where the prevalence of breast-feeding remains high. In Chile in 1960 over 90 percent of infants were breast-fed, and just 8 years later it is reported that fewer than 10 percent were breast-fed. Mortality rates at 3 months of age were 2.5 times higher for both bottle-fed and partially breast-fed, compared with children who were breast-fed only.

In Mexico over 95 percent of infants at 6 months of age were breast-fed in 1960, and this had dropped to about 40 percent in 1966. In Singapore some 80 percent of 3-month-old infants were breast-fed in 1951 and approximately 5 percent in 1971. There is evidence from many other countries of this very rapid transition.[5] It is often accompanied by greatly increased morbidity and mortality due to gastrointestinal infections, malnutrition, and other conditions.

SITUATION IN SOME SOCIALIST COUNTRIES

A country that has undergone rapid industrialization and where this transition from breast to bottle has apparently not occurred is the People's Republic of China. Reports indicate that by far the majority of Chinese infants are breast-fed. The government has taken steps to allow the high number of working mothers to bring their babies to work, to have them well cared for, and to be breast-fed there.[6] Knowledgeable visitors returning from China are impressed by the health and growth of young children, and by reports of incredibly low infant mortality rates from certain cities from which figures are available. Infant and toddler mortality rates for the whole of the People's Republic of China do not seem to be available.

In the Soviet Union and some Eastern European countries, including Poland and Yugoslavia, similar encouragement is given to breast-feeding, but the breast-feeding rates are apparently lower than in China, though much higher than in the countries of Western Europe at comparable stages of industrialization.

REASONS FOR THE DECLINE IN BREAST FEEDING

It is often assumed that a decline in breast-feeding is almost inevitable where there is industrialization and urbanization, where many women are employed in the labor force, and where raised incomes and "modernizing" influences are improving the quality of life. There is a tendency to state that bottle-feeding is an inevitable accompaniment of development. I wish to dispute this dogma before it becomes entrenched.

It is worth examining the reasons commonly given by mothers for discontinuing breast feeding. A partial review of the literature by Almroth[7] is given in TABLE 3. This shows that mothers' employment was given as the reason for weaning the child from the breast in, at most, 6 percent of cases.

An examination of the present pattern of breast- and bottle-feeding in the world shows that there is a poor correlation between, for example, levels of industrialization or of female employment and rates of bottle-feeding. The first five nations in the world to develop nuclear bombs were the U.S., Russia, Great Britain, France, and China. Three of these countries feed most of their infants from the bottle and two from the breast. Peking is as industrialized as Paris; Moscow is as urbanized as Manchester; and Leningrad has a higher rate of working women than does Los Angeles. Yet the majority of infants in Peking, Moscow, and Leningrad are breast-fed, whereas in Paris, Manchester, and Los Angeles the huge majority are bottle-fed.

If factors such as industrialization, urbanization, and women in the labor force are not the major determinants of the shift from breast to bottle, what can we conclude from the different patterns of infant feeding in the world? Clearly in the examples given above the differences are in part at least ideological and political. In general, then, the industrialized countries where bottle-feeding is now the rule are capitalist and those where breast-feeding remains common are socialist. However, some socialist countries are among those in transition from breast to bottle, and in many capitalist countries, all of them developing, breast-feeding predominates. Surely we are not willing to capitulate and state that bottle-feeding with its attendant high rates of infant morbidity and mortality is an inevitable component of a capitalist or non-socialist system. In Norway and Sweden—democratic countries with a free enterprise system— there has been a very significant shift from bottle- to breast-feeding in the period since 1970. In Israel, also, breast-feeding is widely practiced.

Four conditions that are important in the spread of bottle-feeding are:

1. An absence of legislation or government action to ensure optimum care for infants and children of mothers in the labor force.

2. A medical care system that concentrates on curative, not preventive, medicine, where doctors have a strong professional organization that sometimes acts against the public welfare, and where profits from private medical care are high.

TABLE 3

COMMONLY GIVEN REASONS FOR WEANING FROM BREAST *

	Baby Old Enough or Weaned Self (%)	Illness of Mother or Child (%)	Insuff. Breast Milk (%)	Pregnancy (%)	Work (%)	Other (%)
Philippines (Guthrie, 1964) N=245	26	6	7	37	6	18
Colombia (Meija, 1968) N=200	21	9	32	16	3	19
Nigeria (Ransome-Kuti, 1968) N=200	44	4	—	2	0	50
St. Vincent (Greiner, 1976) N=176	42	9	1	7	6	35
Jamaica (Almroth, 1976)	35	15	17	0	6	27

* From Almroth.[7]

3. A system that encourages private industry to act aggressively to change dietary practices in the interests of profits and with disregard for human health and welfare.

4. A government that is unduly influenced by large industrial corporations and is reluctant to control them or their promotion of infant foods even in the public interest.

Developing countries where breast-feeding predominates, and where there is real concern about infant and child health, could take steps to slow, or reverse, the trend towards the bottle, and this would not require a political revolution. A democratic capitalist country could:

1. Examine the system of mass communications and regulate these so that they serve the public good.

2. Take appropriate measures to ensure that the infants and children of working mothers get adequate care, including the right to be breast-fed.

3. Insist that the medical profession exert a positive, not a negative, influence on the practice of breast-feeding.

4. Consider appropriate legislation to control the promotion or even the availability of breast-milk substitutes (for example, newly independent Guinea-Bissau has taken the radical step of making these available only on prescription) and limit the influence and power of transnational corporations and of national food manufacturers.

5. Introduce an education campaign aimed at maintaining high rates of breast-feeding.

ADVERSE RESULTS OF SHIFT FROM BREAST TO BOTTLE

Many of the adverse consequences resulting from bottle-feeding by low-income mothers have been well documented elsewhere.[8, 9] These include:

1. Development of protein-calorie malnutrition, especially nutritional marasmus, due mainly to overdilution of high-cost breast-milk substitutes.

2. A very high prevalence of diarrhea and gastrointestinal infections in bottle-fed infants due to contamination of the formula or bottle in households where facilities are poor and knowledge of hygiene is low.

3. A reduced immunity to disease because no formula provides the immune globulins and white cells of colostrum or early breast milk.

4. A lower level of mother-infant contact and interaction, with consequent effects on behavioral development.

5. An increased risk of obesity.

6. Earlier return of ovulation and therefore greater risk of early pregnancy.

These serious consequences due to inappropriate bottle-feeding, though well described, have not been adequately assimilated by physicians and by health policy makers. In many countries, bottle-feeding may be the major indirect cause of infant morbidity and mortality, yet steps to control it attract little attention, and few health dollars are used for its control. In a large part of the developing world, breast-feeding may be preventing more births than are all other family planning efforts combined, including the pill, IUD, condom, and abortions. Yet breast-feeding is hardly considered in population-control programs, and protection or promotion of breast-feeding figures not at all in the huge family-planning budgets of most countries.

ECONOMICS FOR THE FAMILY AND THE NATION

Among the most serious adverse consequences of the decline in breast-feeding are the economic ones for the family and the nation. These continue to be relatively ignored.

Over 10 years ago, while working in Tanzania, I published evidence to indicate that the cost of adequately bottle-feeding a 6-month-old infant was equivalent to half the minimum wage of that country.[10] The minimum wage in Tanzania, like that in many countries, is higher than the mean family income. How can a family allow over half their income to be spent on the food for their youngest member? It was also estimated in that same year that the production of human milk on the mainland of Tanzania was 40 million gallons, worth perhaps U.S. $22 million, if it had to be replaced with powdered cow's milk, which would have needed to be imported.

The situation has not changed much in 1976. In Kenya this year we worked on a World Bank Study where adult road workers were paid 6 shillings (about 80 U.S. cents per day). The cost of a suitable manufactured milk formula fed in adequate amounts would cost over half this amount (TABLE 4).

Apparently the situation is much worse in India. Reutlinger and Selowsky [11] have undertaken an interesting study on nutrition and poverty. In an examination of data from Calcutta, they suggest that about 50 percent of an employed mother's earnings will be needed to replace breast milk not provided, assuming

TABLE 4

COST OF BOTTLE-FEEDING RELATIVE TO WAGES

	Approx. Monthly Wage	Cost of Formula or Milk	Required Marginal Propensity to Spend on Milk	Percent of Wage
Tanzania * (1964) (Latham)	132 Shs.	68 Shs.	0.51	51%
Kenya * (1976) (Latham)	150 Shs.	88 Shs.	0.58	58%
India * (1976) (Reutlinger and Selowsky)	120 Rs.	91.5 Rs.	0.76	76%

* Tanzania and Kenya data based on cost of manufactured powdered formula; India data on cow's milk.

that she continues to breast-feed while at home. My calculations from their data indicate that if she stopped breast-feeding altogether and used cow's milk, she would spend 75 percent of her income, and if she used a manufactured product, she would have to use her whole income. Why should any woman go to work, often at an unpleasant job, and spend her entire income on a replacement for breast milk? This is an example of all cost and no benefit.

Reutlinger and Selowsky [11] show from these Calcutta data that the marginal propensity to spend on infant foods from additional family income is extremely low and only about 5 percent. This means that for every additional 100 rupees earned, only 5 rupees would be spent on infant foods. They conclude that higher incomes of the kind described not only may fail to reduce malnutrition, but on the contrary may increase infant undernutrition.

It is worth citing another example where employment of mothers, although increasing income, had the result of reducing nutrient intakes of young children. In a vitamin A research project in the Philippines in which we have been following 1700 children in 12 areas for 3 years, we too have found a negative nutritional impact resulting from employment of women in the labor force. Our interest was in consumption of vitamin A by study children. Our findings indicate that employment of mothers increased family income but reduced by almost half the vitamin A intake of young children.

COMMERCIOGENIC NUTRITIOUS FOODS

In 1971 Jelliffe [12] first coined the term "commerciogenic malnutrition" and "commerciogenic nutritious foods." He was referring to the increased production and use of commercially produced foods often high in their protein content being marketed as weaning foods. They include milk products for infant use, semisolid manufactured weaning foods, high-protein snack foods and beverages, various commercial mixtures of cereal, legume, and oil-seed flours, and similar products.

TABLE 5

COST OF PURCHASING 1000 KCAL AND 100 GRAMS PROTEIN
USING SELECTED FOODS

	Rupees per 1000 Cal.	Rupees per 100 g Protein
Processed commercial products		
Uniprotein	2.9	8.0
Proteinex	7.9	9.8
Skim milk powder	1.7	1.7
Multimixes (non-commercial)		
Hyderabad mix	0.3	0.9
Family purchases		
Normal diet	0.2	0.6
(Bottom 30% of incomes)		

We have examined the limitations and dangers of the use of these commercially marketed products by poor families in low-income countries. Clearly, the disadvantages found are not applicable to situations such as famines where there may be a free distribution, or government programs where there is a marked subsidization of these products.

In a simulation study,[13] we investigated the likely nutritional effect of the purchase and use of certain commerciogenic nutritious foods available in India. In the 30 percent of poorest families a survey in Maharashtra showed that 80 percent of income was spent on food and 20 percent on essential nonfood items. It is assumed that if commercial infant or weaning foods are purchased, the money will come from the 80% used for food expenditures. These low-income families using traditional foods purchase 1000 cals. at a cost of 0.2 rupees and 100 grams of protein for 0.6 rupees. The cost of 1000 cals. and of 100 grams of protein from commerciogenic high-protein foods is shown to be 14 to 40 times higher and for 100 grams of protein to be 6 to 20 times higher than in traditionally purchased foods (TABLE 5). Therefore, the diversion of any money spent on traditional foods will result in a reduction of not only calories but also of protein for the family. The purchase of these so-called low-cost/high-protein nutritious foods is apparently having a markedly negative nutritional effect in India. Examination of the situation in Kenya and the Philippines reveals a similar situation. It is likely to be so in nearly all low-income countries where poor families get most of their calories, protein, and other nutrients from locally produced foods.

Yet the rationale for the development of these low-cost nutritious foods has been the need to reduce malnutrition. International and bilateral assistance has been given to help in their development. There are serious dangers in the continuation of such efforts. Again, the commercial advertising and promotion of these products has often been aggressive, they have sometimes been un-truthful, and they have influenced the poor to purchase them. It is often falsely suggested that the commercial product is nutritionally superior to cheaper products that are customarily consumed in the community.

Powerful messages are used to convince parents that product X will result in good health, improved stamina, and increased growth of children. No consideration is given to the fact that the purchasing of product X will result in the replacement of some traditional food. By buying a package of a commercial food the poor are perverting their overall food budget. The replacement as we have shown will all too often result in the availability of fewer calories and of less protein and other nutrients than in their original food purchases.

The beneficiaries, as in the case of infant formulas, are of course the commercial companies, including several of the transnational corporations [14] and sometimes also countries like the U.S. who are the main producers of soybeans, which are often included in these products.

WATER REQUIREMENTS OF INFANTS

It is the practice at many clinics where infants are brought for weighing, for immunization, or for treatment, for mothers to be advised to give water or some other fluid between feeds from the breast or the bottle. In many countries women do fairly early in the infant's life give water, tea or bush teas, glucose water, or other fluids.

Persons concerned with the danger of diarrhea from bottle feeding are also concerned about the contamination of other fluids given to the infant. Clearly products like tea or bush tea, where the water is heated, are safer than plain water. Our interest is greater in breast-fed than bottle-fed infants because the latter are already at high risk from diarrhea.

Little research has been undertaken to determine whether breast-fed babies in tropical countries actually require extra water. Almroth,[7] working with us at Cornell, undertook calculations on water intake, evaporative and fecal water losses, and of water available for excretion of renal solutes. Her data are shown in TABLE 6.

Since the renal solute load was 77 mOSm, the urinary concentration would be 344 mOSm/1000 ml. A baby's kidneys can produce a urine with an osmolar concentration of 1300 to 1400 mOSm per 1000 ml. Therefore, a 4-month-old exclusively breast-fed infant could, in theory, manage without additional water. This has now been tested in the field in Jamaica (by Almroth) under conditions of high temperature. Urine specimens collected for specific gravity in children who were breast-fed but did not receive other fluids were tested. Although the work is not complete, this indicates that breast-fed children do not need additional fluid. Breast milk alone is adequate. Apparently, a similar study in an arid area of Argentina is also underway.[15]

MILK IN THE TREATMENT OF PROTEIN-CALORIE MALNUTRITION (PCM)

There has been considerable concern that because lactose intolerance is prevalent in nonwhite populations throughout the world, milk might be an inappropriate product either in the treatment or prevention of PCM in Africa, Asia, and Latin America. Our research at Cornell,[16] which has been corroborated elsewhere, suggests that most subjects that have flat lactose tolerance curves and evidence of lactose intolerance can in fact consume nutritionally useful quantities of milk without symptoms.

Of more concern has been the appropriateness of milk in the treatment

TABLE 6

WATER LOSSES IN 4-MONTH–OLD INFANT RECEIVING BREAST MILK
TO PROVIDE TOTAL NUTRIENT NEEDS *

A. *Water intake*	980 ml.
B. *Water Losses*	
Evaporative losses	693 ml.†
Fecal losses	63 ml.
Water available for excretion of renal solutes	224 ml.

* From Almroth.[7]
† Maximum likely skin losses.

of children seriously ill with kwashiorkor and nutritional marasmus. These infants and children might have both primary and secondary lactose intolerance (primary due to their genetic inheritance and secondary due to protein-calorie malnutrition and to gastrointestinal infections). We conducted a metabolic study on 12 Ethiopian children to determine whether lactose present in milk tended to aggravate the diarrhea and to retard recovery in children suffering from kwashiorkor.[17]

The metabolic study of each of the 12 male children lasted 11 days and was undertaken in a special unit of the Ethio-Swedish Pediatric Unit in Addis Ababa. Each child was fed two different diets almost identical in their content of calories, fat, protein, and other nutrients. The one diet was milk-based containing lactose, and the second was lactose-free. In this study each child served as his own control, being kept on one diet regime for 3 days, then alternated to the second diet, and then returned to the original diet, with a one-day adjustment period between each change.

There were no significant differences in intestinal transit times nor in the amount of sugars in the stools between the two diets in any period. The mean stool pH did vary significantly, being lower in the lactose-containing diets in the first and last periods. However, the mean pH was always above 5.5, indicating negligible or low fermentation of sugars even on the lactose-containing diet. Stool weights were significantly higher only in the first three days of treatment in those on the milk diet. No clinical evidence was found to suggest adverse effects resulting from the lactose-containing diet. These results suggest that milk products are not contraindicated in the treatment of kwashiorkor.

IMPROVING INFANT NUTRITION

What steps can be taken to improve infant nutrition in developing countries? Clearly any steps to encourage breast-feeding are desirable in those countries and communities where bottle-feeding is a serious cause of increased morbidity or mortality, or is likely to be so. Some possible measures have been suggested. Educational campaigns certainly deserve consideration. Similarly, commercially available weaning foods should be prevented from distorting the food budgets of poor people. Often, locally available cereals, legumes, fruits, and vegetables as traditionally fed provide optimum diets for young children.

If a government accepts that bottle-feeding and processed infant and children's foods are the inevitable pattern in their country, then appropriate steps need to be taken. These products both for infants and young children should be made available free or at highly subsidized costs for poor families or even for all families. Britain took this step after W.W. II, providing free National Milk formula to all families with infants, irrespective of family income, and the Soviet Union takes similar steps. The difference was perhaps that Britain accepted the demise of breast-feeding while Russia does not. The United States, with its WIC Program, is taking rather similar steps to those in Britain but aimed sensibly at low-income families.

In the case of special baby foods, other than infant formulas, if these are to be subsidized rather than issued free, then the level of subsidization should be such that it ensures the availability of the product at a cost per 1000 calories no higher than that of the main staple food and at a protein cost comparable with foods like legumes available in the local market. If this is not done, the the purchase of these nutritious manufactured foods may have a negative effect on child nutrition.

Under-fives clinics and nutrition rehabilitation centers have been increasingly introduced in the last decade as a means of combating malnutrition in young children.[18] The regular weighing of children is useful both as a means of nutritional surveillance and also as a way of eliciting an interest of parents and the community in the growth of their children. The use of a growth chart, appropriately termed a "road to health chart" by Morley [19] working in Nigeria, is now being demonstrated to be effective in a huge nationwide program in the Philippines.

Protein-calorie malnutrition (PCM) is acknowledged to be the major nutritional problem of infants and young children in developing countries. But vitamin A deficiency, sometimes leading to blindness, and iron-deficiency anemias are also important problems. Both conditions should be much easier to control than PCM. Fortification, or nutrification, of appropriate foods offers one such possibility. In Guatemala the use of sugar as a vehicle for vitamin A is being evaluated in a national program. In collaboration with colleagues in the Philippines, we are assessing the effectiveness of adding vitamin A to monosodium glutamate, which was the only consumed product that met accepted criteria for fortification. Sugar and MSG are two items that have not previously been nutrified. Both might also lend themselves to nutrification with iron as well. In this way, two important nutritional problems of infancy and early childhood can be attacked at low cost, and without changing existing food habits. In the control of xerophthalmia, another approach being used in the Philippines project and in some other countries is the provision of a large oral dose of vitamin A every 6 months to all children. This requires a well-organized delivery system. The third method being evaluated in the Philippines is a public health and horticulture intervention.

Conclusions

The control of malnutrition in infants should not be undertaken in isolation. The importance of the interaction between infections and nutrition is well established, although there is still much that is unknown concerning the role of certain parasitic diseases in nutritional status. Clearly the control of infectious and parasitic diseases deserves a high priority and will contribute to improved nutritional status. There seems to be clear logic in having coordinated programs that attempt to control infections, to improve nutritional status, and to make family planning services widely available. These three types of services may themselves be synergistic.

Acknowledgments

The author is grateful to many graduate students majoring in international nutrition at Cornell University whose research results have been used in this manuscript, and whose ideas are a continual source of stimulation. He wishes especially to thank Ted Greiner, Stina Almroth, Deborah Rothman, Barry Popkin, and Lani Stephenson, whose work has been extensively quoted from in this paper. The author wishes to acknowledge, with thanks to Dr. Joe Wray, the prepublication use of his paper "Breast Feeding and the Urban Poor of the Third World." Finally, gratitude is due to Ms. Doreen Doty for typing the manuscript.

References

1. WADE, N. 1975. International agricultural research. Science 188: 585–588.
2. GRULEE, C. G., H. N. SANFORD & P. M. HERRON. 1943. Breast and artificial feeding. J. Am. Med. Assoc. 103: 735–748.
3. ROBINSON, M. 1951. Infant morbidity and mortality. A study of 3266 infants. Lancet i: 788–794.
4. GREINER, T. 1976. Personal communication.
5. BERG, A. 1973. The Nutrition Factor. 1st Edit. The Brookings Institution. Washington, D.C.
6. WRAY, J. D. 1976. Breast feeding and the urban poor of the third world. Mimeograph copy.
7. ALMROTH, S. 1976. Breast feeding practices in a rural area of Jamaica. Unpublished thesis. Cornell University.

8. JELLIFFE, D. B. & E. F. P. JELLIFFE. 1975. Human milk, nutrition and the world resource crisis. Science **188:** 557–560.
9. LATHAM, M. C. 1975. *In* T. Greiner. The Promotion of Bottle Feeding by Multinational Corporations. Cornell Internat. Nutrition Monogr. Ser. Ithaca, N.Y.
10. LATHAM, M. C. 1965. *In* Human Nutrition in Tropical Africa : 40–41. FAO. Rome.
11. REUTLINGER, S. & M. SELOWSKY. 1976. Malnutrition and Poverty. World Bank. Washington, D.C.
12. JELLIFFE, D. B. 1971. Commerciogenic malnutrition? Time for a dialogue. Food Technol. **25:** 55–59.
13. POPKIN, B. M. & M. C. LATHAM. 1973. The limitations and dangers of commerciogenic foods. Am. J. Clin. Nutr. **26:** 1015–1023.
14. GREINER, T. 1975. The promotion of bottle feeding by multinational corporations: How advertising and the health professions have contributed. Cornell Internat. Nutrition Monogr. Ser. No. 2. Ithaca, N.Y.
15. FOMON, S. 1976. Personal communication.
16. STEPHENSON, L. S. & M. C. LATHAM. 1974. Lactose intolerance and milk consumption: the relation of tolerance to symptoms. Am. J. Clin. Nutr. **27:** 296–303.
17. ROTHMAN, D., D. HABTE & M. C. LATHAM. 1977. The effect of lactose on diarrhea in the treatment of kwashiorkor. Fed. Proc. **36:** 1092.
18. LATHAM, M. C. 1976. *In* Textbook of Paediatric Nutrition. D. S. McLaren & D. Burman, Eds. Chap. **18:** 364–374. Churchill Livingstone. Edinburgh.
19. MORLEY, D. 1973. *In* Paediatric priorities in the developing world. Butterworths. London.

KNOWLEDGE AND ACTION IN THE CONTROL OF VITAMIN A DEFICIENCY

V. Ramalingaswami

All-India Institute of Medical Sciences
New Delhi, India

For highly developed or industrialized countries . . . loss of vision is due more to lack of knowledge of cause and process of disease than to the delivery of medical services. In the less industrialized or developed countries, however, the prevention and cure of blindness is frequently more a question of delivery of health care services than it is of the understanding of disease processes.

A. E. Maumenee [1]

INTRODUCTION

It is a little over 60 years since Osborne and Mendel in Yale and McCollum and his associates in Wisconsin discovered that "fat soluble A" present in butter fat, egg yolk, and cod liver oil was essential for growth and for protection against eye lesions in animals.[2] It is 50 years since Wolbach and Howe gave a classic description of the pathology of experimental vitamin A deficiency.[3] It is 30 years since the vitamin has been synthesized and available in unlimited quantities. For as little as 10 cents or less worth of vitamin A, a child can be maintained for as long as a year free from vitamin A deficiency.[4] And yet, vitamin A deficiency continues to be an important cause of corneal destruction and childhood blindness in many parts of the developing world.[5, 6] Although there is no reliable estimate of the worldwide prevalence of vitamin A-related blindness based on valid population surveys, it is generally believed that approximately 100,000 persons, mostly children, are blinded every year, and perhaps an equal number die due to this cause.[7, 8] In India alone, at least 12,000 children are estimated to be going blind each year on account of xerophthalmia; in northeastern Brazil, 1,000 preschool children have gone blind in a one-year period,[9] and in Haiti, two out of every thousand preschool age children carry vitamin A-related corneal scars.[10] The existence of xerophthalmia has been reported in 59 countries, even though only a small area in a given country may have been involved.

Depressing as this picture is, it should be noted, however, that xerophthalmia has been gently on the decline in many parts of the developing world during the past two decades.[6, 8]

Since the discovery of the vitamin and characterization of the effects of its deficiency, impressive advances have been made, albeit in spurts, in our knowledge and understanding of the biosynthesis, absorption, transport, storage, and metabolism of vitamin A.[11-18] At the time of writing, there is a welcome surge of investigative effort in this field from a variety of disciplines that promises to influence frontiers far beyond the immediate realm of vitamin A deficiency and xerophthalmia, out into the fundamental questions of its mode of action at the cellular level, the regulation of cellular proliferation and differentiation, and of neoplasia.[19-24]

There are four deficiency diseases of public health importance that are still widely prevalent: namely, protein calorie malnutrition [PCM], nutritional anemia, xerophthalmia (including keratomalacia), and endemic goitre. Of these, endemic goitre can be readily controlled through iodation of salt—a simple, inexpensive, and effective method.[25] It does not require community participation, and major socioeconomic changes are not essential. Technological solutions have been found to suit particular needs in the use of iodate for fortification of crude, moist salt and iodized oil injections for remote areas. PCM is the most intractable of all, as it is woven into the complex social texture of underdevelopment and poverty. Nutritional anemia and xerophthalmia occupy an intermediate position in terms of tractability.[26] Although iron and vitamin A are inexpensive, the problem is one of an effective delivery system that will provide adequate quantities of these nutrients continuously or intermittently to overcome the deficiency and even to build up reserves. There is a large gap between the possession of knowledge and translation of that knowledge into the reality of the local setting. The former does not mean that the latter will follow automatically. Application of knowledge is more difficult than it is often realized. Preventive technology often requires a social technology in its application and involves significant alterations in the life-styles of people, the roles of health personnel, and active community participation.[27] Fortification of sugar with vitamin A [28] and with iron,[29] like fortification of salt with iodate, offers a technological solution of practical value, but this approach can only be used if a whole set of conditions involving the points of manufacture of sugar down to its consumption by the most needy segments of society together with the distribution channels are fulfilled. Whether an impersonal mass approach or an individual interpersonal approach is used in the delivery system, its success depends upon the degree of understanding of the epidemiology and natural history of the deficiency process. What are the environmental, socioeconomic, and cultural factors that influence the pattern of vitamin A deficiency in an area? How is it expressed in terms of corneal destruction and noncorneal ocular lesions? Which groups are most vulnerable? Is it seasonal or all the year round? What are the geographic variations? Can a profile of high-risk groups be constructed?

EPIDEMIOLOGY AND NATURAL HISTORY OF VITAMIN A DEFICIENCY

The broad picture of the epidemiology and natural history of vitamin A deficiency can be summarized as follows:[30-40] The background against which xerophthalmia arises is multifactorial and wide-ranging, some of which lies within and a large part outside the health system. Deficient intake of vitamin A and its precursor carotenoids lies at the root of the problem. Since foods rich in preformed vitamin A are too expensive for developing countries, it is on the intake of carotenoids from vegetable sources that their state of vitamin A nutrition depends. Knowledge about the value of such foods, affordability, and availability determine the levels ingested. Extrinsic factors such as agricultural and food production policies, pricing policies, food marketing and distribution systems, can profoundly influence the availability of protective foods to vulnerable groups of the poorer segments of society. The diets consumed in areas with endemic xerophthalmia show multiple deficiencies, not only of vitamin A and carotenoids but also often of calories and proteins and of fat. The metabolism of vitamin A is so closely linked to protein nutrition that keratomalacia is seen usually in children who are not only deficient in vitamin A but who also suffer from advanced stages of PCM.

Intercurrent infections and infestations accentuate vitamin A deficiency in a variety of ways affecting absorption, storage, and excretion of the vitamin, depending upon the nature and the acuteness or chronicity of the infection. Living and housing conditions and microbial pollution of the environment are some of the extrinsic factors that influence these events. Measles has been reported to act synergistically with vitamin A deficiency and PCM in precipitating destructive corneal lesions in Kenya,[41] although in El Salvador a reduction of measles following vaccination had no effect on keratomalacia.[42] In northern Nigeria, the frequent admixture of the "measly eye" with xerophthalmia was described.[43, 44] Ascariasis depresses the absorption of vitamin A.[45] The literature is replete with descriptions of frequent association between xerophthalmia and respiratory infections, including tuberculosis. Diarrheal disease preceding xerophthalmia is another association that is quite well known and to which I drew attention years ago.[46] There is strong experimental evidence that vitamin A deficiency itself diminishes immunological reactivity in animals,[47-50] although it would appear that some of this effect is due to accompanying inanition.[49, 50] Despite this clinical and experimental evidence, it is not known with certainty whether vitamin A deficiency in man leads to susceptibility to various infectious agents.[51]

Bio-tradition is a double-edged weapon, sometimes working to the advantage and sometimes to the detriment of the child, depending upon the traditional practice. Literacy, attitudes, and awareness of the mother play a determining role. I have seen mothers with some knowledge, howsoever acquired, about the value of protective foods rear splendid babies in the most desolate conditions of Bangladesh refugee camps in the midst of rampant malnutrition and keratomalacia. Breast-feeding provides much protection, and in impoverished communities prolonged breast-feeding provides prolonged protection. Traditions and taboos sometimes deprive children of green leafy vegetables in spite of their abundance. Oomen [38] talks about the blind survivors of xerophthalmia often being found in the greenest environments.

It is against this multifactorial background that we must look at the phenomenology of xerophthalmia and its evolution. The recommendations of the Joint WHO/USAID Meeting [6] and of the International Vitamin A Consultative Group (IVACG 1976)[52] on the classification of ocular lesions and on the methods of assessment of vitamin A status constitute a significant step forward and should enable a global study to be made of the problem of vitamin A deficiency, although there could still be subjective variations in the recognition of ocular lesions.

Xerophthalmia, in particular keratomalacia, is essentially an affliction of the young growing child somewhat like PCM. Keratomalacia affects children between 1 and 5 years of age, although it can affect infants and older children. In Haiti and northeast Brazil, infants are frequently affected, possibly due to severe maternal malnutrition and early weaning practices. The chronology and sequence of appearance of eye lesions depend upon the severity of the deficiency, the speed of its development, the acuteness or chronicity of associated infections, and the degree of PCM complicating the picture. But in all forms in which the deficiency expresses itself morphologically, the symptom of night blindness is usually elicited or volunteered by the mother, which can be readily verified by the behavior and movement of the child at dusk.[37] A rapidly developing deficiency process may result in keratomalacia without the preceding expression of tell-tale conjunctival lesions in the form of Bitot's spots and conjunctival xerosis. A slowly developing process may result in conjunctival lesions with minimal corneal involvement. The presence or absence of PCM can make a significant difference in the development or otherwise of keratomalacia. Bitot's spots are common in India, Indonesia, and Bangladesh, where keratomalacia is a serious problem, but they are rare in Haiti, where keratomalacia is an equally serious problem. Mild noncorneal xerophthalmia is probably an expression of pure vitamin A deficiency and may have a wide age distribution.[40] The older the child, the more protracted the course and the more frequent isolated conjunctival disease.[38] In an area in the northwestern part of India where dry, semiarid conditions exist and PCM is rare, vitamin A deficiency expresses itself predominantly as seasonal night blindness and conjunctival xerosis over a wide age range, affecting predominantly the adult working population.[53] In a village in West Bengal, marked seasonal variations in night blindness and conjunctival xerosis have been described and attributed to seasonal growth spurts increasing vitamin A requirements following harvest.[54] In adult working populations from tribal areas in India, vitamin A intakes as low as 309 I.U. in daily diets and a high frequency of night blindness and conjunctival xerosis have been reported.[53] Ophthalmologists are located where keratomalacia is least frequent. Active corneal disease, being rapidly destructive and attended by high mortality, the chances of its detection in the field are rare even if there is a sizeable problem of destructive corneal lesions in a community.[10] The significance of Bitot's spots may be a subject of controversy.[10, 51] Lack of knowledge of seasonal variations may lead to pitfalls in the evaluation of control programs. Serum levels of vitamin A decrease only after the liver stores of the vitamin are depleted. Xerophthalmia is a late expression of vitamin A deficiency and is closely associated with depleted liver stores.[34] Studies from Thailand suggest that, from a public health point of view, vitamin A concentration in the liver below 10.0 μg/gm in adults and 20.0 μg/gm in children should cause concern.[55]

The lessons learned over the years are clear: Corneal scars in an appropriate clinical and historical setting are a valuable index of vitamin A-related ocular destruction, even though retrospective.[10] Community surveys are valuable not so much for assessing the magnitude of active corneal disease but to obtain a picture of vitamin A deficiency in the community on the basis of prevalence of conjunctival and "pre-keratomalacic" corneal signs. Serum vitamin A levels and if possible liver levels provide additional information of value for community diagnosis of vitamin A deficiency. Although hospital figures of active corneal disease may not reflect the magnitude of the problem in the population, they can, however, be a useful index of the existence of the problem. The point prevalence rates of xerophthalmic signs and levels of plasma vitamin A to characterize populations at risk suggested by the WHO/ USAID Meeting[6] and the IVACG[52] are of value in the assessment of the magnitude of the problem and evaluation of control programs. It is obvious that intervention strategies should make a careful situational analysis of the problem before plunging into operational activities.

CONTROL OF VITAMIN A DEFICIENCY

Oomen[38, 39] has repeatedly given expression vividly and movingly to the essence of the problem of control of vitamin A deficiency: Keratomalacia is a hidden problem. It is an attackable and preventable problem. It is preventable right up to the onset of liquifaction of the cornea. PCM is usually a partner in the process. The vitcim is often the small child. The expert ophthalmologist comes into the picture when it is too late and sees the survivors of catastrophe with leucoma, phthisis bulbi, or staphyloma. A day may make a difference between cure and permanent blindness. Much depends upon early recognition and prompt action by health auxiliaries. Dietary preformed retinol in requisite quantities is a parameter of prosperity. Promotion of consumption of foods rich in carotenoids is the real solution. As an ophthalmologic issue, xerophthalmia has disappeared from professional journals years ago.

The size, severity, and other epidemiological aspects of the problem of vitamin A deficiency should first be ascertained, on the basis of which a decision is made as to whether control measures should be instituted within the context of available resources and national priorities in health. If the decision is in the affirmative, the objectives of the intervention program should be defined and an appropriate intervention strategy selected. A mechanism for evaluation should be built into the program from its inception, and the evaluation criteria should have relevance to the objectives.[52]

The strategies for the control of vitamin A deficiency can be broadly classified into short-, medium-, and long-term. *Massive dosing with vitamin A* at periodical intervals is a short-term intervention strategy, capable of rapid implementation; it requires personnel of ordinary competence, and the contact between the health agent and the target group need not be more often than once in 6 months or so.[52] On the other hand, the need for repeated administration at least every 6 months can be a disadvantage, the general experience being that coverage tends to decrease with the passage of time; those in greatest need are usually least accessible and the program is dependent upon continued effort and provision of resources for the nutrient, personnel, and their movement.

Fortification of a convenient dietary vehicle consumed uniformly and daily by the entire population, including the very poor and those living in remote far-flung areas, is another intervention strategy that can be short-, medium-, or long-term at will. A number of conditions pertaining to the vehicle, the vitamin, and the industrial process have to be fulfilled before this approach can be considered feasible.[28, 52] There are initial costs for finding technological solutions and for setting up fortification plants and monitoring facilities. The level of the nutrient in the vehicle can be readily altered and so adjusted as to provide it in physiological amounts on a daily continuous basis. Once set in motion, the costs involved in the continuation of the program in terms of personnel and supplies are quite small and no public participation is needed.

The third set of approaches, which are long-term, include *food and nutrition policies and practices at national and local levels, socioeconomic development, and public health measures.* These approaches, clearly the most important of all, with extensive collateral benefits, are generally given lip service, although included regularly in writings on this subject for the sake of tidy completeness. There have been very few sustained efforts to deal with xerophthalmia along these lines. (See the Philippines experiment later.) National food and nutrition policies and ensuing practices specifically designed to meet the needs of the poor and vulnerable segments can bring about lasting improvements over a wide front. Intensive cultivation at the local level of green leafy vegetables in home and school gardens can, by replication, produce a spreading mass effect. Mere expansion in production of protective foods does not automatically reduce vitamin A malnutrition. It must be accompanied by more equitable distribution. The integration of nutritional services into public health services is another knotty problem. Ensuring satisfactory nutrition of the mother during pregnancy and lactation, early detection and appropriate treatment of xerophthalmia in infants and children, the development of adaptive maternal and child health services, prevention and treatment of common childhood infections, use of low-cost weaning mixtures— these are some of the ingredients of a modern indigenous technology for integrated services.[56] Streamlining indigenous channels of community outreach and developing alternative strategies of health care delivery through the use of large teams of simply trained village-level workers are critical factors. Mass immunization, safe water, environmental protection, fertility regulation and nutrition, and health education are essential elements in the strategy. The links between health and socioeconomic sectors need to be strengthened by incorporating health considerations into developmental plans. I believe that relatively high levels of health, including the control of xerophthalmia, are attainable with limited resources.

The present status of the massive dosing program, now in operation in five countries, has been reviewed by the Joint WHO/USAID Meeting.[6] Following the first pilot trial in Jordan and the first large-scale prophylactic trial in India,[57] an oral dosing schedule of 200,000 I.U. of retinyl palmitate in oil, with or without 40 I.U. of vitamin E, once in every 6 months, given to the target population of preschool children is considered optimum for reducing the frequency of xerophthalmia. It should be noted that this schedule is being used on an unprecedented scale for the control of vitamin A deficiency at the present time. In India alone, at the rate of 12 million preschool children a year to be covered during the current fifth 5-year plan, a total of 60 million will be under the program by the end of the plan period (1981). In Bangladesh, all the 15 million children under 6 years of age are to be covered. In Indonesia, 100,000 children are receiving the massive dose. Reports from these countries speak of beneficial effects having been observed on night blindness and non-corneal xerotic lesions, such as Bitot's spots and conjunctival xerosis. There is as yet no evidence that the massive dosing program that obviously had an effect in reducing mild conjunctival evidence of clinical vitamin A deficiency prevented vitamin A-related corneal destruction and blindness. The program failed to reduce the number of hospital admissions with vitamin A-related corneal abnormalities in El Salvador, perhaps partly due to restriction of the program to 1- to 4-year-olds and partly to the children in greatest need being missed.[42] The studies with the massive dosing program had revealed a number of operational difficulties that tend to limit its outreach —increasing dropout rates with time, nonaccessibility of the high-risk groups, poor communications, long distances on bicycle, heavy seasonal rains, shortage of personnel, children being away in the fields at the time of harvest, lack of community interest, poor record keeping, etc. Keratomalacia is often associated with severe PCM in which there are multiple abnormalities in the absorption, transport and release of retinol;[58-61] these factors tend to limit the usefulness of massive dosing with vitamin A alone in such situations without the simultaneous administration of protein.

The efficacy of the massive dosing program has been questioned.[62, 63] It had no clinical or biochemical advantage for children on a moderate carotene diet, whereas on a low carotene diet, xerosis appeared in 8 weeks' time in controls and in 10 weeks' time in those receiving the vitamin A load.[62] Absorption studies of children receiving the massive dose suggest that under the field conditions of absorption and retention of vitamin A, annual or semi-annual massive dosing is unlikely to be effective.[63] There have been criticisms of lack of appropriate controls in studies of this nature where seasonal variations are known to occur and the evaluation of conjunctival xerosis is subject to so much subjective variation. In a controlled study made near Delhi, in which massive doses were given to the entire population, 200,000 I.U. of vitamin A every 6 months gave only marginal benefits over the control placebo group, which also showed improvement over the test period (Tandon et al., to be published). There was no difference between the placebo group and the group receiving 100,000 I.U. of vitamin A every 4 months. The WHO/USAID Meeting [6] concluded that more operational research was needed to judge the effectiveness of the massive-dosing approach.

It will thus be seen that a very extensive program for the control of vitamin A deficiency is already in operation involving millions of children in many developing countries in the midst of doubts about its logistic capabilities in reaching the neediest children and about its effectiveness in controlling the most serious outcome of the deficiency, namely keratomalacia and blindness. I believe that for a nutrient like vitamin A, massive dosing is a theoretically sound intervention [64] and in the absence of better methods, offers a rapid means for the control of vitamin A deficiency in the target population. Vigorous steps should be taken to overcome the difficulties being encountered in order to improve the outreach of the intervention. Taking a lesson from the small-pox eradication program, it would perhaps be more prudent in the future to characterize the high-risk groups for xerophthalmia, especially keratomalacia, and concentrate the limited resources on their intensive coverage.

A process for the fortification of sugar with vitamin A has been developed by the INCAP and the fortified sugar, when ingested in habitual diets, shown to lead to biological effects such as increased concentration of the vitamin in the milk of lactating mothers, raised serum vitamin A levels, and enhanced liver storage.[28] The level of fortification chosen is 15 μg of vitamin A per gram of sugar, which will provide the amount of the vitamin recommended for 1- to 9-year age group children. This intervention strategy is legally approved and is in operation in Guatemala and Costa Rica, and other Central American countries are expected to follow suit.

An interesting public health and horticultural approach is being tried out in Cebu in the Philippines and the results compared with massive dosing and fortification of monosodium glutamate with vitamin A.[65] The outcome of this experiment is awaited with interest.

THE FUTURE

In the future pursuit of knowledge in relation to action, it is essential to make further operational research studies with appropriate controls to evaluate the effectiveness of the massive-dosing program in the control of (1) vitamin A deficiency and (2) the biological spectrum of xerophthalmia from conjunctical xerosis to keratomalacia. The modalities of weaving the massive-dosing strategy into the maternal and child health services should be explored more aggressively.[66] More knowledge about the optimum dosage level and intervals between dosing is desirable. The search for less toxic derivatives of retinol that will enhance storage is necessary. It is not improbable that a single dose of such a derivative can protect a child for 2 years.[64] A single injection of iodized oil can protect a person against goitre for 4 to 5 years.

Epidemiological understanding holds the clue to the choice of strategic intervention, and we must continue to seek new knowledge on causative factors, seasonal variations, and characterization of high-risk groups. The need for new knowledge in this and related areas has been well discussed.[6]

The suddenness with which the cornea liquifies in extreme vitamin A deficiency and the high rate of failure in treating keratomalacia effectively have been a source of great concern. The reduced absorption of vitamin A in PCM, the diminished synthesis of transport proteins—Retinol Binding Protein (RBP) and Pre-albumin in this condition—and the time taken for their regeneration following protein supplementation pose problems in initiating prompt recovery of a liquifying cornea. It is here that basic research on the physiology and mode of action of vitamin A offers some hope. More knowledge of the factors that regulate the synthesis and secretion of RBP, of the storage and release of retinyl esters in the liver, of the role of cell binding sites for RBP and of intracellular receptors for retinol and retinoic acid would be valuable.[16, 17, 67, 68] The experimental finding that xerophthalmic corneas of rats contain an active collagenase and protease,[69] the relation between corneal epithelial disturbance and underlying stromal ulceration and between tear mucus glycoprotein and corneal epithelial integrity,[70, 71] the role of vitamin A in glycosylation reactions and glycoprotein synthesis,[72, 73] the role of serum anti-proteases on corneal proteases and necrosis, are all tantalizing avenues of research of potential practical value. While there is no way of telling whether any of these will yield knowledge that can be applied, we must continue to search for every bit of new knowledge—whether it comes from basic science laboratories, clinical units or field stations—that will enable us to treat and forestall destructive corneal lesions more effectively at the individual level on the one hand and to prevent the deficiency of vitamin A developing at the community level on the other.

"Among the rights of man is the right to see. Between the affirmation of that right and its realization is a long and arduous journey."[74]

REFERENCES

1. MAUMENEE, A. E. 1972. Chairman's opening remarks. Isr. J. Med. Sci. **8:** 1028–1029.
2. FOLLIS, R. H. 1958. Deficiency Disease. C. C Thomas. Springfield, Ill.
3. WOLBACH, S. B. & P. R. HOWE. 1925. Tissue changes following deprivation of fat-soluble A vitamin. J. Exp. Med. **42:** 753–777.
4. BAUERNFEIND, J. C. & M. BRIN. 1974. Vitamin A and E nutrition via intramuscular or oral route. Am. J. Clin. Nutr. **27:** 234–253.
5. OOMEN, H. A. P. C., D. S. MCLAREN & H. ESCAPINI. 1964. Epidemiology and public health aspects of hypovitaminosis A. A global survey. Trop. Geogr. Med. **4:** 271–315.
6. WHO. 1976. Vitamin A Deficiency and Xerophthalmia, Report of a Joint WHO/USAID Meeting. Tech. Rep. Ser. 590. World Health Organization. Geneva.
7. MCLAREN, D. S., W. W. C. READ & M. TCHALIAN. 1966. Extent of human vitamin A deficiency. Proc. Nutr. Soc. **25:** xxviii.

8. DE MAEYER, E. 1976. Xerophthalmia. American Foundation for Overseas Blind. New York.
9. SIMMONS, W. K. 1976. Xerophthalmia and blindness in North-East Brazil. Am. J. Clin. Nutr. **29:** 116–122.
10. SOMMER, A., S. TOUREAU, P. CORNET, C. MIDY & S. PETTISS. 1976. Xerophthalmia and anterior segment blindness. Am. J. Ophthamol. **82:** 439–446.
11. ARROYAVE, G. 1969. Interrelations between protein and vitamin A and metabolism. Am. J. Clin. Nutr. **22:** 1119–1128.
12. OLSON, J. A. 1969. Metabolism and function of vitamin A. Fed. Proc. **28:** 1670–1677.
13. OLSON, J. A. & M. R. LAKSHMANAN. 1969. Enzymatic transformations of vitamin A with particular emphasis on carotenoid cleavage. *In* The Fat-Soluble Vitamins. A. F. DeLuca & J. W. Suttie, Eds. : 213–216. The University of Wisconsin Press. Madison, Wisc.
14. ROELS, O. A. 1970. Vitamin A physiology. J. Am. Med. Assoc. **214:** 1097–1102.
15. WASSERMAN, R. H. & R. A. CORRADINO. 1971. Metabolic role of vitamins A and D. Annu. Rev. Biochem. **40:** 501–532.
16. GOODMAN, D. S. 1974. Vitamin A transport and retinol-binding protein metabolism. Vitam. Horm. (N.Y.) **32:** 167–180.
17. PETERSON, P. A., S. F. NILSSON, L. OSTBERG, L. RASK & A. VAHLQUIST. 1974. Aspects of the metabolism of retinol-binding protein and retinol. Vitam. Horm. (N.Y.) **32:** 181–214.
18. UNDERWOOD, B. A. 1974. The determination of vitamin A and some aspects of its distribution, mobilisation and transport in health and disease. World Rev. Nutr. Diet. **19:** 123–172.
19. FELL, H. B. 1957. The effect of excess vitamin A on cultures of embryonic chicken skin explanted at different stages of differentiation. Proc. R. Soc. London Ser B **146:** 242–256.
20. MAUGH, T. H. 1974. Vitamin A: potential protection from carcinogens. Science **186:** 1198.
21. GANGULY, J. & M. JAYARAMAN. 1975. Possible systemic mode of action of vitamin A. *In* Regulation of Growth and Differentiated function in Eukaryote Cells. G. P. Talwar, Ed. : 287–293. Raven Press. New York.
22. MARCHOK, A. C., M. V. CONE & P. NETTESHEIM. 1975. Induction of squamous metaplasia (vitamin A deficiency) and hypersecretory activity in tracheal organ cultures. Lab. Invest. **33:** 451–460.
23. SPORN, M. B., N. M. DUNLOP, D. L. NEWTON & J. M. SMITH. 1976. Prevention of chemical carcinogenesis by vitamin A and its synthetic analogs. Fed. Proc. **35:** 1332–1338.
24. CHYTIL, F. & D. E. ONG. 1976. Mediation of retinoic acid-induced growth and anti-tumour activity. Nature **260:** 49–51.
25. RAMALINGASWAMI, V. 1973. Endemic goiter in South-East Asia—New clothes on an old body. Ann. Int. Med. **78:** 277–283.
26. WHO. 1972. Nutrition: A Review of the WHO programme-I. WHO Chron. **26:** 160–179.
27. RAMALINGASWAMI, V. 1976. The Leon Bernard Foundation Award address. WHO Chron. **30:** 313–315.
28. INSTITUTE OF NUTRITION FOR CENTRAL AMERICA AND PANAMA, GAUTEMALA. 1974. Fortification of sugar with Vitamin A in Central America and Panama.
29. LAYRISSE, M., C. MARTINEZ-TORRES, M. RENZI, F. VELEZ & M. GONZALEZ. 1976. Sugar as a vehicle for iron fortification. Am. J. Clin. Nutr. **29:** 8–18.
30. COMEN, H. A. P. C. 1958. Clinical experiences on Hypovitaminosis A. Fed. Proc. **17** (Suppl. 2. Part II): 111–124.
31. GOPALAN, C., P. S. VENKATCHALAM & B. BELAVADY. 1960. Studies of vitamin A deficiency in children. Am. J. Clin. Nutr. **8:** 833–840.
32. VENKATACHALAM, P. S., B. BELAVADY & C. GOPALAN. 1962. Studies on vitamin

A status of mothers and infants in poor communities of India. J. Paed. **61:** 262–268.
33. McLAREN, D. S. 1963. Malnutrition and the eye. Academic Press. New York.
34. McLAREN, D. S. 1966. Present knowledge of the role of vitamin A in health and disease. Trans. R. Soc. Trop. Med. Hyg. **60:** 436–455.
35. PATWARDHAN, V. N. 1969. Hypovitaminosis A and epidemiology of xerophthalmia. Am. J. Clin. Nutr. **22:** 1106–1118.
36. REDDY, V. 1969. Vitamin A deficiency in children. Indian J. Med. Res. **57:** 54–62.
37. DOESSCHATE, J. TEN. 1972. Clinical aspects of keratomalacia. Isr. J. Med. Sci. **8:** 1184–1189.
38. OOMEN, H. A. P. C. 1972. Prevention of blindness due to hypovitaminosis A. Isr. J. Med. Sci. **8:** 1195–1198.
39. OOMEN, H. A. P. C. 1974. Hypovitaminosis A as a public health problem. Trop. Geogr. Med. **24:** 344–346.
40. SOMMER, A. 1976. Xerophthalmia: a status report. Trop. Doctor **6:** 87–90.
41. SAUTER, J. J. M. 1976. Xerophthalmia and measles in Kenya. Thesis. University of Groningen, Netherlands. Quoted from Xerophthalmia Club Bulletin, No. 10, June 1976.
42. SOMMER, A., G. FAICH & J. QUESADA. 1975. Mass distribution of vitamin A and the prevention of keratomalacia. Am. J. Ophthamol. **80:** 1073–1080.
43. RODGER, F. C. & H. M. SINCLAIR. 1969. Metabolic and nutritional eye disease : 419. C. C Thomas. Springfield, Ill.
44. OOMEN, J. M. V. 1971. Xerophthalmia in northern Nigeria. Trop. Geogr. Med. **23:** 246–249.
45. SIVAKUMAR, B. & V. REDDY. 1975. Absorption of vitamin A in children with ascariasis. J. Trop. Med. Hyg. **78:** 114–115.
46. RAMALINGASWAMI, V. 1948. Nutritional diarrhoea due to vitamin A deficiency. Indian J. Med. Sci. **2:** 665–674.
47. BANG, B. G., F. B. BANG & M. A. FOARD. 1972. Lymphocyte depression induced in chickens on diets deficient in Vitamin A and other components. Am. J. Pathol. **68:** 147–162.
48. COHEN, B. E. & I. K. COHEN. 1973. Vitamin A: Adjuvant and steroid antagonist in the immune response. J. Immunol. **111:** 1376–1380.
49. KRISHNAN, S., U. N. BHUYAN, G. P. TALWAR & V. RAMALINGASWAMI. 1974. Effect of vitamin A and protein-calorie undernutrition on the immune response. Immunology **27:** 383–392.
50. KRISHNAN, S., U. N. BHUYAN, G. P. TALWAR & V. RAMALINGASWAMI. 1975. Role of vitamin A and protein-calorie undernutrition in immunity and infection. *In* Regulation of Growth and Differential Function in Eukaryote Cells. G. P. Talwar, Ed. : 283–286. Raven Press. New York.
51. SINHA, D. P. & F. B. BANG. 1976. The effect of massive doses of vitamin A on the signs of vitamin A deficiency in preschool children. Am. J. Clin. Nutr. **29:** 110–115.
52. IVACG. 1976. Guidelines for the eradication of vitamin A deficiency and xerophthalmia. A Report of the International Vitamin A Consultative Group.
53. TANDON, B. N., K. RAMACHANDRAN, L. M. NATH, N. N. SOOD, D. K. GAHLOT, M. C. GUPTA, J. P. WALI, S. N. SINHA, P. C. HASTEER & P. R. KUTTY. 1975. Vitamin A nutritional status of rural community of Khol block in Haryana, North India. Am. J. Clin. Nutr. **28:** 1436–1442.
54. SINHA, D. P. & F. B. GANG. 1973. Seasonal variation in signs of Vitamin A deficiency in rural West Bengal children. Lancet **ii:** 228–231.
55. SUTHUTVORAVOOT, S. & J. A. OLSON. 1974. Plasma and liver concentrations of vitamin A in a normal population of urban Thai. Am. J. Clin. Nutr. **27:** 883–891.
56. RAMALINGASWAMI, V. 1976. The anatomy of hunger. *In* Opportunities for Philanthropy. Josiah Macy Jr. Foundation. In press.

57. SWAMINATHAN, M. C., T. P. SUSHEELA & B. V. S. THIMMAYAMMA. 1970. Field prophylactive trial with a single annual oral massive dose of Vitamin A. Am. J. Clin. Nutr. **23:** 119–122.
58. ARROYAVE, G., F. VITERI, M. BEHAR & N. S. SCRIMSHAW. 1959. Impairment of intestinal absorption of Vitamin A palmitate in severe protein malnutrition. Am. J. Clin. Nutr. **7:** 185–190.
59. ARROYAVE, G., D. WILSON, J. MENDEZ, M. BEHAR & N. S. SCRIMSHAW. 1961. Serum and liver vitamin A and lipids in children with severe protein malnutrition. Am. J. Clin. Nutr. **9:** 180–185.
60. SMITH, F. R., D. S. GOODMAN, M. S. ZAKLAMA, M. K. GABR, S. E. MARAGHY & V. N. PATWARDHAN. 1973. Serum vitamin A, retinol-binding protein, and prealbumin concentrations in protein-calorie malnutrition. A functional defect in hepatic retinol release. Am. J. Clin. Nutr. **26:** 973–981.
61. SMITH, F. R., D. S. GOODMAN, G. ARROYAVE & F. VITERI. 1973. Serum vitamin A, retinol-binding protein, and prealbumin concentrations in protein-calorie malnutrition. II. Treatment including supplemental vitamin A. Am. J. Clin. Nutr. **26:** 982–987.
62. PEREIRA, S. M. & A. BEGUM. 1971. Failure of a massive single dose of Vitamin A to prevent deficiency. Arch. Dis. Child. **46:** 525–527.
63. PEREIRA, S. M. & A. BEGUM. 1973. Retention of a single oral massive dose of vitamin A. Clin. Sci. Mol. Med. **45:** 233–237.
64. OLSON, J. A. 1972. The prevention of childhood blindness by the administration of massive doses of vitamin A. Isr. J. Med. Sci. **8:** 1199–1206.
65. SOLON, F. S. Quoted from Reference 6.
66. EBRAHIM, G. J. 1972. Vitamin A deficiency—a continuing health problem in developing countries. Clin. Pediatr. **11:** 610–612.
67. BASHOR, M., D. O. TOFT & F. CHYTIL. 1973. *In vitro* binding of retinol to rat-tissue components. Proc. Natl. Acad. Sci. USA **70:** 3483–3487.
68. WIGGERT, B. O. & G. J. CHADER. 1975. A receptor for retinol in the developing retina and pigment epithelium. Exp. Eye Res. **21:** 143–151.
69. PIRIE, A., Z. WERB & M. C. BURLEIGH. 1975. Collagenase and other proteases in the cornea of the retinol-deficient rat. Br. J. Nutr. **34:** 297–309.
70. DOHLMAN, C. H. & V. KALEVAR. 1972. Cornea in hypovitaminosis A and protein deficiency. Isr. J. Med. Sci. **8:** 1179–1183.
71. SULLIVAN, W. R., J. P. McCULLEY & C. H. DOHLMAN. 1973. Return of goblet cells after vitamin A therapy in xerosis of the conjunctiva. Am. J. Ophthamol. **75:** 720–727.
72. DELUCA, L. M., M. SCHUMACHER, G. WOLF & P. M. NEWBERNE. 1970. Biosynthesis of a fucose-containing glycopeptide from rat small intestine in normal and vitamin A-deficient conditions. J. Biol. Chem. **245:** 4551–4558.
73. DELUCA, L. M., C. S. SILVERMAN-JONES & R. M. BARR. 1975. Biosynthetic studies on mannolipids and mannoproteins of normal and Vitamin A depleted hamster livers. Biochim. Biophys. Acta **409:** 342–359.
74. WILSON, J. 1972. Keynote address. Isr. J. Med. Sci. **8:** 1032–1034.

IRON NUTRITION

Clement A. Finch

*School of Medicine
University of Washington
Seattle, Washington 98195*

This paper is a progress report on our present understanding of iron nutrition in man, particularly in developing countries. We will be concerned with the quantitative aspects of iron balance and in particular with the availability of dietary iron, the recognition of iron deficiency and its prevalence, the effects of iron deficiency on the well being of the individual, and the feasibility of modifying the iron balance of man by dietary means.

Iron Requirements

Iron balance in man begins with a maternal endowment of about 300 mg of iron in the fetus at birth.[1] The iron content of the body increases through childhood and adolescence to about 3 ± 1 g in the adult (Figure 1). More specifically, body iron amounts to about 50 mg/kg in the adult male and 38 mg/kg in the menstruating female. Most of this iron is accumulated in the form of essential body iron and reflects the requirements imposed by growth.

Normal iron requirements include not only those of growth but the amount of iron lost from the body. This has been most accurately measured by injecting normal individuals with ^{55}Fe and determining the loss in activity of the circulating red cell mass with time.[2] This amounts to about 10%/year in the adult male, equivalent to the loss of about 1 mg of iron/day; in the adult menstruating female it amounts to about 20%/year or 1.4 mg/day. Additional losses are incurred by the female during pregnancy, amounting to over 4 mg/day in the third trimester.[3] While iron losses appear to be decreased to about 0.5 mg/day with iron deficiency and increased to about 2 mg/day with iron overload, the overall range is small. Such a restricted loss places emphasis on absorption as the important determinant in iron balance. If iron requirements for both growth and loss are matched against an assumed absorption of 10% of dietary iron (Figure 2), infancy, menstruation, and pregnancy stand out as periods of jeopardy. While additional iron losses may be found, particularly those due to intestinal bleeding from hookworm, it is the basic iron requirements that cannot be met by many individuals throughout the world.

Dietary Iron Supply

Let us now consider how much available iron there is in the diet.[4] Food iron absorption can best be described as occurring along two pathways (Figure 3). The most effective of these involves heme iron, which is taken up and catabolized by the mucosal cell. Its absorption is unaffected by other dietary components. Nonheme iron appears to be absorbed from a soluble pool which is markedly affected by other food articles in the meal. Extensive studies with biosynthetically tagged foods show a low availability of vegetal iron but a better

221

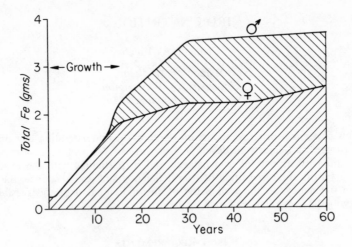

FIGURE 1. Total body iron content as a function of age.

absorption of meat iron. Such studies also show that the absorption of non-heme iron from one food article was affected by the presence of another food article. It was only with the development of the extrinsic tag technique that quantitation of food iron absorption from complex meals could be accomplished.[5] Such studies show that a radioactive iron salt added to a meal is absorbed in an amount identical with that of biosynthetically tagged food

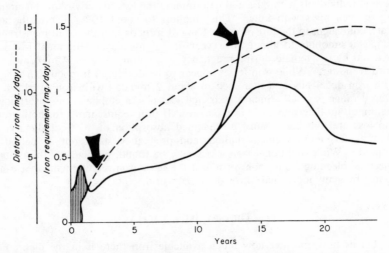

FIGURE 2. Human iron requirements. The daily requirement for growth and to replace losses is shown by the solid line. Available dietary iron on the basis of an assumed absorption of 10% is shown by the dotted line. The shaded area during the first year of life indicates a period of negative iron balance when the infant utilizes iron stores. The black arrows indicate the two critical periods when intake and loss are of similar magnitude. (From Bothwell & Finch.[1])

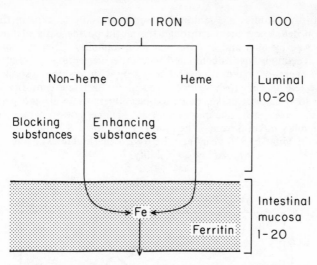

FIGURE 3. Diagram of the two pathways of iron absorption.

articles in the same meal. From studies with the extrinsic tag, it became apparent that the usual absorption of nonheme iron was quite low, i.e., $<5\%$. Its availability could be increased by ascorbic acid or meat but was decreased by tannic acid (tea), phytate, and EDTA. It may be presumed that the diet of each country and different regions of the same country will vary in iron content and availability. If anything, the developing countries have diets somewhat higher in total iron content, but much lower in availability than diets in a country such as the United States.[6] The accompanying TABLE 1 shows the results of food iron absorption carried out by Bjorn-Rasmussen et al. in a group of Swedish men, employing one extrinsic tag for heme and a second for nonheme.[7] The high availability of heme iron is evident. On the other hand, it is the *nonheme iron* that is the most important to an understanding of iron balance in a population since it represents by far the largest portion of food iron ingested. Virtually all of the iron consumed by individuals of low economic status where iron deficiency is so prominent is in that form.

TABLE 1

DIETARY IRON ABSORPTION IN NORMAL MEN *

Type of iron	Amount in diet (mg)	Absorption	
		%	Amount (mg)
heme	1.0	37.0	0.37
non-heme	16.4	5.3	0.88
			1.25

* Data from Björn-Rasmussen et al.[7]

While further studies are required, it seems possible to explain the prevalence of iron deficiency anemia through the world on the basis of the amount of iron ingested by man and in particular its availability. Dietary iron content in man is exceedingly low as compared with other vertebrate species.[8] While a very limited excretion makes it possible to get by with less, the absolute amount of iron ingested appears to have decreased in the last few centuries due to a decrease in total caloric intake, increased cleanliness of food, and perhaps the reduced use of iron pots. The more important change, however, may be related to the availability of food iron. When man ceased to be a hunter and began to cultivate grain some 10,000 years ago, he traded the highly available meat iron in his diet for a grain source of low availability.

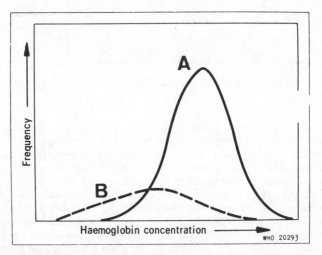

FIGURE 4. Diagram showing the overlap between the distribution of hemoglobin concentrations among a population of normal (curve A) and of iron-deficient individuals (curve B). (From Bothwell & Finch.[1])

PREVALENCE OF IRON DEFICIENCY

In approaching the prevalence of iron deficiency, the first step is to agree on a definition of iron deficiency and to establish the laboratory basis on which the determination will be based. Iron deficiency is considered to be a state in which the iron supply is inadequate to permit normal synthesis of essential iron compounds. In the past, anemia was taken to be the primary indicator of iron deficiency, but this was far from satisfactory. The limited value of hemoglobin as a detector of iron deficiency lies in the difficulty of determining whether any individual does or does not have a hemoglobin below *his* normal level (FIGURE 4). The overlap in a population between the distribution of normal and abnormal values is so great that at the customary value employed to separate normality from iron deficiency, about one-half of anemic individuals will go undetected, and of those identified as anemic, one-half will have values that are normal for those individuals. Thus, large errors are introduced with the use of hemoglobin as an initial screen.

Fortunately, there are more specific measurements of iron deficiency that may be applied to population surveys; these are the plasma transferrin saturation, the red cell protoporphyrin, and the serum ferritin. When transferrin saturation is <16%, serum ferritin <12 μg/liter, and red cell protoporphyrin more than 100 $\mu\mu$g/100 ml red cells, iron supply will be inadequate for erythropoiesis and presumably for other essential tissue iron compounds as well. Since each of these measurements behaves somewhat differently and is subject to different errors, the best criteria to support the diagnosis of iron deficiency in any individual are that two of these three measurements be abnormal.[9] Surveys throughout the world have shown a prevalence of iron deficiency in menstruating women varying from 10 to 50%.[10] These data are sufficient to establish prevalence of iron deficiency of hundreds of millions of people in the world today.

IMPLICATIONS OF IRON DEFICIENCY

What difference does iron deficiency make? In some developing countries where the amount of available dietary iron is extremely low, and particularly when there is also an increase in iron loss from hookworm infestation, anemia of moderate to severe degree is frequent. This interferes with work productivity and results in an increased mortality risk during pregnancy, with infection, and in the presence of other diseases.[11] In developed countries, however, it has been difficult to show any well-defined symptomatology due to mild iron deficiency. It is hard to believe that a deficit of 1 or 2 grams% in circulating hemoglobin could really have any effect in otherwise normal individuals, for powerful mechanisms of compensation exist to ensure an adequate oxygen supply. We have probably been too concerned with the circulating hemoglobin level and not enough with the other effects associated with tissue iron deficiency. Recently, abnormalities in muscle function,[12] immunity, and resistance to infection[13] have been described in iron-deficient animals and man. It seems likely that an element such as iron, involved in so many essential tissue reactions, will be found to be vital to body functions other than oxygen transport. Such tissue effects of iron deficiency need to be examined further.

ACTION AGAINST IRON DEFICIENCY

There are two ways whereby the iron balance of severely deficient populations may be improved: supplementation and fortification.[11] Supplementation (the use of medicinal iron) may be given to special populations such as the pregnant woman or young children. This is required for the individual with severe anemia and when there is no centrally prepared food article that may be fortified. At present, supplementation is required throughout the world for the pregnant woman. The ability of some diets to block supplemental iron absorption is so great that such iron should be administered apart from meals.

Food fortification with iron would seem a better long-term solution to the problem of iron deficiency, but a more difficult one. Attempts have been made to modify iron balance in man through the fortification of foods, but their effectiveness is not well documented. Although food is fortified with iron in the United States and a number of other countries, there is no information as to what effect it has had and, indeed, some of the iron salts previously employed have been shown to be virtually unabsorbable.[14] However, information concerning the adequacy of different iron salts for fortification is now available through the use of the extrinsic tag.[15]

With the development of precise methods for evaluating availability of fortification iron it is now possible to modify available iron in a controlled fashion. The World Health Organization has detailed the sequence of steps that should be taken in a sound fortification program.[11] Since developing countries frequently have ample dietary iron but extremely low availability, it is recognized that an alternative to the increase in iron content may be the addition to the diet of some facilitating substance such as ascorbic acid which will increase the amount of available iron. Essential to such a fortification program is the availability of a convenient method by which iron stores in the population may be assessed so that the effect of any modification on iron balance may be continuously monitored. The serum ferritin method has been shown to be a reliable indicator of iron stores and therefore capable of doing this.[16] With careful planning, with evaluation of proposed changes by extrinsic tag methods, with continuous monitoring of effectiveness as dietary changes are instituted, it seems likely that the iron balance of the population at large can be adjusted to a more optimal level.

REFERENCES

1. BOTHWELL, T. H. & C. A. FINCH. 1962. Iron Metabolism. Little, Brown, and Company. Boston.
2. GREEN, R., R. CHARLTON, H. SEFTEL, T. BOTHWELL, F. MAYET, B. ADAMS, C. FINCH & M. LAYRISSE. 1968. Body iron excretion in man. A collaborative study. Am. J. Med. 45: 336–353.
3. AMERICAN MEDICAL ASSOCIATION/COMMITTEE ON IRON DEFICIENCY. 1968. Iron deficiency in the United States. J. Am. Med. Assoc. 203: 407–412.
4. COOK, J. D. & C. A. FINCH. 1975. Iron nutrition. West. J. Med. 122: 474–481.
5. COOK, J. D., M. LAYRISSE, C. MARTINEZ-TORRES, R. WALKER, E. MONSEN & C. A. FINCH. 1972. Food iron absorption measured by an extrinsic tag. J. Clin. Invest. 51: 805–815.
6. MONSEN, E. R., I. N. KUHN & C. A. FINCH. 1967. Iron status of menstruating women. Am. J. Clin. Nutr. 20: 842–849.
7. BJORN-RASMUSSEN, E., L. HALLBERG, B. ISAKSSON, et al. 1974. Food iron absorption in man. Applications of the two-pool extrinsic tag method to measure heme and nonheme iron absorption from the whole diet. J. Clin. Invest. 53: 247–255.
8. COOK, J. D., C. HERSHKO & C. A. FINCH. 1973. Storage iron kinetics. V. Iron exchange in the rat. Br. J. Haem. 25: 695–706.
9. COOK, J. D., C. A. FINCH & N. J. SMITH. 1976. Evaluation of the iron status of a population. Blood 48: 449–455.
10. WHO. 1972. Nutritional anaemias. Report of a WHO Group of Experts. World Health Org. Tech. Rep. Ser. No. 503.
11. WHO. 1975. Control of nutritional anaemia with special reference to iron deficiency Report of an IAEA/USAID/WHO Joint Meeting. World Health Org. Tech. Rep. Ser. No. 580.
12. FINCH, C. A., L. R. MILLER, A. R. INAMDAR, R. PERSON, K. SEILER & B. MACKLER. 1976. Iron deficiency in the rat. Physiological and biochemical studies of muscle dysfunction. J. Clin. Invest. 58: 447–453.

13. MACDOUGALL, L. G., R. ANDERSON, G. M. MCNAB & J. KATZ. 1975. The immune response in iron-deficient children: impaired cellular defense mechanisms with altered humoral components. J. Pediatr. **86:** 833–843.
14. ELWOOD, P. C. 1968. Radioactive studies of the absorption by human subjects of various iron preparations from bread. Reports on Public Health and Medical Subjects No. 117. H. M. Stationery Office. London.
15. COOK, J. D., V. MINNICH, C. V. MOORE, A. RASMUSSEN, W. B. BRADLEY & C. A. FINCH. 1973. Absorption of fortification iron in bread. Am. J. Clin. Nutr. **26:** 861–872.
16. JACOBS, A. & M. WORWOOD. 1975. The biochemistry of ferritin and its clinical implications. Prog. Hematol. **9:** 1–24.

REPORT FROM THE CLUB OF ROME

W. B. Clapham, Jr. and M. D. Mesarovic

Systems Research Center
Case Western Reserve University
Cleveland, Ohio 44106

One of the key concerns of The Club of Rome for several years has been the state of nutrition in the currently underfed portions of the world and the mechanisms by which problems of maldistribution can be addressed. There are two separate aspects to understanding the problem. The first is descriptive: What is the problem? The second is integrative: How do we solve it? Since other speakers at this conference have addressed the nature of the problem, we will concentrate on the nature of the solution and how we determine what solutions might be feasible. More specifically, what can we as Americans do toward reaching a solution of perhaps the most pressing of all global problems? What courses of action are possible? What goals make sense? What policies will allow us to reach those goals, and how many of those policies are feasible given the political orientation of the country and its decision-makers? Furthermore, once a general policy has been adopted, how do we decide what specific accommodations must be made in order to carry it out, and what kind of *a priori* yardstick exists against which to measure its success? These are not easily answered questions, and yet how well we answer them determines the rationality of public policy planning in the area of global nutrition.

Let us be more specific. Let us concentrate for the moment on a single target region: South and Southeast Asia. This area includes the large region extending from Afghanistan through the Indian subcontinent to Indonesia, the Philippines, and Indochina. It includes over one-quarter of mankind, as well as the largest concentration of hunger in the world. What can be done? Of that which can be done, how much can we as Americans do, how much can be done by residents in the region, and how much must be done in concert? Our team at Case Western Reserve University, working under the auspices of The Club of Rome, has developed a tool that allows us to look at various aspects of the predicament of mankind, including hunger, in considerable detail, to examine the various feasible political and technological approaches to its solution, and to assess the potential for meeting a genuine, long-range solution. This is a computer-based planning tool for the analysis of policy.[1] As such, it has two closely related parts. First, there is the model or the mathematical representation of the system as we have chosen to simulate it. But no less important than the model is the interface between the model and the user. A model designed as a planning tool is limited both by the inherent quality of the model and also by the facility with which it can be used. Model-builders tend to be different sorts of people than decision-makers, and if a model is to be usable for policy planning, a decision-maker must be able to use it as easily as though he had designed it himself. It is not a trivial statement to assert that a model must be used if it is to be useful. As a corollary, different people should be able to ask different questions based on different perceptions and obtain answers and insights relevant to those perceptions. Let us, then, take a closer look, first at the model and then at the way in which it is used. At that point, we shall be able to return to the original question of hunger in South-Southeast Asia and draw some conclusions based on the model.

The food system includes much more than the farmer in his field. It also includes the genetic, ecological, pedological, and hydrological forces that constrain and/or stimulate production. It includes the economic, political, and technological factors that manage the development of the system, allocate resources, and determine patterns of consumption of goods. It includes the value system and the attitudes toward resource development, population, and social stratification that set the guiding forces for the system.[2] All of these factors are important, and all must at least be considered if we hope to be successful in understanding and influencing public policy in the area of food and nutrition.

The world model developed at Case Western Reserve University under the auspices of The Club of Rome provides a comprehensive overview of the food system. Technically, it is a state-variable difference-equation simulation model including sectors comprising economic and population growth as well as production, consumption, and trade of food, energy, raw materials, and investment goods. It divides the world into 10 semi-autonomous regions where supply and demand functions are determined internally but which are interconnected through world trade patterns.[3, 4] Its data bank and set of equations allow several modes of operation. On the most basic level, we can retrieve the data and establish trends by extrapolation into the future (FIGURE 1A). But the future will not be a simple extrapolation of current trends; nor will it even be the result of the extrapolation of observable inputs given a specific structural interaction among factors within the system. Both the inputs to the system and the structural interactions of factors are dynamic and come about as the result of changing public opinion and public perception as well as decisions and policies made by local or national decision-makers. These dynamic changes can be simulated in the model to provide a projection that includes the policy decisions as well as all of the information which was available for the extrapolation (FIGURE 1B). But in areas such as food—especially in the food-poor regions such as Southeast Asia—national policies are not a sufficient basis to determine the behavior of the system. Different regions of the world are interdependent to such a degree that the impact of decisions made at the national level may be altered or even negated by realities at the global level (FIGURE 1C).

SCENARIO ANALYSIS AS A TECHNIQUE

No model is a crystal ball that reads the future, even approximately or erringly. Model outputs are the product of the assumptions that have been made during the modeling process. For some of these assumptions, the data are very good. For others, they are not, either because of uncertainties in measurement, or because the assumption concerns a policy or attitudinal change for which no model would provide an adequate algorithm. For these assumptions that must, in fact, be treated as unknown or inexact, we establish a series of scenarios. A scenario is basically a set of assumptions reflecting the user's belief as to what are "correct" values for uncertainties and what are the most feasible or probable policies that can be carried out. Only as the user makes these assumptions does the model change from its default configuration. Only in so doing is it possible to identify trends or to assess the available options. In essence, the model in its default or baseline condition is a skeleton with little

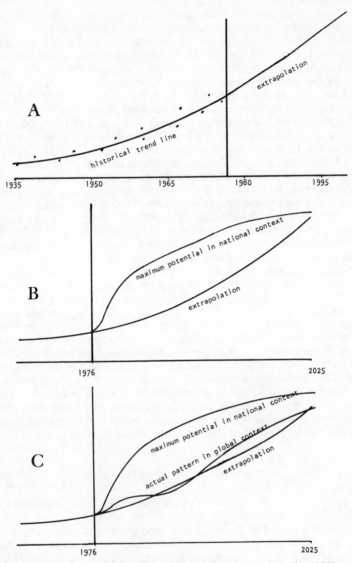

FIGURE 1. Schematic representation of operation of a model using APT-system. *A,* Data (dots) can be represented by historical trend line, which can be entrapolated into the future. *B,* National or regional goals for maximum potential are implemented in computer, assuming constant external conditions. *C,* Scenario implemented in (*B*) is embedded in global context, showing worldwide adjustments which affect or even negate national plans.

significance. It is through interaction with the user that the model takes on meaning. The assumptions made by the user as to changes in policy and public perception represent the input of a critical part of the real-world system. Specific policies are not defined; the mathematical construct requires that the user specify them. The user becomes part of the model; he is, in essence, a model of himself as a decision-maker through his own assessment of what constitutes a feasible policy and how policy and public opinion will respond to the unfolding stream of information.

But who are users? Are they limited to bureaucrats or politicians? Not necessarily. Indeed, anybody who can compose a coherent set of scenarios and assess the trends accordingly is an appropriate user. The public itself is a powerful agent of change through the medium of public opinion. Scientists, engineers, and other professionals have special insight into the nature and the decision-making process, which should be investigated through scenario analysis. And so it goes through the fabric of modern society.

In the section that follows, we will present a set of scenarios established and analyzed by our team at Case Western Reserve University. The scenarios are not all-inclusive, and it must be remembered that the "user" in this instance is one who has the insights of a team of professionals but no special political power beyond that of informed, responsible citizens. The results convey a feeling of uncertainty, but some hope for solution.

SCENARIO ANALYSIS OF THE WORLD FOOD SYSTEM

The question we wish to answer is what must be done in order to alleviate starvation in South and Southeast Asia in the time span of the next 50 years. The first step is to establish the basic nature of the problem through a baseline scenario, expressing a simulation of "no change from present policy" for all identifiable variables. The scenario has several roles. First, it gives a picture of likely consequences of the continuation of the status quo. Secondly, it provides a benchmark against which other scenarios can be prepared. Third, it provides the default assumptions that are used for a run in the event a scenario does not alter the variable in question. FIGURE 2 presents several variables calculated under this scenario. The population of South and Southeast Asia grows continuously for the first 30 years of the run, at which time it levels off. Per capita gross regional product rises very slightly, while the price of food rises markedly. Relative to current levels of starvation, there is no increase until about 1995, at which point starvation deaths rise dramatically to reach a peak of around 30 million per year in the first decade of the twenty-first century. In comparison, per capita GNP of the United States rises dramatically, even faster than the price of food.

The specter of 30 million people per year dying above current levels of starvation is tragic but not totally unexpected. Yet this is under the best of circumstances, where the system is not subjected to major shocks from outside. But shocks do happen. Most notably, there is the weather. There are cycles of weather. Droughts and other disasters on a very wide scale are not impossible. There is considerable evidence that the last 30 years, generally thought of as "normal" climatically, are, in fact, strongly abnormal, and that conditions for crop production are likely to deteriorate in the coming years.[5] Let us postulate an extreme drought in several parts of the world. This represents an ex-

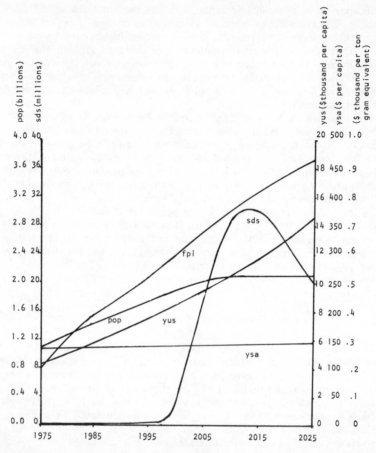

FIGURE 2. Baseline run of world model, showing outputs relating to malnutrition and related areas in South/Southeast Asia: pop=population of South/Southeast Asia, ysa=per capita gross regional product South/Southeast Asia, yus; per capita gross national product United States, fpi=food price index, sds=malnutrition-related starvation deaths.

treme shock, but one that may not be unreasonable, given the potential changes that climatic deterioration might bring. Likewise, 5 years might be too long a time to postulate for a change of this study, but it might also be too short. But this is the essence of a scenario—it is a feasible uncertainty. Let us use it as a way of gaining some insight into the effect on the system of a major shock and also the implications of different responses to that shock. Specifically, let crop yields be reduced by 15% below what they otherwise would have been from 1985 through 1989 in North America, South/Southeast Asia, and eastern Europe and the USSR. Starvation rises markedly. FIGURE 3 shows that even in Africa, which was not a drought-stricken area, starvation reaches demonstrable levels during the drought and goes back to current levels as soon as it is over.

It should be noted that no special response is made to the drought in the United States or in any other country during this scenario. FIGURE 3 also shows the level of investment in agriculture during the drought.

It is conceivable that there would be a policy response on the supply side to widespread drought of this sort. The government might subsidize or otherwise encourage increased investment in the agricultural sector to raise production during the drought years. The effects of increased investment within the United States are shown in FIGURE 4. Food production does rise in response to the increased investment, and starvation deaths in Africa rise sharply at the beginning, but decline to current levels well before the end of the drought.

But it is not sufficient to talk about investment, levels of production, and similar responses in times of crisis. The United States is a surplus agricultural region, and the chances are that it will always remain so. When a region has a surplus, it also has the right to determine who shall purchase it. Thus far, we have assumed that a free market would govern food trade. But food is not traded in a free market. It is traded through long-term contracts, concessional

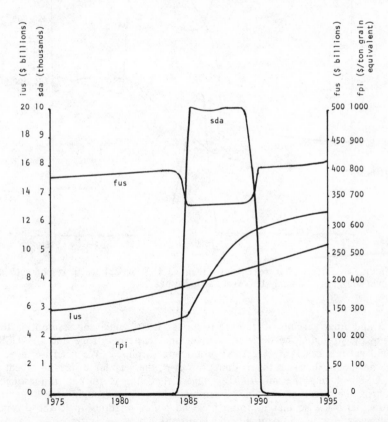

FIGURE 3. Effects of widespread drought on starvation in Africa, an area not affected by the drought (sda), investment in agriculture in the U.S. (ius), food production in the U.S. (fus), and food price index (fpi).

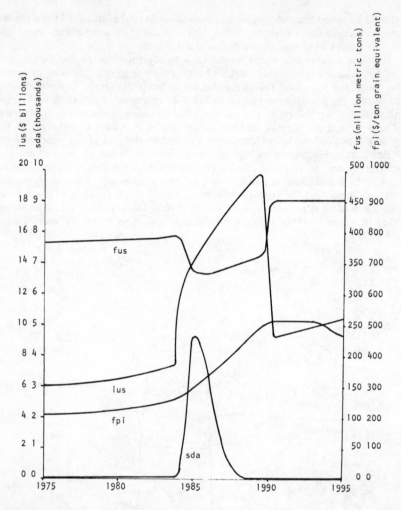

FIGURE 4. Effects of increased investment in U.S. agriculture in response to the drought shown in FIGURE 3. Labels are as in FIGURE 3.

sales, and other variants of trade restrictions. Let us make the assumption that during the drought, the decision is made that eastern Europe and the USSR should get first crack at U.S. food production surpluses. We need not specify for what political reason this is done; however, the very large sales of wheat to the USSR during the mid-1970's suggest that this is not an unreasonable scenario. This decision may have been made before the drought on a long-term contractual basis, so that it would have no policy relationship to the drought whatsoever. FIGURE 5 documents the course of starvation deaths in Africa. We are still assuming that the United States will respond to the drought with increased investment in agriculture. As before, starvation deaths in Africa decline to zero. However, the starvation peak is much higher and lasts much longer. Indeed, the time trend is much more like that of the drought without investment response than the drought with investment response. Thus, it is clear that decisions regarding trade of foodstuffs during a period of stress on the system can be life-and-death matters for large numbers of people.

But there are other life-and-death matters. One factor that has great political significance throughout the world is the price of food. No government anywhere wishes to see food prices rise. The response to noticeable rises in food price may range from boycotts to civil disorders to outright riots. There are few things that are more likely to reflect against a government in terms of public opinion. Let us postulate a scenario, then, in which the price of food in the United States is held constant. The effect of this, of course, is that farmers cannot recover their escalating costs, so that investment is not made, and production goes down. Once again, the U.S. consumer will not pay the price for this policy decision, as even with a somewhat diminished investment,

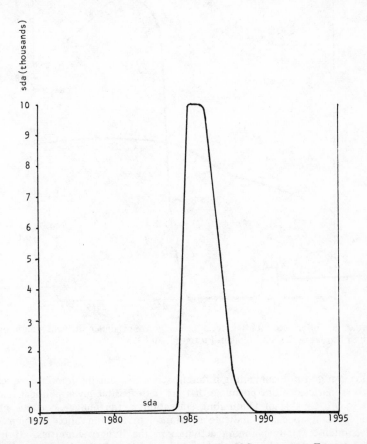

FIGURE 5. Effects of large sales of grain by the U.S. to eastern Europe and the USSR during the drought shown in FIGURE 3, given the investment response shown in FIGURE 4. Labels are as in FIGURE 3.

the U.S. can produce enough food to meet its own domestic needs. The real losers will be those people in the third world who would have bought the food had it been produced. FIGURE 6 shows some of the calculations for this scenario. The peak of starvation in South/Southeast Asia is much sooner than in the baseline scenario, and it is also much higher and lasts much longer. Once again, domestic policies made within the United States can prove to be life-or-death matters in other parts of the world.

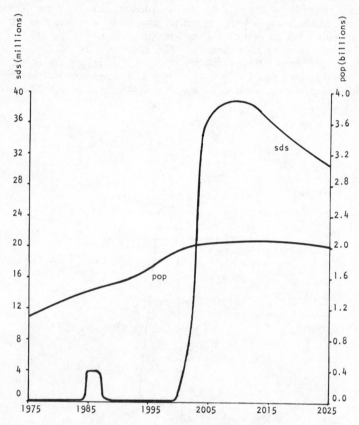

FIGURE 6. Effects of holding food prices constant under drought conditions as shown in FIGURE 3. Labels are as in FIGURES 2 and 3.

One can go on documenting different scenarios, but the important question is what scenarios can one postulate that are both feasible given political realities and also are capable of eliminating starvation in the hungry portions of the world. Several appear to indicate a solution to the starvation problem. All involve intense family planning activities in the hungry countries. It is not possible to postulate a scenario that is successful in reducing hunger in the long run that does not involve family planning. But mere family planning is not enough. Even if fertility were to reach equilibrium (i.e., a net reproductive rate of 1), within 20 years after the beginning of the model run there will still be starvation in the third world unless aid and access to the market are given to the poor countries. But starvation can be reduced to or below current levels through the forseeable future if aid is given at considerably higher levels than is now the practice around the world, and if poor countries commit themselves to reaching fertility equilibrium at an emergency rate.

REPORT FROM THE CLUB OF ROME

This report from The Club of Rome, then, can be interpreted as optimistic or pessimistic, depending on one's outlook or orientation. Its description of the problem is grim, and the kinds of interactions among nations and regions of the world that are needed to reach a solution are prodigious, but they are not infeasible. The problems are grave, but they can be solved. This is nothing new, of course; nor is it the main point. The real points of this report are that the United States is, in fact, in a position to make life-and-death decisions in the area of global nutrition. But these decisions are most likely at the times of extreme stress. During more normal times, there is relatively little that we can do to solve the problem, although we can do much to make it worse. The food system is not a highly controllable one. To change the course of human developments, we as Americans must act in concert with problem regions. Both we and they must make a commitment to act at all levels of the system. Reproductive norms must change to allow effective birth control policies to be adopted in the deficit regions. The foreign aid norms of the surplus regions must be changed to allow effective levels of aid to be given. The allocation of all resources in all countries must be keyed to meeting real-world problems of production and distribution. Resources made available must be translated into the field or the pasture before any increases in production are possible. Only then can the problem be solved—but it can then be solved.

Most importantly, we must recognize that we live on a finite and pluralistic earth. It comprises a vast number of interdependent nations, none of which can completely control its own destiny, all of which can affect the others to one degree or another. We must develop a facility for understanding our problems on a global context and for getting at methods for their solutions. The analysis of policies tool developed by our group at Case Western Reserve University, under the auspices of The Club of Rome, can be a powerful device to reach both of these goals. The job now is to insert it into the arsenal of tools for decision makers, both here and abroad, and to make certain that the kinds of insights that tools of this sort can provide do, in fact, enter into policy process, that decision makers become increasingly aware of the global implications of their decisions, and that the global context to real-world problems becomes a part of the consciousness of every human being.

REFERENCES

1. MESAROVIC, M., E. PESTEL, B. HUGHES, J. RICHARDSON, T. SHOOK & M. GOTT-WALD. 1975. APT-System: A Computer-Based Tool for Assessment of Alternative Policies: An Aid in Planning: A Users Manual. Systems Research Center. Case Western Reserve University. Cleveland, Ohio.

2. CLAPHAM, W. B., JR. 1975. Human Ecosystems: Role of the Social System in the Human Environment. *In* Systems Thinking and the Quality of Life. Blong, C. K., Ed. : 334–338. Society for General Systems Research. Washington, D.C.
3. MESAROVIC, M. D. & E. PESTEL. 1974. Mankind At The Turning Point: Second Report to The Club of Rome. E. P. Dutton & Co. New York.
4. DAYAL, R. 1977. Equations Specification for World Integrated Model: WIM. Systems Research Center. Case Western Reserve University. Cleveland, Ohio.

GENERAL DISCUSSION

Myron Brin, *Moderator*

Roche Research Center
Nutley, New Jersey 07110

DR. BRIN: Our subjects this morning dwelt largely upon technology, problems of intensifying crop production in humid tropics, food energy and nitrogen fixation, and what these hold in store for increasing protein availability, high-frequency irrigation as a means of increasing food production, sources of protein for man, the research needs and specific role of animal proteins, the fortification of foods with vitamins and minerals, and the use and abuse of food technology in the quality of our food supply. All these subjects were discussed this morning, and they are very important to our food environment. This afternoon we concentrated on problems and solutions in developing countries. Protein-calorie deficits, prenatal nutrition, infant feeding in national and international perspective, knowledge and action in the control of vitamin A deficiency, iron nutrition, and beyond the individual nutrients a new approach—a computerized automated approach for trying scenarios of action and trying to predict consequences of these actions.

We are now convening a panel discussion so that speakers can respond to questions that may arise. However, we will begin with three discussants. Immediately on my right, Dr. John Murray, Professor of Medicine, University of Minnesota, Minneapolis; to his right Dr. Les Teply, Senior Nutritionist, UNICEF, New York; and to his right, Dr. Bruce Stillings, Corporate Director for Research of the Nabisco Corporation.

DR. L. J. TEPLY (*UNICEF, New York, N.Y.*): While recognizing the considerable scope for food processing, commercial marketing, etc., I would like to refer to Dr. Latham's indication that a considerable proportion of the families in developing countries, especially, will, for some time at least, continue to depend mainly on home-prepared foods ordinarily available to them. In fact, in many cases they will have to produce whatever foods they have, at least for the most part.

Dr. Behar correctly indicated that Incaparina was only one approach to the problems of Central America and Panama. Simultaneously, there was an important and serious effort on the part of INCAP to educate mothers about the use of home-prepared foods, and getting young children gradually on to the regular family diets. This is a very difficult thing to accomplish. Dr. Ramalingaswami said that for preventive public health action, measures of this sort, including more effective and efficient delivery of basic health services and other basic services, should go along with providing adequate food.

Dr. Ramalingaswami called for social technology, and I submit that this needs encouragement and support just as much as other kinds of technologies that we have been talking about.

I'm sorry Dr. Hardin isn't here to hear me say that last March in India I learned that Dr. Ramalingaswami is one scientist, along with some of his colleagues, who is playing a key role in working with the politicians at the highest levels, with the concerned ministries and the Planning Commission in India, to at least begin to get done some of the things we are discussing.

239

I said that many families will have to raise a good deal (if not all) of their own food for a long time. We heard this morning about the high productivity of small plot production. Dr. Sylvan Wittwer of Michigan State University has pointed out, on a number of occasions, the fact that he has observed that small plot production, particularly of vegetable crops, can be very important both quantitatively and qualitatively, for the nutrition of these families. And quite generally this production is ignored and neglected by agricultural economists and planners. So I would submit that in this interface session we might consider that those in health, agriculture, other sectors, and planning and policy who are concerned with improving nutrition should give more attention to this.

In many developing countries, probably in most, a serious constraint to promotion of small plot production is the lack of a good system of distribution of reliable locally produced seeds. This is something that the industrialized countries are beginning to help with in a few of these countries.

Finally, it seems to me that we've been talking for some decades about the technology of fortifying foods with iron. Quite a few countries are interested in such fortification, using various types of food as vehicles. I wonder if it wouldn't be possible to resolve most of the technological questions with a concerted effort over the next couple of years.

DR. BRUCE R. STILLINGS (*Nabisco, Inc., Fair Lawn, N.J.*): I would like to refer back to the conference objectives that were stated yesterday morning by Dr. Moss and examine how far we've progressed in two days towards answering at least the third objective, which dealt with how technology can and should be used to meet food and nutrition needs.

The sessions this morning were generally concerned with the role of technology, and thus I'd like to briefly mention some of my thoughts and lingering questions based on these presentations. In doing so, I hope to stimulate some thoughts and discussion.

In terms of the role of technology, first let's consider the role in industrialized countries. Certainly technology has resulted in spectacular increases in food production, but I would also submit that, based on energy input-output data, it has also resulted in a high energy-intensive agriculture, as opposed to Dr. Hardy's contention this morning that our agriculture is not energy-intensive.

I think one of the challenges that will face scientists and technologists in the future will be to increase the efficiency of producing and processing food to reduce energy requirements, while still maintaining a high level of productivity. In this regard one has to be encouraged by the exploratory findings presented by Dr. Hardy this morning, in the progress made in abiological and biological nitrogen fixation, increased yields by reduction in photorespiration, and progress made to increase CO_2 fixation.

I wonder, however, and would appreciate Dr. Hardy's comments, on the practicability of these findings, how close we are to obtaining breakthroughs that will lead to practical applications of these findings.

Turning to animal agriculture, I think few would deny that animals will continue to play a key role in meeting food needs in industrialized and developing countries. Certainly, the U.S. will continue to be a meat-eating society for the foreseeable future. We may see some decreases in consumption, but these will be mainly for economic reasons.

The only conflict that I see with plant agriculture is in the tremendous quantities of feed grains that are used in animal production. We must recognize the need for reducing the use of feed grains for meat production: One, it's inefficient; two, it results in meat with a high fat content that probably contributes to many of our most serious diseases. I would like to see (1) clearer recognition of this point and (2) technology applied to reduce dependence on animal production from grains.

In considering productivity and our abundant food supply in the U.S., which we usually take for granted, we should also ponder the sobering predictions made yesterday by Dr. Reid Bryson. If he is right and climatic changes do occur and result in severe droughts, our abundant food supply will be seriously disrupted. Incidentally, the data that he presented are very persuasive on this point. So for this and other reasons, our alternatives must be explored, and the technological research needs outlined by Dr. Milner should receive high priority.

I wonder, however, if the research priorities identified by Dr. Milner will receive the attention and resources they deserve, or whether the exercise will be one in futility, as several others have been in the past. I'd welcome Dr. Milner's comments on how support for these research priorities can and should be aggressively pursued. For example, can a conference such as this be effective in gaining support for this much-needed research?

On the subject of food technology and processing, I certainly can't add to the elegant comments of Dr. Goldblith this morning on progress made in this area. However, in relation to a comment made yesterday, I would submit that the food industry is interested in feeding people wholesome food and is not in business for the sole purpose of making a profit.

In regard to fortification programs, discussed by Dr. Mertz this morning, I think some caution must be exercised. For example, as Dr. Mertz mentioned, in 1974 the NAS recommended broadened fortification levels in flour, including the addition of zinc, but not copper. Now we're finding that copper intake is also low, and that zinc fortification may aggravate the copper deficiency. I'd appreciate Dr. Mertz's comments on this particular issue.

Turning briefly now to developing countries, the question is not only how to transfer our technology but also whether it should be transferred. I wonder if we should encourage high energy-intensive agriculture in the Tropics, as discussed by Dr. Greenland this morning, if these countries cannot ultimately afford to pay for the energy that would be required once hooked on this system.

These high energy systems that have worked so well here may not be the answer to stimulate food production in developing countries. For example, Dr. Teply mentioned that small plot production may offer another alternative.

We must also exercise some caution in the marketing of western-type foods to developing countries, and in encouraging nutrition intervention programs. Dr. Latham mentioned some of the problems that have resulted in negative impacts on nutritional status in developing countries. As he pointed out, however, there is a place for cooperative programs between government and industry in developing countries. What is needed, I believe, are commitments by governments to carry out sound food and nutrition programs. To date, few governments have been willing to make commitments and give high priority to feeding their people.

What we come back to, I think, is the point made yesterday—food and nutrition problems are not only technical but are also highly political. This would indicate that qualified technologists and nutritionists must somehow become involved in the political process if we are to use our present technology effectively.

DR. BRIN: Well, today we've had about 15 presentations, some of which were provocative and others very pragmatic. Perhaps the purpose of open communication is to convert the controversial into the pragmatic. Dr. Murray, do you have any specific questions for any of the speakers?

DR. JOHN MURRAY (*University of Minnesota, Minneapolis*): I'd like to ask Dr. Finch if he's really convinced that iron deficiency encourages development of infections. There is a body of evidence published from East Africa, at least, that would say the contrary, at least as far as malaria is concerned. What are your reactions to that?

DR. C. A. FINCH: I think it's very hard, upon examining the clinical reports, to feel that they have been sufficiently controlled for the many variables present, to allow me to conclude that iron deficiency either protects against infection or makes a person more vulnerable to it. I have had the conviction that these questions may need to be studied much more specifically in an animal model under very controlled conditions.

I would like to quote some studies dealing with muscle disability. Recently it was shown that iron-deficient animals, corrected as far as their low hemoglobin was concerned, were able to run only 2 minutes in a treadmill, as compared with 20 minutes with control animals. This defect of muscle function was probably due to a specific enzyme dysfunction resulting in lactic acidosis but was not really visible as long as anemia confused the picture.

I think likewise with infection, there are two series of arguments. One has to do with the low transferrin, perhaps protecting against infection because it prevents bacteria from having as much access to iron. The other is that a number of defense mechanisms in the body that require iron—lymphocyte transformation, granulocyte function, and so forth—are impaired in iron deficiency. These can probably be pursued in animal experimental systems to a point where they can be carefully tested and then transferred to man.

DR. STILLINGS: Could Dr. Milner give us his prognosis on the research priorities and proposals that were submitted to NSF? I know you mentioned this morning that there was encouragement for a modest increase, but is this really the commitment that's going to be needed if we're going to make significant progress in this area?

DR. MAX MILNER: To a large extent I think we can all agree that the answer to Bruce's question relates to the statesmanship-like posture that Congress may assume towards science in general. The lovely panorama that I presented this morning of needed research, in protein resources, which was put together with the help of some of the best specialists in this country, can be counted on as extremely reliable in terms of its relevance.

It depends not just on the National Science Foundation alone, but to a large extent on what priorities Congress is willing to follow in research.

Now, you heard me mention at the last, in response to a question, that as long as wheat is $2.50 a bushel and corn $2.40 a bushel, from the short-range point of view people can very rightly ask why bother? Those are extremely cheap prices considering today's cost. Even soy beans today at $6.50 a bushel, as I indicated, isn't too bad, and the prices are probably headed down.

But this, as I contended this morning, is really not the true state of affairs in terms of what the world's food needs are at the moment. It is a completely artificial and false situation. The world is hungrier, and yet in international markets there aren't many people who are prepared to buy products even at those prices.

I think, frankly, that there is a new look in Congress towards agriculture and food research. And I think that Walter Wilcox, my colleague from the Office of Technology Assessment, is going to address himself to that point as to what the feelings seem to be developing in Congress towards a greater concern for the future, in terms of research needs both in food supply and agriculture, etc. I don't want to anticipate what Walter will say, but we do know that there are some straws in the wind. In the Foreign Assistance and Food Emergency Act—I forget the exact title—passed in 1975 in Congress, there is the now famous Title 12, which presupposes an entirely new look, a new ordering of priorities in food and agriculture research, at least in terms of the needs of developing countries. A council on food and agricultural policy has been set up under Title 12, with Dr. Clifford Wharton as Chairman. That group, now pulling itself together, will presumably recommend a whole new look in agricultural and food research priorities.

In addition to that, there were in the past Congress additional efforts—the Wampler Bill (after Congressman Wampler, who had some original inputs). There was this initiative that at the moment is quiescent; without any question it will come up again in the new Congress for an additional approach to agricultural and food research.

For the first time, rather than formula funding of state university and land grant college research, there is a whole new approach being contemplated there. So unless my colleague from OTA, who knows this field much better than I, has something more to say, I am optimistic that Congress will indeed take a statesmanship-like approach, notwithstanding that the short-term need seems to be quite in the other direction.

DR. STILLINGS: I think that's true, Max. However, we have conferences year after year on food and nutrition. Maybe the emphasis is somewhat different, but can a conference such as this be effective in gaining support for programs such as we're talking about in the protein research area?

DR. MILNER: Yes, I think so. Dr. Moss asked me precisely the same question: How did I conceive that the followup could be made more effective, other than by simply publishing the proceedings, tossing it out, and forgetting about it in the future. I did make the point that in my work in OTA—which is not a perfect instrument but has, at least, done some useful work and will, I am sure, continue to—the question is constantly asked by Congress: Is there a better way that Congress can be apprised of the emerging impacts of science and technology? They always seem to kick us in the back of the head in terms of their impact on society, and we've reacted to them rather than planned for them.

And I made this point to Dr. Moss—that this is a question which OTA is also now considering. Is there a better method whereby Congress, the policy-makers and legislators in this country, can approach the coming impacts of science and technology? In other words, what is going on in the laboratories, what is coming out of the laboratories that Congress should be apprised of by the scientists themselves in terms that the Congressmen can understand and presumably crank into their policy and planning at the legislative level.

I made that point to him, that a conference of that kind is eminently timely right now, and perhaps that might be the kind of conference that The New York Academy should set up at a very early date.

DR. BRIN: I think that one of the valuable results of our current conference could be the development of subsequent conferences to elaborate on specific issues that are of scientific importance and need.

DR. STILLINGS: One other point that we touched upon briefly was related to food fortification. I think it is an important point, particularly if we are thinking of continued intervention programs in this country, as well as transferring this kind of program to the developing countries.

The question I raised is how much information do we need before we embark on an extensive fortification program. I gave the example of the NAS recommendations in '74, which in the light of current data may aggravate a problem rather than totally correcting one. Do you have any comments Dr. Mertz?

DR. WALTER MERTZ: Thank you for asking that question. Let me first answer the question of zinc-copper relation. You can never be completely satisfied that you have all the knowledge that you need when you make a decision. In the case of the recommendation for zinc enrichment, the evidence was based on good studies showing a substantial incidence of marginal zinc levels and zinc deficiency in children. I think the decision was a very good one because there is a problem, and if the recommendation is implemented it will do some good.

At that time, however, nobody had been particularly interested in the copper situation. And we now know that according to the latest analyses the average American diet does not need, doesn't even come close to needing, the USRDA of 2 mg of copper. However, I would not be prepared at the present time to talk about a situation that now demands a change of our policies. I would not recommend now starting a copper enrichment program, because I have to have two questions answered.

The first one is this: If, indeed, the old methods that determined a copper content in our diet between 2 and 5 mg were incorrect, then they were also incorrect when they were used to determine the 2 mg in the diet of subjects that were necessary to produce balance. In other words, if they overestimated the dietary content of a free living population, they might have very well overestimated the amount in the diet of the experimental subject. In other words, it is possible, if the analysis is the explanation, that the real amount as measured with modern methods required to obtain copper balance is only 1 mg.

This is why we have to start some new copper balance studies, and these are being planned in the human nutrition laboratory.

The second question that I have to have answered is very similar to that of our iron situation. We know very well from Mill's work in Scotland that there are quite remarkable differences in biological availability of iron compounds, those of plant extracts being entirely different from those of salts. We don't know—at least I don't know at the present time—what diets were used to produce these copper balances. We have now let a contract to investigate that question through a search of the literature.

Once it is clearly shown that 2 mg are indeed needed, in a typical, representative diet, and that our diet does not indeed furnish this, then I would very strongly recommend consideration of copper enrichment.

DR. BRIN: The previous discussion by Dr. Mertz and Dr. Stillings clearly exemplifies the complexity of hematopoiesis. Some years ago there were a number of papers in the animal literature on meat anemia and osteoperosis caused by feeding experimental animals red meat as a sole diet (no other ingredients). This meat anemia was relieved by the administration of copper.

And it raises another question: I'm not familiar with any good collection of papers on nutrient-nutrient interrelationships. There have been conferences on drug-nutrient relationships, on nutrient needs and excesses and so on. Perhaps this too can be a subject for a future conference to be held under the auspices of The New York Academy of Sciences. There are many of these interrelationships that are highly significant, in animal as well as in human nutrition.

DR. V. RAMALINGASWAMI: I would like to make a very brief comment on Professor Murray's very provocative discussion. The area of nutrition and infection is in fact a very complex one, and I agree with Clem Finch that when you are analyzing a multifactorial situation in the clinic, the administration of a particular intervention and the result that follows are not necessarily connected since there may be a number of intermediate links.

The only comment that one can make at this stage is that with the modern immunological techniques that are now available, there is an opportunity to at least somehow clarify as much as possible the linkages between nutritional deficiencies and various types of immunological reactivities. And when one does this in an experimental model, I think the recent evidence is reasonably conclusive that when you are dealing with fairly severe protein energy deficiencies in animals, you do end up with a substantial deficit in cell-mediated immune reactions. But how this is going to be reflected in the clinical community horizon with multiple infections and antigenic loads, etc., is something that needs to be resolved.

I think the point about the optimal defense is the ideal for us. What are the nutrient intakes that would enable us to have a balanced optimal defense against a wide variety of antigenic stimuli, ranging from a virus to a multicellular parasitic infection? And as Dr. Behar has said in his paper, it is alright to talk about extreme forms of protein-calorie malnutrition, whereas, in fact, the bulk of the problem is under the tip of the iceberg. An functional correlations of milder and moderate degrees of protein-calorie malnutrition in terms of host-defense reaction are the kind of research effort that I see in the future that might illuminate some of the questions that Professor Murray has raised.

Finally, to comment on Dr. Stillings question, on how far has this conference really shown to what extent Dr. Moss's third criterion has been satisfied —the technology as help: There were many examples given in Dr. Mertz's paper of ways in which technology has helped.

But I would try to look into the future and see the possibilities where technology or scientific solutions could help in very, very difficult circumstances. If the massive dosing program at periodic intervals for the control of vitamin-A-related blindness is not going to succeed, it would not be because it has any fault in its theoretical formulation but simply because of our channels of community outreach, the way our societies and our health service system are organized today. They are just not in a position to reach out to those who are in greatest need.

Well, if that is the case, we must look for new avenues. I am reminded of what happened in the eradication of small pox recently in my country and seven others. We know that it may be essential for at least several years for the vaccine against small pox to work. But the strategy that was adopted was to have a surveillance system, to identify a case, and to have an immunological barrier built around that case. This is how it has been eradicated, and not by 100% primary immunizations in the susceptible group.

For example, we may be able to use a vital stain, a vital dye that could be simply dropped into a child's eye. If it could be shown that there is a patch there of a dystrophic conjunctival or corneal epithelium, then we have identified a child who must somehow be taken in hand and treated.

Many other approaches are possible. Metabolites in the urine that could be readily identified through a simple field estimation that might indicate the state of nutrition for the vitamin of that particular child might be a great help.

DR. BRIN: Your perspectives are certainly very pertinent, and we appreciate them.

DR. MOISES BEHAR: Only a very short observation in regard to the data presented by Dr. Widdowson this afternoon: She indicated that there are no control studies on the effect of nutrition and birth weight in developing countries, and that's why she was making most of her representation on the experience in some disaster situations of developed countries. I would like to mention that in the last few years a very well controlled study was done at INCAP. It was very clearly shown that the addition of a relatively small amount of calories in the diet of mothers during pregnancy resulted in a very significant increase in the birth weight of their babies. The addition of 200–1,000 calories during pregnancy resulted in an increase in the average birth weight from 2800 g to 3100 g as an average.

More significantly, the production of babies that weighed less than 2500 g was reduced from 18% to 5%. The other point is in agreement with Dr. Widdowson. By analysis it was shown that the reason that the correction of the nutrition of mother during pregnancy was only able to increase the weight from 2800 to 3100 g, and not to 3500, was due primarily to the small size of the mothers. That was primarily due to poor early nutrition of those mothers.

So, the point is that we need at least two generations in order to correct the effect of undernutrition on the size of babies. In those studies it was also very clearly shown that the underweight babies had a very, very high mortality, not only during the perinatal period, which is well known, but during their whole infancy. Dr. Widdowson was saying that if the child is born small and he is well taken care of afterwards and raised in a good environment, it is not very much of a handicap. But this is unfortunately not the situation in most developing countries, because they are not taken care of properly, they don't live in a good environment, so the very high infant mortality in developing countries is contributed in very great proportion, by the children who are born small, and primarily as a result of inadequate nutrition of the mothers.

DR. E. M. WIDDOWSON: Yes, I had made that last point you made, at the end of my paper. So far as the supplement to pregnant women is concerned, I'm afraid this is one of the things I had to cut out of my paper to shorten it. I felt that the studies in the developed countries were more clear-cut as a scientific study, perhaps. But I do agree with you.

DR. BRIN: Thank you very much. We can now open the discussion to the audience participators.

DR. PAUL LACHANCE (Rutgers University, New Brunswick, N.J.): I'd like to agree and disagree. First of all I'd like to congratulate Dr. Behar on his making very clear that the FAO-WHO document, which has misled so many Americans, including some of the speakers at this program, expressed that calories are the only problem and you can solve all the other things by giving them more food, which in another step is very important. It is not just an issue of calories, or just an issue of food, or just an issue of protein.

However, I would like to disagree with his conclusions, and I think particularly the one that says that just going back and increasing the social and economic factors in a village or something like that or putting in more sanitation, as Dr. Murray has suggested, is going to solve our problems. That's just so costly you'll never get it done—you'll never be able to solve your problem that way. And if you are really realistic, you'll realize that the change has to take place from the inside, and that we must increase the productivity of the individual. You can do that only if you change the number of cells that he has, including the number of brain cells.

I then would like to point out, being a party to this Santa Maria study which he quoted, that—and he did not mention this—although protein fortification of tortillas resulted in a 30% decrease in morbidity, it also produced a 50% decrease in infant mortality. I think that is highly significant. It is more significant than any study has ever revealed in a two-and-a-half year period that I am aware of. On top of that, the appetites of the pregnant women were increased by 120 calories per day. We had no explanation for that; we only know that it is real, that it did take place.

The fact that the babies did not increase in size doesn't mean very much, I think. Maybe we're using the wrong benchmark. And I listened to Dr. Widdowson very carefully. You know, small babies are just as beautiful, and some women are very small and really can't afford big babies.

Now, if they resist disease better, maybe we have to create a new hypothesis that says that you may need the right ratio of protein. Remember, we were adding some calories and some vitamins. We, in fact, are in completing this data, observing that they now have a better resistance to disease. There is no other explanation for a decrease in mortality and morbidity.

Now, in the case of Dr. Murray, he has to recall that in all his cases his people are already infected. And if you're going to feed the host you're going to feed the pathogen, and that's why they take off. Whereas when they are treated *in utero* they've got a chance. I think that that has to be brought about and discussed also.

DR. DANA RAPHAEL (*Human Lactation Center, Westport, Conn.*): I run the Human Lactation Center. It's the only research center in the world on human lactation, which is a very tragic statement that Dr. Latham brought out.

We have a constituency of two billion women, and nobody seems to think it significant enough to really make a statement and start a proper series of centers as you suggested. What bothers me is the discrepancy between what we know and what we can do about it.

We have 12 anthropologists out in the field trying to determine this particular problem of reduced months of breast-feeding that Dr. Latham has talked about. In that situation we have tried to get women to understand what's going on, and we haven't used the sophisticated terms that you used this morning. We said look—breast feeding is best, now come on, it's economically good, breast-feed. And they say, what do you mean it's economically good? We're not cows.

Then we say to them, things like—well, breast-feed for a little while. Recently Dr. Shantigosh has shown that breast-feeding is not in fact sufficient for 6 months only, but she claims it is only sufficient for 4 months.

Now we have a problem, and it's just been brought up, about government subsidizing and government supplementing food. I'd like to throw it open to those of you who supplementing food. I'd like to throw it open to those of you who work with government because I am afraid this is where we're going to get to. Dr. Teply,—well, anybody who wants to answer this.

What do you think are the potentials in having governments of Third World countries really get concerned with the weaning food patterns and with breast-feeding enough so that they will interact in some form?

DR. BEHAR: I think there is no basic disagreement with Paul Lachance on my presentation. I was forced to shorten it so much that many of the points that I wanted to make were not clear. I do agree that we cannot wait until socioeconomic development, and there are some interventions that we can and should do immediately. I am also in agreement with him on the fact that the study of protein fortification of tortillas did provide extremely useful information.

The problem is that this type of information is not applicable to immediate solution of the problem in terms that there is not a possibility of fortifying tortillas right now. I mean that was done for experimental purposes in a highly controlled condition, but there is no possibility of doing it right now.

But he did express the point that I want to make clear, that it is not only food which is the factor responsible for malnutrition. There are many other factors associated with it that should be taken into consideration.

DR. MICHAEL LATHAM: Just a very brief comment to the important points that Dr. Raphael made. I think we are all delighted to hear that there are a number of anthropologists around the world looking at the questions of breast-feeding. I think this is terribly important. As she said, there is a very big constituency out there.

I don't think, though, that we should judge how things are going by the response of people in developing countries being told, especially being told by Americans, that they should be breast fed or that they should be breast-feeding in this particular way. It seems to me that up until 100 years ago nearly the whole world was breast-feeding, and in most of the developing countries they now are breast-feeding. We don't need people to tell them how to breast-feed, and we shouldn't have people telling them how to breast-feed anymore than we should be telling people how to urinate or copulate. It seems to me that these are fairly normal things that are going on.

The problem is that there has been too much interference, there has been too much of people coming in and saying this is how you should breast-feed and this is what you should do. And we are singularly unsuccessful as a people in Europe and North America as successful breast-feeders.

In regard to the length of breast-feeding, I think most of us agree that four or five months is probably the maximum amount of time that a woman should breast-feed only; that after that the child, the infant, needs other foods introduced into the diet. But this does not mean that they should then stop breast-feeding. I think if she goes on for two years, so much the better. But she should introduce other foods, just in the same way as the young puppy goes on suckling from its mother at the same time it is getting other foods. So breast-feeding should continue for as long as is desireable and and possible. Other foods should be introduced at perhaps four months of age.

DR. GENE CALVERT (*American Public Health Assoc., Washington, D.C.*): I was particularly struck by the data that Dr. Latham presented showing the percentage of women in selected countries—Philippines, Colombia, Jamaica, Nigeria—who has discontinued breast-feeding, and the reasons why. He indicated that 6% or less had stopped because of work. Were those percentages based on the percent of women who were working with children at the age for breast-feeding? Or was it based on the percentage of total women within each of the samples?

DR. LATHAM: To respond to that question, I think it is regrettable that there is so little information. This was taken from five or six countries; we could find about 10 or 12 studies in which this question had even been asked. The data are very variable. On the whole, this is asking women, some of whom are working women and some of whom are not, some rural and some urban, the reasons why they they stopped breast-feeding their child at a particular age. Obviously these are not good data, and there is inadequate research, and we really don't know enough about the reasons why women do breast-feed and why they don't. The data are variable; they give a very general indication and I don't think should be taken as ideal information.

DR. RABIN: My area is clinical nutrition. Clinical nutrition covers everything from infancy to adultery. The difference between our meeting here and radio or TV is that when the speaker appears on radio or TV, we don't always get a chance to answer back. But I have some comments and questions for several of the speakers.

First of all I would like to say I agree wholeheartedly with the comments of Dr. Murray, our first discussant. I have been in various countries and have learned a great many things. And what you say Dr. Murray is quite true.

We have become so wedded to drug therapy that we can see little else. It has been said that those who live by the sword will die by the sword. We can paraphrase that to say those who live by chemicals will die by chemicals.

And so I would like first of all to enter the area of infant feeding. I don't know whether you people have ever noticed how close you've gotten to a diaper. The bowel movement of a baby is acid and does not have an offensive odor. As soon as you give that baby cow's milk or a formula, the bowel movement becomes alkaline and has an offensive odor. And then there are the problems of constipation or diarrhea—caused by the amount of dextro-maltose. The proper sugar for milk is lactose, and the difference between the two is about a dollar a pound.

As far as breast-feeding is concerned, we have strayed so far from natural living and become such artificial animals that we forget what parts of our body are for. And the sooner we return to the ways of our fathers, the sooner we'll get rid of a lot of troubles.

You'll recall that vitamin A deficiency was mentioned. I'd like to give you a case that will probably illustrate something or other to you. We were taught that vitamin A deficiency results in all of the eye problems that you've been told. I'd like to cite the case of a young man, 28 years old, who had an injected sclera, bitot spots, and night blindness. He had to give up driving his taxi at night. We are supposed to give him vitamin A, of course. I never gave him vitamin A. I put him on a high protein diet, the same foods that people ate 40, 50 years ago before we became the sickest nation in the world. We gave him the proper hormones to balance his endocrine system, which controls the metabolism, and everything disappeared.

Now, from what we have heard about requirements for food, it seems that pretty soon before we sit down to eat a meal we'll need a computer to tell us how much of each to eat and in how many of the different elements. This makes eating a chore, not a pleasure, as it used to be.

MARY GOODWIN: (Rockville, Md.): My question deals with fortification. I want to question the addition of iron to infant formula for babies from birth to, say, the 3-month period, whether this is necessary.

Also, we know there can be a dependency on certain nutrients. I wonder if any research had been done on the possibility of giving infants excessive iron early in life through formula, through iron drops, through fortified cereal, and what the potential consequences of this might be. Has any research been done on it?

Adding to the suggestion of a symposium, seminar, or conference on imbalances and excessives—attention should also be directed toward dependency on nutrients which may develop through our arms race of nutrients, so many foods are being fortified with the same hit parade of popular nutrients.

DR. C. A. FINCH: I'm glad to have the opportunity to make a comment about fortification. I tried to indicate that recent evidence suggests that the present diet that man has is far from the form in which the genetic behavior of his intestinal mucosa is adapted, in terms of heme iron versus non-heme iron.

Furthermore, man is operating at an extremely low level, if you compare him with the rat, who has 100–200 times more iron per kilogram per day in the food he eats. We are at an exceedingly low threshold. There is nothing that would make us believe from evidence available that one can produce iron "overload." Infants are usually operating at the top of their absorptive capacity to take in enough iron to meet needs and build up some stores. There is every reason to believe that they would shut off iron absorption to a degree that would prevent overload.

So that I think the evidence would indicate that iron overload is no problem, that it hasn't been seen in infants, and that there is abundant evidence of iron deficiency.

Now, whether that is important or not is the real question. Dalman has now shown that certain enzymes in the brain are decreased in an iron-deficient animal in the early part of its life, who when then fed with iron does not replete these enzymes. I think it's going to be very important to try to determine whether effects that are produced due to iron deficiency may continue for some time, and if they can have identifiable effects.

I think infancy is the opportune situation for doing something of a fortification type; with adults the complexity of fortification is much more than had been appreciated. And yet we now have techniques that both allow us to evaluate the potential of fortification changes in diet and monitor it as it goes along. So I'm very optimistic that we can be more effective in our manipulation of what I regard as a highly artificial diet in terms of the adult. And I guess we have to say artificial in the infant, but we're adjusting it as we think is best.

DR. BRIN: Thank you very much, Dr. Finch. I know that many of you have more questions but the hour is very late and we must reconvene at eight o'clock, not giving very much time for alimentation, which is what it's all about. So we will close this session and thank you very much for your cooperation.

NUTRITION FORUM—OPENING REMARKS

Howard Schneider

Institute of Nutrition
University of North Carolina
Chapel Hill, North Carolina 27514

We're about halfway through the Conference, and this evening's session is a kind of pause that will allow for a little stock taking and a better perspective. I propose to begin this Nutrition Forum, as your program says, focusing on the nutrition of the American people. To our foreign visitors that may seem a little chauvinistic. But, after all, this *is* the Bicentennial, and you are here, in the United States.

I propose to begin by asking, "Why are we here?" If you can answer that question you will have come a long way with us. Why, indeed, are we here?

The Conference thus far has dealt almost exclusively with what I would say is correctly titled, "global concerns." I suppose the day now must be regarded as fully passed when the United States of America could consider anything, really anything, in terms of its own native and domestic economies. But rather, we are indeed one world.

These global concerns have reminded me now of something that I wish I'd thought of earlier. I thought of it only a few hours ago, and there has been no time to rush to the library to do any checking. But I'm going to attempt it anyway as far as I can, because, I'm told, Benjamin Franklin has a very good press in this town.

I would allude to the fact, because this is the Bicentennial, that 200 years ago when the Founding Fathers assumed their roles the only man who was really known in Europe was Benjamin Franklin, a member of the Royal Society, a recognized scientist, and discoverer of electrical phenomena that had the world agog. This man, a Renaissance Man of the 18th Century, was more visible in Europe than any other citizen from these shores.

We have other heroes—Thomas Jefferson, for one—but in European eyes Thomas Jefferson was a rustic compared to the sophistication, the knowledge, the expertise of a Benjamin Franklin. I think Franklin would have approved the fact that in this scientific conference we have attempted to grapple with issues in terms of a political and economic context, and have not been narrowly confined to what we all would be more at home with, the details and functions of molecular structures.

Franklin was not only a scientist, he was a bon vivant. The wine that sparkled in the glass pleased his eye. I think, too, that attention to food was something he enjoyed full well.

Now, the 200 years of this nation's existence include three distinctive features of philosophical development in the history of nutrition. The first phase, which lasted 2,000 years, beginning with Hippocratic notions, and lasting really until about the middle of the 18th century, made one simple presupposition about the whole phenomenology of nutrition: that foods contained one item called nutriment. And if there were any distinctions to be made between foods, it was that they had more or less of nutriment. As so often happens, the ghost of that idea, that simple idea that was current for so many years, is still in our minds.

When we ask, "Is it nutritious?," we mean, "Does it contain nutriment?" But the meaningfulness rests in terms of the totality of what else is eaten. But, no, we are asked, "Is this apple nutritious?" Is this loaf of bread nutritious? All this without any regard, most of the time, alas—as to what else is being eaten.

Now, about the time when political ferment had begun in the colonies we came into the second phase of a science of nutrition, a chemico-analytical period, epitomized by the beheading eventually of the genius, Lavoisier, who founded the science of chemistry. Before we had a chemistry we really could not begin an analysis of foodstuffs, eventually developed through the genius of Liebig. By the middle of the 19th century there was, we realized, more than one thing called nutriment. There were four things: minerals, fats, proteins, and carbohydrates.

For awhile we were satisfied with that, and we entered into the chemical analysis of food with great abandon. The literature is filled, if you look back to those early days, of lists and lists, analyses compounded upon analyses. But the test of application of these analyses in such a rigorous, demanding industry as the animal industry, the rearing of animal life for consumption by human beings, gave only trouble. The chemist's analyses were no help.

It was only the genius of a McCollum that began the biological era around the turn of this present century. We turned away from chemical analysis and asked the question biologically. This is the biologic era in nutrition history. We used laboratory animals that guided us into a whole new world that we never knew existed and the chemists knew nothing of, a world of micronutrients: vitamins and trace minerals. The nutrient entries increased to 50.

Well, we've come, in other words, from one nutrient to four, to 50. I think we've also had another thing happen recently, and that is a lot of us have become aware of the fact—if we've forgotten it—that agriculture is "THE" basic industry. Without agriculture there is nothing. And if, as speaker after speaker has demonstrated to you, the number of people involved in this enterprise diminishes as our mechanization is increased, but, as others have pointed out, at tremendous costs in the squandering of fossil energy, this is only to emphasize that it may well be that agriculture will be the next revolutionary growth industry. I have read in the *New York Times* of the increasing enrollment in colleges of agriculture, the interest of young people in careers in agriculture, and I think this all bodes well.

I think, however, it would be simplistic to say that all is well. For we still have no nutrition policy in the U.S.

I think a national policy demands two things: (1) the goal addressed; and (2) a politically acceptable mechanism to reach the goal. What, in this world of all sorts of constraints, is realistically possible?

Now, when you have those two features, you have policy. Before that you have lists of aspirations, of goals. Many of these are pious, well-meaning, etc., but the list must be reduced in terms of that second constraint, of some means of arriving at it. And I would now like to take just a few minutes to show four ways in which "food policy" in the United States has been put together piecemeal, with resulting contradictions, because of very real need of addressing demands in a politically acceptable fashion.

For example: The Secretary of Agriculture is admonished by law to see to it that the American people have an adequate diet at fair prices. Now, you see the operative word is "fair." What is a fair price? The Secretary of Agriculture really has two constituencies. The first, are the farmers. If their prices are benign for them, the consumer pays more. But it happens that the consumer is the great American public, which is also the Secretary's constituency for he is a member of a politically elected administration. So tensions arise. We have not yet resolved these although we have "policy" in place, and the Secretary of Agriculture has to live with it, whoever he is, and as best he can.

The second point is that the Secretary of Agriculture is admonished also to see to it that we have a nourishing diet for all. On this our Food Stamp system is based and all of the other food supplement systems that we've added on to that. Here again we find ourselves torn in trying to decide whether indeed the food-supplementing systems that we have provided do that with nutritional goals in mind, or whether they are, from the political standpoint, another matter, namely, an incomes-transfer program so that dollars are freed for individual purchases of other things. Whether we continue to address these programs solely in terms of their nutritional impact is a matter which is open to doubt. And that's the reason why tension exists, because of a failure to clearly specify what is indeed the case.

A third point is that the Secretary of Agriculture, as a result of the Great Depression, is admonished to assist the farmers of this country to have access to world markets. And that is accelerated to a point now where it is the largest single component of our earning of foreign exchange. We have, in the last two years, exported in agricultural products something of the order of $22–23 billion, which go to pay the oil bills; whereas heretofore this was of the order of $7–8 billion. We have moved into this very rapidly under the impact of the watershed events of '72 and '73.

And lastly, in place, is a Food for Peace program, which was once begun actually in order to dispose of surplus commodities. Political advantages were seen, and the program became a very palatable thing indeed. But we see Congress continuing to struggle to define who is a friend, who an enemy, whether this program should be solely humanitarian, or whether we should make some kind of a fractionation thereof: so much for humanitarian reasons, so much for political reasons, so much for military reasons. The struggle continues.

These are the tensions that are built in to what, under a general rubric, one would call a kind of food policy. So in the United States, today, in the Bicentennial year, having come this long way, having seen the rise of an agriculture of tremendous productivity, we remain left with some of these decisions in which the U.S. citizenry has a stake, and find ourselves buffeted by the tensions that I have indicated.

Tonight we will attempt to address this general problem in some useful way so that you can walk out of here feeling that you've got some sort of a package out of this. I've given a brief historical synopsis of some of the difficulties which now enmesh us, but we will have the help of experts. I will introduce these gentlemen as they appear. Let me give the schema of our program. First we will be told of some of the probabilities of what the new administration may well put into place as nutrition policy.

The second consideration is that the only way in which we can relate nutritional goals in terms of normative social theory is against a set of standards.

And who makes the standards? We will have here someone who is well equipped to describe to us how the standards are arrived at, and their true significance.

And then last, when it's all put together, we still are operating, not in a Marxist society, but in a society of free enterprise in an American system. And in that system of free enterprise we must acknowledge, as some other speakers have already done, our dependency upon the free and efficient functioning of our food industries.

In this there are ideals and there are realities, harsh ones, that have to be dealt with. And one of our speakers will deal with that.

So now, that's the outline of what we hope to do tonight. But our speeches are going to be short. I hope mine has not been unduly long. Our speakers will have 15 minute presentations. The idea is that when we have given a kind of précis in the way in which I have described, there will be adequate time for free and open discussion. You will be invited to come to the microphone—this meeting is open to the public—and have your say. The panel and other participants in the conference may want to be responsive. We will hopefully conduct a dialogue which will improve our understanding.

ALTERNATIVE U.S. FOOD POLICIES

Walter W. Wilcox

Office of Technology Assessment
Washington, D.C. 20515

A brief review of the changes that have occurred in U.S. food supplies and prices in the recent past will help in setting the stage for a consideration of alternative U.S. food policies.

As recently as 1971, the Government was holding large stocks of grains, and a major policy objective was to achieve their liquidation.

It was in August 1971 that President Nixon announced a wage-price freeze, followed by wage and price controls in 1972 and 1973.

The value of the dollar in international exchange was devalued in 1971, and again in February 1973.

Energy prices increased sharply in 1973 and have continued at sharply higher levels since that time.

U.S. and world grain reserves were pulled down to minimum levels in 1972 and 1973 by unprecedented exports to the U.S.S.R. and to other countries that had experienced partial crop failures. This is the first year since 1973 that world crops have been large enough to permit some rebuilding of stocks.

These events have had the cumulative effect of increasing prices in grocery stores for food used in the home by 51 percent since December 1971.

Also, in the last few years the public has become so much concerned about the pollution of the environment and the hazards of using agricultural chemicals that food producers and processors are now restrained in many ways by broad new Federal regulatory programs.

Another essential aspect of the current setting for alternative food policies is the difference in philosophy and thrust of the new Administration as compared with the one that closes its books on January 20th. Although some may disagree, I would characterize the philosophy and thrust of the Nixon-Ford Administration as one of very reluctantly interfering, and then as little as possible, with the functioning of the free enterprise system. I would characterize the philosophy and thrust of the incoming Carter Administration as one of recognizing the central importance of the free enterprise system, with a confidence that in important aspects its functioning can be improved by appropriate government policies.

With this background, let us look at alternative food policies in the years immediately ahead. We will not only have a new administration beginning next year, but for the first time in four years, we will finish the season with adequate grain stocks after restoring the normal flow of livestock products to consumer markets.

The 95th Congress, which opens January 4, must amend and extend four major pieces of legislation dealing with food policies. These are:

1. The Agriculture and Consumer Protection Act of 1973, which authorizes farm and food supply and price stabilization activities, expires at the end of the 1977 crop year.

255

2. The Public Law 480 Food for Peace Act, which authorizes concessional food sales and grants to foreign countries, expires December 31, 1977.
3. Authorization for the Food Stamp Program, which provides additional food for 18 to 19 million Americans, expires in September 1977.
4. The Federal Insecticide, Fungicide, and Rodenticide Act administered by the Environmental Protection Agency also expires in 1977.

My 25 years of experience in working with Congress leads me to observe, however, that new legislation is not required for many substantial changes in food policies. The Agriculture and Consumer Protection Act of 1973, which expires in 1977, grants a wide range of discretionary powers to the Secretary of Agriculture. I would not be surprised to see it extended for a year with only minimum amendments. Yet I would expect a Secretary of Agriculture appointed by President Carter to follow sharply different policies with respect to grain reserves and level of producer price supports than those followed in recent years by President Ford and Secretary Butz.

Congress may enact enabling legislation, but it has little control over the administration of the programs authorized. For this reason, as we consider alternative food policies in the years immediately ahead, the prospective administrative policies of Carter appointees are fully as important as the prospective legislative actions of Congress.

Since the opening remarks of the panel members will be followed by a discussion period, let me quickly list some of my personal views as to the likelihood of specific food policy changes in the next few years.

We have already acquired fully adequate reserves or stocks of wheat in the United States and Canada. We also expect to have minimum adequate feed grain stocks at the close of this marketing season. The policy issue in the United States no longer is whether or not reserve stocks should be accumulated. We have them. The question is whether they will be managed as reserve stocks or as burdensome surpluses. The Executive could develop adequate policies under an extension of the 1973 legislation. It is likely, however, that Congress will enact more specific guidelines than are contained in the expiring legislation. I expect the 95th Congress and the Carter Administration to develop a positive grain reserve policy, with producers holding most of the stocks.

With respect to the extension of Public Law 480, I am again inclined to expect more changes in the administrative policies developed by the new Administration than in the congressional authorizations for Food for Peace programs.

As we have gained experience with concessional food programs for developing countries, we have become increasingly aware of shortcomings that offset a part of their benefits. All too often, substantial Food for Peace imports under long-term loans or grants have adverse effects on indigenous food production. I have been told that in the past few months, Public Law 480 programs have been negotiated primarily to increase our exports of wheat and rice, with relatively little attention given to their contribution to long-term accelerated food production programs in the recipient countries.

I will be surprised if the new Administration does not develop additional guidelines for administering Public Law 480 programs, which integrate them more fully into the accelerated food production programs of the developing countries.

In the extension of the Food Stamp Program authorization, there may be some changes in program eligibility, but here again the more significant changes are likely to be made by a new administrator of the program.

It is my understanding that the Environmental Protection Agency has gained valuable experience in administering the National Insecticide, Fungicide, and Rodenticide Act, which expires in 1977. Adverse reaction to a number of the regulations that were promulgated in recent months almost surely will cause Congress to provide more restrictive guidelines for the EPA administration of the new legislation. It is probable that food producers and processors will not find compliance with EPA regulatory policies as difficult in the years immediately ahead as in the recent past.

Agricultural research and development is another issue that merits consideration. Several congressional committees and several executive agencies have studied the reasons for the decline in public support for food and agricultural research in recent years and the implications of this decline. The Wampler Bill, which authorized an expanded research program, was approved by the House of Representatives last fall but was not even considered by the Senate. It is highly probable that an improved and expanded food and agriculture research bill will be introduced early in the 95th Congress. The new Administration is expected to support such legislation. New legislation of this type would increase formula funds for research and would authorize a substantially new competitive grants program for high-priority research, including high-priority basic research to enhance food production.

In closing these brief remarks, I want to call attention to the continuing uncertainty regarding the adequacy of future world food supplies. Eighty percent of the variability in international trade in wheat in the past decade has been due to the variations in U.S.S.R. imports. The U.S.S.R. also accounted for 50 percent of the variability in international trade in feed grains. The U.S.-U.S.S.R. long-term grains purchase agreement negotiated in 1975 is expected to reduce the year-to-year variations in our sales to the Soviet Union. Its effectiveness will be reduced, however, if the Soviet Union fails to follow similar policies with its other major suppliers.

I note that climatologists have already addressed your meetings this year. I doubt that they promised you less variability in the weather in the years ahead. If we cannot reduce the fluctuations in crop yields due to variations in the weather, one means of achieving increased stability in annual food supplies would be an expansion in international trade. Another would be an international system of grain reserves, which could be utilized to offset regional or worldwide shortfalls in crop production.

I am not hopeful of rapid progress in removing current barriers to international trade in foodstuffs; primarily, they are national policies that insulate individual countries, and groups of countries, from world market prices. But I am hopeful that in the future, the food-importing countries, as a result of their recent experiences, will carry larger stocks. The importing countries in the past have depended on a stability of supplies in the exporting countries, which was assured primarily by the large stocks carried by the North American exporters. The short supplies and high prices encountered by these countries in 1973, 1974, and 1975 almost surely will cause them to hold larger stocks now that supplies are again more plentiful.

Although the 1974 World Food Conference recommended the establishment of world grain reserves to be managed and controlled by a new international institution, little progress has been made in resolving the many problems encountered in their establishment. In part, this was due to the position taken by United States representatives. It is possible that under the Carter Administration, United States representatives will be given new negotiating instructions, and a system of international grain reserves will come into being. The problems encountered are so complex, however, that each country may have to hold its own reserve stocks, rather than depend on the availability of internationally managed reserves.

HUMAN NUTRITION NORMS

Gilbert A. Leveille

Department of Food Science and Human Nutrition
Michigan State University
East Lansing, Michigan 48823

Ideal nutrition norms or standards have been sought for a long time, and although several standards have evolved, it is fair to say that none have been found to be perfect. This stems in part from the fact that standards are used for different purposes, that needs of individuals vary, and that significant variations exist in the nutrient content of foodstuffs. These factors make the establishment of precise standards difficult, if not impossible. Consequently, all standards involve a number of compromises. In this presentation, I will attempt a brief review of those standards that are currently in use and consider their value as well as misuses. Also, I will attempt to indicate the significance of the various norms to the average consumer. Additionally, I will touch on existing information needs.

The standard that has been used most extensively is the RDA, or Recommended Dietary Allowance, established by the Food and Nutrition Board of the National Research Council, National Academy of Sciences. The RDA's represent the best estimate of nutrient needs arrived at by a select committee of distinguished nutritionists. It has been recognized from the start that the establishment of a definitive requirement is rarely possible. Therefore, the RDA represents the best possible *estimate* of nutrient needs plus a safety factor to compensate for individual variability. Thus, the values reported as recommended dietary allowances are designed to meet the needs of over 95% of the population. The values were originally designed to serve as a guide in planning food supplies. They were not and are not today designed to be used as individual requirements. In spite of this, the Recommended Dietary Allowances are often used in this way, and it should be recognized that while they are not requirement values to be used in evaluating the diets of individuals they do serve as a guide for this purpose and are probably as good as any available. However, it should be clearly recognized that failure of individuals to meet the Recommended Dietary Allowances does not necessarily indicate a state of deficiency or inadequate nutrition.

Another value to which the consumer is frequently exposed is the U.S. RDA or U.S. Recommended Daily Allowances. These values, derived from the Recommended Dietary Allowances of the National Research Council, are used by the Food and Drug Administration in food labeling. They serve as a guide to consumers in evaluating the nutritional quality of food products. Clearly, they are not requirement levels. These values appear on foods that are nutritionally labeled according to food and drug regulations. This information can be extremely useful to the consumer in learning more about the nutrient composition of foods. It is very unlikely, however, that these values will be used in a compulsive way by consumers to establish that 100% of one's nutrient needs are met on a daily basis.

Another nutrition guide that has been in use for many years and is a

259

useful "rule of thumb" for consumers, is the so-called basic four food groups. The four food groups are represented by milk and dairy products; meat, poultry and fish products; fruits and vegetables; and cereals and cereal products. By selecting an appropriate number of servings from each of the food groups, it is presumed that individual nutrient needs will be met. This system is relatively simple and has proven useful in various nutrition education programs. Nonetheless, the system has received severe criticism in recent years as being overly simplified and not necessarily insuring an adequate diet. To be sure, it is possible to devise a diet that, while meeting the objectives of the four food groups, is nutritionally inadequate. This, however, is rather unlikely, and the four basic food groups remain a useful consumer guide to the planning of adequate diets.

It should be noted that the U.S. food supply is extremely varied and abundant. As a consequence, deriving an adequate and nutritious diet from this food supply should present no particular problem. In fact, most individuals consuming a variety of foods are very likely to meet their nutrient needs. Nonetheless, in this age of enlightened consumerism, one would hope that the public could be educated to make wiser food selections to ensure that nutritional needs are being met. Two of the standards alluded to are extremely useful in this regard. The simplest is the basic four food groups; the other is the use of nutrition label information that lists the U.S. RDA of selected nutrients per serving. The nutrition labeling system, with adequate consumer education, should prove to be a very effective nutrition education tool. Unfortunately, little progress has been made thus far. Most surveys indicate that consumers make little use of the information found on nutrition labels. The challenge to the professional community, therefore, remains one of educating consumers to utilize nutrition information available to them. This has not proven to be an easy task, and increased efforts in this area are needed.

Numerous schemes have been tried to inform consumers about their nutritional needs and how these needs can be met through wise food selections. A number of various scoring systems have been tried, but all have been discarded as ineffective. The food group concept, currently in use, has evolved from one that included seven basic groups, and other efforts along these lines have been tried, including as many as 11 food groups. The present system of four food groups appears to be as effective as any of the other more complicated approaches involving food groups. A standard that has been extensively used in labeling foodstuffs in the past, the so-called MDR or Minimum Daily Requirement, has also been eliminated. The difficulty with establishing MDR values relates to the lack of available information on nutrient needs and to the expected variation between individuals.

Another topic I would like to touch upon is the need for assessing the nutritional status of our population. The yardsticks currently available are far from ideal; nonetheless, there are biochemical and other techniques available that can provide a reasonable assessment of food and calculated nutrient intakes and of nutritional status. Unfortunately, even in an affluent country like the U.S. we have not evolved an ongoing system of monitoring nutritional status and food intake of our population. I recognize that we have some limited efforts—the USDA household survey, a decennial survey of food intake, and the HANES survey. The USDA household survey, while useful, fails to provide an updated, moving assessment of what is happening to food and nutrient intakes in various segments of our population. The latest information we have available is that for the 1965 survey, and it is unlikely that any new information will be available before 1980—a 15-year lag. Many changes are likely to have occurred in this period. The HANES survey represents the first effort at an ongoing survey, but is in its infancy and certainly is not without serious limitations. There is a definite need to establish, as part of a national policy, a mechanism of assessing the nutritional status of our population on a continuous basis in order to alert us early of potential problems so that corrective action can be taken.

It is very clear, as one examines the available information, that considerable effort will be required in the future. Specifically:

1. More precise nutrient standards that can be applied to individuals and groups must be established.
2. Information is badly needed on the nutrient requirements of man. The requirements for many nutrients, particularly trace minerals, remain unknown.
3. A continuing and vigorous program of nutrition education is needed to bring to the attention of consumers the latest information in the field of nutrition, which can be applied to improve their nutritional status and thereby their health and well-being.
4. Food consumption and nutritional status surveys must be established on an ongoing basis to alert us of emerging nutritional problems.

IDEALS AND REALITIES IN FOOD SYSTEMS

S. M. Cantor

Sidney M. Cantor Associates
Haverford, Pennsylvania 19041

A few years ago, an English woman, who must be most interesting, wrote a book called *Consuming Passions*.[1] It is a history of the progress of civilization in England as reflected in English appetites. While behavior with respect to food is the main theme, sexual behavior, luxurious indolence, and abuse of the poor are included by legitimate association. Along with these, the author shows that such items as cannibalism, wet nursing, politics, prostitution, housekeeping, aphrodisiacs, and witchcraft are also related. She records the inequities in the distribution of food and other needs and pleasures, but most importantly at the same time she accepts and celebrates the humanness of her subjects, particularly as she criticizes the "mass produced artifically flavored frozen fare that people eat in England" today. "Something," she mourns, "has gone out of us."

The point here, of course, is that food is more than just survival. In the vernacular, food is soul and everyone, everywhere, has a soul food. Food is inextricably related to all human activities, passionate and otherwise. Poets and painters, in their roles as social commentators, have been saying this for centuries.

Such works speak eloquently of the intimate relationship of man and food—of feast and famine, of mystical rites, of acts of grace, of celebration, of sacrifice, of hunt and harvest, of food as decoration or as symbolic of rise and fall, and of the sharing of food as power, pleasure, and pain. They provide a humanistic dimension to statistical data.

Recognizing this inextricable relationship and the unique role of food in human activities, what has this got to do with food systems and what is a food system?

In simplest terms, food procurement by the consumer began as a tribal hunting and gathering activity with all its concomitant ceremonies and symbolism, developed as a first phase through a succession of household technologies and crafts, a separation of these into guilds and then trades—farmer, dairyman, butcher, miller, baker, confectioner, greengrocer—which were put together into a personal or family food preparation system by the housewife or, if affluent, her designated agents. This was a food system, and it was substantially finished by the close of W.W. II, at least in the U.S. Development continues, and currently we are in the midst of a second phase. Indeed, we may be well passed the midst. As an index of change, sweetener delivered to the food industry, as distinguished from direct consumption, crossed in the mid-fifties and is currently at the 75% level.

This second or current phase is the shift of food preparation and service from the household to the factory and—significantly, but to a somewhat lesser extent—the restaurant or public eating place, and to institutional services. Further, it is marked by different commercial entities such as the supermarket chain, by the activities of food scientists and technologists, by large-scale

262

factory farming, by sophisticated commodity processing (interconvertability of source of foods, i.e., textured vegetable protein, high fructose corn syrup, single-cell protein), by multinational food companies, and by expanded government bureaucracies that exercise control over various aspects of this evolving and dynamic new food system.

In a relatively few words, we have skipped over several thousand years in going from man's hunting and gathering period to an almost totally commercialized food system in a highly industrialized society. One reflects the other, and it should not be surprising to recognize that, rates of change in various areas of human activity being different, vestiges of past habits are carried forward or otherwise persist. Advanced technologies clearly show their craft origins, ethnic and regional food identities are apparent as they should be, as are health and food associations. Human food behavior, for the most part being especially slow to change, confounds those who seek simple relationships.

We can put together a useful model of today's food system. It consists of a chain of activities or subsystems. First is *agricultural production,* that is, raw-material procurement, and this must include imports as well as domestic production. It also includes directly or indirectly matters related to water, land availability, fertilizers, energy, environment and international marketing, hedging, and related practices. This is followed by *processing* (including such activities as drying and storage and other preparations for conversion to finished food products). Processing includes packaging, sterilization, quality assurance, and adherence to food regulations and nutritional norms. It also includes shelf-life considerations, as does the next part of the model or subsystem, which is labeled *distribution.* Distribution is concerned with transport, also with packaging and shelf life, with marketing in general, including advertising and promotion, and with all the problems of competition in a free market, to name a few. Finally, the last subsystem is *consumption.* This subsystem is concerned generally with all of the knowledge about the consumer that is pertinent to acceptance of the final food product. In a marketing-dominated system, such as ours, it is the consumption subsystem that represents the point of departure for initiating the forward action in the total system.

What I have described quickly is the U.S. food system and some of its modifying influences (by no means all of them). When the food system stopped at supplying the consumer with food ingredients from which she prepared the final product, the food industry was relatively simple. It is infinitely more complicated today.

With the advent of change in the social structure resulting from continuing industrialization and urbanization, which in turn has created the requirement as well as desire for more family members to contribute to family income, has come the popular acceptance of convenience foods, the fast food system, and the shifting of food preparation responsibility to the food industry.

The complications of the current food system attract comment. If we consider the number of transfer points in the system outlined, that is, points where an intermediate or final product or idea changes hands, so to speak, the compromises between offerer and accepter that are necessary to keep the process going are staggering. So the process is not concerned with the consumer alone but also with many intermediate accepters. Obviously, the consumer is dominant or else the viability of the process ceases, but the decisions are always compromises. Acceptability is the key to continuity.

The model obviously also is not perfect because the system isn't perfect. An ideal system requires quantitative knowledge at every step. The role of food in health alone is complicated by tradition, mystery and ancient as well as current beliefs, and by lack of knowledge. The anxieties among consumers thus created constantly generate new problems. These problems create opportunities for both honest and objective intervention, as well as opportunistic intervention. This pluralism is characteristic of our society. The clamor gets louder, but the understanding does not necessarily expand.

Do we return to older practices? There is little evidence that we will do so, economic pressures being what they are. Instead, we are busily engaged in building the food system of the future by a trial-and-error process.

What is the relationship between nutrition and this imperfect food system? One very specific association is an apparent increase in fat and sugar consumption which in Western socioeconomic terms is usually related to urbanization and industrialization. This is the most profound change in food behavior that has occurred in the U.S. and generally in Western food systems. It has developed over a period of about 50 years.

In the United States our economy is already classified as being in a post-industrial stage, with concomitant exurbanization continuing rapidly and changes in family structure and life style being particularly apparent and reflected in our food. However these changes are described, affluence is a commonly used term, and affluence in life-style is frequently reflected as richness in diet as well as in "eating out." Moreover, richness in diet can be associated with fat and sugar in the diet, and "eating out" with fast foods and snack foods consumed "on-the-go." The latter also are not only identified with high fat and high sugar but reflect "fast" as part of life-style and, in some respects, reinforce fast living. This matrix of change incorporates an increasing incidence of degenerative and stress-related diseases which, in turn, are associated with overconsumption and the affluent diet that again signifies high fat and sugar consumption. These diseases include obesity, cardiovascular disorders, diabetes mellitus, and dental caries. I emphasize "associated." A causal relationship except in caries has yet to be demonstrated.

It is within this dynamic complex that nutritionists are examining nutrients and disease relationships and epidemiologists are seeking statistical data to help identify causal relationships between food components and disease. But, as Hegsted [2] has pointed out, "this is an oversimplification" for "we have entered into a new era in nutrition"—from emphasis on essential nutrients in the diet to concern for food-related problems that have little to do with essential nutrients and much to do with factors that affect food intake. *These factors affect quantity.* They include cultural background, textural qualities of food, and marketing pressures, and they relate to continuing industrialization of the food system. Industrialization emphasizes mass markets, tends to create limited choices, and can accordingly accentuate particular food components. And so this cycle can aggravate the problems.

The increasing recognition of this situation demands efforts to understand more about the food behavior of humans. The goal is to provide more effective ways of equating food consumption and individual need, both with respect to energy requirements and nutrient balance. The rewards include an increase in the quality of life and substantial reductions in the cost of public health maintenance.

How do we get more quantitative information about food intake? It is most significant that our food information statistics, largely generated by the U.S.D.A., are somewhat antiquated and devoted largely to disappearance data, which are referred to as "consumption." Such data are characteristic of a production system in which the goal is to regularly increase production and therefore necessarily consumption. In a marketing-dominated system, the goal is theoretically to meet the "need" of the consumer. When need is fulfilled in a consumption-dominated society, new needs must be "perceived" to "expand the demand structure." These, when properly merchandised, expand the markets and the gross national product. There must be, accordingly, serious concern about treating food as any other consumer item subject to all the wiles of merchandising practices. This is legitimate concern and is as much a concern of industry as of the consumer and consumer advocates.

Our food system is a remarkable structure. Daily, it makes available to every person on average about 3200 calories. It faithfully reflects the social structure and reciprocally influences change. When Betty Furness said recently in a television documentary that she did not remember asking for antioxidants in her food (which was part of an anti-additive statement) she was wrong, figuratively speaking. By the nature of her work and her reflection of the rapidly changing role of women, she was asking to be released from household responsibilities. Antioxidants in foods which prolong shelf life are part of a technological answer to women's liberation. Abdication of responsibility is a serious problem. Who fills the gap? The food industry in our system operates according to net profitability, and social profit is not yet interchangeable with economic profit. This is an area for change that needs special investigation. If the food industry is to be responsible for nutrition in our society, according to some norms to be established and regulated from a central authority, then it ought to be paid for its services. Without reimbursement for added responsibility, the system doesn't work. Nor does it work if the instrument that is to supply the service is under constant suspicion.

Aside from such concerns, however, I worry about central authority and the imposition of regulations derived from an *ideal* systems model on an imperfect real world. Norms of human food intake and human food behavior vary greatly, and these variations and differences in individual practice need to be protected against the homogenization already too apparent. We are just beginning to understand the need for true consumption data which can set limits of food behavior. The practice of relying on food disappearance for consumption data encourages excesses. We do need a national food policy, but we need one that respects and encourages individual and regional differences in food behavior. It is too easy to substitute an oversimplified model for reality. Moreover, we need a food policy that recognizes the unique consumer product that food represents. Eating is to be enjoyed, and not to become a practice so surrounded by negative admonitions that anxiety about disease becomes the basis for choice of food.

REFERENCES

1. PULLAR, P. 1970. Consuming Passions. Little, Brown & Co. Boston, Mass.
2. HEGSTED, D. M. 1975. Health: summary of evidence. *In* Sweeteners: Issues and Uncertainties : 86. National Academy of Sciences. Washington, D.C.

GENERAL DISCUSSION

Howard Schneider, *Moderator*

Institute of Nutrition
University of North Carolina
Chapel Hill, North Carolina 27514

Mr. Jack Iacano (*Agriculture Research Service, USDA, Falls Church, Va.*): I should like to make a comment relative to nutritional surveillance of the United States. This is information that I'm sure Dr. Leveille has not been privy to, and hence will add a little to what he has given.

I think, as has been pointed out, we need considerably more nutritional surveillance in the United States. The USDA has been aware of this and been pressing for this, at least in all the time that I've been with the USDA. I know that Willis Gortner has pressed for this also.

But I must say this: Congress is very anxious now, in the light of the problems with the Food Stamps program, to increase the activity in nutritional surveillance, and in the past six months we've seen our budget rise from $600,000 a year to $3.2 million—a very healthy step in the right direction.

But, even more importantly, Congress has recommended that USDA and HEW get together to discuss USDA's household food consumption survey on the one hand, and HEW's HANES Survey, on the other to see what areas of overlap exist and where we may move forward together on the surveillance. We have had several meetings now between these two agencies, and there appears to be a very positive step forward in the direction of settling some of the issues between the two agencies in terms of individual programs.

The next survey is signed. Contracts have already been placed—

Dr. Schneider: This is the household consumption—

Mr. Iacano: This is the household consumption survey of the USDA, which is the 10-year survey. This will commence in April 1977. At least half of the information that will come from this total survey of 50,000 households should be available by September 1978. The funds that are coming into this program are recurring; that is, this will mean that as we proceed through this first survey, that beyond that we will move according to needs. There is already indication from Congress that there will be more money forthcoming to combine the efforts of this survey to include not only the recall survey, but also the nutritional survey aspect.

There is, however, a great need for research to devise better methods for proceeding with surveys from every point of view. Although these have been called consumption surveys, as has been pointed out, they are not. They are based on recall and we should make every effort in the future to try to determine how best to go about making actual consumption surveys.

Dr. Schneider: Can you tell us why the survey was held last in '65. We're now standing in '76. You're mentioning '77, and by '78 we'll really have the next one. That's 13 years. What happened?

Mr. Iacano: I think that question has already been responded to by the first gentleman who spoke this evening. It takes money to do these surveys. Congress must provide it.

266

DR. SCHNEIDER: And the Executive must furnish the drive to see to it that it is done, right?

DR. GILBERT A. LEVEILLE: Jack, before you sit down, one point of clarification. Did I understand you correctly that you anticipate that the first half of the data will be calculated out and available within a year?

MR. IACANO: For distribution by the September of 1978.

DR. LEVEILLE: I certainly hope your optimism is warranted.

DR. SCHNEIDER: Do you feel that funds would be continuing? How can you be sure of that? Congress changes, you know. We have a new one on the deck now.

MR. IACANO: This is true, but under this continuing law that we have at the present time, these are referred to as "recurring funds," which means that they will be allocated to the Agricultural Research Service on a yearly basis, along with our regular budget. And these monies are earmarked specifically.

DR. SCHNEIDER: OMB agrees to that?

MR. IACANO: Yes.

DR. LEVEILLE: Do you have plans now to conduct these surveys more frequently than every 10 years, Jack?

MR. IACANO: As I've pointed out, we're involved in a very massive survey now. This will include all 50 States and Puerto Rico. We hope to get to Guam, the Virgin Islands, and other outlying areas. And we are in the midst of making plans for the future in terms of combining not only the recall-type of survey but also the nutrition health survey. Based upon the discussions and plans which emerge from the combined HEW-USDA planning groups, we hope that this will be an ongoing activity in our country.

DR. SYDNEY CANTOR: I assume this means that the pilot has been completed.

MR. IACANO: The pilot is in effect right now. The contracts were signed approximately one month ago, and the pilot is in effect now.

DR. CANTOR: And it means that the objections that the OMB had to the technology have been answered satisfactorily.

MR. IACANO: That's correct. In fact the very last questions that arose were settled last week.

DR. CANTOR: What's your objection to recall data?

MR. IACANO: I had no objection to it except that as you've pointed out this tells not only what we eat but what we throw out. And therefore we do not get a real estimate of food intake.

DR. CANTOR: Well, it's a lot better than dividing what's available by the population, by a questionable population figure.

MR. IACANO: Well this, in effect, was what we had dealt with. I mean, we end up with a recall survey of individuals and households, but we do deal with individual data.

DR. CANTOR: Well, having been involved with a very extensive recall data collection system in India, I'll tell you we got more information out of that than had ever been obtained before in any particular situation. We found that there was a calorie problem and not a protein problem, for example. And we also found some other interesting things, like how food was divided among members of a family. It all came out of recall data, which were checkable.

MR. IACANO: I agree that is a very good approach. However, I think that we should work toward better techniques for determining food intake.

DR. SCHNEIDER: Thank you very much. I should explain to members of the general public, who may wonder why this sudden flurry of excitement, it's because scientists live on data. It's their life blood. What you're seeing here is a new jugular that's been exposed. This is the kind of information that appears in mind-numbing tables. But in the end, through appropriate means, it comes forth in a kind of intuitive understanding, which becomes the basis of communication, which in the end results in convincing some Congressman that he should vote for it.

DR. LEVEILLE: I think it's important for the audience to point out that we've been talking about two different surveys which might be quite confusing. One is the Decennial Survey, which is a recall survey, of actually trying to find out what people have consumed in the previous 24 hours. Another survey, which Sid Cantor spoke to, is conducted on an on-going basis by the Economic Service of USDA by simply looking at the total available and dividing it by the population. This is availability data and not consumption data.

DR. VICTOR BARBERO (*Johns Hopkins School of Public Health, Baltimore, Md.*): My question is directed to Dr. Wilcox. You mentioned that Public Law 480 had some adverse effects. I was wondering could you describe those adverse effects and elaborate on how they could be remedied in the future?

DR. WALTER W. WILCOX: The adverse effects I had in mind were the temporary lowering of the price of food in the receiving country and the consequent discouragement of home production; also, the feeling on the part of the country that they could depend on food gifts from abroad and therefore did not have to develop their own food production capacity. There was a seminar at the Brookings Institute just a few weeks ago which focused on this particular aspect of the PL/480 program. The discussions that I've heard around Congress are that this is going to be a more important consideration in the years ahead because we are now of the firm opinion, for the countries that are seeing big deficits ahead, the most important thing they can do is increase their own food production. They cannot depend upon PL/480 programs to supply their needs.

DR. MAX MILNER: Not a question, a point of information: I think it would be extremely useful if Dr. Wilcox would continue his discourse. I was disappointed that he stopped as soon as he did, to tell us Congress' initiative in finding out how to establish priorities for all these requests for new food and agriculture research. How are they going to reach priorities on what to fund first?

DR. WILCOX: I'm not sure I can tell you as much as you'd like to know. I have been working for the past year with two different projects in the Office of Technology Assessment on agricultural research and development. One deals with organizing and financing high-priority basic research to enhance food production. Another one deals with increasing U.S. assistance to developing countries in strengthening their national research programs for food crops.

Out of this activity some of our staff are working hard with members of the Committee staffs on a new agricultural research bill that would set up some new committees for advising on what are the most important items that should be taken up and how to move forward more rapidly in getting research on the more important aspects of our various food systems. I don't believe I can be much more specific than that.

I might say that one of the reasons Mr. Cordaro * could not be here is that he's been spending a lot of time on the phone the last few days talking to all different parts of the country with people that are interested in this bill, and they want to know will it do this, will it do that, won't it do this, or so on. We can't be sure what it will be like when it gets introduced, but it will probably have two aspects:

One, it will provide more funds for research, more emphasis on basic research, more emphasis on nutrition. And it will set up some new committee systems for advising on changing research programs.

DR. SCHNEIDER: Dr. Wilcox, is this to take the place of the Wampler Bill?

DR. WILCOX: Yes.

DR. SCHNEIDER: There is a yeasty ferment that's now going on in Congress, and a sensitivity towards this issue, that was exemplified by the success of the Wampler Bill in passing in the House of the old Congress. For the first time agricultural research was to be identified as a mission of the Department of Agriculture, and it would have an Assistant Secretary, who would be assigned to run the show.

DR. WILCOX: Let me say that I think there were political things involved. The Administration did not want to spend extra money that was proposed there, and so opposed the bill for a substantial part of the time. This is primarily the reason why it didn't go through the Senate.

DR. SCHNEIDER: Alas. The game starts all over again. There will be a new House, we've got some of the Senators back with us, and some new ones there too. What you were discussing before, if I understand you correctly Dr. Wilcox, was the thrust and continued inclusion in the new bill of further inputs from the various constituencies across the country.

DR. WILCOX: There isn't much change in Congress. There will not be much change in basic legislation that comes from Congress. The basic change will be in the help that they get from the Executive.

DR. SCHNEIDER: Remember you heard it here first.

DR. MICHAEL RABIN: First, I'm wondering how you make these surveys, on what basis? I've been taking dietary histories for 25 years, and my results don't quite agree with what I've read.

Second, why don't you push just putting everything on the label that the food contains in plain English?

DR. SCHNEIDER: Does anyone have any comments to make on this?

DR. LEVEILLE: Let me take a stab at the first question. I would not expect your results, Dr. Rabin, to agree with the results of the U.S. survey, for several reasons. You are dealing with quite a different population. The U.S.D.A. survey attempts to take a cross-section of the American population, cutting across all economic levels, sex levels, age levels, etc. Hopefully, it does give us a basis for intakes.

One of the very important elements that has been missing, however, is that all of the data provided are averages for each group. We have no idea of what the distribution of intakes is, and this is a very important element of information to get at.

Your second point regarding labeling I think we would all agree with.

* J. B. Cordaro, Food Program Manager, Office of Technology Assessment, Washington, D.C.

There are some extremely difficult constraints when one attempts to develop a label, as I'm sure many of the representatives from industry here could point to. It is one thing to say that we should simply put things on the label in plain English that everyone can understand. Achieving that is something else again. And there may be some individuals, some industry, who'd like to comment on that.

I don't think—at least it's my impression after speaking to many people from the food industry—that it is an attempt on the part of the industry simply to deceive the consumer by not telling what's in the food. We, in fact, now have great problems with ingredient labels that do tell, perhaps not in plain English, what is in the food product.

Ms. MARY GOODWIN (*Rockville, Md.*): I was particularly fascinated with Dr. Cantor's talk. I felt he outlined the problems that we face very succinctly and clearly. But I wondered if he had any solutions, how do we get around the homogenization of our food supply. How do we build in ethnicity and regionality into foods? What do we do about a new emerging group of foods that I call the 5-F's: fabricated, formulated, frivolous, fortified, fake foods, which seem to be making inroads into the basic four food groups. Gil, you didn't put those into perspective when you were dealing with the basic fours. But foods are being diluted somewhat. We read ads saying "Use our tomato extender, cut your tomatoes in half or why not eliminate them?" Are we getting tomatoes in a pizza, are we getting imitation cheeses, which have been approved for use in school food service programs? What about spreadables, what's in them?

I wanted to know how we dealt with this. When we looked at some of the questions raised by consumer groups pushing for more local self-reliance, is this realistic? Can we get back to maybe Green Belts around our cities that could produce food at less energy, or does it cost more to do this?

DR. CANTOR: Let me try to pick it apart. I'm very sympathetic to your point of view, which may not by any means answer the question. Let me say this: I tried to point out that in a complicated system, such as the American food system represents, that the thing that keeps it going is acceptability. Every time we move over a transfer point somebody has to give and somebody has to accept. And one of the consumer's best weapons is not to accept.

On the other hand, the fabricated foods that you're talking about probably have a place. One can draw all kinds of attention to, let's say, negative aspects of dairy products. The fact that milk is being taken apart to the extent that it is and reconstituted into a whole series of other products is testimony to that. Little by little, things are happening. Consumption of milk is going down, consumption of dairy products is going down.

The use of vegetable proteins as sources for extenders of cheeses is a very legitimate kind of thing. It certainly doesn't decrease the protein value of the material, nor does it have a major effect on acceptability apparently.

In other parts of the world the protein system is not based on animals; it's based on soy, let's say, in a very acceptable way and people do survive on the stuff and like it. I'm not saying that the Chinese system can be superimposed on the American system with complete success. But there certainly has been an increase in Chinese food around the world.

But that's beside the point also. Local effort, it seems to me, is the kind of innovative activity that can make inroads into what you object to. Besides, it will keep people busy. And that's a very good thing to have happen, as I think you would agree. It provides a focus for local enthusiasm. I know some people who are involved with gardening. They spend as much time gardening as they previously spent playing golf. I don't offer the two things as alternatives, by any means. But what I'm saying is that we need that kind of enthusiasm about a return to some kind of active participation in the production of food or in the processing of food, or at whatever level that happens to be.

Ms. MONA DOYLE (*Pantry Pride Supermarkets*): The question is for Dr. Leveille. What's the state of the research art when it comes to minimum daily requirements, especially in the trace minerals area? What would be your prognosis of how much time is going to elapse before we really have information on what those minimum needs are? Because that's very related to the kind of information that is going on the label and the kinds of frivolous foods that Mary is talking about.

DR. LEVEILLE: I wish I could give you a definitive answer. It's related I think in part to what Dr. Wilcox was talking about, and what's been mentioned several times already in these sessions. It depends upon the availability of resources to do the necessary research. There has been a fantastic lag in research and establishment of human nutrient needs. And without that information obviously we can't come up with realistic estimates of recommended allowances.

Some of that research is going on. It's going on slowly, and it can be speeded up with the availability of additional resources. However, we must keep in mind that the other factor that is going to very significantly influence the rate at which we can move, and the kinds of information that we can obtain, is some of the very serious constraints that are now being put on almost any kind of research involving humans. In many cases it is simply not possible to do the kind of research that is needed, and we must extrapolate from a variety of other studies involving model systems other than man himself.

Now, Dr. Mertz may want to make some estimates since he's attempting to come up with at least the best guesses that we now have available of where we are particularly in terms of trace mineral needs.

DR. WALTER MERTZ: I agree with what Dr. Leveille has said. We have a good amount of information now for those trace elements for which we suspect there might be a problem nutritionally, that is zinc, particularly, and iron. For both of those we have recommended allowances, and for both we have actual suggestions to the public as to how to implement those allowances.

Now, nutrition science has made some very remarkable progress in the past six or seven years by identifying about six or seven new trace elements that we never suspected before to be essential. But all this information comes from very sophisticated animal experiments. The only thing that we can say—and this is very sincere now—we know roughly what the signs and symptoms of deficiency for those new elements look like. And these signs and symptoms do not exist in the population. We can also make a very rough estimate of what the animals need, and we can make a rough estimate of how much is in our diet. When we put all this together, the best and most sincere advice that we can give you is get your foods from as large a variety of individual food items as possible. By doing this you greatly increase the chances that you will get an abundant supply of even those new exotic trace elements. This is really the best advice that we can give. I think it's a very valid one, until in the years to come we can give you more exact ones.

MR. TOM NICHOLSON (*Germantown, Pa.*): I find it very hard to believe that information is hard to come by these days. I found through my own readings and research that there are basic questions we can ask ourselves for our own personal nutrition. And there are certain things we can come up with, stating, for instance, whether we should eat certain things or not. I feel that just as scientists have proposed different theories for the creation of the universe, they should also postulate to us the fact that certain foods have indeed been shown not to be good for us.

If we eat nothing but natural foods we are following the basic principles of nature, and the basic process of evolution over thousands of years. If we tend to increase our consumption of artificial foods, we are going against the basic laws of nature. Very few of us today, I am sure, would deny the theory of evolution. So why is it that the basic tendency today is for science to hold back until we have definite proof? I feel that nutrition is one area where we cannot do this. We do know enough about certain foods, certain chemicals, and certain pesticides that are definitely harmful to us.

My question is, do you feel that you have to wait until we have definite proof on the harmful substances that we all are now consuming? Or should we give advice right now on as much information as we have right now and let the consumer choose for himself.

DR. LEVEILLE: When you say what do we do about the harmful elements that we're all consuming, I don't know what those are. I think you'll find a diversity of opinion amongst the scientific community as to what's good and what's bad, what food should be eliminated, and what food should be included.

I think the important point is that all foodstuff can play an important role as part of a complete diet. Individually we make different choices, for a variety of reasons. So a food which may be harmful in some ways in a given diet is not harmful in others. It would take a number of examples to demonstrate this; I'll use just one:

Many people in the consumer's movement attack one of the meat products on the market that is widely consumed—the frankfurter—because 80% of its calories come from fat and because it contains nitrite. I'm not very concerned about nitrites, and I think this morning we had a pretty good discussion of the fact that the benefits derived from nitrites exceed the potential risk the public may be exposed to.

Now, the fat question is one that there has been considerable debate over. Certainly no one would agree that we should consume 80% of our calories from fat. However, a product supplying 80% of calories from fat, when diluted with other foods, presents no particular problem at all. So it is a total diet concept that we need to deal with.

Secondly, let me try to address the general concern that you were getting at, and I think people in the scientific community would agree with you, although we don't really know how to come to grips with it: the whole question of benefit-risk. We think it is important to be able to inform consumers about the hazards of certain components of the food supply. Nothing is 100% safe, and I think we have to dump the concept of a food supply that is 100% safe.

On the other hand, the risks involved from anything that is in the present food supply are very small. But we don't know how to put a figure on that, so that a consumer would be able to make a truly intelligent evaluation of whether or not they want to consume a given product. I think the whole area of benefit-risk evaluation is something that we need to address ourselves to, in terms of having a system that will permit consumers to make reasonable judgment.

That obviously doesn't answer your question, but I think it puts it in a form that we can begin to address.

JOHN VANDERVEEN (*Food & Drug Administration, Washington, D.C.*): I guess I ought to respond to that. I think there are two things implied there. One, that we are holding back information from the public. Under the Freedom of Information Act any information that the government has is available to the public. We don't hold information back on the safety of products in our food supply.

I would say categorically that the standards that are set for approval of things in the food supply are extremely strict, and it is very, very hard for me to conceive that there is any real, serious problem from that point of view.

Now, there are a number of food products that have been on the market for many, many years, some of them up to a thousand years. Some occur naturally in many products and people don't recognize this, although they are now being bandied around as being detrimental. Perhaps the thing most people don't realize is that of the ingredients of the food supply that are the most dangerous in terms of excessive intake are the nutrients themselves. The toxicities of all the trace elements are well known.

Of course we can't do without them, and the misjudgement being made in this regard by well-meaning people in our society is perhaps more shocking than the effects of food additives per se.

I would like to emphasize that I know of no data, hidden away in closets, that support the notion that certain things that are toxic continue to be put in the food supply and that the public is being deceived in any way, shape, or form on that score.

Ms. ANN POTTMAN (*Simon Fraser Univ., Vancouver, British Columbia*): I would like to come to the support of the consumer at this point. I feel that consumers are not adequately represented at this meeting. And, of course, it's not a conference designed for the average consumer. I think this is part of the problem that we've been experiencing in the past.

This evening we've been discussing the fact that the decision lies with the consumer, and granted that is true. Every consumer who goes into a supermarket has the choice of buying white bread or whole wheat bread and so on. But there is also the problem that consumers are experiencing an abysmal lack of knowledge in the field of nutrition. And people who are knowledgeable in the field of nutrition, nutritionists, scientists, whatever you want to call them, have, I feel, failed to provide the public with an adequate and reliable source of information.

This void has been present for many years. There has been an evident increase in awareness and in knowledge by the general public in their state of health and in their food supply. When you have this increased awareness without an adequate source of knowledge, well then you're leaving yourself wide open for food faddism, people following unusual dietary habits, losing faith in the traditional nutritionists, losing faith in the food industry, losing faith in government. And that seems to be the stage where we are right now.

From today's proceedings it has been obvious that food technology still does have a lot to contribute in solving many of the food problems in North America, many of the food problems in the world. But how are you going to convince a public that has no faith in the food industry or in government that there are good things that can still be done for them?

The question that I would like to pose is why have nutritionists and the scientific community allowed this void to exist for so many years? Why have we been so elitist about our knowledge? Why have we not provided it in a manner that the general public can understand? I would like somebody on the panel to support the scientific community. I would like them to explain why they have failed the general public.

DR. SCHNEIDER: You want somebody to support the scientific community in its record as, in your view, having been inadequate in informing the public. Okay, who would like to try this one?

DR. CANTOR: Let me take two positions. The first position will be that of the supporter for the scientific community. In 1954 there was a very interesting book published by a very prominent psychologist, Ann Rowe, who examined the psyche, the lifestyle, of 60 scientists who were judged to be prominent by their peers. She put them through very, very rigorous tests, and they were from all phases of science. She came up with a rather remarkable report, which has had all kinds of reverberations in the 20-odd years since it was published.

One of the things that she came up with is that scientists, generally speaking, seek the sciences and research in the sciences because they choose to organize their own worlds. They organize worlds which appeal to them. Out of the process of investigating these worlds come some of the advances in science.

They are very energetic people, they are very ambitious people, but they concentrate their efforts in fields which interest them, and they generally step back from espousing issues of one kind or another. They try to solve problems, and they don't pretend to address issues which arise from the problems.

Now, let me take the other side. That side has been addressed in a series of forums at the National Academy of Sciences in Washington in which an effort has been made to get scientists to understand the issues which are generated by the problems that they are working on, to understand the anxieties which exist in the minds of the public, and to address those anxieties in a fashion which will help to alleviate them.

I can tell you, having participated in one of these, that it always starts with a kind of private meeting in which the scientists are admonished by people who have a lot to say on the subject, who are very much concerned about the subject. The reason they are concerned is largely because oversimplification of answers has lead to erroneous conclusions and erroneous information going to the public.

People who oversimplify situations and take a sympathetic view to the anxieties of the consumer can attract a lot of attention and become the focus of a great deal of action and power. As one very eloquent lawyer who's been following this whole problem said, "You people are talking to yourselves. [This is in addressing the scientists.] You don't talk to anybody else. And in effect you are painting yourselves into a corner and if you don't stop doing it, you're not going to have any place in the resolution of public problems at all. Other people will do it for you, other people will speak for you."

I happen to be a member of the committee that organized this meeting, and this program tonight was addressed to exactly that kind of a situation and for that reason. Some of us said this is a great meeting. A lot of people who have been talking to each other for a number of years are going to get together again and talk to each other, but there ought to be the kind of program that addresses the public problems, and the issues created by the very problems that we're all working on. And that's the basis of this forum. Whether it is successful or not, it's up to you to say.

I think you have a very good point and you have addressed a very sore subject. What I've tried to tell you is that I agree with you on the one hand, but that I can offer apologies for myself on the other.

DR. BERNARD L. OSER (*Consultant (Food & Drug), Forest Hills, Queens, N.Y.*): I think that if you haven't gotten the impression from the meetings here today, yesterday, that nutrition is a very complex subject, we—those of us who have been present as scientists and those who have been participating in the program—have not made the point clearly. Several speakers have raised the question of why isn't more of this nutrition information conveyed to the public. I was on one of the panels of the White House Conference several years ago when it was contended that dog foods were more accurately labeled than human foods. Now, no nutritionist believes that, and no nutritionist really believes that foods are accurately labeled, even today, when they merely describe the content of protein, of fat, of calories, and of ash and so on.

The reason for it is that every one of these nutritional components is exceedingly complex. It is misleading, not to say simplistic, to evaluate a food on the basis of the percentage protein it contains unless one knows something about that protein, what it is, what its quality is. The same is true of fat. Percentage means nothing in today's nutritional context. It's the quality of that fat in terms of degree of saturation, polyunsaturation, the presence of sterols and so on. It's just impossible to put accurate nutritional information on labels for an audience not professionally and technically qualified to understand all the nuances.

We talk about ash. Well, here we've heard that minerals are necessary in the diet in great number. That will be ten or fifteen minerals ought to be declared on the label of food if one is to be provided really accurate and educational nutrition information. Yet we know that some of this information is not really available and we don't have enough information to be able to make qualified judgments.

So it's wishful thinking to expect labeling to educate consumers to the extent that has been expressed here tonight.

Ms. GRETCHEN GILMAN (*Morris County Nutritional Council, Convent Sta., N.J.*): In the last few days the term has been whispered, "junk foods." Tonight for the first time someone actually uttered "sugar." I wonder, what would happen if we were to accept as a premise that sugar doesn't directly hurt anybody and go ahead on the assumption that it is only a displacement factor. It's already been mentioned that we have lowered our intake of nutrients because of our lowered calories requirement. What part does sugar consumption play in reducing our intake of other foods wherein we would be given perhaps more worthwhile nutrients? Has any research ever been done or will it ever be done on this?

DR. CANTOR: Would you define something for me, please? When you say sugar what do you mean? Do you mean sucrose? Do you mean sweeteners?

Well, if one accepts the idea that it is sucrose that is meant by the term sugar, then it's pretty clear that the amount of this that is circulated in the food system is going down. Sucrose, that is, but not total sugars, total sweeteners.

We've always been told that sugar consumption was 100 pounds a year per capita in the United States. The statistics that we've been talking about, of the United States Dept. of Agriculture, were started in 1909. Starting in 1909 the rate got up to 100 pounds very quickly and it stayed there, fluctuating a little until 1974—a very interesting year in the history of sucrose consumption.

A new product appeared on the market then and began to penetrate total sweetener consumption. Also the price of sugar went to 74¢ a pound, an important factor. That combination of events dropped the consumption of sucrose in 1974 very considerably, and that downward consumption has been going on ever since. In 1975 it was 87½ pounds a year per capita.

Now, let me turn you around and talk about total sugars. The advancing industrialization of our food system has created an increasing market for other sweeteners, notably those made from corn starch—glucose, syrup and dextrose, crystalline dextrose and, recently, a new and sweeter product—high fructose corn syrup. The total of all of those products has been going up consistently. At the present time it is somewhere around 120 lbs. That is total of all sweeteners added in the food system.

Now, the other thing that has happened that is of critical interest to this major behavioral change is that *total* carbohydrate consumption in the diet has been going down consistently since 1909. We used to eat about 500 grams a day of total carbohydrates, including sugars. Today we eat about 380 grams a day of total carbohydrate, but the percentage of sugar has gone up relatively. So we are eating more of the simpler carbohydrates and less of the polymeric carbohydrates, like starch.

At the same time our consumption of fat has increased. There is something very mysterious about the combined consumption of sugar and fat.

Now to get to your question, after having given the data. You asked whether that situation had been responsible for unbalancing the food system. The answer to that is, probably so. The reason, of course, is that it's so acceptable to the public, the combination of sugar and fat, equating to richness, that it is quite conceivable with the changing behavior—that is, people eating outside the home, more fast foods, whatever—that the total caloric requirement, which is relatively non-elastic, can be satisfied from that source, which is a relatively unbalanced source, rather than a balanced diet. That's the major reason for the request or for the suggestions that all major foods in the diet be nutritionally valid.

The answer to that question after all that rigamarole is yes.

DR. DANIEL ROSENFIELD (*Miles Laboratories, Inc., Elkhart, Ind.*): Begging the panel's indulgence, I want to overstate and perhaps oversimplify a concern, but it will I hope illustrate the problems of public policy.

Now, Dr. Leveille clearly expressed tonight one fact of nutrition when he talked about allowances, requirements. Naturally if you dislike deficiencies, you want assurance that we Americans get all the micronutrients and protein and so forth that we need. Dr. Cantor touched eloquently on what I call overages, and a topic that I know Dr. Wynder will discuss in great detail tomorrow. This concern of overages—whether we're talking about fat or sugar or what-have-you—it would seem that there is a certain problem here. If you do your surveillance, and depending upon how you read the results, if you try to perhaps increase micronutrients because you might find there are some deficiencies, you might also tend to increase the overages in our diet, which we don't want. Or vice versa; if you try to decrease the overages you might have some problems with assuring adequate consumption of micronutrients.

I've overstated that just a little bit, but perhaps you could comment on that.

DR. GILBERT A. LEVEILLE: I'm not quite sure how to respond to that. I guess what I was pointing to in talking about the need for surveillance is to have an awareness of what is happening at any point in time with regard to nutrient-intake of the general population. Hopefully, that would alert us to any problem which was occurring in terms of inadequacy of specific nutrients, or overages in terms of some nutrients if we know that to be detrimental.

What we do about it once we recognize the problem is obviously something that we really can't decide upon tonight because it would depend upon the nature of the problem. But one of the points that Dr. Mertz alluded to this morning was the possibility of increasing the nutrients with which we fortify our foods, or enrich our foods, such as zinc and perhaps copper. If we find that there is indeed a need for these nutrients, then we have some basis on which to develop a rational enrichment formula, or to change an existing formula. And I think that's really what I'm saying. Right now we have no basis for making any of those decisions.

MS. SUSAN GRANBERT (*Simon Fraser Univ., Vancouver, British Columbia*): I would like to recall a point that was made earlier. Someone brought up the possibility of a ban on food advertising. I would like to ask the panel if you would care to offer an opinion or speculation on the possibility and perhaps the plausibility of food advertising to being replaced by a type of nutritional advertising. What I mean by nutritional advertising is that the product would be advertised by its nutrients or by its components and their interactive effects in the body. Does anyone have any comments on that? *

DR. T. R. HENDERSON (*Lovelace Biomedical & Environmental Research Inst., Albuquerque, N. Mex.*): I think there is a point that Dr. Leveille slides over very easily, and the rest of you didn't comment on it at all. What about the individuality of human nutritional requirements? What do we really know about that, and how can we ever untangle any of these things. That's the thing that we haven't really discussed here.

DR. SCHNEIDER: It's not for lack of trying.

DR. HENDERSON: But how can we ever untangle any of these problems? Maybe, as you say, some of the minimum daily requirements we have estimated do cover 95% of the people. But how do we know?

DR. SCHNEIDER: We will need more research.

I'm sorry. Our time is running out. I think, however, that you must now all be aware, consumer advocates, people from Albuquerque, and all across the country, that this is a complicated business. And I think you've also found out that scientists don't always speak with one voice. The complaint is made that as far as government advice goes they would prefer to have one-armed scientists because a scientist is forever saying, "on the one hand," but then "on the other." If we were just only one-armed, maybe we would get some answers.

I'm going to tell you a little now, in the remaining two minutes before this

* No answer was forthcoming.

meeting closes, of an exercise in politics that is addressed to food. I participated in it, I have just emerged from it, and I want to share it with you.

Earlier on in this conference I made so bold as to ask whether or not we would have a U.S. nutrition policy and whether or not we ought to be driving toward one. I was lectured that pluralism was the answer, and we will somehow all muddle through. I don't believe one word of that. Although we all drown in a sea of paper—I suppose that's true of everyone in this room—Congressmen drown in oceans of paper. Now, when the Carter/Mondale people asked some of the people of the nutrition-science community to devise a position paper a dialogue began and emerged with a long laundry list of all possibly desirable goals, a long list which I doubt will ever get read.

I protested against this. The election went as you know. Two days after the election I drafted my position paper. It's on one page. This is my United States nutrition policy.

Like clean air and pure water, adequate and nourishing food for the citizenry is a prime responsibility of government. In the United States American agricultural productivity, fairly rewarded in the marketplace, can supply our needs. But the consumer too must be considered in the prices he has to pay. Further, if he cannot pay, subsidies of various kinds must be furnished so that he can pay and enter the marketplace in the name of economic and social justice.

Add on to all this the fact that the United States is the food nation of last resort in a world of hungry people, and the outline of the complexity of the present problem of human nourishment becomes evident.

To advance towards solution of this important problem, high on the Nation's agenda, and to accommodate dynamically the ever-shifting tides of conflicting factors, the Office of Science & Technology Policy shall be charged to advise the President on a continuing basis of appropriate means to improve and insure the nourishment of the citizenry. In accepting the charge the Office of Science & Technology Policy shall have the benefit of a Permanent Advisory Commission on Human Nutrition, which shall include representatives of the many diverse aspects of the American food system, including the consumer, so that satisfactory nourishment of all Americans can be assured.

That is, I believe, a politically acceptable device. What I am saying now of course is not engraved in granite. I have suggested to you a device for a continuing dialogue between all the participants in the American food system, which would include consumers, so that we could, at low profile, continue the dialogue and provide the Executive branch with the kind of inputs that will arrange on a continuing basis, a dynamic, adapting food policy. Dr. Moss has a few words to say at this time.

DR. HENRY MOSS: First of all I'd like to commend the panel and thank them very much for participating. I also would like to ask the panel whether they have any very precise or specific recommendations as how this conference can be helpful in some of the concerns that were expressed tonight, that the public be more adequately informed. Also, we have not really adequately considered the void created by the medical profession, which I am sad to say has not taken a very active role in this area. Medicine leaves a void because many people look to their own doctors for this kind of leadership. It has been lacking in the past, but we hope that will be corrected in the future.

I wonder whether the panel has precise and specific recommendations as to how the conference itself can be helpful on some of the points raised tonight?

DR. CANTOR: Can we start out, Henry, by educating the medical profession about nutrition?

DR. SCHNEIDER: I agree with that. The suggestions I hear should not be lost here—some one said, teachers, all the allied health sciences, in general.

DR. LEVEILLE: I think the conference, and particularly this evening's session, has served a useful purpose in at least raising a number of issues. I don't think any of us are wise enough to have any simple solutions that can be immediately implemented. However, I think one other point that has come up that is extremely important, and I hope we don't lose sight of, is the need for education. Reference was made earlier to the fact that the scientific community has failed to address this. That is unwarranted in the sense that there has been a tremendous effort going on for a long time trying to educate consumers. It's not a simple task. We must keep trying and we must keep trying to find better methods of doing it. But, as has been brought out, we're dealing with an extremely complex subject. Trying to simplify it to a few slogans and a few catch words is not going to be an effective solution.

EARLY MALNUTRITION AND SUBSEQUENT BRAIN DEVELOPMENT

Myron Winick and Jo Anne Brasel

Institute of Human Nutrition
College of Physicians and Surgeons
Columbia University
New York, New York 10032

Malnutrition early in life has been shown to retard brain growth,[1] reduce the rate of cell division in both animal and human brains,[2] slow the rate of myelination,[3] reduce the number of dendritic arborizations [4] and alter the synthesis and secretion of certain neural hormones.[5]

Concomitant with these results, data have accumulated demonstrating that severe early malnutrition in animals will affect subsequent behavior and that malnutrition coupled with the other elements present in the usual environment of the malnourished child results in a later deficit in learning ability.[6] Other data in the human, however, suggest that malnutrition per se may not permanently affect subsequent learning ability. For example, children with cystic fibrosis,[7] who were extremely malnourished early in life, tend to develop normally; the same is true of children with pyloric stenosis. Results from the Dutch famine studies also suggest that severe prenatal malnutrition when imposed on a well-nourished population, and followed by return to a "normal" environment, will not result in retarded mental development.[8] By contrast, studies in Guatemala and in other developing countries have demonstrated that not only do severely malnourished children returned to the environment from which they came do poorly but also that food alone is not enough to prevent the sequelae.[9]

Critical examination of these data led Levitsky and Barnes to postulate that early malnutrition functionally isolates an animal or infant from its normal environment, producing its effects on subsequent behavior by that mechanism. They further postulated that by "enriching the environment" they might be able to prevent and perhaps even overcome the effects of malnutrition. Their initial experiments suggested that their theory might be valid.[10]

We have examined the effects of environmental stimulation on the subsequent development of malnourished infants both in animals and humans. Our data demonstrate that environmental enrichment, supplied by even as simple a method as handling the animals for two minutes a day, each day, for the first 21 days of life, is sufficient to reverse the effects of neonatal malnutrition. For example, for one behavioral characteristic—attention to a novel stimulus (i.e., how much an animal simply plays with a rubber ball on a string introduced into the cage)—handling results in increased attention both in the malnourished and in the well-nourished animal. In these experiments, not only were the behavioral effects reversed by handling the animals, but also some of the biochemical effects were reversed as well. Although cell number was still reduced, the content of protein and RNA per cell was increased in both the malnourished and the well-nourished groups.

Encouraged by these results, we began an investigation of the effect of environmental enrichment on a group of previously malnourished children. We studied three groups of Korean orphans subsequently adopted by United States families. One group, the "Well Nourished," was above the 50th percentile for height and weight on admission to the adoption agency under age one. A second group, the "Moderately Nourished," was between the 25th and 3rd percentile for height and weight on admission. And a third group, the "Malnourished," was below the third percentile for height and weight on admission. All children were adopted before age 2. These children's physical growth and school records, in the United States, were examined for I.Q. and achievement scores when all the children were between age 7 and 12. The results indicated:

1. All children exceeded expected Korean norms for weight. None reached U.S. norms, and there were no differences between groups.
2. All children exceeded expected Korean norms for height. None reached U.S. norms and there was a small, but significant, difference between the previously malnourished and previously well nourished children.
3. The average I.Q. of the malnourished group was 102—right at U.S. norms. The well-nourished children, however, did even better—112— and the difference was significant.
4. The average I.Q. of the moderately nourished children fell right in between.
5. Finally, the results in achievement were exactly the same as for I.Q.

Thus, a remarkable amount of recovery can occur if a stimulated environment is introduced early—before age 3. We know from other studies that if these children had been returned to the environment that produced the malnutrition, their I.Q.'s would have ranged about 30 points less and their school achievement would have also been significantly retarded.

But how early is early? When do we have to start this stimulation to get the desired results? To attempt to answer this question, a second study was undertaken. The same three groups of children were studied, except that all were adopted after age 3 but before age 5. The results demonstrate that the malnourished group, in regard to both I.Q. and achievement, performed below the expected norms. A comparison of the data in the two studies demonstrates a reduced I.Q. and school achievement of roughly equal magnitude in all three groups of children adopted after age 3. Again, however, the I.Q. and achievements, even in the malnourished group, exceed what we would expect if they were returned to their original environment. Thus, environmental enrichment at any time up to age 5 would seem to improve the learning ability of previously malnourished children. If the environment is "enriched," at least by adoption before age 3, almost complete recovery can occur.

How great must the change in environment be? Other studies are beginning to suggest that total environmental change, such as adoption, may not be necessary. McKay et al. in Colombia are demonstrating results similar to those of the Korean children in a pre-Head Start Program in progress at present in Cali.

We seem to have come full cycle—from the feeling that there was no problem—to the feeling that the problem was one in which there was no hope for those already malnourished—to our present recognition that although the best solution is to prevent malnutrition from occurring, we can still salvage many of the children who were malnourished as infants. What still remains is to learn the most efficient and effective ways of accomplishing this.

References

1. DICKERSON, J .W. T., J. DOBBING & R. A. McCANCE. 1966–67. The effect of undernutrition on the postnatal development of the brain and cord in pigs. Proc. R. Soc. London B **166:** 396.
2. WINICK, M. & A. NOBLE. 1966. Cellular response in rats during malnutrition at various ages. J. Nutr. **89:** 300.
3. DAVISON, A. N. & J. DOBBING. 1966. Myelination as a vulnerable period in brain development. Br. Med. Bull. **22:** 40.
4. SIMA, A. 1974. Cited in studies on calibre growth of nerve fibres and perinueral permeability in normal, undernourished, and rehabilitated rats. Neuropathological Laboratory, Institute of Pathology, University of Goteborg. Goteborg, Sweden.
5. SHOEMAKER, W. J. & R. J. WURTMAN. 1971. Effect of perinatal undernutrition on the development of the brain catecholamines in the rat. Science **171:** 1017.
6. WINICK, M. 1976. Malnutrition and Brain Development. Oxford University Press. New York.
7. LLOYD-STILL, J. D., P. H. WOLF, I. HORWITZ & H. SCHWACHMAN. 1972. Studies on intellectual development after severe malnutrition in infancy in cystic fibrosis and other intestinal lesions. Presented at IX International Congress of Nutrition. Mexico City.
8. STEIN, Z., M. SUSSER, G. SAENGER & F. MAROLLA. 1972. Nutrition and mental performance. Science **178:** 708.
9. CRAVIOTO, J., E. R. DeLICARDIE & H. G. BIRCH. 1966. Nutrition, growth and neurointegrative development: An experimental ecologic study. Pediatrics **38:** (Suppl. No. 2, Part II) 319.
10. LEVITSKY, D. A. & R. H. BARNES. 1972. Nutritional and environmental interactions in the behavioral development of the rat: Long-term effects. Science **176:** 68.

DIETARY FIBER: WHAT IT IS AND WHAT IT DOES *

David Kritchevsky

The Wistar Institute of Anatomy and Biology
Philadelphia, Pennsylvania 19104

There is no concise, fully descriptive definition of dietary fiber. Trowell [1] has defined it as "the skeletal remains of plant cells that are resistant to digestion by enzymes of man." He later broadened his definition to include structural polysaccharides, lignin, and other substances.[2] Spiller and Amen [3] have tried further to systematize the nomenclature, but the search for a really adequate definition continues.

Several substances make up the bulk of what we call fiber. Among these, cellulose is the best known and most widely distributed. Cellulose is primarily an unbranched polymer of $1-4\beta$-D-glucose which may contain from 3000 to 100,000 glucose units. Hemicellulose is a much more complicated molecule than cellulose. The term was proposed by Schulze [4] to describe a family of compounds that were easily soluble in hot dilute mineral acid. In general, the hemicelluloses consist of a xylose backbone that exhibits varying degrees of substitution and branching. Most hemicelluloses contain two to four different sugars; those most commonly occurring are (besides xylose): arabinose, mannose, galactose, glucose, rhamnose, as well as glucuronic and galacturonic acids. The pectins are present in the cell walls as well as in the intercellular layers of plants. This class of materials exhibits molecular weights in the 60,000–90,000 range. The basic structural component is a polymer of $1-4\beta$-D-galacturonic acid, but this class of substances also contains D-galactose, L-arabinose, D-xylose, L-rhamnose, and L-fucose. Another group of polysaccharides that are generally classified as fiber are the plant gums, mucilages and storage polysaccharides. Chemically, these substances are highly branched uronic acid (galacturonic or glucuronic) containing polymers that contain xylose, arabinose, and mannose. Lignin is the only substance included under the heading of fiber that is not carbohydrate in nature. Lignin is a phenylpropane polymer, and the three major polymeric chains are derived from 4-hydroxyphenylpropane, 4-hydroxy-3-methoxyphenylpropane and 3,5-dimethyl-4-hydroxyphenylpropane. The lignin polymer generally has a molecular weight of 1000–4500.

Other substances generally associated with fiber are phytic acid (inositol hexaphosphate), waxes, cutins (hydroxylated fatty acids), some protein, and other minor components. Cummings [5] and Southgate [6] have recently written excellent descriptive reviews of fiber chemistry.

The scheme of fiber analysis that, until recently, had been in widest use is known as the Weende method [7] and dates to 1860, although it has been attributed by Van Soest [8] to Einhoff in 1806. This method consisted of treatment with solvent, acid, and base. However, with the recognition of the structure of cell walls, more complete methods have been introduced. These methods permit determination of celluloses, hemicelluloses, pectins, and lignins. The two most

* Supported, in part, by grants (HL–03299 and HL–05209) and a Research Career Award (HL–0734) from the National Heart and Lung Institute.

widely used methods are those of Southgate [9, 10] and Van Soest.[8, 11] Southgate [12] has recently reviewed methods of fiber analysis.

Cleave,[13] in his book *The Saccharine Disease,* postulated that the diseases common to present-day Western (or developed) populations were due to ingestion of refined flour and sugar, in contrast to the earlier experiences of these populations or those of countries subsisting on a high fiber diet. In a review article that has been widely cited, Burkitt et al.[14] pointed out that certain disease conditions prevalent in the United States were virtually unknown in Africa and attributed this difference to the difference in fiber intake between American (low) and African (high) populations. The eight conditions specifically cited by Burkitt et al.[14] were: ischemic heart disease, appendicitis, diverticular disease, gallstones, varicose veins, hiatus hernia, hemorrhoids, and colon cancer. This point of view has been amplified in a recent book edited (and largely written) by Burkitt and Trowell.[15]

The data cited are indirect, and association is not to be confused with causality. Some of the differences cited by Burkitt may be related to life-span as well as to life-style. Eastwood et al.[16] have pointed out the possible additive effects of co-existing disease states. In the case of appendicitis, Mendeloff [17] has shown that, in the United States, there has been a marked drop in incidence since 1940—this despite the reduced intake of dietary fiber. Scala [18] reports that the intake of dietary fiber in the United States fell by 42% between 1964 and 1974.

The most evident effect of dietary fiber is in decreased intestinal transit time and increased fecal bulk. This one effect can possibly explain the influence of fiber on diverticular disease, varicose veins, hiatus hernia and hemorrhoids, all of which can be related in some way to straining at stools.

Burkitt [19] quotes Hippocrates who observed, "To the human body it makes a great difference whether the bread be made of fine flour or coarse, whether of wheat with the bran, or without the bran." Hakim, a Persian physician of the ninth century, made a similar observation.[19] More recently, Cowgill and his co-workers [20, 21] noted that bran exerted a distinct laxative effect. Burkitt [19] has summarized the effects of diet on transit time and stool weight (TABLE 1).

TABLE 1

INFLUENCE OF DIET ON INTESTINAL TRANSIT TIME AND STOOL WEIGHT *

Population	Diet †	Transit Time (hrs)	Stool Weight (g)
Uganda Villagers	U	35	470
So. Africa Rural Pupils	U	33	275
So. Africa Rural Pupils	I	45	165
Uganda Boarding School	I	47	185
Indian Nurses	I	44	155
English Vegetarians	I	42	225
So. African White Pupils	R	54	150
English Students	R	70	123
Royal Navy	R	71	124

* After Burkitt.[19]
† U=unrefined carbohydrates; I=intermediate carbohydrates; R=refined carbohydrates.

TABLE 2

EFFECT OF A HIGH-FIBER DIET (17 DAYS) ON PLASMA GLUCOSE AND LIPIDS IN 13 DIABETIC MEN *

	Diet	
	ADA †	Fiber ‡
Weight	158±8	156±8
Glucose (mg/dl)	183±11	136±13 (p <0.005)
Cholesterol (mg/dl)	198±11	151±7 (p <0.001)
Triglycerides (mg/dl)	165±24	140±8

* After Kiehm et al.[29]
† 2200 calories; 234 g carbohydrate; 128 g protein; 83 g fat; 4.7 g fiber.
‡ 2200 calories; 414 g carbohydrate; 86 g protein; 23 g fat; 14.2 g fiber.

In two populations ingesting a diet containing unrefined carbohydrates, the transit time and stool weight were 34 hours and 373 grams, respectively; in four populations eating carbohydrates of an intermediate level of refinement, the values were 45 hours and 183 grams; and three groups subsisting on refined carbohydrate exhibited an average transit time of 65 hours and average stool weight of 132 grams.

These differences may be attributable to one specific property of fiber, namely, its water-holding capacity. McConnell et al.[22] have shown that a number of vegetable products have a high water-holding capacity. Painter et al.[23] reported that addition of bran to the diet could overcome the symptoms of diverticular disease. Williams and Olmstead [24] fed a series of bulking agents to human subjects and tried to correlate their laxative effects with composition, but no simple correlation was possible. This, too, suggests that the water-holding capacity of the test substances rather than their chemistry was the basis of their action. Mitchell and Eastwood [25] report on a small study (9 patients) in which persons with slow (62.8 hours) or rapid (24.7 hours) intestinal transit times (p < 0.005) were compared. The fecal net weight (g/24 hr) was 24% higher in the rapid transit group, but dry fecal weights were identical. However, this study had few patients, and their past dietary history may have had an effect.

Cleave [13] and Trowell [26] have argued that eating fiber-depleted carbohydrate represents a risk factor for onset of diabetes. Their argument suggests that replacement of fiber-rich foods with fiber-poor, processed foods results in increased consumption of fat, sugar, and calories and that this dietary pattern increases the risk of diabetes. Rats [27] and mice [28] have been reported to develop hyperglycemia when fed low-fiber, high-calorie diets. Recently, Kiehm et al.[29] have shown that a high-carbohydrate, high-fiber diet fed to hyperglycemic, diabetic men lowered plasma glucose and lipid levels. Several of the men who were on sulfonyl-ureas or insulin (<30 units/day) were able to discontinue therapy (TABLE 2). The changes in plasma lipid levels may also be attributable to the reduced fat content of the fiber diet.

Burkitt [14, 30, 31] attributes the high rate of colon cancer in the Western world to lack of dietary fiber. On the other hand, Drasar and Irving [32] have found practically no correlation between incidence of colon cancer and dietary fiber. In their study, total fat and animal protein showed the best correlation with colon cancer. Leveille [33] reviewed the correlation between diet and colon cancer in Connecticut males and found a high positive correlation with beef consumption ($r = +0.905$) and consumption of other meat, poultry, and fish ($r = +0.941$). He also found high negative correlations with consumption of cereals ($r = -0.974$) and potatoes ($r = -0.968$).

Hill [34] has postulated that colon cancer is due, in part, to the action of intestinal bacteria which can convert bile acids to potential carcinogens. Hill et al.[35] obtained a straight-line relationship when plotting total fecal dihydroxycholanoic acid content versus incidence of colon cancer in six different populations. They also found a greater population of the bacteria which can produce chemical alterations in the feces of the populations with high rates of colon cancer. Burkitt [36] has pointed out that, on the average, the three high cancer populations ingest 295% more fat, 320% more protein, and at least twice as much fiber as do the low cancer ones.

How can fiber affect the level of bile acids in the colon, other than by decreasing intestinal transit time, hence decreasing the residence time of potential carcinogens or co-carcinogens?

Eastwood and Hamilton [37] observed that some cereal grains had the ability to bind various bile acids. In a systematic study of bile acid binding, we [38, 39] have found that each bile acid or salt has a specific binding capacity for certain types of fiber. As TABLE 3 shows, lignin has the greatest general binding ability and cellulose the least, but specific substrates may exhibit greatest binding to substances other than lignin.

How fiber affects the spectrum of intestinal flora remains to be determined.

Insufficient dietary fiber has been implicated as an etiologic factor in ischemic heart disease.[1, 40-42] Walker and Arvidsson [43] were the first to suggest that crude fiber might be the factor that protected the African Black from heart disease. Assigning a protective role to only one dietary component in a disease of multi-factored etiology is an oversimplification. Fat intake is considered to be one dietary risk factor in heart disease and, in general, populations that ingest a high fiber diet eat relatively little fat and vice-versa. Which factor is it?

Alfalfa [44, 45] and pectin [46] have been shown to protect rabbits and chickens, respectively, from cholesterol-induced atherosclerosis. Kritchevsky [47] has sum-

TABLE 3

PERCENT BINDING OF BILE ACIDS AND BILE SALTS TO FOUR TYPES OF FIBER *

Bile Acid or Salt	Binding Agent			
	Alfalfa	Bran	Cellulose	Lignin
Cholic Acid	20	10	3	44
Taurocholic Acid	7	1	3	22
Glycocholic Acid	12	4	1	23
Chenodeoxycholic Acid	25	18	2	23
Taurochenodeoxycholic Acid	15	10	0	25
Glycochenodeoxycholic Acid	15	21	0	25
Deoxycholic Acid	10	5	0	17
Taurodeoxycholic Acid	11	3	1	31
Glycodeoxycholic Acid	28	8	5	53

* After Story and Kritchevsky.[39]

marized the data which show that when saturated fat is added to a semipurified, cholesterol-free diet it is atherogenic for rabbits but when added to stock diet it is without effect. It was shown [48, 49] that the protective effect of stock diet was due to its fiber content. Different types of fiber have been shown to exert various levels of protection.[50, 51]

A summary of 10 studies has concluded that bran exerts no effect on serum lipid levels in man.[52] Pectin,[53-55] guar gum,[55] and bengal gram [56] do exhibit hypocholesteremic properties.

Approaches to the mechanism of action of fiber have shown that semipurified diets decrease cholic acid and neutral steroid excretion in rats.[57] Pectin increases bile acid but not neutral steroid excretion in cholesterol-fed rats,[58] and alfalfa increases neutral steroid excretion in rats.[59] The observed effects are obviously a function of the composition of the fibers being fed, and more has to be learned about this phenomenon.

Dietary fiber also affects the action of certain toxic materials. Chow et al.[60] first showed that rats fed a high sucrose diet plus 5% Tween 60 exhibited greatly reduced weight gain (40% below control), but when the diet contained half as much sucrose and a high level of soybean meal weight gain was only 5% below normal.

Ershoff [61] repeated this experiment using Tween 20 and showed that alfalfa meal reduced the observed weight loss and mortality. Ershoff also showed that stock ration protected rats from the weight loss occasioned by addition of 0.1–0.2% 2.5-di-t-butylhydroquinone (DBH) to their diet.[62] He also showed that stock ration could reduce the toxic effects of 2.5–10% sodium cyclamate.[63] Ershoff and Thurston [64] fed rats a semipurified diet containing 5% Amaranth (FD and C Red #2) and observed no survival beyond 14 days. Addition of 10% pectin, cellulose, or alfalfa to the diet completely overcame the dye's toxicity (TABLE 4).

Does fiber have any deleterious effects? Phytic acid is present in some grains. This material impairs absorption of iron [65] and zinc [66] and may induce

TABLE 4

INFLUENCE OF DIETARY SUPPLEMENTS ON AMARANTH (FD AND C RED #2) TOXICITY IN RATS *

Diet	Average Weight Gain (g)		
	7 days	14 days	21 days
Basal (B)†	30 (6)‡	63 (6)	90 (6)
B+5% Amaranth (BA)	3 (5)	3 (1)	—
BA plus §			
5% cottonseed oil	2 (5)	13 (3)	26 (20)
10% casein	4 (5)	24 (1)	42 (1)
10% pectin	16 (6)	44 (6)	71 (6)
10% cellulose	24 (6)	61 (6)	87 (6)
10% alfalfa	30 (6)	65 (6)	93 (6)

* After Ershoff and Thurston.[64]
† Sucrose, 66; Casein, 24; Salt Mix, 5; Cottonseed oil, 5.
‡ Number of rats surviving, starting with 6 per group.
§ Added at expense of sucrose.

negative zinc balance.[66, 67] Another unpleasant side effect of a high fiber diet is volvulus of the sigmoid colon. This condition is the most common cause of colonic obstruction in India,[68] where the incidence is higher in vegetarian Hindus than in nonvegetarian Moslems or Sikhs. Sigmoid volvulus is also prevalent in East Africa [69] and Scandinavia,[70] but rare in the United States or the United Kingdom.

In summary, the data relating to the effects of dietary fiber in man are still largely epidemiological in nature. Some beneficial effects are observed when fiber is added to the diets of animals fed special diets. Work on the action of dietary fiber is an area of research well worth pursuing. We must also learn to identify the individual components of fiber so that we may properly attribute the observed effects to the appropriate constituent.

REFERENCES

1. Trowell, H. C. 1972. Atherosclerosis **16:** 138.
2. Trowell, H. C. 1974. Lancet **i:** 503.
3. Spiller, G. A. & R. J. Amen. 1975. Am. J. Clin. Nutr. **28:** 675.
4. Schulze, E. 1891. Ber. Deutsch. Chem. Ges. **24:** 2277.
5. Cummings, J. H. 1976. In Fiber in Human Nutrition. G. A. Spiller & R. J. Amen, Eds. Plenum Press. N.Y.
6. Southgate, D. A. T. 1976. In Fiber in Human Nutrition. G. A. Spiller & R. J. Amen, Eds. Plenum Press. N.Y.
7. Mangold, D. E. 1934. Nutr. Abstr. Res. **3:** 647.
8. Van Soest, P. J. & R. W. McQueen. 1973. Proc. Nutr. Soc. **32:** 123.
9. Southgate, D. A. T. 1969. J. Sci. Food Agric. **20:** 326.
10. Southgate, D. A. T. 1969. J. Sci. Food Agric. **20:** 331.
11. Van Soest, D. J. & R. H. Winde. 1967. J. Animal Sci. **26:** 940.
12. Southgate, D. A. T. 1976. In Fiber in Human Nutrition. G. A. Spiller & R. J. Amen, Eds. Plenum Press. N.Y.
13 Cleave, T. L. 1974. The Saccharine Disease. John Wright and Sons, Ltd. Bristol, England.
14. Burkitt, D. P., A. R. P. Walker & N. S. Painter. 1974. J. Am. Med. Assoc. **229:** 1068.
15. Burkitt, D. P. & H. C. Trowell. 1975. Refined Carbohydrate Foods and Disease. Academic Press. London.
16. Eastwood, M. A., J. Eastwood & M. Ward. 1976. In Fiber in Human Nutrition. G. A. Spiller & R. J. Amen, Eds. Plenum Press. N.Y.
17. Mendeloff, A. I. 1975. Nutr. Rev. **33:** 321.
18. Scala, J. 1975. In Physiological Effects of Food Carbohydrates. A. Jeanes & J. Hodge, Eds. Am. Chem. Soc. Washington, D.C.
19. Burkitt, D. & N. Painter. 1975. In Refined Carbohydrate Foods and Disease. D. P. Burkitt & H. C. Trowell, Eds. Academic Press. London.
20. Cowgill, G. R. & W. E. Anderson. 1932. J. Am. Med. Assoc. **98:** 1886.
21. Cowgill, G. R. & A. J. Sullivan. 1933. J. Am. Med. Assoc. **100:** 795.
22. McConnell, A. A., M. A. Eastwood & W. D. Mitchell. 1974. J. Sci. Food Agri. **25:** 1457.
23. Painter, N. S., A. Z. Almeida & K. W. Colebourne. 1972. Brit. Med. J. **2:** 137.
24. Williams, R. D. & W. H. Olmstead. 1936. Ann. Int. Med. **10:** 717.
25. Mitchell, W. D. & M. A. Eastwood. 1976. In Fiber in Human Nutrition. G. A. Spiller & R. J. Amen, Eds. Plenum Press. N.Y.
26. Trowell, H. 1975. In Refined Carbohydrate Foods and Disease. D. P. Burkitt & H. C. Trowell, Eds. Academic Press. London.

27. HACKEL, D. B., L. A. FROHMAN, E. MIKAT, H. E. LEBOVITZ, K. SCHMIDT-NIELSEN & T. D. KINNEY. 1966. Diabetes **15:** 105.
28. GLEASON, R. E., V. LAURIS & J. S. SOELDNER. 1967. Diabetologia **3:** 175.
29. KIEHM, T. G., J. W. ANDERSON & K. WARD. 1976. Am. J. Clin. Nutr. **29:** 895.
30. BURKITT, D. P. 1971. J. Nat. Cancer Inst. **47:** 913.
31. BURKITT, D. P. 1971. Cancer **28:** 3.
32. DRASAR, B. S. & D. IRVING. 1973. Brit. J. Cancer **27:** 167.
33. LEVEILLE, G. A. 1975. J. Animal Sci. **41:** 723.
34. HILL, M. J. 1977. *In* The Bile Acids. Vol. 3. P. P. Nair & D. Kritchevsky, Eds. Plenum Press. N.Y. In press.
35. HILL, M. J., B. S. DRASAR, V. C. ARIES, J. S. CROWTHER, G. HAWKSWORTH & R. E. O. WILLIAMS. 1971. Lancet **i:** 95.
36. BURKITT, D. 1975. *In* Refined Carbohydrate Foods and Disease. D. P. Burkitt & H. C. Trowell, Eds. Academic Press. London.
37. EASTWOOD, M. A. & D. HAMILTON. 1968. Biochim. Biophys. Acta **152:** 165.
38. KRITCHEVSKY, D. & J. A. STORY. 1974. J. Nutr. **104:** 458.
39. STORY, J. A. & D. KRITCHEVSKY. 1976. J. Nutr. **106:** 1292.
40. TROWELL, H. C. 1972. Am. J. Clin. Nutr. **25:** 926.
41. TROWELL, H. C. 1973. Proc. Nutr. Soc. **32:** 150.
42. TROWELL, H. C. 1973. Plant Foods for Man **1:** 11.
43. WALKER, A. R. P. & V. B. ARVIDSSON. 1974. J. Clin. Invest. **33:** 1358.
44. COOKSON, F. B., R. ALTSCHUL & S. FEDOROFF. 1967. J. Atheroscler. Res. **7:** 69.
45. COOKSON, F. B. & S. FEDOROFF. 1968. Brit. J. Exp. Path. **44:** 348.
46. FISHER, H., W. G. SOLLER & P. GRIMINGER. 1966. J. Atheroscler. Res. **6:** 292.
47. KRITCHEVSKY, D. 1964. J. Atheroscler. Res. **4:** 103.
48. KRITCHEVSKY, D. & S. A. TEPPER. 1965. Life Sci. **4:** 1467.
49. KRITCHEVSKY, D. & S. A. TEPPER. 1968. J. Atheroscler. Res. **8:** 357.
50. MOORE, J. H. 1967. Brit. J. Nutr. **21:** 207.
51. STORY, J. A., S. A. TEPPER & D. KRITCHEVSKY. 1976. Fed. Proc. **35:** 294.
52. TRUSWELL, A. S. & R. M. KAY. 1976. Lancet **i:** 367.
53. KEYS, A., F. GRANDE & J. T. ANDERSON. 1961. Proc. Soc. Exp. Biol. Med. **106:** 555.
54. PALMER, G. H. & D. G. DIXON. 1966. Am. J. Clin. Nutr. **18:** 437.
55. JENKINS, D. J. A., A. R. LEEDS, C. NEWTON & J. H. CUMMINGS. 1975. Lancet **i:** 1116.
56. MATHUR, K. S., M. A. KHAN & R. D. SHARMA. 1968. Brit. Med. J. **1:** 30.
57. PORTMAN, O. W. & P. MURPHY. 1958. Arch. Biochem. Biophys. **76:** 367.
58. LEVEILLE, G. A. & H. E. SAUBERLICH. 1966. J. Nutr. **88:** 209.
59. KRITCHEVSKY, D., S. A. TEPPER & J. A. STORY. 1974. Nutr. Rep. Int. **9:** 301.
60. CHOW, B. F., J. M. BURNETT, C. T. LING & L. BARROWS. 1953. J. Nutr. **49:** 563.
61. ERSHOFF, B. H. 1960. J. Nutr. **70:** 484.
62. ERSHOFF, B. H. 1963. Proc. Soc. Exp. Biol. Med. **112:** 362.
63. ERSHOFF, B. H. 1972. Proc. Soc. Exp. Biol. Med. **141:** 857.
64. ERSHOFF, B. H. & E. W. THURSTON. 1974. J. Nutr. **104:** 937.
65. BJORN-RASMUSSEN, E. 1974. Nutr. Metab. **16:** 101.
66. REINHOLD, J. G., K. NASR, A. LAHEMGARZADEH & H. HEDAYATI. 1973. Lancet **i:** 283.
67. MCCANCE, R. E. & E. M. WIDDOWSON. 1942–43. J. Physiol. **101:** 44.
68. GULATI, S. M., N. K. GROVER, N. K. TAGORE & O. P. TANEJA. 1974. Dis. Colon Rectum **17:** 219.
69. SHEPHERD, J. J. 1968. Brit. Med. J. **1:** 280.
70. PETERSON, H. I. 1967. Ann. Surg. **166:** 296.

AGING, NUTRITION, AND THE CONTINUUM OF HEALTH CARE

Donald M. Watkin *

*Office of State and Community Programs
Administration on Aging
Office of Human Development
Office of the Secretary
Department of Health, Education and Welfare
Washington, D.C. 20201*

The Aging-Nutrition-Health Triad

Aging, nutrition, and the continuum of health care are three agglomerates forming a triad whose integrity is the essence underlying human aspirations for long, successful, and happy lives.

Concern about components of the triad is widespread. Concern about the integral triad is less widespread, largely because proponents of any one component have little knowledge of the ingredients of the other two and little understanding of the complex reciprocal dependencies among all three.

Two Categories of Issues

Public concern has led to many issues. These comprise, first, the still unknown realms of the basic and applied sciences relevant to the triad. These have been the subject of many presentations by myself and others.[1-14] Second, however, they comprise the application of presently known science and technology to human problems associated with the triad in both technically advanced and developing societies.

In consideration of the themes of this Bicentennial Conference, the suggestions of the Conference's Nutrition Advisory Committee and my own recent professional experiences, I will focus on issues of the second category, i.e., those concerned with the application of presently known scientific knowledge and technology to human problems associated with aging, nutrition, and the continuum of health care.

An Issue Defined

First, let me define an issue. An issue is a problem of broad public concern under discussion, debate, or dispute to which there are one or more possible and effective solutions. In the light of this definition, consideration of issues requires the identification of problems. Obviously, also, in dealing with three agglomerates—any one of which comprises knowledge derived from all the

* On detail from the Veterans Administration's Department of Medicine and Surgery.

natural, biologic, clinical, social, economic and political sciences—the potential number of problems is incredibly large.

In the interests of time, I will confine my remarks to four issues whose resolutions are in my judgment crucial to the successful survival of mankind in the next half century.

Four Issues

Each of these may be stated as a question:

1. How can present-day societies be convinced that aging, nutrition, and the continuum of health care are inseparable triad components, no one of which can be treated independently or neglected without jeopardizing the welfare of the affected societies?

2. How can these societies be convinced that the integrity of the aging-nutrition-health triad is critical at all chronological ages?

3. How can these same societies be convinced that promotion of the aging-nutrition-health triad concept is an effective approach to improving current life-styles that have been identified as agents most responsible for human misery and waste of resources in the world today?

4. How can these societies be convinced that promotion of the aging-nutrition-health triad concept is cost-effective in assuring steady economic development?

The Summarizing Issue

An issue summarizing all four may be stated as "how can societies be convinced?"

The issue in 1976 is not "should they be convinced?"; it is not "is the price affordable?"; it is not "can it be done?" If any qualification is required, it is "how can societies be convinced in the shortest possible time?"

The Time Factor

Time is critical because of demographic considerations with serious economic and social implications for both technically advanced and developing societies. In its Bicentennial Year, the United States already has 32 million people aged 60 or over. Population samples of this age category drawn from among participants in various health and nutrition surveys suggest that over half have from one to six illnesses and/or disabilities, many of which are unknown to or misunderstood by their human hosts.[15] Surveys of nutritional status among those 60 and over suggest that disease and disability compounded by economic deprivation often stemming from the high financial cost of disease and disability initiate vicious cycles through which disease and disability are further aggravated by malnutrition. If conditions remain unaltered, this 1976 tragedy in the United States will be worsened appreciably in the next half century, especially as those born during the post-World War II baby boom reach late maturity and old age.

While time is crucial in the United States, it is even more critical in developing societies where population growth has led to situations where as many as 75 percent of national populations are now under 25 years of age. As these enormous young populations age and themselves become victims of present-day life-style diseases and disabilities, the demand placed on resources for their care will exceed supply by many times the ratio present today.

CONVINCING SOCIETIES REQUIRES CONVINCING LEADERS

Convincing societies to accept application of an integrated aging-nutrition-health triad to life-style-related problems requires first conviction by national leaders of the validity, universal applicability, effectiveness, and cost-effectiveness of the triad concept.

CONVINCING LEADERS/SOCIETIES REQUIRES PROFESSIONAL LEADERSHIP

Breeding such conviction among charismatic political leadership should be a prime function of government, academic, and industrial professionally trained leaders. The examples professionally trained American leaders and their colleagues around the world set for their peers who have assumed political leadership roles are prime ingredients in this breeding process.

Other ingredients in the recipe include articulate presentation of scientific convictions before elected legislators and elected officials of executive branches of government. This can be done by appearances of professionally trained scientists at hearings and also by their influence on articulate spokesmen of consumer and other well-organized pressure groups.

Breeding such conviction must not stop with politicians. Powerful and presently unenlightened leaders exist among various professions, among Federal, State, and local government bureaucrats, among representatives of the news media, among representatives of advertising and industrial enterprises, among leaders of our labor movements, and among our religious leaders. As is the case with political leaders, reaching these leaders can also be achieved via consumer and pressure groups, via legislative actions, and by mass media public service announcements. Such maneuvers, however, are time-consuming. A more practical approach may be to complement all other efforts by personal contacts and to use these to extract from leaders in all categories commitments to use their influence in behalf of promotion of the aging-nutrition-health triad concept.

THE ISSUES

Let me now return to the four specific issues listed above and urge all of you to remember that, in dealing with issues involving the interrelations of three exceedingly complex agglomerates, each issue may have pluralistic as opposed to single answers.

Issue Number One

Issue number one, how to convince societies that aging, nutrition, and health are intimately related, suggests the need to articulate in detail on every possible occasion the influence of appropriate nutrition on aging and health but also, and perhaps even more important, to stress the influence of the continuum of indicated health care at all ages on nutritional status, on prevalence rates for morbidity, and on effective longevity.

A major obstacle to successful resolution of this issue is the veritable avalanche of overt food fad promotions, of promotions of medical quackery often vested in nutritional raiment, and of slick and effective product promotions via mass media designed to augment profit margins of the sponsors but unconcerned with the simultaneous augmentation of life-style diseases and disabilities. Even among highly educated professionals, the concept of malnutrition secondary to disease and disability is virtually unknown. The concept of nutrition's having, during infancy, childhood, youth, and early maturity, positive impact on the incidence of life-style diseases and disabilities of late maturity and old age and on longevity itself is even less understood. Instead, many highly educated but non-science-oriented professionals seek guidance and solace from afflictions and anxieties from the promotional material of faddists and quacks.

The scientific community has failed to meet this obvious challenge among the well-educated, not to mention other less fortunate persons around the world. Although dietary caloric restriction has been known for over 40 years [16] to enhance longevity in animals and fish, no scientifically acceptable explanation of its mechanism of action has yet been established.[17] Wanting such, counterattacks against faddism, quackery, and profit-oriented promotions lack the infrastructure of firm conviction. The lack is equally apparent with respect to nutrition's role in the pathogenesis of most life-style diseases and disabilities. Obviously, more basic and applied research is needed to ameliorate this situation.

But, at a more pragmatic level, fault must also be assigned to educators for their failure to provide students in both initial training and continuing education sufficient insight into the unity of aging, nutrition, and the continuum of health care based on what is already known.

To summarize in respect to issue one, measures must be taken to augment our ability to convince population groups that aging, nutrition, and the continuum of health care are inseparable components of all effective measures to decrease morbidity and increase effective longevity.

Issue Number Two

Issue number two, how to convince population groups that the unity of the aging-nutrition-health triad is critical at all chronological ages, suggests the need to develop effective measures for inducing change in current short-term attitudes toward life-style diseases and disabilities and the need to disseminate effectively information on the critical role nutrition plays in the management of acute illness and injury at all phases of the life cycle.

Attacking the *carpe diem* philosophies in youth-oriented societies requires building a new image for the latter half of life. The joys of late maturity and old age need reinforcement based on real achievements by the natural, biologic, clinical, social, economic and political sciences. No one will strive to be alive in the latter half of life if that epoch holds forth only an image of illness, disability, loneliness, poverty, and indifference by family, society, and government. Integration of all components of the agglomerates of the aging-nutrition-health triad and application of the integrated whole at all levels of the age cycle requires dynamic leadership charismatic in nature and, particularly, active, inspiring leadership from among the elderly themselves.

Obtaining desired respect for the critical role nutrition plays in management of illness and injury at all phases of the life cycle requires reinforcement by constant repetition of data on the lives spared and the time and money saved by minimizing periods of disability through emphasis on appropriate nutrition. Among persons in late maturity and old age, reserves characteristic of younger adults are generally lacking, giving high priority to the requirements for prompt fulfillment of fluid and nutrient needs during the early hours of acute illness or injury.

What has been said for the elderly is equally true for infants and children, with the added proviso that their infirmity (short of death resulting from faulty nutrition during illness) may lead to disease and premature aging in mature adult life.

Let me reemphasize that nutrition can not resolve problems even in the short term without health care and aging receiving appropriate consideration.

Issue Number Three

Issue number three, how to convince population groups that promotion of the aging-nutrition-health triad is an effective approach to improving current life-styles, which are identified as being most responsible for human misery and waste of resources in the world today, suggests the need for an effective, honest promotional campaign.

With application of scientific knowledge, recently exemplified by the World Health Organization's proclamation of worldwide erradication of variola (small pox),[18] infectious disease has become the lesser of two major preventable disease and disability groupings afflicting mankind. The greater is that associated with life-styles. Marc Lalonde, Canada's Minister of National Health and Welfare, recently [19] spotlighted its importance by describing how his Ministry is giving priority in planning and funding during his tenure of office to an assault on life-style diseases and disabilities. Belloc and Breslow, reporting on a 1965 survey of 6,928 adults in Alameda County, Calif.,[20] noted seven components of life-style associated with disease, disability, and diminished longevity and observed that four were related directly to nutrition.

If life-style diseases and disabilities are attacked using the aging-nutrition-health triad, all seven are approachable through the integrated concept. According to interpretations of the Belloc and Breslow data,[21] success of such an approach could increase life expectancy for the man of 45 by 11.5 years.

The effectiveness of life-style changes induced by application of the integrated triad approach need not be accepted on faith alone. Data on the effects of smoking, alcoholism, drug abuse, gluttony, lack of scheduled recreation, uncontrolled hypertension, lack of adequate sleep and appropriate exercise, high-speed driving, gunshot wounds, etc., can leave trained observers only with the impression that life-style diseases and disabilities are major obstacles to better lives for all. More subjectively, observers of technically underdeveloped societies are appalled at the apparent premature aging of less privileged segments of their populations.

This issue, in summary, becomes how to convince people that life-style changes induced by application of the integrated aging-nutrition-health triad are effective. Certain approaches seem mandatory, e.g., collection and dissemination of more data, revision of certain laws, and recruitment of disciples among persons with qualities of leadership. Promotion of the concept by all possible means is the *sine qua non* of success.

Issue Number Four

Issue number four, how to convince population groups that promotion of the aging-nutrition-health triad is cost effective in assuring steady economic development, is probably the issue on which more than any other a better life for all mankind depends.

A few years ago, the Science and Education Staff of the United States Department of Agriculture released a table [22] indicating the billions of dollars that might be saved annually were known and proven nutrition practices and more nutrition research implemented in the United States alone. These projections recently resurfaced in a report prepared by the Senate Select Committee on Nutrition and Human Needs. [21]

During recent years, the news media have reported growing concern over the fiscal integrity of the Social Security Administration in the United States, especially in view of the ever-increasing numbers of elderly and disabled persons looking to Social Security payments not as complements to other income but as their one and only source of cash. Among the solutions proposed has been increasing the age of retirement so that a person may contribute more to and draw less from Social Security than is possible at the present time. Such a solution would require better health, fewer disabilities, and greater effective longevity than exist now if it were to fulfill present and projected needs. Hence, greater attention to aging, nutrition, and the continuum of health care throughout life offers one resolution of a serious economic concern.

Health care costs in the United States have doubled—from $60 billion to $120 billion—in only five years. These data more than other considerations have made imperative new solutions and have given new prominence to the potential value of the aging-nutrition-health triad.

In all societies, deficiencies in nutrition and health care lead inevitably to disease, disability, premature aging, and tremendous wastes of societal and individual monetary and human resources. These wasted resources inhibit economic development by restricting capital available for investment in agricultural and industrial expansion. They also have another unfortunate byproduct with terrifying implications for the welfare of mankind—the population explosion. By emphasizing the aging-nutrition-health triad and thereby assuring longer, healthier, more secure lives to all population groups, we can by indirection complement other efforts to correct a trend that contains every harbinger of political, economic, and social disaster.

Finally, let me leave you with a dramatic example of how emphasis on the aging-nutrition-health triad exemplifies cost-effectiveness. An 18-year-old—overweight, muscularly underdeveloped with suboptimal bone structure, under the influence of alcohol, and driving in excess of the speed limit while not wearing a seat belt—fails to navigate a turn, collides with a fixed object, is thrown from the vehicle and sustains a fracture of the fourth cervical vertebra with cord compression, paralysis, and neurogenic dysfunction of the bladder and bowel.

This youth is the victim of instant aging, since in a few milliseconds he has acquired the physical, physiologic, biochemical, psychologic, social, and economic characteristics often associated with those few persons alive at ages 110 and over.[23] Society will pay over the course of the ensuing 50 years $2½ million (1976 dollars) to provide for his health care alone. Assuming he could, barring the accident, have worked 50 years at an average annual income of $30,000 (1976 dollars), his income alone would have totalled $1½ million (1976 dollars). Assuming his services were worth at least twice his annual income to his employer, the waste of another $1½ million (1976 dollars) is apparent. In other words, his failure to heed concepts embodied in the aging-nutrition-health triad results in a total loss of $5½ million (1976 dollars).

While certain accidents are inevitable, avoiding risk factors contributing to accidents (speed, alcohol, drugs) and acquiring and maintaining a physical condition (ideal weight, good muscular development, sound bone structure) capable of withstanding the forces of trauma can do much to spare society and its individual members such grevious losses.

SUMMARY

The interrelations of aging, nutrition, and the continuum of health care have been discussed in terms of four issues, all of which focus on how to convince modern societies that meaningful attention to the triad is not only desirable but, in the light of the alternative, practically mandatory.

The action steps required consist by and large of convincing societal leadership who in turn can convince their followers that meaningful attention to the aging-nutrition-health triad can produce better lives for all. The attention must be directed at all human life from conception to death. Properly applied throughout life, the attention can dramatically decrease the misery and waste currently imposed by life-style diseases and disabilities.

To highlight the tangible and appeal to the pecuniary qualities of mankind, attention has been focused particularly on the cost-effectiveness of such attention. The fractionation of the triad's components into individual units each furthered by its own proponents is not only wasteful of scarce resources but dangerous to individuals and their societies.

Professionally trained scientists concerned with nutrition are keys to the catalysis of societal comprehension of the triad's interrelations. They have the education, training, experience and contacts at all levels to lead the leaders who in turn will convince societies worldwide that integration of aging, nutrition, and the continuum of health care at all phases of the life cycle is desirable, mandatory, effective, and economically sound.

REFERENCES

1. WATKIN, D. M. 1958. The assessment of protein nutrition in aged man. Ann. N.Y. Acad. Sci. 69: 902–913.
2. WATKIN, D. M. 1964. Protein metabolism and requirements in the elderly. In Mammalian Protein Metabolism. Chap. 17. H. N. Munro & J. B. Allison, Eds. Lea & Febiger. Philadelphia, Pa.
3. WATKIN, D. M. 1966. The impact of nutrition on the biochemistry of aging in man. Eighth Annual Ciba Foundation Lecture on Research on Aging, Glasgow, 1964. In World Review of Nutrition and Dietetics. G. Bourne, Ed. Vol. 6: 124–164. S. Karger. Basel/New York.

4. WATKIN, D. M. 1966. Nutrition and aging. *In* Nutrition: A Comprehensive Treatise. Chap. 4, Vol. 3. E. W. McHenry & G. H. Beaton, Eds. The Academic Press. New York.
5. WATKIN, D. M. 1968. Nutrition problems today in the elderly in the United States. *In* Vitamins for the Elderly: Report of the Proceedings of a Symposium held at the Royal College of Physicians, London, on 2nd May 1968. A. N. Exton-Simth & D. L. Scott, Eds. : 66–77. John Wright & Sons. Bristol, England. (Distributed in the United States by The Williams & Wilkins Co., Baltimore.)
6. WATKIN, D. M. 1970. A year of developments in nutrition and aging. Med. Clin. N. Am. **54:** 1589–1597.
7. WATKIN, D. M., Ed. 1972. Symposium on Nutrition and Aging, Part I. Am. J. Clin. Nutr. **25:** 807–859.
8. WATKIN, D. M. 1973. Improving the nutrition of those most vulnerable to hunger and malnutrition: the aged. *In* U.S. Nutrition Policies in the Seventies. Chap. 7. J. Mayer, Ed. W. H. Freeman & Co. San Francisco.
9. WATKIN, D. M. 1973. Nutrition for the aging and the aged. *In* Modern Nutrition in Health and Disease, Fifth Edition. Chap. 25. R. S. Goodhart & M. E. Shils, Ed. Lea & Febiger. Philadelphia, Pa.
10. WATKIN, D. M. & G. V. MANN, Eds. 1973. Symposium on Nutrition and Aging, Part II. Am. J. Clin. Nutr. **26:** 1091–1162.
11. WATKIN, D. M. 1974. Viewpoint: nutritional needs of the elderly are intertwined with other factors and attitudes affecting health. Geriatrics **29:** 40–42.
12. WATKIN, D. M. 1977. Nutrition and aging: the Nutrition Program for Older Americans—a successful application of current knowledge in nutrition gerontology. *In* World Review of Nutrition and Dietetics. G. Bourne, Ed. **26:** 26–40. S. Karger. Basel/New York.
13. WINICK, M., Ed. 1976. Nutrition and Aging. *In* Current Concepts in Nutrition. Vol. **4:** 1–208. John Wiley & Sons. New York.
14. ROCKSTEIN, M. & M. L. SUSSMAN, Eds. 1976. Nutrition, Longevity and Aging. : 1–284. The Academic Press. New York.
15. LINTZ, L. P. 1975. Weber County Health Screening Project. Weber County Department on Aging. Ogden, Utah.
16. MCKAY, C. M., M. F. CROWELL & L. A. MAYNARD. 1935. The effect of retarded growth upon the length of life span and upon the ultimate body size. J. Nutr. **10:** 63–79.
17. WATKIN, D. M. 1976. Biochemical impact of nutrition on the aging process. *In* Nutrition, Longevity and Aging. M. Rockstein & M. L. Sussman, Eds. : 47–66. The Academic Press. New York.
18. TIME MAGAZINE. November 29, 1976 : 66.
19. LALOND, M. 1976. The Fourth Annual Matthew B. Rosenhaus Lecture. 104th Annual Meeting of the American Public Health Association. Miami Beach, October 18, 1976.
20. BELLOC, N. B. & L. BRESLOW. 1972. Relationship of physical health status and health practices. Prev. Med. **1:** 409–421.
21. MCGOVERN, G. 1976. U.S. Senate Select Committee on Nutrition and Human Needs. Hearing on Diet Related to Killer Diseases, July 27–28, 1976. Committee Print 76–554. U.S. Government Printing Office. Washington, D.C.
22. WEIR, C. E. 1971. Benefits from human nutrition research. Science and Education Staff, U.S. Department of Agriculture. Washington, D.C.
23. WATKIN, D. M. 1972. Practical solutions to malnutrition in spinal cord dysfunction. *In* Proceedings of the Joint Meeting of the 18th Spinal Cord Injury Conference of the Department of Medicine and Surgery of the United States Veterans Administration and the International Medical Society of Paraplegia, Boston, October 5–7, 1971. : 231–233. U.S. Government Printing Office. Washington, D.C.

OBESITY AND THE SOCIAL ENVIRONMENT: CURRENT STATUS, FUTURE PROSPECTS *

Albert J. Stunkard

Department of Psychiatry
University of Pennsylvania
Philadelphia, Pennsylvania 19104

This report describes the impact of the social environment on the prevalence of obesity. Its four sections describe what we have learned about (1) the influence of unplanned and uncontrolled factors such as social class, (2) the planned and controlled influence of behavioral therapies upon individual persons, and (3) the first applications of these therapies to very large groups of people. The last section looks to the future and to some social forces that it may be possible to direct more effectively for the control of obesity and of other health problems associated with life styles.

THE INFLUENCE OF SOCIAL FACTORS UPON OBESITY

The first evidence of how the large-scale social environment influences obesity was obtained by the Midtown Study, a comprehensive survey of the epidemiology of mental illness.[23] The population under study consisted of 110,000 persons, adults between the ages of 20 and 59 years of age, in an area of Manhattan selected so that it represented extremes in socioeconomic status, from extremely high to extremely low. A cross-section of 1,660 persons was selected as representative of the 110,000 by systematic probability sampling. Two-hour interviews were conducted with these subjects in their homes by trained observers, who obtained information about social and ethnic background and a number of items designed to assess psychological and interpersonal functions as well as height and weight.

This study showed a striking association between socioeconomic status and the prevalence of obesity, particularly among women.[12] Socioeconomic status was rated by a simple score based upon occupation, education, weekly income, and monthly rent. FIGURE 1 shows the strong inverse relationship between socioeconomic status and the prevalence of obesity. Fully 30 percent of women of lower socioeconomic status were obese, compared to 16 percent among those of middle status, and no more than 5 percent in the upper status group.

Among men the differences between social classes were similar, but of a lesser degree. Men of lower socioeconomic status, for example, showed a prevalence of obesity of 32 percent, compared to that of 16 percent among upper class men.

One notable feature of these studies was that they were designed to permit causal inferences about the influence of socioeconomic status. This was achieved by ascertaining not only the socioeconomic status of the respondents at the time of the study, but also that of their parents when they were 8 years old. Although

* Supported in part by Grant MH28124 from the National Institute of Mental Health.

a subject's obesity might influence his social class, it is unlikely that this disability in adult life could have influenced his parents' social class. Therefore, associations between the social class of the respondent's parents and disability can be reviewed as causal. FIGURE 1 shows that such associations were almost as powerful as those between the social class of the respondents and their obesity.

The impact of these findings increased as additional social variables were considered, for it is a remarkable fact that, in Midtown at least, every single social variable investigated was related to the prevalence of obesity, with the relationship usually stronger for women than for men. In addition to socioeconomic status and socioeconomic status of origin, these variables included social mobility, generation in the United States, and ethnic and religious affiliations.

Obesity was more prevalent among downwardly socially mobile subjects (22 percent) than among those who remained in the social class of their parents (18 percent), and far more prevalent than among those who were upwardly

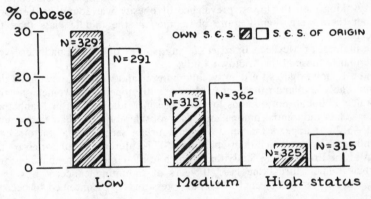

FIGURE 1. Decreasing prevalence of obesity with increase in socioeconomic status (SES). (From Goldblatt et al.[12] By permission of Journal of American Medical Association.)

socially mobile (12 percent).[12] Generation in the United States was also strongly linked to obesity. Respondents were divided into one of four groups on the basis of the number of generations that their families had been in the country. Of first-generation respondents, 24 percent were overweight, with the prevalence falling to 22 percent, 6 percent, and 4 percent during succeeding generations.

The presence of nine different ethnic groups in the Midtown Study permitted assessment of the influence of ethnicity upon obesity.[26] The strongest evidence of this influence was found among persons of lower socioeconomic status, with wide variability about a mean of 30 percent. Ethnicity was not quite as strong a predictor of obesity as socioeconomic status, with its 6 to 1 differential between lower and upper classes. Nevertheless, when only lower class respondents were considered, the 40 percent prevalence among Hungarians and Czechs meant that there was a 3 to 1 differential between them and the least obese group, fourth-generation Americans, who showed a prevalence of only 13 percent.

Religious affiliation is still another social factor linked to obesity.[27] Again the sample size precluded adequate control of all relevant variables. Nevertheless, the findings closely fitted the expected pattern. The greatest prevalence of obesity was found among Jews, followed by Roman Catholics and Protestants. Among Protestants, the pattern was further exemplified: the largest amount of obesity was found among Baptists, with a decreasing prevalence among Methodists, Lutherans, and Episcopalians.

Is this relationship between social factors and obesity exclusively an American phenomenon? Or is it more broadly applicable? Two studies have assessed the relationship between socioeconomic status and obesity in London. It should be noted that these studies were correlational ones. No study since the Midtown one has gone to the immense pains to determine the social class of the respondent's parents. The close correspondence between the socioeconomic status of respondents and that of their parents in Midtown, however, makes it likely that causation underlies at least part of the correlations described below.

Silverstone et al.[22] found a twofold greater prevalence of obesity among women of lower socioeconomic status than among those of upper socioeconomic status. Among men the lowest prevalence of obesity was found in the upper class, but there were slightly more obese men in the middle class than the lower class.

The findings of McClean Baird et al.[3] in a survey of 1,334 Londoners were quite similar to those of the Midtown Study.

TABLE 1 shows figures for obesity among lower and middle class women that are remarkably similar to those of Midtown, with upper class women showing lower rates, although not quite as low as those in Midtown. As in Manhattan, the social class differential among men was considerably less than that among women—3:2. It appears that in a Western, urban setting social factors have more influence upon women than upon men. This inference is supported by the findings of the Framingham Study that women in the United States have become somewhat thinner during the last 20 years of mounting concern over their weight, whereas men, subjected to far less pressure, have continued to become fatter.

Onset of Social Influences

The consistent and striking relationship between social factors and obesity has led three groups to investigate the vital question of the age at which this influence makes itself felt. The first of these studies, by Huenemann,[14] found the same inverse relationship between socioeconomic status and obesity well

TABLE 1

PREVALENCE OF OBESITY (PERCENT) IN LONDON SURVEY

	A & B	C	D & E
Women	16	18	36
Men	12	16	18

Figures are the percentage of obese persons in each social class. A & B=upper, C=middle, D & E=lower social classes. (From Baird.[1])

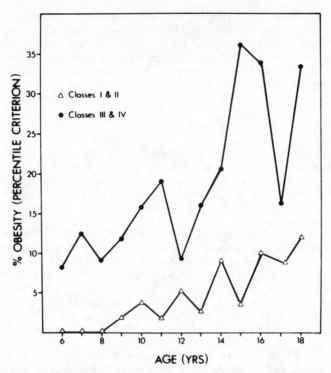

FIGURE 2. Greatly increased prevalence of obesity among lower class white girls compared to upper class white girls. (From Stunkard *et al.* By permission of *Journal of American Medical Association.*)

established by adolescence. Among girls, 11.6 percent in the lower class were obese compared with 5.4 percent in the upper class. Comparable figures for boys were 6.2 and 2.3 percent.

Whitelaw [33] also found a decrease in obesity with increasing social class in London schoolboys age 7 to 15. Skinfold thickness measures revealed that 8.5 percent of lower class boys were obese, compared with a 5.1 percent prevalence of obesity in middle class boys and 4.9 percent among those of upper social class. Interestingly, he found no relationship between social class and mean skinfold thickness, suggesting that there is no general increase in fatness among lower class boys but rather an increased proportion of definitely obese individuals.

A study of 3,344 white schoolchildren in three Eastern cities in the United States provided conclusive evidence for the influence of social class upon obesity in children and further disturbing indications of just how early this influence is exerted.[30]

FIGURE 2 shows that at age 6 the lower socioeconomic group contained 8 percent obese girls, whereas the upper class group had no obese girls at either ages 6 or 7. This difference was maintained until age 18, with an increase in the prevalence of obesity with increasing age in both groups. The slopes for the upper and lower classes differed, with the greater yearly increment in the percentage of obese in the lower class girls. Obesity is thus not only more prevalent among lower class girls, but its greater prevalence is established earlier and increases at a more rapid rate than among upper class girls. Lower class boys showed a greater prevalence of obesity than did those of the upper class, but the differences were neither as large nor as consistent.

Influence of Social Factors in Less Affluent Societies

Until recently we have had no information on the relationship between social factors and obesity in a non-affluent, developed society. This lack is unfortunate, for such information is essential to an understanding of this most potent force. Are the obesity-controlling effects of increasing socioeconomic status in New York a general phenomenon or only a special case in an affluent society?

There is highly suggestive evidence that the relationship of New York *is* a special case. Scattered information on the relationship of social factors and mean body weight or mean skinfold thickness (not obesity) in developing countries reveals a relationship that is the precise opposite of that in Western urban society. Among adults in India,[20] Latin America,[32] and Puerto Rico and among children in South China[5] and the Philippines an increasing standard of living is associated with increasing mean body weight or skinfold thickness. The first data on the relationship of social factors to obesity (as contrasted to mean body weight) in a less affluent society—the Navaho Indian—have been obtained recently. They show that in this setting, affluence is *directly* related to the prevalence of obesity, in sharp contrast to the relationship found in Western urban societies.[10] This influence is stronger among Navaho boys than among girls, as is an equally strong inverse relationship between affluence and the prevalence of thinness.

Comparison of the standard of living of these Navaho children and those in the study of Western city children revealed that the least affluent city children enjoyed a considerably higher standard of living than did the most affluent Navaho children. These findings permit us to construct a general proposition relating affluence and its associated social factors to the prevalence of obesity. FIGURE 3 shows a maximum prevalence of obesity occurring among the poor members of Western urban society. This prevalence decreases with both decreasing and increasing affluence, but the reasons for the decreases differ dramatically. With decreasing affluence, the constraint upon the development of obesity is a lack of food. With increasing affluence, fads and fashions exert the control. Information on the relationship of affluence to thinness, although less detailed, shows a pattern that is the mirror image of that for obesity.

The full implications of these findings for our understanding of obesity and for its control have yet to be realized, for they mean that whatever its genetic determinants and its biochemical pathways, obesity is to an unusual degree under social environmental control. And they suggest that a broad-scale assault on obesity need not await further understanding of its biochemical determinants. Understanding of its social determinants may be sufficient. Such understanding has been greatly advanced by recent studies of the influence of the behavioral therapies.

INFLUENCE OF THE BEHAVIORAL THERAPIES UPON INDIVIDUALS AND SMALL GROUPS

It is unconventional to look at therapy as a form of the social environment, but introduction of behavior modification for the control of obesity in 1967 has made such a view entirely appropriate. For behavior modification is an attempt to construct a special kind of environment—social and material—to help obese persons gain control over their eating.

The distinguishing characteristic of the various methods called behavior modification is the belief that behavior disorders of the most divergent type are learned responses and that modern theories of learning have much to teach us regarding both the acquisition and extinction of these responses. Furthermore, proponents of behavior modification have been distinguished by

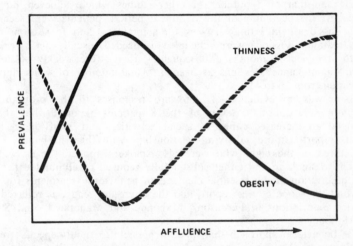

FIGURE 3. Schematic representation of the relationship between affluence and prevalence of obesity and thinness. (From Stunkard.[27] By permission of Newman Publishing Co.)

their explicit statements of methods and goals, and by their willingness to put their results on the line for comparison of different methods of treatment. Behavior therapists, for example, were among the first to recognize the power, as a dependent variable in psychotherapy research, of weight change in pounds, and they have turned to the treatment of obesity in increasing numbers in order to utilize this measure. No other dependent variable in psychotherapy research comes close to the sensitivity, reliability, and validity of weight change.

It has been, in the past, fairly easy to assess the effectiveness of any out-patient treatment for obesity because the traditional results have been so uniformly poor and the treatments so obviously inadequate. (In-patient treatment, with its potential for greater control over the patient, has, of course, been more successful in weight reduction. Its usefulness has been limited, however, by the almost invariable regaining of weight after discharge. Intestinal bypass surgery shows great promise for treatment of severely obese persons, but the number and severity of side reactions severely limits its applicability). Only 25 percent of persons entering conventional out-patient treatment for obesity lose as much as 20 pounds, and 5 percent as much as 40 pounds.[28]

Against this background, Stuart's report on "Behavioral Control of Overeating" [24] stands out. It describes the best results yet obtained in the out-patient treatment of obesity and constitutes a landmark in our understanding of this disorder. Even the absence of a control group does not vitiate the significance of its findings. The 8 patients who remained in treatment out of an original 10 lost large amounts of weight: 3 lost more than 40 pounds and 6 more than 30 pounds.

Certain features of this report highlight its significance. First, the expenditure of time was not exorbitant. In fact, time spent in treatment was no greater than that of a number of other studies which achieved far poorer results. At the beginning of the treatment period, patients were seen in 30-minute sessions held 3 times a week for a total of 12 to 15 sessions. Thereafter, treatment sessions were scheduled as needed, usually at 2-week intervals for the next 3 months. Subsequently, there were weekly sessions and finally "maintenance" sessions as needed. Total number of visits during the year varied from 16 to 41.

There was no evidence of untoward responses to the program or of "symptom substitution." Seven of the 8 patients reported that they had developed an increased range of social activities, and 3 of the 6 married patients reported more satisfying relationships with their husbands. Furthermore, three of the eight who were also smokers applied the same general program to smoking and either substantially reduced or eliminated it.

A description of the essential elements of behavioral treatments for obesity is beyond the scope of this report, and the interested reader is referred to the extended descriptions in Ferguson,[8] Mahoney and Mahoney,[18] and Stunkard and Mahoney.[31]

The behavioral approach that made it possible to rigidly specify treatment conditions and the dependent variable of weight change that made possible fine dissection of the results have resulted in an explosion of research on behavioral control of obesity. Soon after Stuart's landmark program, a controlled outcome study based upon it reported an average weight loss of 10.5 pounds among moderately overweght women college students.[13] Subjects in a no-treatment control group gained 3.6 pounds, a difference significant at the 1 percent level.

A no-treatment control group was quite acceptable in psychotherapy research in 1969. Yet it has serious disadvantages. For refusing treatment to someone who has come seeking it is far from a neutral event. And deterioration in the condition of members of a control group that has been disappointed in its expectation of treatment could give the false impression that a treatment was effective. The problem calls for the use of a placebo control group to match the attention and interest received by patients in the active treatment program. An elaborate study by Wollersheim [25] provided precisely such controls and opened up new vistas of psychotherapy research.

Wollersheim's elegant factorial design contained four experimental conditions:

1. "Focal" (behavioral) treatment.
2. "Non-specific therapy" to control for factors such as increased attention,

"faith," expectation of relief, and presentation of a treatment rationale. Treatment was carried out in groups that explored psychological issues related to the patient's obesity but avoided specific behavioral considerations.
3. "Social pressure" was patterned after that of the self-help group TOPS (Take Off Pounds Sensibly) and included such TOPS procedures as a weigh-in, followed by praise for weight loss, and encouragement for failure to lose weight.[29]
4. A no-treatment weight control condition of persons promised treatment but receiving it later.

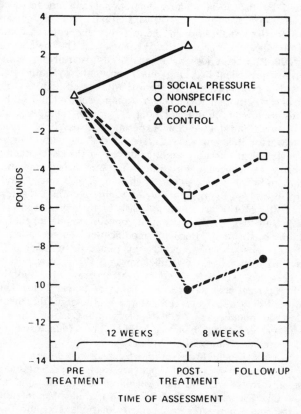

FIGURE 4. Mean weight loss of the food (behavioral) treatment group, the two alternative treatment control groups, and the no-treatment control group. (From Wollersheim.[35] By permission of *Journal of Abnormal Psychology*.)

The study thus contained three treatment conditions (1, 2, and 3) and three control conditions (2, 3, and 4) for behavior modification. The 80 subjects were mildly (29 percent) overweight female college students. Four therapists each treated one group of five subjects in each of the three treatment conditions for 10 sessions over a 3-month period.

Wollersheim's findings are illustrated in FIGURE 4. At the end of treatment, and at 8-week followup, subjects in the behavioral treatment condition had lost more weight than those in the no-treatment condition. In addition, they had lost significantly more weight than those in the two placebo control conditions, which had themselves both achieved respectable weight losses. Clearly, the behavioral treatment contributed something to the outcome, which was over and above the usual effects of psychological treatment.

This contribution seems to have resulted from the specific effects of the behavioral intervention, because a detailed eating-patterns questionnaire revealed that subjects in the "focal" therapy condition showed major changes in self reports of eating behavior. Statistically significant differences between the "focal" therapy and the other three conditions were found in four of the six factors assessed by the questionnaire: "emotional and uncontrolled eating," "eating in isolation," "eating as a reward," and "between meals eating." Whatever caused the weight loss in the two placebo control conditions apparently did it without affecting these behaviors. The behavioral therapy apparently produced weight loss by means of its ostensible rationale.

Wollersheim's precedent-breaking study brought psychotherapy research face to face with a problem resulting from the increased maturity of the field: experimenter bias. Although the placebo therapy controlled for the patient's expectations of treatment, it did not control for the therapist's, and this is not a trivial matter. The double-blind experiment in psychopharmacology has shown how powerful this influence can be in dealing with drugs, and it is surely more powerful in the more emotional case of the psychotherapies.

The problem of experimenter bias was approached in an ingenious manner in the study by Penick et al.,[21] which was also one of the very few to deal with severely (78 percent) overweight persons. Therapists were selected to treat the control group on the basis of their great skill in the treatment of obesity and their use of the entire conventional therapeutic armamentarium, including medication. Behavior modification, on the other hand, was carried out by persons with no previous experience in treatment. Fifteen patients were treated with behavior modification and 17 by conventional therapy, both on a once-a-week basis for 2 hours over a period of 3 months.

The results of treatment favored the behavioral approach. Thus, weight losses of the control group were comparable to those in the medical literature: none lost 40 pounds and only 24 percent lost more than 20 pounds. By contrast, 13 percent of the behavior modification group lost more than 40 pounds and 53 percent lost more than 20 pounds.

Variability in the weight losses of the behavior modification subjects was considerably greater than that of the patients treated by traditional methods. The five best performers were in the behavior modification condition, as was the single least effective patient. Such greater variability has in other circumstances been associated with greater specificity of treatment, and this explanation of the findings seems reasonable. It appears that for half of the patients, behavior modification seemed to offer something specific that resulted in greater than usual weight loss. For another half it seemed of considerably less value.

The most important implication of the Penick study lies in its promise of greater applicability of the behavioral therapies. For it showed that behavior modification, devised by a team with little experience in the modality, was more effective in the treatment of obesity than was the best alternative program that could be devised by a research team with long experience in treatment of this disorder. In fact, the inexperienced therapists achieved about a twofold increase in the effectiveness of treatment over conventional measures. Lesser increases in effectiveness have brought about major changes in the management of other disorders. The question arose, "How can the advantages of behavior modification be exploited most effectively?"

INFLUENCE OF BEHAVIORAL THERAPIES AND OTHER MEASURES UPON LARGE GROUPS

Self-Help Groups

A century and half ago, deTocqueville described the proclivity of Americans to organize in informal groups to achieve ends that are the responsibility of government in other societies. Nowhere is this proclivity more impressively expressed than in the organization of patients to cope with common illnesses. Patient self-help groups, pioneered by Alcoholics Anonymous, are favored by increasing numbers of persons suffering from an increasing variety of conditions. One of the largest and most effective of these groups is TOPS (Take Off Pounds Sensibly), a 25-year-old organization that enrolls over 300,000 members in 12,000 chapters in all parts of the country.[11, 29] TOPS would appear to offer a promising vehicle for the introduction of behavioral techniques. A recent feasibility study confirmed this promise.[16] The study involved all 298 female members of 16 TOPS chapters, situated in West Philadelphia and its adjacent suburbs.

The average subject was a 45-year-old woman who had been a member of TOPS for 3 years and who had lost 11 pounds during her membership. She currently weighed 180 pounds, 42 percent above her ideal weight. The homogeneity of TOPS membership permitted remarkably close matching of subjects in the different conditions.

Four treatment conditions, each containing four TOPS chapters, were employed for a total of 12 weeks:

1. Behavior modification carried out by professional therapists.
2. Behavior modification carried out by the TOPS chapter leader and co-leader, each of whom had received brief training in the procedures and who utilized the same manual as that used by the professional therapists.
3. Nutrition education provided by chapter leaders who had received an amount of training in this area comparable to that provided the chapter leaders in behavior modification.
4. Continuation of the standard TOPS self-help techniques.

TOPS shares with the medical treatment of obesity the problem of very high drop-out rates. The first major finding of this study was that far fewer subjects dropped out of the behavior modification programs. FIGURE 5 shows that the attrition rate in the two behavior modification conditions was lower during treatment and significantly lower at 1-year followup. At followup, 38 percent and 41 percent of subjects had dropped out of the behavior modification programs, compared to 55 percent for the nutrition education and 67 percent for the standard TOPS program.

Despite the bias against behavior modification resulting from the differential attrition rates, behavior modification produced significantly greater weight loss than did the control conditions. Professionally led chapters lost 4.2 pounds, compared to a loss of 1.9 pounds in the TOPS-leader-led chapters. The nutrition education chapters showed no change in weight, whereas chapters receiving the standard TOPS program actually gained 0.7 pounds. The relative superiority of the behavioral treatments increased at 1-year followup. Chapters that had professional leadership continued to show lower attrition rates and also to lose weight, to a total of 5.8 pounds. The initial weight of the subjects in the behavior modification program conducted by TOPS leaders was not maintained during followup, but these subjects did better than those in the nutrition education and control groups, who gained significant amounts of weight.

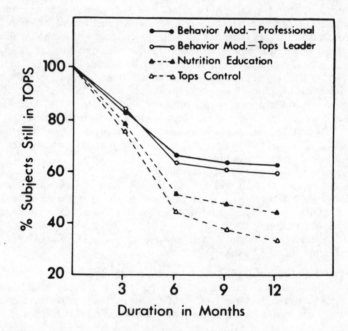

FIGURE 5. Attrition rate of TOPS subjects over a 1-year period under four experimental conditions. (From Levitz & Stunkard.[16] By permission of *American Journal of Psychiatry*.)

This has been an important feasibility study. We now know that behavior modification can be introduced into large population groups through appropriate institutional auspices. The next step is to improve the performance under these conditions and to find institutions receptive to introduction of the techniques.

TOPS, it appears, is not to be such an institution. It has made no effort to capitalize upon the program to which it made such a significant contribution, and, ironically, the chief beneficiary may well be TOPS' arch rivals, the commercial organizations such as Weight Watchers.

Commercial Enterprises

There has been little scientific investigation of commercial weight reduction enterprises, and what we know about them is largely anecdotal and impressionistic. This situation is now changing, and the next few years will doubtless bring us an objective appraisal of this rapidly developing area.

By far the largest and most successful of the commercial enterprises is Weight Watchers International, which has grown from its establishment in 1963 to an organization that now serves over 400,000 people each week in the United States and 25 foreign countries.

The vast Weight Watchers organization is operated on a decentralized basis through a number of semiautonomous franchises. It retains much of its operating format as developed by its founder, Mrs. Jean Neditch. Its program content has been strengthened over the years with the addition of a medical director, professional nutritionists, and a psychological director. Its members meet weekly for a period of about an hour in groups of varying size. They are weighed privately and then participate in a class lead by a Weight Watchers employee who has herself achieved weight loss.

The food plan used by Weight Watchers originally followed Dr. Norman Jolliffe's, New York Department of Health, diet very closely. In the late 1960's this diet was substantially modified to increase the volume and number of foods permitted. It has recently been further modified to provide a greater variety of foods in a nutritionally balanced diet with specialized food plans offered to those who reach plateaus in weight loss and to those who have achieved their weight-loss goals. In 1974, after a period of careful planning, a program of behavior modification was introduced into Weight Watchers on a very broad scale by Dr. Richard Stuart, who had initiated the explosion of research in this area 9 years before. The program is presented in 18 general-purpose and 5 special-purpose "modules." Each module contains a rationale, several specific behavior change recommendations, and a means of charting progress in making these changes. Modules are presented in class one week, and members' progress in taking the recommended steps is discussed the following week. Introduction of the modules is reported to have increased average weekly losses in groups selected for special study.[25]

The application of the behavioral weight management program on such a large scale stands as one of the major social experiments of our time, and the first approach to the control of obesity that is sufficiently broad to warrant description as a public health measure.

Traditional public health efforts in the field of weight control have been conspicuous for their absence until quite recently. Within the past year, however, a pilot study of a highly integrated health change program that included weight control has been reported by the Stanford Heart Disease Prevention Program.

Medical Auspices

The program was carried out in three California towns of 14,000 persons each, remarkably well matched on a variety of demographic variables.[6, 17] One town served as a control. The two others were subjected over a period of 2 years to a highly sophisticated media campaign, which contained about 50 television and 100 radio spots, 3 hours of television, and several hours of radio programming, columns, stories, and advertisements in the weekly newspapers, posters and billboards, printed material sent via direct mail to participants, and other assorted materials. The dominant characteristic of the media campaign was its organization as a total integrated information system based at first on data gathered from preliminary surveys, and later upon the information gathered during the course of the programs. In one of these towns the media campaign was supplemented by a face-to-face instruction program directed at two-thirds of the participants identified as being in the top quartile of risk of coronary heart disease. These 107 men underwent a behavior modification program once weekly for a 10-week period during the first year and a less intense effort during the second year.

The goal of the program was to reduce the risk of cardiovascular disease by changing information, attitudes, and behavior that would lead not only to weight reduction but also to reduction in intake of saturated fats, cholesterol, and salt, cessation of smoking, and increase in physical activity.

Both alone and combined with face-to-face instruction, the media campaign produced highly significant changes in all three areas: knowledge, attitudes, and behavior. And by the end of the second year, risk of coronary disease had decreased by 17 percent in the treatment communities, whereas it increased by more than 6 percent in the control community. Knowledge of risk factors increased proportionately with the intensity of the instruction, and it was highly correlated with improvement in "harmful behavior," consisting of a composite of dietary intake of saturated fat and cholesterol and smoking. FIGURE 6 shows the progression of improvement in the treatment compared to the lack of change in the control community. The high-risk subjects who received face-to-face instruction showed a remarkable, 30 percent, decrease in Cornfield risk factors during the first year of treatment, compared with a lesser, but still statistically significant, decrease in the persons who received only the media program. By the end of the second year, however, the media-only treatments had produced continuing rapid decrease in risk factors in their populations, reaching a statistically insignificant difference from the face-to-face subjects, whose rate of decrease had asymptoted.

The magnitude of the effects of this study is suggested by the fact that a 30-percent reduction in Cornfield risk factors is equivalent to a 5-year increase in life expectancy. Such an increase is unprecedented in this kind of (relatively) large-scale intervention effort, and compares favorably with the 4-year increase in life expectancy at age 40 that has been the fruit of all our medical efforts between the years 1900 and 1970. Clearly, major health benefits can be achieved by this kind of ambitious campaign. Its costs, however, are high. Can comparable results be achieved by other, less costly, and more effective means? The prospects are good. Many promising possibilities exist; if no more than a few are realized, they could transform the American health scene.

THE MANY POTENTIAL INFLUENCES OF THE FUTURE

The developments of the very recent past make it clear that leadership in broad-scale efforts to control obesity is passing to nonmedical agencies. As we look to the future it appears that this trend may accelerate; the most promising new methods for controlling obesity seem to lie almost entirely outside the province of the medical profession. For obesity is, in very large part, a result of the way we live, of our life styles, and the most effective means for controlling obesity today may lie in alterations in our life styles. Such an undertaking as altering the life styles of a nation is far beyond the capability of a profession such as medicine. It will require changes in those powerful social and economic forces that have given rise to these life styles and that sustain them.

These forces are powerful indeed. Consider just the impact upon our nutritional practices of the amount spent each year by the food industry to

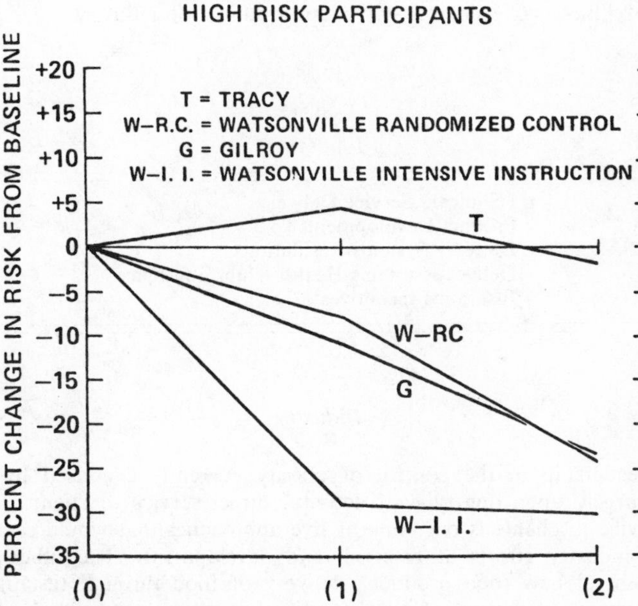

HIGH RISK PARTICIPANTS

FIGURE 6. Percent change from baseline (0) in risk of coronary heart disease after 1 and 2 years of health education in various study groups from three communities. Cardiovascular risk is measured by a multiple logistic function of risk factors (From Farquhar et al.[6])

advertise its products—$1.2 billion![19] Efforts by physicians to treat individual patients on a one-by-one basis are puny in comparison with these forces. They might be likened to exhortations to a swimmer to persevere against a raging current. What are the possibilities of swimming *with* the current?

Changing the social and economic forces that maintain our life styles is by no means as overwhelming a task as it might at first appear. In the first place, relatively small changes in each of the institutions could, by their cumulative— and perhaps potentiating—effect bring about considerably larger changes in the end product. Second, these forces are not simply blind, economic ones. They involve human beings in positions of responsibility that enable them to make choices between alternatives. Within their constraints, people choose what helps over what hurts. Finally, there is the possibility of generating powerful new social forces that can change the existing pattern. Interest in personal health can be precisely this kind of force.

Just as in the past the nation has taken special interest in particular afflictions—poliomyelitis and mental retardation—so in the future it seems likely to take an increased interest in general health, especially as it bears upon prevention of illness. Obesity seems likely to be a prominent focus of any such interests. The recent "Perspective on the Health of Canadians" [15] and the subsequent activities of the Long-Range Planning Committee of the Canadian Department of Health and Welfare [4] illustrate how many different agencies might be mobilized in the interest of improved health and the prevention of illness. Consider first the contribution of industry.

TABLE 2

INDUSTRY

(Clinical) Service Delivery
Product Development
Delivery Systems-Restaurants
Delivery Systems-Health Clubs and Spas
Insurance Incentives

Industry

The leadership in the control of obesity currently exercised by industry depends largely upon one type of activity: direct service to clients. But such direct service to clients is only one of five approaches that would seem ideally suited to industry efforts at research and development. The other four are development of new food products, delivery of food through restaurants and catering services, provision of opportunities for exercise through health clubs, health spas, and sporting goods manufacturers and, finally, insurance incentives. Each of these five approaches can be effective as a free-standing enterprise; integration of various combinations of them could multiply this effectiveness.

1. Direct service to clients. We have considered at some length the rise of commercial programs of direct service to clients, and this area needs no elaboration. Clearly established trends would seem to insure a strong and continuing role for commercial endeavors: the research-based increase in the efficacy of behavioral measures, the feasibility of their application by persons with progressively fewer educational qualifications, and the growing acceptance of nonmedical agencies.

2. One of the first and perhaps the most notable of the foods developed for weight reduction purposes was Metrecal, adapted from the "Rockefeller Diet" of the mid 1950's. Metrecal was taken up by the public with an enthusiasm that astonished its pharmaceutical manufacturer, and it quickly broke all kinds of sales records before its poorly understood and inexorable

decline. Diet foods have become increasingly popular in the period since
the introduction of Metrecal, and Weight Watchers, in particular, has capital-
ized upon this interest to sponsor a variety of franchised diet foods, quite
independent of its program of lectures. Low-calorie beverages have occupied a
significant part of the soft drink market. But the potential for development
of new products for weight control still seems virtually unlimited.

3. The third component of an integrated industry approach to weight
reduction could be the restaurant and food service industries. Despite the
widespread concern with body weight on the part of vast numbers of persons
who eat out, most find it awkward or impossible to secure satisfying low-
calorie, non-atherogenic foods in restaurants. Even when restaurants serve
low-calorie dishes, all too frequently the choice is limited and the selection
uninspired. There is great need for restaurants that serve an assortment of
attractively prepared low-calorie dishes. This need could be met either by the
establishment of specialty restaurants or by modifying some of the items on
the menus of traditional restaurants.

Speciality (health) restaurants need not be explicitly identified with programs of direct service to clients, an identification that might well limit the
number and diversity of their customers. And, they could serve a vital function
for both members and non-members of these client-service programs. Imaginative promotion of these restaurants, capitalizing upon the nation's growing
interest in nutrition and health, could give birth to a vital new industry.

Modifying the menus of traditional restaurants could have an impact upon
the nutrition of the American people even greater than the development of
speciality restaurants. For traditional restaurants will presumably always attract vastly greater numbers of customers, and even small improvements in
their offerings could affect the eating habits of tens of millions of persons.
Furthermore, such improvements could begin on a modest basis, involving no
more than two or three items, thus permitting restaurants to explore the
potential market before making a major commitment. And, if this exploration
showed that specially prepared items could return at least as good a profit as
traditional ones, it would not take long for the self-interest of industry to
enlist it in the campaign for improved nutrition. Already one pilot study has
produced encouraging results. A small restaurant chain in Houston, Texas has
begun to list the calorie content of a few items on its menu, selected for their
limited fat and calories and prepared with polyunsaturated oils.[9] The first
response was an increase in consumption of these items sufficiently promising
to induce the company to expand their number and introduce a special menu
to describe them.

The growth of large catering agencies that furnish complete food services
for schools, businesses, and other institutions provides an important strategic
opportunity for nutritional intervention. Large and increasing numbers of
young people eat in facilities served by these agencies, and the nutritional education they receive in the process doubtless carries over to meals eaten elsewhere
and to their future eating practices. Any improvement in the nutritional quality
of the foods provided by these agencies would thus benefit vast numbers of
people now and, hopefully, in the future. And such improvement need not await
the uncertain outcome of efforts at building a market in the highly competitive
restaurant business; it could flow directly from management decisions involving
a small number of experts in the relevant disciplines.

4. Health clubs and spas have already demonstrated their appeal to a large

and growing market, even as free-standing enterprises. They in particular, might be more effective, and less costly as part of an integrated network of weight-reduction agencies that also included restaurants for eating out, food products for eating at home, and nutritional-behavioral programs of direct service to clients. Enlisting the sporting goods industry in such enterprises is an unexplored area of possibly great effectiveness.

5. The greatest potential for health behavior change by industry may lie in an almost totally unexplored agency—life and health insurance. Assessment of the risk of death and disability lies at the heart of the insurance industry, and the industry has achieved remarkable accuracy in predicting such outcomes for population groups and in modifying predictions on the basis of changing health contingencies. It has, however, with rare exceptions, not attempted to alter these contingencies. In that direction may lie an unparalleled promise for the future. The insurance companies may well possess the most powerful incentives for health behavior change in our society today.

Automobile insurance provides an instructive example. Premiums for young persons are routinely reduced solely on the basis of attendance at Driver Education courses, with no requirement for demonstrated effectiveness of this education in the case of the individual driver. The experience of population groups is sufficient insurance. Surely Health Education programs can be as actuarially sound. And making reduction in premiums for individuals contingent upon concrete evidence of health behavior change, such as reduction in weight or blood pressure, would provide a powerful new incentive. The power of such incentives can hardly be overestimated. Recent research on contingency contracting has shown that, for reasons which are not entirely clear, the symbolic value of relatively small rebates can be very great. And the potency of such rebates can be further increased by the imaginative use of incentives from other areas of industry. Membership in a health club or reduced rates for a vacation in a health spa could not only reward people for improved health behavior, the rewards could themselves become stimuli for further improvement in health behavior.

Almost alone among the agencies of our society, the insurance industry benefits from improved prevention of disease. The change in life expectancy produced by the Stanford Three-Community Study, if achieved more widely, would have enormous impact upon the life insurance industry. The prospects of bringing about even a small part of that change could well warrant intensive efforts. Similarly health insurance programs could be immeasurably affected by simple preventive measures. Health insurance could have a more direct impact upon health behavior than life insurance and if possible, a stronger one. As health insurance becomes more closely associated with the providers of medical care, particularly with health maintenance organizations, it can furnish a powerful stimulus for the introduction of health behavior programs into medical care settings. In fact, this stimulus alone could finally make health maintenance an integral part of medical care.

The Media

Although properly viewed as a form of industry, the media have sufficient special characteristics to merit separate consideration. The results of the Stanford Three-Community Study show the potential of an integrated mass media campaign. Such integration might be more difficult to achieve on a national or even a regional basis. But any such disadvantages would be more than offset by the economy of scale and the relatively low costs once the initial materials are developed. Furthermore, we can expect continuing improvement in the capacity of the media, and particularly of live and videotape television, to influence health behavior.

Much of the power of the media derives from their ability to influence all three factors of a behavior change program: knowledge, attitudes, and skills. Television is a shining example. The ability of television to impart information is well established; suitably programmed it could teach information about weight reduction with perhaps greater effectiveness than any other method. Attitude change is the second well-established capability of television, particularly well exemplified by the changing of attitudes towards commercial products through advertising. Measures to develop favorable attitudes toward health behavior, towards exercise and decreased food intake, for example, are well within the capability of the medium that has dictated American buying practices. Even small changes in the character of food advertising, with its $1.2 billion budget, could have a significant impact.

In contrast to its acknowledged power in imparting knowledge and changing attitudes, the development of skills has generally been felt to be beyond the capabilities of television and a measure that requires direct person-to-person interaction. The development of videotapes designed to show step-by-step procedures for behavior change has reversed this assessment and has brought training in health behavior skills—how to stop smoking, for example—within the range of anyone with access to a videotape viewer. And live television is being increasingly used for its potential for teaching skills. A recent program on Los Angeles commercial television combined a step-by-step description of a weight loss program by an attractive newscaster who modelled the requisite behaviors while reporting her own progress in the program. An unofficial estimate suggested that Los Angeles lost 700,000 pounds during the course of the program.

Education

A major neglected area in the control of obesity is our schools. Tens of millions of school children are fed each day in our schools, and their nutrition and what they learn about nutrition is inexorably determined by the policies of their schools. Nutritious hot school lunches are more and more giving way to machine-dispensed junk foods, with a deterioration in both nutrition and nutrition education. Vigorous advocacy of both improved nutrition and of sound nutrition education by parent-teachers associations and school boards could reverse this trend and could make a major impact upon childhood obesity, with its legacy of stubborn persistence throughout adult life.

Failures of nutrition education do not stop at the elementary school. The low state of nutrition education in higher education, and notably in schools of medicine, must play a part in the nutritional problems—including obesity—of our nation.

Government

The fourth great agency that could play a role in the control of obesity is our government, and its potential has been realized as yet to only a limited degree. The taxing function could be used to powerful effect in modifying health behavior. Just as improved health behavior might lead to lowered insurance premiums, so might it also lead to tax rebates. Such a proposal seems just. Our enormous medical costs are not generated equally across the population. Disproportionate costs are generated by the excess illness of those who eat too much, drink too much, and exercise too little. It would seem appropriate to build incentives for them to improve their health behavior by lightening their tax burden contingent upon loss of weight.

A second area where the government could have a major impact is in improvement of the nutrition of the millions of government employees that it feeds every day—in and out of the military. Improved nutrition could be coupled with nutrition education in each cafeteria and mess hall. And the uncertainties about what kinds of food constitute good nutrition have been resolved in part by the action of another arm of the government—the report on "Dietary Goals for the United States," [19] prepared by the Staff of the Select Committee on Nutrition and Human Needs of the United States Senate.

The Federal regulatory agencies have a long and distinguished history of service on behalf of the nation's health. Years ago Frances Kelsey's celebrated refusal of Food and Drug Administration approval for the marketing of thalidomide saved this country the epidemic of malformed infants that afflicted our neighbors. More recently the Federal Trade Commission's regulations requiring disclosure of nutritional content of packaged foods and its efforts to promote truth in advertising [7] make it a major force in promoting nutrition education.

The climax of a vigorous, integrated governmental program of obesity control could be capped by the promotional capabilities of prominent government figures. Remember Franklin Roosevelt and his impact in transforming poliomyelitis from a fearsome plague to a national challenge. Here is a power that can be exercised with remarkably little cost to remarkably great effect.

Work Site Training

A very promising opportunity for changing health behavior is provided by the use of work sites for the conduct of programs of direct service to clients. "On the job training" has a long and honorable history in American industry. On the job training for the improvement of health behavior can be as rewarding, to worker and employer alike. Better health easily repays the costs of the program by improved work performance, decreased absenteeism and, particularly, decreased hospitalization.

Fortunately, the potential of the work site as a locus for the provision of long-term care has recently been demonstrated in a pilot project in a related area. Hypertension, like obesity, is rarely cured, but it does respond to effective and available treatment. A large percentage of hypertensive persons, however, do not receive treatment for their hypertension and of those who do, the treatment of a large percentage is inadequate.[34] Thus, in the pilot project, carried out under union auspices in New York City, less than half of the hypertensives in conventional treatment had achieved satisfactory results. By contrast, the specially designed work site program achieved long-term control of blood pressure in over 80 percent and radically reduced days of hospitalization for cardiovascular causes.[1, 2] The health benefits and cost savings have been sufficiently encouraging to induce the union to expand services to 1500 persons among 15,000 employees at 10 work sites.

Work site programs have many advantages. First, time away from work is kept to a minimum—an hour a week for 20 weeks is sufficient for a serious program of weight reduction. Second, work site programs obviate the high overhead costs of hospitals and the lower, but still substantial, costs of rented space. Third, they greatly decrease the probability of missed appointments and treatment dropouts. A program carried out with the collaboration, and in part at the expense, of the employer exerts far stronger sanctions for attendance than one conducted during leisure time and with varying degrees of personal or family commitment. Fourth, job site programs tap potential for health behavior change heretofore unexplored in this country. Accounts from the People's Republic of China have given hints of how much can be achieved when concern for the health of individuals is complemented by a concern for the health of working groups. Efforts at making unions and industries, or subgroups of them, the focus of efforts at health behavior change programs can generate high morale and strong group effort. The organized support and encouragement of fellow workers can constitute an unprecedented stimulus for weight loss. Rewards given to groups for improving their collective health could be even more effective than those given to individuals. And these rewards might become even more effective as prizes for a competition between, for example, members of union locals for number of excess pounds lost.

The potential population for job site health programs is enormous. Current executive and union health programs have no more than scratched the surface. The vast numbers of persons in the employ of the government—particularly those in the armed forces—provide attractive targets for health behavior intervention.

Voluntary Agencies

Some religions inculate an enviable series of health behaviors in their members and offer assistance to others in changing health behaviors. The Smoking Cessation Clinics conducted by the Seventh Day Adventists were landmarks in such endeavors. It seems entirely reasonable to expect that, in a favorable climate, other health promotional activities could be carried out under other religious auspices. Weight control could qualify as a prime candidate.

Fraternal organizations have often taken a special interest in health care. The activities of the Lions on behalf of visually impaired children and of the Shriners with crippled children are notable examples. Other fraternal organizations might well develop an interest in other health problems, and an enlightened membership might decide to deal with its own health problems, overweight, for example, as well as those of its beneficiaries.

Recreational organizations have traditionally had a strong interest in health behavior. The gymnasiums of the Young Men's Christian Association are among the important health facilities of many communities. Encouragement of the work of these organizations and facilitation of further efforts would capitalize upon one of the traditional health promotional agencies of our society.

The voluntary health agencies such as the American Cancer Society and the American Heart Association occupy a special place in the American health care system. They have carried out extensive programs of health education, and the

American Heart Association has already devoted some effort towards weight control. These agencies show great promise for disseminating new information about weight control and new techniques for achieving it.

Youth groups have traditionally had a major concern for health, and the camps and outings of the Boy Scouts and Girl Scouts have provided the major opportunities for physical activity for many boys and girls. Youth is a promising time of life, and youth groups are promising vehicles for intensified efforts at preventing and treating obesity.

Permutations and Combinations

To this point we have considered what might be called single factor approaches to the control of obesity. But future approaches are not likely to be confined to such inefficient, one-by-one, forms of intervention. Combinations of different forms of intervention seem particularly promising. For combining interventions may accomplish more than simply adding their effects; it may actually multiply them. We have earlier discussed combinations of measures

TABLE 3

VOLUNTARY AGENCIES

Religious: Seventh Day Adventists, Mormons
Fraternal Organizations: Lions, Shriners
Recreational Organizations: YMCA, YWCA, YMHA, YWHA
Voluntary Health Agencies: American Cancer Society, American Heart Association
Youth Groups: Boy Scouts, Girl Scouts, 4-H Clubs, Future Farmers of America

that industry has taken in the past and could take in the future, and the prospects of effectively integrating diverse strategies under commercial auspices seem bright. But such integration need not be confined to purely commercial ventures. Insurance carriers, for example, could require hospitals and Health Maintenance Organizations to provide health education programs, including ones for obesity, as part of their contract. And if the insurance companies lagged in this enterprise, they could be encouraged towards greater efforts by judicious use of governmental regulations.

The voluntary agencies are in an excellent position to develop comprehensive programs of weight control. School-based programs could serve as a promising starting point. One or more voluntary health agencies could produce the syllabus and media materials, recruit volunteers for face-to-face teaching, and negotiate for time on public or even commercial television for weight control programs. These agencies are well situated to enlist the President, movie stars, and famous athletes to increase the impact of the media messages and to reward achievement of both groups and individuals with low-cost symbols such as certificates, banners, and plaques. Once individual intervention strategies have been devised, the only limitations to their effectiveness would seem to be those imposed by limitations in the creativity with which they are deployed.

SUMMARY

Systematic studies have shown that social forces such as socioeconomic status exert a powerful influence upon the prevalence of human obesity. This susceptibility of obese persons to social forces has been utilized by behavior modifiers to construct programs of obesity control that are more effective than traditional ones. These programs have quite recently been successfully utilized with large population groups in the first approach to the control of obesity that is sufficiently broad to warrant description as a public health measure. But this is only a beginning. A variety of agencies and institutions stand at the threshold of major new capabilities of controlling obesity. Industry is the most developed; no less than five different potential intervention strategies can be identified. But government, education, and numerous voluntary agencies are not far behind. Each could multiply its effectiveness by developing the enormous unused capabilities of the media for weight control. The prospects of job site health training programs are almost entirely unexplored. Development of the capabilities of any of these agencies will contribute significantly to the control of obesity. Combining their capabilities in integrated programs of weight control could bring as yet unimagined benefits.

REFERENCES

1. ALDERMAN, M. H. 1976. Organization for long-term management of hypertension. Bull. N.Y. Acad. Med. **52:** 697–717.
2. ALDERMAN, M. H. & E. E. SCHOENBAUM. 1975. Detection and treatment of hypertension at the work site. New Engl. J. Med. **293:** 65–68.
3. BAIRD, I. M., J. T. SILVERSTONE & J. J. GRIMSHAW, et al. 1974. The prevalence of obesity in a London borough. Practitioner **212:** 706–714.
4. BOUDREAU, T. 1976. Personal communication.
5. CHANG, K. S., M. M. LEE & W. D. LOW et al. 1963. Height and weight of southern Chinese children in Hong Kong. Am. J. Phys. Anthropol. **21:** 497–509.
6. FARQUHAR, J. W. & W. MACCOBY et al. 1977. Community education for cardiovascular health. The Lancet. In press.
7. FEDERAL TRADE COMMISSION. 1976. Federal Register. March 2. **41:** 8980.
8. FERGUSON, J. 1975. Learning to Eat, Leader Manual and Student's Manual. Bull Publishing Co. Palo Alto, Calif.
9. FOREYT, J. 1977. Personal communication.
10. GARB, J. L., J. R. GARB & A. J. STUNKARD. 1975. Social factors and obesity in Navaho Indian children. In Recent Advances in Obesity Research. A. Howard, Ed. : 37–39. Newman. London.
11. GARB, J. R. & A. J. STUNKARD. 1974. A further assessment of the effectiveness of TOPS in the control of obesity. Arch. Intern. Med. **134:** 716–720.
12. GOLDBLATT, P. B., M. E. MOORE & A. J. STUNKARD. 1965. Social factors in obesity. JAMA **192:** 1039–1044.
13. HARRIS, M. B. 1969. Self-directed program for weight control: A pilot study. J. Abnorm. Psychol. **74:** 263–270.
14. HUENEMAN, R. L. 1969. Factors associated with teenage obesity. In Obesity. N. L. Wilson, Ed. F. A. Davis Co. Philadelphia, Pa.
15. LALONDE, M. 1975. A new perspective on the health of Canadians. Information Canada, Ontario.
16. LEVITZ, L. & A. J. STUNKARD. 1974. A therapeutic coalition for obesity: Behavior modification and patient self-help. Am. J. Psychiat. **131:** 423–427.

17. MACCOBY, N. & J. W. FARQUHAR. 1975. Communication for health: Unselling heart disease. J. Commun. **25:** 114–139.
18. MAHONEY, M. J. & K. MAHONEY. 1976. Permanent Weight Control. Norton. New York.
19. McGOVERN, G. 1977. Dietary Goals for the United States. Report of the Select Committee on Nutrition and Human Needs of the United States Senate. January 1977.
20. MAYER, J. 1955. The role of exercise and activity in weight control. *In* Weight Control. E. S. Eppright, P. Swanson, C. A. Iverson, Eds. Iowa State College Press. Ames, Iowa.
21. PENICK, S. B., R. D. L. FILION, S. FOX & A. J. STUNKARD. 1971. Behavior modification in the treatment of obesity. Psychosom. Med. **33:** 49–55.
22. SILVERSTONE, J. T., R. P. GORDON & A. J. STUNKARD. 1969. Social factors in obesity in London. Practitioner **202:** 682–688.
23. SROLE, L., T. S. LANGNER & S. T. MICHAEL, *et al.* 1962. Mental Health in the Metropolis: The Midtown Manhattan Study. McGraw Hill. New York.
24. STUART, R. B. 1967. Behavioral control of overeating. Behav. Res. Ther. **5:** 357–365.
25. STUART, R. B. 1977. Self help approach to self management. *In* Behavior Self Management: Strategies and Outcomes. R. B. Stuart Ed. Brunner Mazel. New York. In press.
26. STUNKARD, A. J. 1968. Environment and obesity: Recent advances in our understanding of the regulation of food intake in man. Fed. Proc. **27:** 1367–1373.
27. STUNKARD, A. J. 1975. Obesity and the social environment. *In* Recent Advances in Obesity Research. I. A. Howard, Ed. : 178–190. Newman. London.
28. STUNKARD, A. J. & M. McLAREN-HUME. 1959. The results of treatment of obesity: A review of the literature and report of a series. Arch. Intern. Med. **103:** 79–85.
29. STUNKARD, A. J., H. LEVINE & S. FOX. 1970. The management of obesity: Patient self-help and medical treatment. Arch. Intern. Med. **125:** 1367–1373.
30. STUNKARD, A. J., E. D'AQUILI, S. FOX & R. D. L. FILION. 1972. The influence of social class on obesity and thinness in children. JAMA **22:** 579–584.
31. STUNKARD, A. J. & M. MAHONEY. 1976. Behavioral treatment of the eating disorders. *In* Handbook of Behavior Modification and Behavior Therapy : 45–73. Prentice Hall. Englewood Cliffs, N.J.
32. WEST, K. M. 1974. Epidemiology of adiposity in regulation of the adipose tissue mass. Proceedings of the IV International Conference Meeting of Endocrinology, Marseilles, 1973. Excerpta Medica : 202–207.
33. WHITELAW, G. L. 1971. Association of social class and sibling number with skinfold thickness in London school boys. Hum. Biol. **43:** 414–420.
34. WILBER, J. A. 1973. The problem of undetected and untreated hypertension in the community. Bull. N.Y. Acad. Med. **49:** 510–520.
35. WOLLERSHEIM, J. R. 1970. The effectiveness of group therapy based upon learning principles in the treatment of overweight women. J. Abnorm. Psychol. **76:** 462–474.

NEW ASPECTS IN THE CONTROL OF FOOD INTAKE AND APPETITE

Robert I. Henkin

Center for Molecular Nutrition and Sensory Disorders
Georgetown University Medical Center
Washington, D.C. 20007

One of the challenges expressed as an important goal of this meeting relates to defining the technology required to meet the food and nutrition needs of the world community. Problems of the control of appetite and food intake are primarily those of the developed, affluent countries of the world rather than those of developing countries. Although in the United States the poor may exhibit a proportionately higher rate of obesity than among the affluent, problems of food intake control in our country, in Western Europe, and in other affluent countries relate primarily to people who have readily available access to food, to those people who, by choice, consume too many calories. This differs from the problems in the developing countries, where malnutrition is readily common and readily available access to food is limited.

To define the above challenge further involves the seeking out and finding of comprehensive solutions for specific problems. The first step in this process is to state and define the specific problem clearly so that a technological approach can be formulated. The second step in this process is to develop the technology to be applied to satisfy and solve the problem. Two examples of the success of this approach have already been offered at this meeting: one, relating to Dr. Hardy's discussion of CO_2 and N_2 fixation as a technique for increasing plant production, the second relating to Dr. Rankin's application of high-frequency irrigation as a unique solution to the watering of some plants in an arid environment.

One problem faced by the obese, stated in a rather oversimplified manner, can be formulated out of questions asked of me many times as I have traveled across the United States speaking about taste, smell, and sensory dysfunction. The question commonly arises in the discussion period after the scientific presentation and is usually raised by a middle-aged, moderately obese person who asks, "Doc, can you take away my taste so that I won't eat so much?" This question implies a self-awareness on the part of the questioner of a lack of self control, and an awareness that somehow, with the ability to control taste and food intake, will come the successful reduction of excess body weight. Since this approach also represents my own bias in this problem I am always pleased to receive such questions. However, the answer is not usually satisfactory to the questioner since it is necessary to separate taste control from appetite and food intake control; while these control processes are related by some metabolic parameters, they can have different antecedents and the timing of their interrelationships can vary greatly.

The problems I wish to define in this paper may be classified as those of overnutrition and undernutrition. In overnutrition the subject consumes more calories than expended as energy and hence, gains weight. The reasons for the increased caloric consumption are commonly multifactorial, involving social, emotional, psychological, and metabolic interactions. These subjects choose to consume excessive amounts of food and when this occurs obesity is a common result. Although the incidence of obesity in the United States may not be known with certainty, it has been estimated that at least 25% of our population weighs more than ideal standards indicate for their body height and habitus. The hazards of obesity are multiple. Associated with obesity is an increased incidence of hypertension, coronary artery disease, other forms of cardiovascular diseases, diabetes mellitus, and, perhaps, even some forms of cancer. Obesity is a serious public health hazard in our country and, as such, it must be appreciated as an important parameter of several disease states.

On the other hand, undernutrition may be defined as the consumption of fewer calories than expended as energy. These subjects also have free access to food and drink but choose not to consume it. As with overnutrition this problem is multifactorial, involving many of the same factors observed with overnutrition. Cachexia is a severe form of undernutrition and is associated with various forms of cancer, anorexia nervosa, and with some severe malabsorptive processes. Simple anorexia may be considered a less severe form of this problem and is associated with various forms of taste and smell dysfunction, x-irradiation to the head and neck, xerostomia, and some less severe malabsorptive processes. Although the incidence of these problems may be less than those associated with overnutrition, because of the usually serious nature of the pathology underlying the anorexia these problems are important and deserve careful consideration as to etiology and treatment.

From the work of the many investigators studying these problems, food intake and appetite appear to be controlled by many complex social physiological, biochemical, and psychological factors. These factors may act independently or in concert to produce the daily intake of food and drink. Whether or not there is a continuum upon which these factors can be plotted is not known, so that instead of a systematic approach to these problems we are faced with fragments of information related to specific techniques to increase or decrease food and/or fluid intake.

Much of the knowledge we possess about over- and undernutrition has come from therapeutic attempts to influence the pathological state. Various techniques have been used in humans in an attempt to decrease appetite as a treatment for obesity (TABLE 1) or to increase appetite as a treatment for anorexia (TABLE 2). The production of anorexia has involved mechanical, surgical, psychological, hormonal, and drug therapies; each of these approaches has some value and some success, but unwanted side effects or long-term failure of the therapy has limited the usefulness of each of these approaches. In addition to the better known interventions, it is also of interest that timing of meals may play some role in this complex interaction of variables.[1] On the other hand, attempts to treat anorexia, particularly in the cachexic cancer patient, have involved various procedures that may result in some short-term improvement, but little success in dealing with the multiple factors in this complex problem has been encountered.

In our laboratory over the past 10 years we have been studying zinc metabolism and its relationship to various aspects of sensory physiology and body homeostasis. Other laboratories have also been involved in the same process for even longer periods of time. Through careful evaluation of these data, collected over the last 15 years, it has been possible to attempt a systematic evaluation of one aspect of food and fluid intake that seems to underly both overnutrition and undernutrition. Although the data collected have been substantiated among

TABLE 1

METHODS OF DECREASING FOOD INTAKE AND APPETITE

Method	Technique	Effect
Mechanical	Jaw wiring closure	↓ food intake
Surgical	Jejunoileal bypass	↓ GI absorption
Psychological	Behavior modification	↓ food intake?
	Acupuncture	?
Diet	Bulk addition	↑ gastric filling?
	Food deprivation	↓ food intake
	Low caloric intake	↓ caloric intake
Hormonal	Human chorionic gonadotropin	?
	Thyroid hormone	↓ appetite?
Drug	Sympathomimetic amines and their derivatives	{ ↓ appetite? / Other CNS effects?
	Cationic exchange resins	?
	Histamine	↓ appetite
Vitamin Depletion	↓ B_6	↓ appetite
Zinc Depletion	Oral L-histidine	↓ appetite
	↓ histidine decarboxylase	↓ appetite

TABLE 2

METHODS OF INCREASING FOOD AND APPETITE

Method	Technique	Effect
Surgical	Gastrostomy	↑ calories, nutrition
	Parenteral Hyperalimentation	↑ calories, nutrition
Psychological	Behavior Modification	↑ food intake
	Psychiatric counseling	?
	Conditioned response to food	?
	↑ Dietary "moreishness"	↑ food intake
Diet	Food modification	↑ food interest
	↑ textural interest	
	↑ color interest	
	↑ taste/flavor interest	
	Δ in diet character	↑ nutritional intake
	↑ caloric, nutritional content of traditional foods (e.g., bread)	
	↑ caloric, nutritional content of new foods (e.g., liquids, new proteins)	
	Δ in meal size	↑ food intake?
	{ ↓ meal size / ↑ meal frequency	
	Δ in timing meal intake	↑ food intake?
Hormonal	Insulin	↑ appetite
	Δ in gastrointestinal hormones	↓ satiety?
Mineral	↑ Dietary Zinc	↑ appetite

several groups of investigators, the basic mechanisms underlying these results are still unclear. Thus, attempts to establish a common, unifying principle as a foundation for both increased and decreased food intake have not yet been successful. However, the results of these studies suggest that an approach may be possible that deserves careful consideration.

In studies carried out at the Rowett Laboratories in Scotland, zinc deficiency in rats was associated with the rapid onset of anorexia as the initial symptom of the deficiency.[2, 3] In FIGURE 1, in work carried out in our laboratory, rats fed an *ad libitum* diet consumed approximately 3–4 times as much food as did rats fed zinc-deficient rations,[4] confirming the earlier work carried out at Rowett.[2, 3] This decrease in food intake, however, was peculiar in that the zinc-depleted rats exhibited wide fluctuations in their meager food intake, the zinc-replete rats consuming a more constant intake of food (FIGURE 2). In spite of this variation, the food intake of the zinc-depleted rats was always below that of the zinc-replete rats, which caused the zinc-depleted rats to remain static in their gain of body weight during the time they took in small amounts of food (the food being normal in terms of adequacy of all essential nutrients, carbohydrates, fat and protein, except for the omission of zinc;[4] see FIGURE 3). Following the administration of very small amounts of zinc to these zinc-deficient rats their food intake increased significantly, and they increased their body weight. In another series of studies, following the onset of the zinc-related anorexia, the rats were offered a choice between two solutions, one usually avoided, e.g., hydrochloric acid or quinine sulfate, and one that was neutral, e.g., water. The zinc-depleted rats could not distinguish well between the normally avoided solutions and water, indicating that subsequent to the onset of zinc deficiency and the onset of anorexia they exhibited loss of taste acuity or hypogeusia.[4] Following administration of zinc to these rats they once again rejected solutions of hydrochloric acid and quinine sulfate, as occurs with normal body zinc status. This second series of studies emphasized the timing

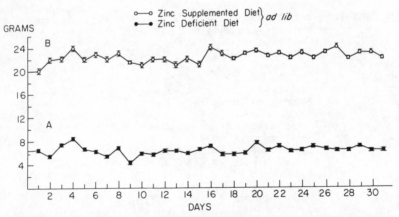

FIGURE 1. Comparison of food intake in rats fed zinc-deficient (A) and zinc supplemented (B) diets, *ad libitum*. Each point represents the mean ± SEM of 12 rats fed each diet. Mean intakes of the rats fed the zinc deficient diet were approximately ⅓–¼ those of the rats fed zinc-supplemented diet. (After McConnell & Henkin.[4])

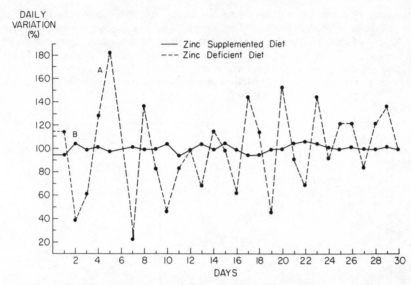

FIGURE 2. Daily variation in food intake in rats fed zinc-deficient (A) and zinc-supplemented (B) diets *ad libitum*. The values are expressed as a percentage of the daily mean intake for each group of rats. Rats fed zinc-deficient diet exhibited marked variation in their daily intake of food, whereas the rats fed zinc-supplemented diets exhibited a much more constant intake of food. (After McConnell & Henkin.[4])

relationships in zinc depletion such that the first sensory indication of the development of zinc deficiency was anorexia, the second, the onset of hypogeusia.

We then considered how to produce these changes in humans on an experimental basis. In this respect, biochemical information proved very helpful. We had previously been studying the interrelationships between zinc and its major carrying protein in blood, albumin.[5] These studies and others[6] demonstrated that there existed in blood an equilibrium between zinc, albumin, and amino acids and that addition of amino acids, particularly cysteine and histidine, caused the zinc that is normally bound to albumin to be stripped from that protein and to bind with the amino acid moieties. In the physiological state in man histidine, an essential amino acid, was a more commonly encountered amino acid than cysteine, and it was chosen to be given in these experimental studies. Knowledge of the *in vitro* studies suggested that administration of L-histidine would not only strip the zinc from its binding sites on albumin, but the small histidine-zinc moieties would be rapidly excreted from the body in the urine, causing acute zinc loss. Since the basis of these chemical effects lay in mass action our hypotheses also predicted that little or no tachyphylaxis would occur with these effects.

To study these phenomena L-histidine was administered orally in graded doses to normal volunteers and to patients with scleroderma. The first sign of L-histidine administration was hyperzincuria, which occurred immediately after the L-histidine was administered[7, 8] (FIGURE 4). With graded increases in L-histidine dose, graded increases in urinary zinc excretion were observed[7, 8] (FIGURE 4). Subsequent to the urinary loss of zinc there was a gradual decrease in serum zinc concentrations, which eventually fell below the lower limit of normal in each subject studied (FIGURE 4). That these studies indicated total body loss of zinc rather than body redistribution of the metal came from two sources: (1) with graded increases in L-histidine administration there were graded increases in urinary zinc excretion (FIGURE 5), and (2) following oral administration of ^{65}Zn prior to the administration of L-histidine, subsequent

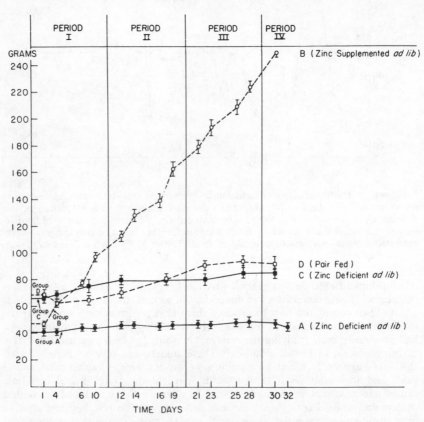

FIGURE 3. Changes in body weight (±1 SEM) in rats fed zinc-deficient (Groups A and C), zinc-supplemented diet (Group B), and pair-fed controls fed zinc-supplemented diet (Group D). There were 12 animals in Group A and B, 10 in Group C, and 8 in Group D. Means of the body weights of rats in Groups A and B, the rats reported in this study, were essentially the same at the start of the study prior to feeding specific diets.

oral administration of L-histidine produced a significant decrease in the total body half time of ^{65}Zn, indicating that it was being lost from the body at a more rapid rate during L-histidine administration than during administration of no agent or during administration of zinc ion (FIGURE 6). Indeed, subsequent to the rapid excretion of ^{65}Zn during L-histidine, if no agent were administered there was an apparent compensatory diminution of ^{65}Zn excretion, which was

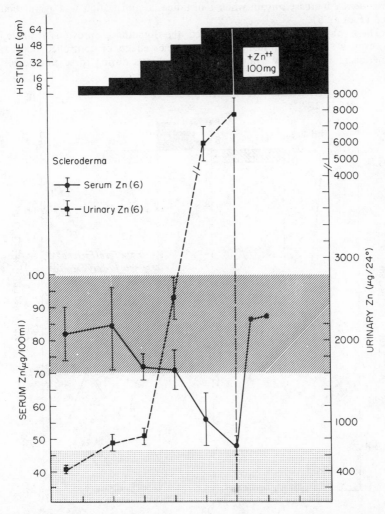

FIGURE 4. Effects of graded increases in oral L-histidine administration on urinary excretion and serum concentration of zinc in six patients with untreated scleroderma. The lower, hatched area, using the scale on the right side of the figure, indicates the range of normal urinary zinc excretion. The upper hatched area, using the scale on the left side of the figure, indicates the range of normal serum zinc concentration. The uppermost part of the figure indicates the doses of L-histidine administered. Each point represents the mean ±1 SEM of all patients studied during the last full day of L-histidine administration at the dose indicated. L-histidine was given at each dose level for periods of 2–4 days. Exogenous oral zinc sulfate, 100 mg daily, was added to the treatment regimen after the highest dose of L-histidine was attained and given along with the L-histidine (at the dark and the dotted perpendicular line through the middle of the figure). Subsequent to zinc administration, serum zinc levels returned to the normal range, even though L-histidine administration continued.

subsequently increased again when L-histidine administration was again reinstituted (FIGURE 6).

These physiological data supported the hypotheses previously made.[7, 8] However, we were interested in studying other effects of controlled body zinc depletion as well. Daily evaluation of the subjects during these zinc-depletion

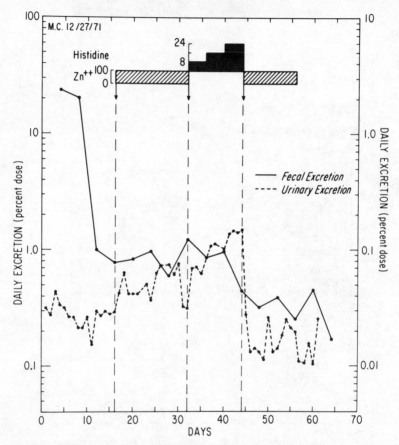

FIGURE 5. Fecal and urinary zinc excretion in one subject during oral administration of exogenous zinc sulfate and graded doses of L-histidine. Scale for fecal zinc excretion is on left side of figure; scale for urinary zinc excretion is on right side of figure. During L-histidine administration there was a graded increase in urinary zinc excretion in relationship to graded increases in dosage of administered L-histidine.

studies demonstrated that within 4–6 days after L-histidine was instituted the subjects spontaneously complained of onset of anorexia (TABLE 3). This was quite interesting in view of the fact that the normal volunteers studied constituted young college men who had "never missed a meal in their lives." Yet, they spontaneously noted a decrease in their appetites and had to be encouraged as vigorously as possible to continue to eat their meals. In some subjects it

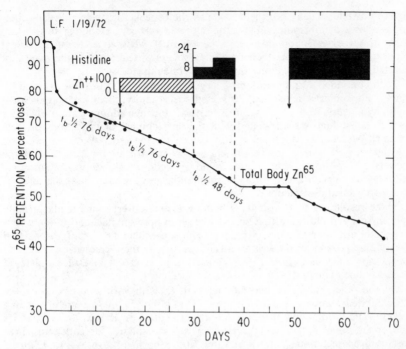

FIGURE 6. Changes in total body half time ($Tb_{1/2}$) of ^{65}Zn in one subject during administration of exogenous zinc sulfate and graded doses of L-histidine. During administration of no agent or oral zinc ion $Tb_{1/2}$ was 76 days. During administration of oral L-histidine $Tb_{1/2}$ decreased to 48 days, indicating a more rapid loss of total body zinc. Immediately after L-histidine was stopped there was a compensatory retention of ^{65}Zn indicated by the flattening of the retention curve. When L-histidine was once again administered, rapid loss of total body zinc began once again and continued throughout the administration of L-histidine.

TABLE 3

L-HISTIDINE-INDUCED ANOREXIA IN NORMAL SUBJECTS

Subject	L-Histidine (mg)	Anorexia Onset (Days)	Urinary Zinc ($\mu g/24$ hrs)
1	8.1 *	6 †	1,490 ‡
2	4.2	4	765
3	8.1	5	950

* L-histidine was given orally in divided doses twice daily.

† Onset of anorexia in days after first dose of L-histidine.

‡ $p < 0.01$ with respect to pretreatment values. There were no changes observed in serum zinc values obtained at the time of anorexia onset compared to pretreatment values.

was not possible to convince them to finish their meals. In these normal volunteers on doses of L-histidine of 8 g the anorexia was severe enough to produce weight losses of 2–3 pounds over a period of 1 week in spite of persistent encouragement to complete their meals. In general, breakfast was the meal best tolerated, lunch next, and dinner the least tolerated meal.

With continued administration of larger quantities of L-histidine, 16 and 32 g daily, all subjects developed decreased taste acuity, then decreased smell acuity, hypogeusia and hyposmia, respectively. Further administration of larger doses of L-histidine was associated with the development of distortions of taste and smell perception, dysgeusia and dysosmia, respectively.[8] With the addition of exogenous zinc, even in the presence of continued administration of large amounts of L-histidine, there was a rapid and complete abolition of anorexia within 24 hours with a concomitant diminution and eventual disappearance of all taste and smell dysfunction.

These results were consistent with the previous observations made in zinc-depleted rats and indicated that zinc depletion in both animals and humans was associated with anorexia and taste loss. The subsequent finding of the parotid salivary zinc protein gustin was useful in quantifying these changes in humans,[9] and measurement of parotid salivary zinc has been useful in estimating rapid changes in body zinc status.[10]

On the other hand, we had studied patients with various types of cancer who exhibited anorexia and hypogeusia (TABLE 4). In these patients median detection and recognition thresholds for representatives of four taste qualities (salt, sweet, sour, and bitter) carried out by a standard forced choice-three stimulus drop technique,[11] were elevated above normal (TABLE 4). Each of these subjects was also subjectively aware of taste loss, and four of seven exhibited dysgeusia. Measurement of serum and urine zinc levels by atomic absorption spectrophotometry [12] revealed significantly lower mean levels of serum zinc in the patients ($p < 0.01$), compared with those of normal volunteers and patients with other diseases who did not exhibit hypogeusia (controls); however, there were no differences between the groups in serum concentration of copper or in urinary excretion of either zinc or copper. Treatment of each of these patients with zinc sulfate in various doses for various periods of time (TABLE 5) was successful in assisting the restoration of taste acuity to or toward normal, as indicated by the return to or toward normal in the median detection and recognition thresholds measured; mean serum zinc concentration increased to normal levels or slightly above normal, and urinary zinc excretion increased significantly ($p < 0.01$) over pretreatment values. Somewhat prior to the return toward normal of taste acuity there was a diminution in the anorexia of these patients and a decrease in the dysgeusia among those patients in whom this symptom was present.

If serum zinc levels in this small sample of patients reflected body zinc status, then the hypogeusia, anorexia, and dysgeusia observed in them could be related to zinc depletion. The return of serum zinc levels to normal and the remission of the abnormal symptoms following administration of exogenous zinc are consistent with this hypothesis. However, many factors may be involved in this complex process, and serum zinc does not always provide an accurate estimate of body zinc status. This provocative, uncontrolled study suggests that some forms of anorexia may be improved by administration of exogenous zinc, particularly if the anorexia were related to body zinc depletion,

TABLE 4

TASTE THRESHOLDS AND SERUM AND URINE ZINC AND COPPER LEVELS IN PATIENTS WITH CANCER BEFORE ZINC THERAPY

Patients	Taste Thresholds (mM/L)				Serum Metals (µg/dl)		Urinary Metals (µg/24 hr)	
	NaCl	Sucrose	HCl	Urea	Zn	Cu	Zn	Cu
1	300/S*	300/1000	30/30	800/800	81	113	205	51
2	500/500	90/90	15/60	2000/2000	65	123	161	32
3	300/300	60/90	30/>500	>8000/>8000	83	66	607	17
4	90/90	60/60	15/30	800/1000	69	84	441	36
5	150/800	150/500	150/>500	1000/5000	77	93		—
6	300/∞	300/300	30/>500	>8000/>8000	68	106	413	24
7	300/∞	150/150	60/500	800/>8000	47	119	187	14
Median‡	300/800	150/150	30/500	1000/5000	70 ± 5 ‡	100 ± 8	339 ± 76	29 ± 6
Controls	30/60	30/60	3/6	120/150	99 ± 2	100 ± 2	419 ± 25	34 ± 3

* Numerator of fraction, detection threshold; denominator of fraction, recognition threshold; S, ability to recognize a saturated solution; >500 or >8000, inability to detect or recognize a 500 mM solution of HCl or an 8000 mM solution of urea. ∞, inability to recognize a saturated solution of NaCl.

† Median, median detection and recognition thresholds.

‡ Mean ± 1 SEM.

TABLE 5

TASTE THRESHOLDS AND SERUM AND URINE ZINC AND COPPER LEVELS IN PATIENTS
WITH CANCER AFTER ZINC THERAPY

Patients	Taste Thresholds (mM/L)				Serum Metals (μg/dl)		Urinary Metals (μg/24 hrs)		Treatment*	
	NaCl	Sucrose	HCl	Urea	Zn	Cu	Zn	Cu	mg	Months
1	150/150 †	60/90	6/6	120/120	110	125	819	57	25	2
2	60/60	30/60	3/3	120/120	122	133	657	21	100	6
3	60/60	60/60	3/15	150/150	160	73	1794	41	100	3
4	30/30	30/30	6/6	300/300	85	98	553	44	25	2
5	90/150	30/30	15/>500	120/2000	—	—	—	—	100	4
6	150/500	12/30	15/60	150/150	150	93	1500	24	100	6
7	150/150	60/60	15/15	120/150	—	—	—	—	100	3
Median	90/150 ‡	30/60	6/15	120/150	125±14 §	104±11	1065±246	37±7		
Controls	30/60	30/60	3/6	120/150	99±2	100±2	419±25	34±3		

* Treatment consisted of oral administration of graded doses of zinc sulfate for 2–6 months; all zinc doses are given in terms of zinc ion, in mg. All values were obtained at the end of each respective treatment period. The same patients, 1–7 were studied before and during treatment with zinc.

† Numerator of fraction, detection threshold; denominator of fraction, recognition threshold; >500, inability to detect or recognize a 500 mM solution of HCl.

‡ Median, median detection and recognition thresholds.

§ Mean ± 1 SEM.

and is consistent with the previous data which indicated that anorexia could be produced by body zinc depletion.

The role of zinc as a factor in the control of appetite and food intake has been observed in both animals and man. Its importance, however, has not been previously emphasized, even though its action has been recognized for several years. The mechanisms through which these effects occur are not known and also those that are known are not well studied. L-histidine can rapidly and easily cross the blood brain barrier,[13] and thus it is possible that it can mobilize and thereby possibly deplete the brain of zinc; in that manner it may produce central effects influencing appetite and food intake. The specific nature or loci of these possible central effects are unclear, but their presence is supported by the finding of several central nervous system changes following severe acute body zinc depletion [8] and the rapid return to normality in these changes following oral administration of exogenous zinc, even in the presence of continued administration of L-histidine. The importance of peripheral or metabolic effects of zinc in the control of food intake and appetite is also unclear, although zinc is known to play an important role in several systems that impinge upon the appetitive processes. For example, zinc is an integral part of the taste system, playing a role in gustin, the protein which influences taste bud nutrition,[9] and it is also involved at the level of the taste bud membrane.[14, 15] At the taste bud membrane, zinc is an integral part of the key enzyme alkaline phosphatase, which appears prominently in the isolated and partially purified taste bud receptor membrane.[14] It also plays an important role in the binding of tastants to the membrane, as indicated by decreased specific binding following zinc chelation and a return toward normal binding following zinc replacement.[15]

The future of this new approach toward understanding some of the important characteristics of food intake and appetite and the application of this knowledge in the control of these systems is encouraging; however, much more work is required to understand the multiple variables involved in this complex system. In the case of obesity studies, double blind trials to confirm the efficacy of L-histidine as an anorectic agent need to be undertaken. In the case of anorexia treatment, particularly as associated with cancer patients, carefully controlled and defined studies are necessary to understand the nature of the anorexia before treatment designs can be instituted, although the provocative and promising early observations reported in this work may provide useful models. With the performance of these studies it may be possible to attempt to define the mechanisms of action of zinc in these systems more clearly.

REFERENCES

1. HALBERG, F. 1974. Protection by timing treatment according to bodily rhythms. Chronobiologia 1(Suppl. 1): 27–68.
2. WILLIAMS, R. B. & C. F. MILLS. 1970. The experimental production of zinc deficiency in the rat. Brit. J. Nutr. 24: 989–1003.
3. CHESTERS, J. K. & J. QUARTERMAN. 1970. Effects of zinc deficiency on food intake and feeding patterns of rats. Brit. J. Nutr. 42: 1061–1069.
4. McCONNELL, S. D. & R. I. HENKIN. 1974. Altered preference for sodium chloride, anorexia and changes in plasma and urinary zinc in rats fed a zinc-deficient diet. J. Nutr. 104: 1108–1114.
5. GIROUX, E. L. & R. I. HENKIN. 1972. Competition for zinc among serum albumin and amino acids. Biochim. Biophys. Acta 273: 64–72.

6. GIROUX, E. L. & R. I. HENKIN. 1972. Macromolecular ligands of copper, zinc and cadmium in human serum. Bioinorg. Chem. **2:** 125–133.
7. HENKIN, R. I. 1974. Metal-albumin-amino acid interactions: Chemical and physiological interrelationships. *In* Protein-Metal Interactions. Mendel Friedman, Ed. : 299–328. Plenum Publishing Co. New York, N.Y.
8. HENKIN, R. I., B. M. PATTEN, P. RE & D. BRONZERT. 1975. A syndrome of acute zinc loss. Arch. Neurol. **32:** 745–751.
9. HENKIN, R. I., R. E. LIPPOLDT, J. BILSTAD & H. EDELHOCH. 1975. A zinc-containing protein isolated from human parotid saliva. Proc. Nat. Acad. Sci. **72:** 488–492.
10. HENKIN, R. I., C. MUELLER & R. WOLF. 1975. Estimation of zinc concentration of parotid saliva by flameless atomic absorption spectrophotometry in normal subjects and in patients with idiopathic hypogeusia. J. Lab. Clin. Med. **86:** 175–180.
11. HENKIN, R. I., P. J. SCHECHTER, R. C. HOYE & C. F. T. MATTERN. 1971. Idiopathic hypogeusia with dysgeusia, hyposmia and dysosmia: A new syndrome. JAMA **217:** 434–440.
12. MERET, S. & R. I. HENKIN. 1971. Simultaneous direct estimation by atomic absorption spectrophotometry of copper and zinc in serum, urine, and cerebrospinal fluid. Clin. Chem. **17:** 369–373.
13. OHLENDORF, W. H. 1971. Brain uptake of radio-labeled amino acids, amines and hexoses after arterial injection. Am. J. Physiol. **221:** 1629–1639.
14. LUM, C. K. L. & R. I. HENKIN. 1976. Characterization of fractions from taste bud and non-taste bud enriched filtrated from and around bovine circumvallate papillae. Biochim. Biophys. Acta **421:** 362–379.
15. LUM, C. K. L. & R. I. HENKIN. 1976. Sugar binding to purified fractions from bovine taste buds and epithelial tissue: relationships to bioactivity. Biochim. Biophys. Acta **421:** 380–394.

THE NUTRITIONAL EPIDEMIOLOGY OF CARDIOVASCULAR DISEASE

Willard A. Krehl

Department of Community Health and Preventive Medicine
Jefferson Medical College
Philadelphia, Pennsylvania 19107

INTRODUCTION

Cardiovascular diseases, particularly atherosclerotic coronary heart disease and stroke, are the leading causes of mortality in the United States, and it is further estimated that nearly 29 million Americans have some form of heart and blood vessel disease producing significant morbidity. It is estimated that nearly 24 million people have hypertension (one in six adults); nearly 4 million have evidence of coronary heart disease; and approximately 1.7 million are affected by stroke [1] (see TABLE 1 and FIGURES 1, 2, 3).

It is generally recognized that arterial atherosclerosis involving the principal target organs of the heart, brain, and kidney is the basic underlying pathological process that gradually develops until a major cardiovascular catastrophe occurs, leading either to sudden death or to significant morbidity.[2, 3]

A major stimulus to the use of traditional epidemiological tools in the analysis of the development of atherosclerotic cardiovascular disease arose from the extensive observations of a most significant reduction in their incidence associated with the serious food restrictions involving huge populations in a number of countries as the result of the catastrophe of World War II.[4, 5] Since then, an accelerating avalanche of a variety of fundamental epidemiological studies involving many countries and population groups, extensive basic science research, clinical investigations and more recently intervention trials have been published or are currently in progress.

In the United States two major efforts have provided particularly valuable epidemiological information, i.e., the Framingham Heart Study [6] devoted to the detection of factors increasing the risk of coronary disease and their epidemiological evaluation and the National Cooperative Polling Project,[4] a study of coronary proneness in more than 11,000 men in selected and representative areas of the United States.

It would be a Herculean task, quite beyond the limited scope of this paper, to give adequate review and citation of the many excellent contributions aimed at unravelling the etiology of the atherosclerotic process and its contribution to the development of cardiovascular diseases. Much of this work has been the subject of numerous review articles published elsewhere.[2-6]

A major significant concept has evolved, particularly from the numerous epidemiological investigations, that identifies coronary risk factors involving habits, traits, and abnormalities that when identified are associated with a considerable increased risk of developing cardiovascular disease in middle age or young adulthood, in comparison with individuals that do not exhibit such traits, habits, or abnormalities.[4-7] The major benefit of identifying and focusing on "risk factors" has shifted the emphasis to the potential primary prevention

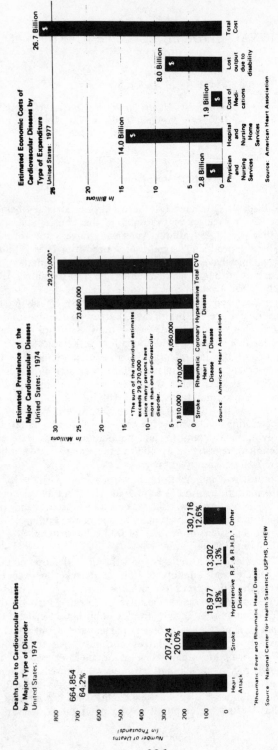

FIGURE 1. The magnitude and scope of the cardiovascular problem. (From American Heart Association.[1])

of cardiovascular diseases, as opposed to the direct treatment of individuals already ill (FIGURE 4). It is significant to emphasize that the major coronary risk factors that have been identified are associated with at least a doubling

TABLE 1

SELECTED HEART FACTS *

CVD COST—$26.7 billion (AHA est.) in 1977.

PREVALENCE—29,270,000 Americans have some form of heart and blood vessel disease.
- Hypertension—23,660,000 (one in six adults).
- Coronary heart disease—4,050,000.
- Rheumatic heart disease—1,770,000.
- Stroke—1,810,000.

CVD MORTALITY—1,035,273 in 1974 (54 percent of all deaths). 1977 (AHA est.): 1,036,900 (52 percent).
- One-fourth of all persons killed by CVD are under age 65.

ATHEROSCLEROSIS—contributed to many of the 872,278 heart attack and stroke deaths in 1974.

HEART ATTACK—caused 664,854 deaths in 1974.
- 4,050,000 alive today have history of heart attack and/or angina pectoris.
- 350,000 a year die of heart attack before they reach hospital—average victim waits 3 hours before decision to seek help.
- Over a million Americans will have a heart attack this year, and about 650,-000 of them will die.

STROKE—killed 207,424 in 1974; afflicts 1,810,000.

HYPERTENSION (HBP)—23,660,000 adults have it, but more than 7 million don't know it.
- Of those who do know they have it, many are untreated or inadequately controlled.
- Only a minority have it under adequate control.
- For 90 percent of those with high blood pressure, science doesn't know the cause; but it is easily detected and usually controllable.

MAJOR RISK FACTORS
    BLOOD PRESSURE—man with systolic pressure over 150 has more than *twice* the risk of heart attack and nearly *four* times risk of stroke of man with systolic pressure under 120.
    CHOLESTEROL—man with blood cholesterol of 250 or more has about *three* times the risk of heart attack and stroke of man with cholesterol level below 194.
    CIGARETTE SMOKING—man who smokes more than one pack a day has nearly *twice* the risk of heart attack and nearly *five* times the risk of stroke of a non-smoker.

* From American Heart Association.[1]

of the risk of an adverse event occurring in the order of 100 or 200 percent or more.[5]

It has been amply demonstrated that three major risk factors exist for the premature development of atherosclerotic coronary heart disease and stroke,

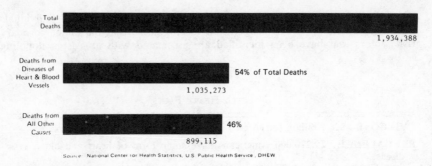

FIGURE 2. Diseases of the heart and blood vessels. Number 1 cause of death—
United States: 1974. (From American Heart Association.[1])

i.e., hyperlipidemia (especially hypercholesterolemia), hypertension, and
cigarette smoking (FIGURE 5). Other identifiable risk factors that have been
implicated are: glucose intolerance, ECG abnormalities (left ventricular
hypertrophy), elevated uric acid levels, and lack of exercise or sedentary life
style.[4, 5] The potential of obesity as an isolated risk factor is still a matter of
some debate, but since it is so commonly associated with other major risk
factors, particularly hypertension and often with hyperlipidemia, its significance
assumes importance.[4-7]

It is also evident from the major epidemiological studies that atherosclerotic
cardiovascular diseases have a predilection for the technically developed and
affluent societies and are commonly identified with life styles associated with
"luxious" food consumption, with excessive caloric intake particularly of high
caloric density diets and possibly "sweets," an excessively sedentary life style

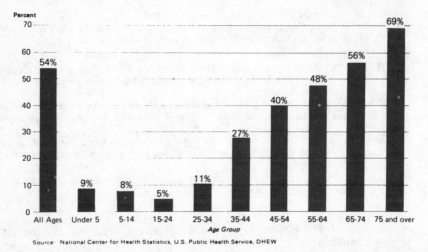

FIGURE 3. Percentage of all deaths due to cardiovascular diseases by age—United
States: 1974. (From American Heart Association.[1])

PERIOD OF LITTLE OR NO RISK	VULNERABLE TO RISK	PREDISPOSING FACTORS — NO EXPRESSED PRECURSORS	EXPRESSED PRECURSORS PRESENT	OVERT SIGNS PRESENT	SYMPTOMS PRESENT	MANIFEST DISABILITY AND DISEASE
FOCUS OF PROSPECTIVE MEDICINE				FOCUS OF CRISIS MEDICINE		

FIGURE 4. Prospective medicine—spectrum of the natural history of disease.

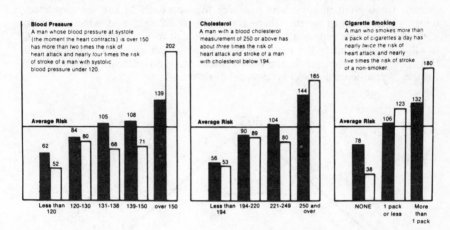

These charts show the extent to which particular risk factors increased the risk of heart attack and stroke in the male population, aged 30-62 of Framingham, Mass. For each disease, columns below the black horizontal line indicate lower than average risk; columns above the line, higher than average risk.

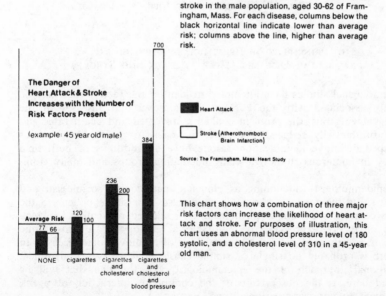

This chart shows how a combination of three major risk factors can increase the likelihood of heart attack and stroke. For purposes of illustration, this chart uses an abnormal blood pressure level of 180 systolic, and a cholesterol level of 310 in a 45-year old man.

FIGURE 5. Risk factors in heart attack and stroke. (From American Heart Association.[1])

with a lack of appropriate exercise, possibly the abusive use of alcoholic beverages, and possibly related to the so-called stresses of high-technology living.[4]

Of the three major risk factors that have been unequivocally identified as highly significant, emphasis will be given to hyperlipidemias (i.e., hypercholesterolemia, hypertriglyceridemia, and hyperlipoproteinemias) and hypertension, particularly since these have been identified as being related to dietary habit and nutrient intake.[4, 8, 9]

The principles of epidemiology will be applied to the evaluation of these factors, since epidemiology best provides the approach to the circumstances under which diseases occur, where they tend to flourish, and where they do not. Although this represents a simplistic approach to a most complex subject, it will serve to identify the major contributions of diet and food nutrients and their potential implication in the development of atherosclerosis and ultimately to atherosclerotic cardiovascular diseases (FIGURE 6).

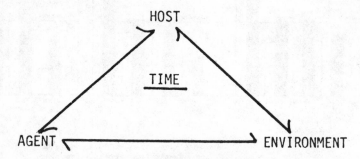

FIGURE 6. The epidemiology triad.

THE PRINCIPLES OF EPIDEMIOLOGY APPLIED TO CARDIOVASCULAR DISEASES (HEART ATTACK AND STROKE)

Epidemiological studies have attempted to identify the factors that may be significantly associated with the etiology of cardiovascular diseases in the hope that knowing this, the problem could be prevented and death rates and morbidity substantially reduced. To date, the cause or more likely causes have escaped definitive identification despite huge expenditures of both time and money in numerous studies of many population groups and many countries.[4, 5, 6, 10, 11]

The epidemiologist functioning as clinician, pathologist, sociologist, and statistician shifts the focus of the study of disease in a single patient to the study of a complex spectrum of phenomena in a selected population in which disease is or is not expressed. A multifactorial etiology of atherosclerotic disease is manifestly evident in the epidemiology of cardiovascular disease. In short, there is probably no single or simple cause, at least as yet identified. The traditional approach of the epidemiologist, and the one that will be emphasized here, is the observation of the continuous interaction of agent, host, and environment over a period of time (FIGURE 6).

The significant *host factors* that are of concern in the epidemiology of cardiovascular disease are: age, sex, race, or ethnic group and, most specifically, familial or genetic characteristics that enhance susceptibility in the host. With regard to *agents* that impact on the host and interact with the environment to produce atherosclerotic cardiovascular disease, a major emphasis has been placed upon dietary components with an overwhelming emphasis on fat (saturated fat vs. polyunsaturated fat), carbohydrate, simple sugars vs. complex polysaccharides, which are factors that have been incriminated in the development of hyperlipidemia and hence atherosclerosis.[12-14]

Other dietary agents such as salt (sodium) and excessive caloric intake leading to caloric imbalance and obesity are of concern and probable significance in the development of hypertension—a major risk factor for the development of heart attack and stroke.[4, 8, 9]

More recently, a variety of macro- and micro-mineral elements have been considered as agents or a part of the multifactorial system contributing to the development of atherosclerotic disease.[15,16] A whole host of other positive agent factors have been studied, such as coffee drinking,[17] soft water,[18, 67] stress," [4] etc. Cigarette smoking emerges as the major non-dietary stimulating agent (risk factor) relating to the causation of atherosclerotic cardiovascular diseases.

With regard to environment, factors such as national, local, urban, rural, and climatic have been studied, and as indicated above, the major observation emerges that the development of atherosclerotic cardiovascular disease flourishes in technically developed and affluent societies, and further, there has been noted a changing pattern in ischemic heart disease and mortality.[18, 19]

THE LIPID THEORY IN THE EPIDEMIOLOGY OF ATHEROSCLEROSIS

The body of evidence that links lipids, particularly cholesterol and saturated fat, with the development of atherosclerosis has evolved from four areas of evidence: [2-5, 10, 11]

1. Experimental atherosclerosis can be produced in a variety of animals by feeding diets containing cholesterol.

2. The atherosclerotic lesions found in blood vessel plaques associated with experimental atherosclerosis are heavily laden with lipids.

3. In the preponderance of all epidemiological studies as well as clinical investigations, there exists a strong correlation between high levels of serum cholesterol and the occurrence of clinical atherosclerotic cardiovascular disease in human beings.

4. There is, however, an uneven distribution of atherosclerotic coronary disease among different cultural groups and even within individuals of the same group, and overall the disease tends to affect most seriously those most highly placed in the socioeconomic system.

Whether or not triglycerides as an isolated factor and unrelated to cholesterol levels have a significant predictive value in the development of atherosclerotic disease remains a debated problem.

Overall, the above facts have led to a very effective working theory, which can be summarized as follows:

Diet (nutritional factors)
  a. excessive consumption of saturated fat vs. polyunsaturated fat
  b. large intake of dietary cholesterol (derived exclusively from animal food sources)
  c. character of carbohydrate intake (excessive sucrose use as compared to starches)

Hypercholesterolemia (? hypertriglyceridemia) (hyperlipoproteinemia)

Atherosclerosis (primarily of heart, brain, kidney)

Atherosclerotic coronary heart disease and stroke

An abbreviated review of the extensive report of the Framingham Study [6] will serve as an admirable prototype to identify the lipid profile and its sequential development related to diet and nutritional components and the development of cardiovascular disease, i.e., heart attack and stroke. Kannel has emphasized that, "it is a mistake to conceptualize the atherosclerotic diseases as the product of any single etiological agent. It is clear that in different populations, such as those in the United States, everyone has enough lipid to manufacture atheromata, but the rate of its development appears to depend upon multiple contributing factors as well as the degree of elevation of the blood lipid content." [20] Kannel further points out, and this is most important, that "as regards atherogenesis—it is hard to specify where normal leaves off and abnormal begins for any of the major atherogenic coronary precursors including lipid, blood pressure, and impaired carbohydrate tolerance. Most are continuously distributed in the population with no bimodality to designate where abnormal begins." [20] Despite this nebulous continuum, the risk of becoming a victim of cardiovascular disease can be estimated over as much as a 30-fold range. Blood lipid, particularly cholesterol, unquestionably plays a key role in atheroma formation. Thus, the determination of total cholesterol in the serum continues to be of major importance in the study of the epidemiology of this problem, despite the sophistication and biochemical refinements afforded by lipoprotein analysis whether by electrophoresis or ultracentrifugation. The Framingham data further suggest that elevations of indigenous triglycerides associated with the triglyceride-rich pre-β-lipoprotein fraction are significantly associated with an increased risk of coronary heart disease only when accompanied by an increased cholesterol level.[20] This observation is particularly relevant to men, and the role of triglyceride-rich pre-β-lipoprotein in the potential development of coronary heart disease in women remains of considerable interest. This observation may be significantly affected by the common use of oral contraceptives. Of further interest is the observation that the risk of coronary heart disease increases progressively in proportion to serum cholesterol values at all ages in men, whereas no similar relationship is observed in women beyond the age of 55.[20] Of particular interest from the Framingham data is the observation that it is still difficult to pinpoint the "major determinants" producing the generally high cholesterol values observed. Neither the Framingham nor any other epidemiological study assessing free-living, affluent, general population samples has succeeded in demonstrating at the high nutrient intakes encountered that the nutrient composition of the diet is related either to blood cholesterol concentration or to coronary disease status.[20-22]

Kannel emphasizes that it is not to be interpreted that diet has no connection with blood cholesterol values; rather it is considered that from the liberal supply of nutrients in the United States food supply [22] there exists a general nutritional overload of saturated fat, cholesterol, and refined carbohydrate, and particularly the high percentage of calories derived from fat, thus influencing the metabolic energy balance with a potential inability to cope with this overload and which combines to influence and determine the resulting generally excessive blood cholesterol levels that are observed. It certainly should not be concluded that an individual's diet is not related to or responsible for evident blood lipid abnormalities if such are noted and, most importantly, that diet modification cannot help to reduce cholesterol and triglyceride levels and potentially to reduce the risk of coronary disease.

Many studies have provided evidence that dietary manipulation with regard to total fat, saturated fat, and dietary cholesterol can reduce serum cholesterol values predictably in humans and, in the case of experimental animals, can cause the regression of established atherosclerotic lesions, at least moderately.[23-26, 10, 11]

Continued caloric excesses resulting in weight gain may often be associated with increases in serum cholesterol levels, and weight loss results in their reduction. A diet plan reducing the caloric density, particularly from saturated fat and refined carbohydrate, is a reasonable approach to weight reduction, maintaining leanness, and achieving more desirable levels of blood lipids, particularly cholesterol. Unfortunately, at the present time in technically developed countries, affluent societies greatly enjoy the "luxious" consumption of diets containing much animal protein contributing both excessive amounts of saturated fat and cholesterol in a highly caloric concentrated diet. Sadly, we are not about to change our dietary habits. Most of us then appear to have sufficient serum lipid levels to produce atherosclerosis—hence the epidemic, since the risk is proportional to serum lipid levels, particularly cholesterol.

Although epidemiological evidence strongly supports the developmental hypothesis relating diet to blood lipids to atherosclerosis and ultimately to the epidemic of atherosclerotic cardiovascular disease, the most important facts are still lacking. We simply do not have conclusive evidence to show whether or not in man a consistent correction of a particular lipid abnormality, i.e., hypercholesterolemia or hyperlipoproteinemia particularly in the general asymptomatic population, will produce a better prognosis for a reduction in the excessive incidence and prevalence of atherosclerotic lesions or the ultimate development of atherosclerotic disease. It is hoped that prospective studies and well-programmed intervention trials will provide this final link to complete this story.[20] Perhaps then, an even bigger challenge will follow, i.e., how do you influence individuals or populations to change a set and established life style? None of this, however, alters the fact that elevations of serum lipids and cholesterol, particularly, significantly identify the coronary-prone profile and can be useful in estimating the risk in predicting atherosclerotic disease.[20]

One of the most practical outcomes of the epidemiological information derived from the Framingham studies as well as others is the development of the Coronary Risk Handbook. With this the practicing physician can estimate the risk of coronary heart disease in patients seen in medical practice, after the major risk factors have been identified.[68] Certainly, individuals are not easily persuaded to make life-style changes until their risks can be identified and their predictive importance explained—thus the practicality of this predictive guide.[68]

While it has been possible in small group studies under carefully controlled clinical conditions to demonstrate the effects of dietary management as a means of reducing serum cholesterol concentrations and the potential risk of cardiovascular disease, broadly based epidemiological studies still do not provide sufficient support of the hypothesis that changes in diet decrease risk.[20] At best, only modest reductions in blood cholesterol have been observed, i.e., approximately 10 percent when low-fat, low-cholesterol diets have been applied in epidemiological studies. This leaves open the question whether or not there should be a broadly applied recommendation to persuade the general population to modify their diet with respect to total fat, saturated fat, and cholesterol.[9] The fact is that the American people at least are so persistently addicted to the traditional high-fat, saturated fat, and cholesterol-containing diet provided predominately by animal protein that it is most difficult even under the application of epidemiological rules to effect significant dietary modifications sufficiently to alter the lipid patterns of a generally atherogenic-prone population. This in no way suggests that individuals with elevated serum lipids should not be strongly advised to modify their diet, since effective diet modification will lower lipids and decrease (we hope) the risk of cardiovascular disease.

The International Cooperative Study on the Epidemiology of Cardiovascular Disease, a prospective study of 18 population samples in seven countries—Finland, Greece, Italy, Japan, The Netherlands, The United States, and Yugoslavia—has produced very interesting results.[77] Investigators compared the incidence of heart disease among 12,000 men between the ages of 40 and 59 at the beginning of the study. These men were then studied for 10 years. Very interestingly, the mean rates of heart disease varied four-fold, with the highest rates being noted in the United States and Finland and the lowest in Japan. The rates were significantly correlated with serum cholesterol concentrations and also with the saturated fat intake of the respective population. It is most difficult in such a study to assess the impact of the differing genetic backgrounds and habits, and of course, the independent effects of diet and cholesterol are hard to evaluate.

It would appear that when many answers rather than a single answer are given to explain a question, an adequate explanation is not available. Overall, however, the general consensus among epidemiologists is that there are some very plausible if not certain links between the diet and its nutrient composition, serum cholesterol, and atherosclerotic coronary heart disease.

The Role of Polyunsaturated Fats

It has been shown that the replacement of saturated fat in the diet with sources supplying polyunsaturated fatty acids is effective in lowering serum cholesterol.[3-5, 25, 26] Despite extensive studies by many investigators, we still do not know the mechanism of this effect of polyunsaturates on cholesterolemia. There still remains a controversy whether it is more effective to lower the total fat content of the diet or retain the current, rather excessive level, of total dietary fat and significantly alter the ratio of polyunsaturated: saturated fatty acids to as much as 1.5 to 1.

Population studies, particularly in areas of the world where there is low incidence of atherosclerotic coronary heart disease, the diet is low in total fat and many believe that high "polyunsaturate" diets are not required but rather it is more important to lower the total fat content of the diet. There certainly is no observable or identifiable nutritional deficiency related to fat in huge populations where the total fat content may range from 15 to 20 percent of the total calories and where the ratio of saturated to polyunsaturated fats is approximately equal. It is doubtful that adding polyunsaturated fatty acids to a currently high fat diet will effectively promote a reduction in the risk of atherosclerotic heart disease; rather it is more appropriate to lower total fat intake along with modest shifts towards increasing polyunsaturated fatty acids as a percentage of this lower total fat intake. Again, these rather significant dietary modifications are difficult to implant in huge populations where traditional high-fat and saturated-fat dietary patterns are so firmly established. Again, individual patient dietary pattern changes, while difficult to modify, are indicated, can effect lipid level changes and may be more effective, especially effected through nutritional and diet counselling programs.

THE CARBOHYDRATE THEORY AS A FACTOR IN PRODUCING ATHEROSCLEROSIS

Yudkin has studied the sugar intake in various countries and believes that sucrose is more closely related to mortality from coronary heart disease than any other nutrient.[27] Further, studies by Yudkin provided the mechanism of taking diet histories and concluded that men with myocardial infarction or peripheral artery disease consumed twice as much sugar as did controls and indicated that high sugar consumption was an important factor in the development of these two disorders.[27] These studies have obviously stimulated considerable interest, and other studies have been conducted and reviewed. The working party on the relationship between dietary sugar intake and arterial disease established in England conducted an extensive review of the relationship between dietary sugar intake and men with myocardial infarction. They reported that "the sugar consumption of men with myocardial infarction was compared with that of matched controls in four centers. The average sugar consumption was slightly greater in the patients with myocardial infarction than among the controls, but the differences were not statistically significant. Findings in one center suggest that the slightly higher sugar intake in patients with myocardial infarction was likely to have been due to an association between the consumption of sugar and the smoking of cigarettes." [28] In another epidemiological field study (the seven-country study) a rather good correlation of sugar intake with a five-year coronary heart disease incidence was demonstrated, but in those countries sugar intake was also highly correlated with the intake of saturated fat.[10] Relationships between dietary carbohydrates and serum cholesterol have been reviewed based on studies by the former ICNND Nutritional Program and surveys of 16 different countries with respect to food consumption and the nutrient intake of fat, simple sugars, and complex carbohydrates. The average fat intake was found to be associated in a significantly positive fashion with the intake of sugar. It was also observed that there was a negative association between the average concentration of cholesterol in the blood and the average intake of complex carbohydrates as represented by cereals, vegetables, and the like. It is of particular interest that the actual cholesterol values reported in these multi-country studies average less than 200 mg per 100 cc, except in two countries—Chile (231 mg/100 cc) and Venezuela (212 mg/100 cc). It is hardly anticipated that the cholesterol levels noted in these countries studied would be sufficiently high to have a significant atherogenic effect.[29]

Ahrens has reviewed the extensive literature relating sucrose, hypertension, and heart disease and in general does not support the concept of a significant role for sucrose in the etiology of atherosclerosis.[30] Other studies [31] have suggested that the fructose component of sucrose may have a significant effect in the elevation of serum triglycerides, but in many instances this elevation appears to be rather transient and as indicated from many epidemiological studies, triglycerides as an isolated predictive factor, not associated with cholesterol, are of dubious value as a risk factor for the development of atherosclerotic coronary heart disease.[4, 30, 34, 35] One significant point posed by Ahrens and supported by a study of Michailov is the possibility that sucrose might increase the concentration of lipids in the blood by increasing blood pressure.[30, 32] It has been found that hypertension induced experimentally in rats produced notable changes in the fatty acid spectrum of the blood serum triglycerides, with a marked elevation in the levels of the essential fatty acids. This has been attributed to a reduced ability of the liver to form triglycerides with proportionately more serum triglycerides arising directly from the dietary fat in the intestinal wall.

Obviously, the sucrose theory in the etiology of atherogenesis remains a matter of considerable debate as well as some confusion. It might be well to recall the words of Dr. William Stark, who in 1769 wrote "does not an excess in sweets give a greater shock to the system then an excess in fat? Is there any article of food so hurtful as either when taken immoderately?" [33] Evidently, history does have a way of repeating itself.

There must be great nutritional concern, however, regarding the fact that the per capita consumption of sucrose, at least in the United States, appears to be in excess of 110 pounds per year, which calculates to provide approximately 20 to 24 percent of the average daily caloric intake. Adding to this, the "adult" caloric intake from alcoholic beverages of about 10 percent of total calories, it is readily understandable that the nutritional quality of the diet becomes diluted with non-nutrient containing calories that must contribute very significantly to the huge incidence of obesity so common in our modern technically developed society.

The Role of Genetics in Developing Atherosclerosis

Of great significance has been the development of a much better understanding of genetic factors that enhance hyperlipidemias and particularly hypercholesterolemia with associated increases of low density lipoproteins (LDL) and very low density lipoproteins (VLDL) (pre-β-lipoproteins.[36-38] The frequency of familial hypercholesterolemia in the general population has been estimated to range between 0.2 and 0.5 percent. It is important to emphasize, however, that most individuals with hypercholesterolemia, i.e., whose serum cholesterol levels fall in the upper 5 percent of the urban United States population, do not have this condition. With a frequency of familial hypercholesterolemia at a level of 0.2 percent, only 1 of 25 persons with a cholesterol value in the upper 5 percent of the population would have this disorder. This is most important to identify since, obviously, dietary factors that contribute to elevations of cholesterol and triglycerides become further magnified in the genetically influenced person. When serum cholesterol exceeds 350 mg per 100 cc, a genetic contribution should be suspected. The early development of xanthomas, xanthelasmas, arcus corneai, and possible hepatomegaly should further lead to the suspicion of familial hypercholesterolemia.

When such a situation is noted, it is most important to evaluate all family members to identify the extent of this problem. This genetic condition is inherited as an autosomal dominant disorder. Patients are heterozygote, and on the average 50 percent of the children of an affected parent carry the gene. This makes it particularly important to identify this problem as early in life as possible, and it can be done at birth by the analysis of umbilical cord blood and of course in later childhood as well. In this circumstance, a determination of cholesterol in low-density lipoprotein (LDL) may be a better identification marker than plasma cholesterol determination alone. Certainly, this disease is a predictor of early coronary atherosclerosis and mortality.

Homozygotes for familial hypercholesterolemia are found with the frequency expected from matings between two affected parents, i.e., about one case per million population. In those individuals who have extreme hypercholesterolemia, i.e., over an excess of 600 mg per 100 cc, all of the complications previously noted, as well as very early development of atherosclerotic coronary heart disease and death, are anticipated. The obvious treatment of such individuals is extreme reduction of dietary cholesterol and saturated fat intake; cholestyramine resin may also help reduce cholesterol levels.[37]

Familial hypertriglyceridemia is characterized by elevations of triglycerides alone and may rarely be associated with chylomicronemia. This problem appears to be transmitted as an autosomal dominant trait, but only 10 to 20 percent of children and adolescents express the trait with hypertriglyceridemia. Homozygotes in this circumstance have not been identified. Diabetes, insulin resistance, obesity, and hyperinsulinemia have been more frequently reported associated with this problem. Genetic studies have indicated that familial hypertriglyceridemia is inherited independently from diabetes. The basic defect at a biochemical level of familial hypertriglyceridemia remains unclear.[36]

Familial combined hyperlipidemia is evident by the occurrence of hypercholesterolemia and hypertriglyceridemia or one or the other alone in approximately one-third each of affected patients in the family. In this instance, premature coronary atherosclerosis has been documented with hypertriglyceridemia alone, with hypercholesterolemia alone, or with elevation of both lipids. It has been suggested that a single autosomal dominant gene affecting triglyceride metabolism is responsible for this problem.[36] The genetic unravelling of this problem is still a subject of study and not fully elucidated. Treatment predominately with dietary measures aimed at lowering both cholesterol and triglyceride levels, if present, is the treatment of choice.

Lipoprotein lipase deficiency is identified in Type I lipoproteinemias and is a very rare defect transmitted genetically, as in autosomal recessive, and affected patients are homozygotes for the enzyme deficiency. Severe hypertriglyceridemia with excessive chylomicronemia, usually appearing in very early childhood, is often associated with multiple episodes of abdominal pain, and eruptive xan-

thomatosis is typical. It has been postulated that some patients with hypertriglyceridemia alone are heterozygotes for this chain.

Type III hyperlipidemia or "broad-β disease" is a very rare condition associated with premature atherosclerosis and frequent peripheral vascular disease,
and is associated with a unique "floating pre-β-lipoprotein." It is identified by an
abnormal β-band on a electrophoresis of isolated VLDL, and with a VLDL
cholesterol to plasma triglycerides of greater than 0.3. Inheritance appears to
be autosomal dominant. It is a very rare problem and is best treated by a dietary
and/or drug treatment.[38]

The diagnosis of genetic lipoproteinemias utilizes the phenotyping system
which may utilize lipoprotein electrophoresis or ultracentrifugation techniques.[38]
Certainly, variations of these problems are noted, such as Type IIa and Type
IIb hyperlipoproteinemia. Naturally, cholesterol and triglyceride determinations
are essential components of the diagnostic procedure.[38]

Retrospectively, a high frequency of coronary heart disease has probably
always existed in the monogenic hyperlipidemias. The low incidence of genetically influenced hyperlipidemias, however, cannot be blamed for the tremendous excess of atherosclerosis that exists in our broadly atherogenic population; certainly our traditional diet enhances the risk of the genetically influenced
hyperlipidemias.

PEDIATRICS AND ATHEROSCLEROSIS

Certainly, the observations outlined above regarding the genetic influences
in the development of hyperlipidemias have increased the focus of looking for
hyperlipidemias in the pediatric age group.[39-41] In fact, atherosclerosis must
be viewed as a pediatric problem, and if the appropriate approach of primary
prevention is to be developed, a much broader emphasis must be given to
identifying elevated blood lipids, particularly cholesterol in the pediatric age
group. This, in fact, should become a basic component of a pediatric evaluation,
and of course, specifically so in families with a strong history of premature
atherosclerotic coronary heart disease and/or stroke.

Screening for risks of cardiovascular disease in children has indicated a
significant percentage of youngsters whose levels of serum cholesterol are too
high.[39] One report on Viennese school children between 11 and 12 years of
age indicated that 38 percent had an increased concentration of cholesterol in
their serum and 3 percent had an increased serum triglyceride concentration.[42]
No one, however, is quite set on what should be the normal or the desired level
of serum cholesterol, although it has been recommended that the serum cholesterol value in children not exceed 160 mg per 100 cc.[43]

As numerous studies are developed in the pediatric age group, it is increasingly evident that a significant percentage of this group have levels of serum
cholesterol that may predict premature development of atherosclerosis, and quite
possibly early atherosclerotic coronary heart disease. In our experience with
Iowa teenagers in a nutrition survey study, 15 percent of those evaluated had
serum cholesterols in excess of 220 mg per 100 cc, and half of these were well
above 250 mg per 100 cc; quite likely some were genetically influenced hypercholesterolemias, although these concepts were not adequately understood at the
time this study was done.

A basic question has arisen as to what should be done regarding general dietary changes for the pediatric age group. No one questions the desirability of appropriate identification and treatment of genetic hyperlipidemias in children, or in fact, acquired hyperlipidemias if they are noted. Fundamental argument comes as to whether or not there should be a widely applied recommendation of significant dietary modification applied at the early pediatric age. There are very strong proponents for a much more broadly based dietary modification for children, with the assurance given that marked modifications in dietary fat and sweets in the diet can be made without impairment of their normal physical and mental development. The other side of the argument asks why involve everyone in the pediatric age group, particularly when the total diet of our affluent population is so difficult to change, modify, and to accept, and since convincing evidence that these changes (mostly very modest) really alter the excessive impact of early atherosclerotic disease is lacking.

Genetically influenced hyperlipidemias in children have been treated with modest success, although evidently very disappointing from the long-term point of view.[40] One might ask if it is reasonable to expect a child to go on a rigid dietary modification when parents have traditionally failed to change life styles and dietary patterns. "Like father—like son" becomes all too evident in the real dynamics of everyday living.

Certainly, prospectively from a preventive medicine point of view, the potential for change in reducing the epidemic of atherosclerotic disease seems most promising if we can start early in life, at the pediatric age level.

BIOCHEMICAL ENRICHMENT OF NUTRITIONAL EPIDEMIOLOGY

The study of the biochemical aspects of the metabolism of cholesterol and other lipids, and particularly the very sophisticated investigations involving lipoproteins that carry blood lipids, has tremendously enriched our knowledge of the mechanisms involving lipid transport particularly, and potentially our knowledge of the developing atherosclerotic process. This basic biochemical approach, done both at the basic science and clinical levels, promises to give new and direct insight into the very complicated process of atherosclerosis and also provide a more accurate understanding of the effects of dietary modification and various drug therapies involved in altering serum lipid levels (FIGURE 7).

Very significantly, new insights have been provided regarding the receptor-mediated control of cholesterol metabolism. A mechanism has been detailed and supported with elegant experimental studies using mammalian cells, such as cultured human fibroblasts, to identify a receptor mechanism for low-density lipoprotein (LDL).[43a] The LDL receptor mechanism binds the major cholesterol-carrying lipoproteins of plasma and hence regulates the rate at which this lipoprotein specifically transfers its cholesterol into the cell. Furthermore, the LDL receptor itself is under feedback regulation in the cell so that its activity and, therefore, the amount of cholesterol that may enter the cell are inversely proportional to the cellular content of cholesterol.

Very importantly, the establishment of the LDL receptor model and an understanding of its complex actions have also provided a firmer appreciation of the mechanism of familial hypercholesterolemia. It has been noted that a defective cell surface, LDL, binding is the principal deficiency in the homozygous familial hypercholesterolemic circumstance. Furthermore, a study of fibroblasts from heterozygotes with familial hypercholesterolemia shows approximately one-half the normal number of LDL receptors. These most important discoveries involving mutations in a single gene involving the LDL receptor mechanism can result therefore in a series of biochemical lipid transport abnormalities that are seen and measured as varying degrees of serum cholesterol in these familial hypercholesterolemias. Other genetic diseases involving cholesterol have also been identified in the intracellular processing of cholesterol and cholesterol esters involving a deficiency in lysosomal acid lipase

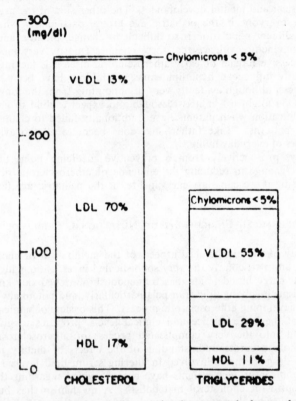

FIGURE 7. Contribution of each lipoprotein class to total plasma cholesterol and triglycerides in the normal subject. Most of the plasma cholesterol is present in LDL, and most of the triglycerides are in VLDL in the fasting state.

activity. Such a defect permits intact LDL-derived cholesterol esters to accumulate in the cell proximal to the metabolic block within the lysosome itself.

The evolution of this information, regarding the LDL receptor mechanism, gives credence to the concept that plasma lipoproteins function not only to solubilize lipids but also may contain within their protein structure specific information that dictates the body sites to which each lipid is to be delivered.

Also of considerable interest is the developing concept that serum high density lipoprotein may be an important factor in reducing the risk of atherosclerotic coronary heart disease. It has been demonstrated that serum high density lipoprotein concentration is significantly lower in men with coronary heart disease than in control subjects.[44] Such information suggests that high levels of high density lipoprotein, although carrying cholesterol, may protect to some degree against the development of atherosclerotic heart disease. This obviously is a major subject for current biochemical investigation.

INTERRELATIONSHIPS BETWEEN PHYSICAL ACTIVITY, DIETARY INTAKES, AND SERUM LIPIDS

In view of the fact that obesity and excessive weight may variously contribute, or at least be associated with hyperlipidemias, and that exercise is an effective mechanism for lowering the serum cholesterol particularly, it is proposed that too little attention has been given to the potential value of exercise in minimizing the development of atherosclerotic heart disease.[45] Population groups that do exercise significantly, and whose traditional diets are very rich in saturated fat and cholesterol, have been shown to have low serum cholesterol levels and also a low incidence of atherosclerotic heart disease.[46] Exercise is not costly, can and should be fun, and is both mentally and physically stimulating; most importantly, it may be a significant protective factor against atherosclerotic heart disease and the lowering of serum lipids. Appropriate training programs have been developed to provide graduated exercises, taking into consideration the cardiovascular status of the individual,[47, 48] and unquestionably such programs should be pursued and studied under controlled surveillance to demonstrate that exercise might have important value in reducing the epidemic of heart attack currently present in the United States.

A specific study on the interrelationship between serum lipids, dietary intakes, and physical exercise in medical students has been reported,[49] and most significantly, there was noted a marked decrease in triglyceride rich pre-β-lipoproteins, a significant decrease in the cholesterol-rich β-lipoproteins, and perhaps, most importantly, a marked increase in cholesterol rich α-lipoproteins (HDL), which may have protective implications against atherosclerotic development. This biochemical approach to the evaluation of a physiological activity is most important since a measurement of total cholesterol alone exhibited either little change or only a slight decrease, but significantly a shift was noted in the cholesterol carrying character of the lipoproteins.

DIET AND HYPERTENSION, THE SODIUM CONNECTION

With hypertension affecting approximately 24 million people in the United States, it is the most common of the chronic diseases and one of the three major risk factors contributing to the excessive and premature mortality of atherosclerotic heart disease and stroke.

Kempner clearly demonstrated the effectiveness of diet in relation to hypertension. In 1939 he originated a rice, fruit, sugar diet regimen for the treatment of chronic glomerulonephritis with uremia and hypertension.[50-54] This basic "rice diet" was most simplistic, containing nothing but rice, sugar, fruit, and fruit juices providing 2400 calories, less than 150 mg of sodium, less than 200 mg of chloride, less than 5 g of fat, no cholesterol, and about 25 g of protein derived from rice and fruit. The diet was supplemented with appropriate vitamins, and while it has been criticized regarding its borderline protein quantity and quality, no dietary regimen has been more effective, not only in the treatment of severe hypertension, but obesity, and a variety of cardiovascular difficulties including the complications of advanced diabetic retinopathy,[55] and very likely was most protective prospectively in the management of atherosclerotic disease. There is no doubt that this is a most difficult diet regimen both to administer and to tolerate. It requires extreme diet discipline, and in the Kempner regimen is coupled with an emphasis on progressively accelerated levels of exercise. There is perhaps no practically applied clinical dietary regimen that has been more effective in the reduction of both blood pressure and serum cholesterol and in the general management of cardiovascular diseases. If the caloric intake from this diet is not excessive, and it generally is not, there is no significant accumulation of triglycerides, at least over extended periods of time. The major problem for such a rigid dietary regimen is of course continued compliance—this is most difficult. Concerning its effectiveness, there is absolutely no doubt.

One of the major concerns in our current society is the evident excessive use of salt, possibly related to a marked increase in the use of processed foods, food technology, and the availability and sale of a whole host of so-called ready-to-serve meals.

Dahl has reviewed the extensive literature that has accumulated regarding the possible role of salt intake in the development of essential hypertension.[8] From these observations, it is quite clear that the average salt intake is grossly greater than the salt need, considering the tremendous renal capability of conserving sodium. Many studies have been done with animals clearly implicating salt and sodium specifically as an etiological factor in the development of hypertension and excessive early mortality.[8] Epidemiological studies in population groups also strongly suggest an etiological role for sodium in the development of essential hypertension.[8] In our experience, it is rare indeed to find an individual in whom hypertension is identified who does not add salt excessively to the food at the table or during cooking. These practices can be clearly demonstrated by measuring sodium excretion in the urine—perhaps the most accurate way of determining excessive salt usage.

From the prospective preventive medicine point of view great concern has evolved relative to infant feeding practices in which salt has been used in a great variety of foods fed to babies.[56] This practice has come under surveillance, and in general the salt intake of baby foods has been reduced. This would seem to be a worthwhile objective.

MACRO AND TRACE METALS IN THE DEVELOPMENT OF ATHEROSCLEROSIS

The role of trace elements in relation to cardiovascular diseases has been a subject of a World Health Organization publication,[15] and Sellig has reviewed the role of magnesium and the effects of magnesium deficiency on the arteries and on the retention of sodium, potassium, and calcium.[16] It may be premature to attribute a major contribution of macro and trace minerals in the development of atherosclerosis, but experimental models have been developed that show that magnesium deficiency produces changes in the arterial vasculature that resembles the earliest signs of human atherosclerosis.[57, 58] With magnesium deficiency there appears to be an excessive retention of calcium and sodium that relates to the intensification of the lesions. The cardiovascular lesions of experimental magnesium deficiency are similar to those seen in comparable circumstances in infants and children in which they usually entail fibroblastic intimal proliferation and degeneration of the internal elastica and focal degeneration of the tunica media generally in the small coronary arteries.[16] Plaque formation, of course, is not usually seen until later on in the disease and may reflect a superimposition of lipids or other dietary factors.

Of great interest has been the observation in epidemiological surveys that there is an inverse association between indices of water hardness and cardio-

TABLE 2

SUMMARY OF CURRENT CONCEPTS RELATING MINERAL DEFICIENCES
TO ATHEROSCLEROTIC HEART DISEASE

Metal Deficiency	Measured Biologic Effect
Calcium	Decreased excretion of fatty acid, if fat intake is largely saturated fat. Increased serum lipid. Depletion of cardiac calcium promotes infarction. Myocardium is more excitable. Endothelium and platelets are more adhesive.
Cadmium	May be a positive factor in development of hypertension.
Chromium	Glucose tolerance is impaired.
Lithium	A possible negative lithium-AHD correlation may be significant protective factors in hard water.
Magnesium	Depletion of cardiac magnesium promotes myocardial infarction. Failure of protection against cardiotoxins. Clotting time tends to be decreased. Endothelium and platelets are more adhesive.
Vanadium	Hepatic synthesis of cholesterol is not controlled. The oxydation of brain monoamines and their precursors is not catalyzed. Fatty acid is not desaturated.
Zinc	Atherosclerosis is promoted. Cadmium-induced hypertension is not prevented.

vascular death rates; the softer the drinking water the higher the death rate.[59-62] This association has been found in Japan, in the United States, in the United Kingdom, in Sweden, Ireland, and in other countries. The similarity of findings in the largest studies were those done in the United States and the United Kingdom. It is not clear at this time what the significant factor is in hard water that functions in a protective manner, although lithium has been suggested as a possibility.[15] This remains unproven. Of interest, also in view of the importance of hypertension as a risk factor, is the observation that cadmium may be a positive factor in producing hypertension in experimental animals.[57] TABLE 2 lists metallic factors that have been implicated, predominately in experimental animals, in the evolution of atherosclerosis. There is as yet insufficient evidence to indicate that these factors have an importance in man, although it is quite evident that magnesium deficiency is far more common in human beings than has been previously suspected and that, in fact, magnesium deficiency should be looked at under appropriately controlled studies to determine its role in the development of atherosclerotic disease.[16]

COFFEE DRINKING AND DEATH DUE TO CORONARY HEART DISEASE

This is a classical representation of the difficulties of evaluating prospective and retrospective studies in the estimation of the contribution of a given factor in the etiology of a disease. Conflicting results have been reported about a potential role of coffee in the etiology of coronary atherosclerotic disease. Two prospective studies have shown no association between coffee drinking and coronary heart disease,[63, 64] while a control study of survivors of myocardial infarction showed positive associations.[65] Recent studies limited to low-risk and middle-risk patients suggest that the risk, if any, of death from coronary artery disease associated with coffee drinking is small indeed.[17] Whether or not putting large amounts of sugar and/or cream in coffee and the associated practice of cigarette smoking with coffee drinking contributes to the "coffee question" is difficult to unravel.

SOME PRACTICAL DIETARY CONSIDERATION, OR WHAT DO WE ADVISE

It is most interesting that there has been a distinct reduction in cardiovascular disease mortality starting in 1963 and especially since 1968. Between 1970 and 1975 this decrease was approximately 13 percent, which appears most significant, although it is still not established whether this is only a trend and may reverse itself [66] (TABLE 3).

A contributing and probably favorable factor has been the increased emphasis on the early identification and more aggressive treatment of hypertension: Is this related to the decrease in mortality from stroke? It is difficult to say, but it would appear that progress is being made. A practical example of this progress is the fact that one major insurance company has adjusted its dividend payouts because the insurer figures that heart disease, the nation's number one killer, has started to decline. This of course is a most positive and practical recognition of the favorable downward trend currently being experienced.

What is the optimum level of serum cholesterol is a question often asked and often poorly answered.[43] The traditional pathology laboratory reports list a normal range, usually of 150–300 mg per 100 cc. From all of the epidemiological evidence, a more desirable and certainly achievable level for the retardation of atherosclerosis is probably 200 mg per 100 cc or less. In populations with significantly low levels of atherosclerotic coronary heart disease, serum cholesterols range between 150 and 175 mg per 100 cc. A *practical* upper limit for a patient goal is certainly not above 220 mg per 100 cc—better if less than 200 mg per 100 cc. This is achievable through appropriate diet manipulation and especially with the help of nutrition counselling. One harkens back to the positive benefits of the rice, fruit diet but questions whether or not this has a practical utility except in individuals who have obvious disease and are strongly motivated, even though compliance is difficult. A more recent and severely rigid diet proposal has been the Pritikin diet, which is utilized by the Longevity Research Institute in Santa Barbara, Calif., and also by researchers at the University of Southern California, in their investigative program under the supervision of Blankenhorn. Here again, such a rigid dietary approach will not have broad practical appeal or application except under circumstances in which there exists evidence of severe cardiovascular atherosclerosis that is clinically manifested.

Overall, the nutritional quality and quantity of our diet appears to be one of the most critical continuing environmental factors that influences our health. Disregard of this obvious fact, along with a neglect of other major risk factors, will certainly lead to a continuous epidemic of atherosclerotic heart disease and stroke.

TABLE 3

AGE-ADJUSTED DEATH RATE FROM ISCHEMIC HEART DISEASE PER 100,000 POPULATION IN THE UNITED STATES *

| Year | \multicolumn{6}{c}{Age, years} | | | | | |
	35–44	45–54	55–64	65–74	75–84	>85
1958	58.0	232.7	658.4	1,628.8	3,364.8	7,069.3
1959	57.6	233.7	655.3	1,642.6	3,359.2	7,321.0
1960	57.7	238.0	665.5	1,553.7	3,434.8	7,296.5
1961	57.9	235.2	649.4	1,541.4	3,360.6	7,383.3
1962	58.7	238.4	660.4	1,586.7	3,449.2	7,922.2
1963	61.0	240.3	668.4	1,619.1	3,495.6	8,165.6
1964	61.0	235.8	660.3	1,586.7	3,388.6	7,885.7
1965	60.0	236.6	657.4	1,584.0	3,422.0	8,088.2
1966	59.6	236.4	661.4	1,609.9	3,413.6	8,037.7
1967	60.1	231.4	645.0	1,568.8	3,334.2	7,941.8
1968	56.9	216.8	624.1	1,552.2	3,441.7	8,496.7
1969	55.4	210.3	598.4	1,500.3	3,367.6	8,400.2

* From *Vital Statistics of United States*. Rates for 1958 to 1967 multiplied by 1,1457 to make comparable to 1968–1969 rates. (From Walker.[66] By permission of *Journal of The American Medical Association*.)

$$\text{Age-specific death rate} = \frac{\text{No. of deaths in given age group in area in year}}{\text{No. of people in same age group in area in year}} \times 1000.$$

SUMMARY

A basic review of the extensive literature focusing on the major risk factors of atherosclerotic coronary heart disease and stroke, i.e., elevation of blood lipids related to diet, blood pressure elevation, and genetic factors using the traditional epidemiological model of interaction between host, agent, and environment, has strongly supported the concept that diet and particularly saturated fat and/or cholesterol are significant contributors to the elevation of blood lipids, especially cholesterol, and contribute importantly to the premature development and mortality of atherosclerotic coronary heart disease. Certainly genetics exert an important impact on this process. To date it remains unclear whether or not major changes in the dietary pattern of huge population groups can be practically effected. The minor dietary modifications so far studied in the average atherosclerosis-prone population cannot be anticipated to make a major dent in the epidemic proportions of atherosclerotic coronary heart disease.

It is quite clear that prospective preventive medicine must be implemented at a very early age in the pediatric age group, in which atherosclerosis is now recognized by many as the number one pediatric problem.

Tremendous biochemical advances have provided new insights in knowledge regarding the transport of blood lipids, particularly cholesterol, and the regulatory mechanisms at the cellular level for cholesterol under normal circumstances and in the genetic influenced hyperlipidemias (TABLE 4). A bright future lies ahead for the reduction of the epidemic of atherosclerosis which could be greatly enhanced by a greater personal responsibility for health care and a much more careful and prudent diet selection and exercise management.

TABLE 4

CHARACTERISTICS OF HYPERLIPIDEMIAS

C—Cholesterol (*free* and *esterified*)
TG—Triglyceride (esters of *glycerol* and *fatty acids*)
Hyperlipidemia (excess C or TG or both)
Chylomicrons—Particles of newly absorbed fat
FFA—Free fatty acids
HDL—High-density lipoproteins (γ-lipoprotein)
LDL—Low-density lipoproteins (β-lipoprotein)
VLDL—Very low density lipoprotein (pre-β-lipoprotein)

REFERENCES

1. AMERICAN HEART ASSOCIATION. 1976. Heart Facts. Dallas, Texas.
2. HAIMOVICI, H., Ed. 1968. Atherosclerosis: Recent Advances. Ann. N.Y. Acad. Sci. 149: 585–1068.
3. BORTZ, W. M. 1974. The pathogenesis of hypercholesterolemia. Ann. Int. Med. 80: 738–745.
4. BLACKBURN, H. 1974. Progress in the epidemiology and prevention of coronary heart disease. *In* Progress in Cardiology. P. N. Yu & J. F. Goodwin, Eds. 3: 1–36. Lea and Febiger. Philadelphia, Pa.
5. STAMLER, J., J. A. SCHOENBERGER, H. A. LINDBERG, R. SHEKELLE, J. M. STOKER, M. B. EPSTEIN, L. DEBOER, R. STAMLER, R. RESTIVO, D. GRAY & W. CAIN. 1969. Detection of susceptibility to coronary disease. Bull. N.Y. Acad. Med. 45(12): 1306–1325.
6. KANNEL, W. B. & T. GORDON, Eds. 1969. The Framingham study: an epidemiological investigation of cardiovascular disease. Section 24. Diet and the regulation of serum cholesterol. Natl. Inst. Health. Bethesda, Md.
7. DOYLE, J. T. 1966. Etiology of coronary disease: Risk factors influencing coronary disease. *In* Modern Concepts of Cardiovascular Disease. E. S. Orgain, Ed. XXXV(4): 81–86. Am. Heart Assoc., Inc. N.Y., N.Y.
8. DAHL, L. K. 1960. Effects of chronic excess salt feeding, elevation of plasma cholesterol in rats and dogs. J. Exp. Med. 112(4): 635–651.
9. JAMA. 1972. Diet and Coronary Heart Disease. A Council Statement. Joint statement of the AMA Council on Foods and Nutrition and the Food and Nutrition Board of the National Academy of Sciences. JAMA 222: 1647.

10. KEYS, A. 1970. Coronary heart disease in seven countries. Circulation **41** (Supp. 1): 1–211.
11. KEYS, A., N. KIMURA & A. KUSAKAWA. 1958. Lessons from serum cholesterol studies in Japan, Hawaii and Los Angeles. Ann. Int. Med. **48:** 83–94.
12. YERUSHALMY, J. & H. E. HILLEBOE. 1957. Fat in the diet and mortality from heart disease. A methodologic note. N.Y.S. J. Med. **57:** 2343–2354.
13. FIDANZA, F. 1972. Epidemiological evidence for the fat theory. Proc. Nutr. Soc. **31:** 317–321.
14. STONE, M. C. 1972. The role of diet in the management of hyperlipoprotein-aemias. Proc. Nutr. Soc. **31:** 311–316.
15. MASIRONI, R., Ed. 1974. Trace Elements in Relation to Cardiovascular Disease. WHO Offset Pub. **5:** 1–42. Geneva.
16. SELLIG, M. S. & H. A. HEGGTVEIT. 1974. Magnesium interrelationships in ischemic heart disease: A review. Am. J. Clin. Nutr. **27:** 59–79.
17. HENNEKENS, C. H., M. E. DROLETTE, M. J. JESSE, J. E. DAVIES & G. B. HUTCHISON. 1976. Coffee drinking and death due to coronary heart disease. N. Engl. J. Med. **294**(12): 633–636.
18. ANDERSON, T W. 1973. The changing pattern of ischemic heart disease. C.M.A. J. **108:** 1500–1504.
19. ANDERSON, T. W. 1973. Mortality from ischemic heart disease. JAMA **224:** 336–338.
20. KANNEL, W. B. 1971. Lipid profile and the potential coronary victim. Am. J. Clin. Nutr. **24:** 1074–1081.
21. NICHOLS, A. B., C. RAVENSCROFT, D. E. LAMPHIEAR & L. D. OSTRANDER, JR. 1976. Independence of serum lipid levels and dietary habits. JAMA **236**(17): 1948–1953.
22. FRIEND, B. 1967. Nutrients in United States food supply. A review of trends. Am. J. Clin. Nutr. **20:** 907–914.
23. CARLSON, L. A. & L. E. BOTTIGER. 1972. Ichemic heart disease in relation to fasting values of plasma triglycerides and cholesterol: Stockholm prospective study. Lancet (April) : 865–868.
24. ANDERSON, J. T., F. GRANDE & A. KEYS. 1973. Cholesterol-lowering diets. J. Am. Dietet. Assoc. **62:** 133–142.
25. SHAPER, A. G. 1972. Diet in the epidemiology of coronary heart disease. Proc. Nutr. Soc. **31:** 297–302.
26. VEGROESEN, A. J. 1972. Dietary fat and cardiovascular disease: possible modes of action of linoleic acid. Proc. Nutr. Soc. **31:** 323–329.
27. YUDKIN, J. 1972. Sucrose and cardiovascular disease. Proc. Nutr. Soc. **31:** 331–337.
28. PLATT, L., K. P. BALL, W. W. BRIGDEN, R. DOLL, M. F. OLIVER, D. D. REID, J. P. SHILLINGFORD, A. M. THOMSON & T. B. BEGG. 1970. Dietary sugar intake in men with myocardial infarction. Lancet **7686:** 1265–1271.
29. LOPEZ, A., R. E. HODGES & W. A. KREHL. 1966. Some interesting relationships between dietary carbohydrates and serum cholesterol. Am. J. Clin. Nutr. **18:** 149–153.
30. AHRENS, R. A. 1974. Sucrose, hypertension and heart disease: a historical perspective. Am. J. Clin. Nutr. **27:** 403–422.
31. MACDONALD, I. & C. M. BRAITHWAITE. 1964. The influence of dietary carbohydrates on the lipid pattern in serum and in adipose tissue. Clin. Sci. **27:** 23.
32. MICHAILOV, M. L. 1972. Alteratien des Spectrums der veresterten fettsauren (triglyzeride) im blutplasma bei experimenteller hypertonie an der ratte. Acta Med. Jugoslav. **26:** 169.
33. SMITH, J. C. 1788. The works of the late William Stark, M.D. Revised and published from his original manuscripts, printed for J. Johnson, St. Paul's Church-Yard, London.
34. GRANDE, F., J. T. ANDERSON & A. KEYS. 1974. Sucrose and various carbo-

hydrate-containing foods and serum lipids in men. Am. J. Clin. Nutr. **27:** 1043–1051.

35. KEEN, H. 1972. Glucose tolerance, plasma lipids and atherosclerosis. Proc. Nutr. Soc. **31:** 339–345.

36. MOTULSKY, A. O. 1976. Current concepts in genetics: the genetic hyperlipidemias. New Engl. J. Med. **294:** 823–826.

37. LEVY, R. I., D. S. FREDRICKSON, R. SHULMAN, D. W. BILHEIMER, J. L. BRESLOW, N. J. STONE, S. E. LUX, H. R. SLOAN, R. M. KRAUSS & P. N. HERBERT. 1972. Dietary and drug treatment of primary hyperlipoproteinemia. Ann. Int. Med. **77:** 267–294.

38. FREDRICKSON, D. S. 1972. A physician's guide to hyperlipidemia. *In* Modern Concepts of Cardiovascular Disease. R. C. Schlant, Ed. Am. Heart Assoc., Inc. N.Y., N.Y.

39. FRIEDMAN, G. & S. J. GOLDBERT. 1973. Normal serum cholesterol values. Percentile ranking in a middle-class pediatric population. JAMA **225**(6): 610–612.

40. WEST, R. J. & J. K. LLOYD. 1976. Coronary heart disease. The paediatrician's approach to prevention. R.S.H. **5:** 201–204.

41. WILLIAMS, C. L. & E. L. WYNDER. 1976. A blind spot in preventive medicine. JAMA **236**(19): 2196–2197.

42. MARKTL, W. & B. RUDAS. 1976. Screening for risks of cardiovascular disease in children. A preliminary report. Brit. J. Nutr. **35:** 223–227.

43. WRIGHT, I. S. 1976. Correct levels of serum cholesterol, average vs. normal vs. optimal. JAMA **236**(3): 261–262.

43a. BROWN, M. S. & J. L. GOLDSTEIN. 1976. Receptor-mediated control of cholesterol metabolims. Science **191:** 150–154.

44. BERG, K., A. BORRESEN & G. DAHLEN. 1976. Serum-high-density-lipoprotein and atherosclerotic heart disease. Lancet **7958:** 499–501.

45. MANN, G. V., H. L. GARRETT & A. LONG. 1971. The amount of exercise necessary to achieve and maintain fitness in adult persons. Southern Med. J. **64:** 549.

46. MANN, G. V., A. SPOERRY, M. GRAY & D. JARASHOW. 1972. Atherosclerosis in the Masai. Am. J. Epidem. **95:** 26.

47. MANN, G. V., H. L. GARRETT, A. FARHI, H. MURRAY & F. T. BILLINGS. 1969. Exercise to prevent coronary heart disease: an experimental study of the effects of training on risk factors for coronary disease in men. Am. J. Med. **46**(1): 12.

48. MANN, G. V., R. D. SHAFFER, R. S. ANDERSON & H. H. SANDSTEAD. 1964. Cardiovascular disease in the Masai. J. Atherosclerosis Res. **4:** 289.

49. BALART, L., M. C. MOORE, L. GREMILLION & A. LOPEZ. 1974. Serum lipids, dietary intakes, and physical exercise in medical students. J. Am. Diet. Assoc. **64:** 42–46.

50. KEMPNER, W. 1944. Treatment of kidney disease and hypertensive vascular disease with rice diet. II. N.C. Med. J. **5:** 273–274.

51. KEMPNER, W. 1944. Treatment of kidney disease and hypertensive vascular disease with rice diet. I. N.C. Med. J. **5:** 125–133.

52. KEMPNER, W. 1945. Compensation of renal metabolc dysfunction. Treatment of kidney disease and hypertensive vascular disease with rice diet. III. N.C. Med. J. **6:** 61–87, 117–161.

53. KEMPNER, W. 1946. Some effects of the rice diet treatment of kidney disease and hypertension. Bull. N.Y. Acad. Med. **22:** 358–370.

54. KEMPNER, W. 1948. Treatment of hypertensive vascular disease with rice diet. Am. J. Med. **4:** 545–577.

55. KEMPNER, W., R. L. PESCHEL & C. SCHLAYER. 1958. Effect of rice diet on diabetes mellitus associated with vascular disease. Postgrad. Med. **24:** 359–371.

56. GUTHRIE, H. A. 1968. Infant feeding practices—a predisposing factor in hypertension. Am. J. Clin. Nutr. **21**(8): 863–867.

57. SCHROEDER, H. A., A. P. NASON & I. H. TIPTON. 1969. Essential metals in man: Magnesium. J. Chron. Dis. **21:** 815–841.
58. HELLERSTEIN, E. E., M. NAKAMURA, D. M. HEGSTED & J. J. VITALE. 1960. Studies on the interrelationships between dietary magnesium, quality and quantity of fat, hypercholesterolemia, and lipidosis. J. Nutr. **71:** 339–346.
59. CRAWFORD, M. D. 1972. Hardness of drinking water and cardiovascular disease. Proc. Nutr. Soc. **31:** 347–353.
60. ANDERSON, T. W., L. C. NERI, G. B. SCHREIBER, F. D. E. TALBOT & A. ZDRO-JEWSKI. 1975. Ischemic heart disease, water hardness and myocardial magnesium. Can. M. A. J. **113:** 199–203.
61. CRAWFORD, M. D., M. J. GARDNER & P. A. SEDGWICK. 1972. Infant mortality and hardness of local water supplies. Lancet **1:** 988–992.
62. HANKIN, J. H., S. MARGEN & H. F. GOLDSMITH. 1970. Contribution of hard water to calcium and magnesium intakes of adults. J. Am. Dietet. Assoc. **56:** 212–224.
63. DAWBER, T. R., W. B. KANNEL & T. GORDON. 1975. Coffee and cardiovascular disease: observations from the Framingham study. N. Engl. J. Med. **291:** 871–874.
64. KLATSKY, A. L., G. D. FRIEDMAN & A. B. SIEGELAUB. 1973. Coffee drinking prior to acute myocardial infarction: results from the Kaiser-Permanente epidemiological study of myocardial infarction. JAMA **226:** 540–543.
65. BCDP. 1972. Coffee drinking and acute myocardial infarction: report from the Boston Collaborative Drug Surveillance Program. Lancet **2:** 1278–1281.
66. WALKER, W. J. 1974. Coronary mortality: what is going on? A special communication. JAMA **227:** 1045–1046.
67. CRAWFORD, T. & M. D. CRAWFORD. 1967. Prevalence and pathological changes of ischaemic heart disease in a hard water and in a soft water area. Lancet **1:** 229–232.
68. GORDON, T. & W. B. KANNEL. 1973. Coronary Risk Handbook. Estimating Risk of Coronary Heart Disease in Daily Practice. *From* Coronary Heart Disease, Atherothrombotic Brain Infarction, Intermittent Claudication—A Multivariate Analysis of Some Factors Related to Their Incidence: Framingham Study, 16-year followup. American Heart Association. N.Y., N.Y. 1–35.

NUTRITIONAL CARCINOGENESIS

Ernst L. Wynder

American Health Foundation
New York, New York 10019

INTRODUCTION

It seems fitting at this Bicentennial event to address ourselves to one of the Nation's primary concerns—health. As has been stated so often, no individual and no society can accomplish its best in the absence of mental and physical well-being.

During the past two centuries many diseases have been eradicated primarily by preventive measures. If some of these past diseases were to occur today they would still be incurable. Other diseases, however, have taken over: heart disease, cancer, and stroke have replaced the major illnesses of the past: small-pox, typhoid, and cholera. In this Bicentennial year, these main causes of death in both men and women—heart disease, cancer, and stroke—have been shown by extensive epidemiologic evidence not to be inevitable consequences of aging.

It is obvious that differences in life style distinguish today's society from that of our founding fathers. We need to ask whether present-day excessive behaviors related to eating, drinking, and smoking do not overburden modern man's metabolic capability. We need to inquire whether the ever-increasing intake of foods, often high in calories, by an ever-increasing sedentary population, does not represent a situation antagonistic to our bodies. From an evolutionary point of view, it is unlikely that the metabolic capacities of man developed millions of years ago were designed to withstand the present-day challenges and assaults to his respiratory and digestive tracts. Today we deal with diseases of "excess"—largely related to our life-style—diseases that are unfortunate byproducts of modern civilization.

The specific subject we were asked to review is nutritional carcinogenesis, of which excessive nutritional intake represents a vital part.

NUTRITION AND CANCER

The impact of nutrition on the pathogenesis of human cancer may be divided into three areas: (1) additives and contaminates; (2) deficiencies; and (3) excesses.

Additives and Contaminants

The first area deals with food additives and contaminants that have been suggested to relate to the occurrence of cancer in man (TABLE 1). These components include mycotoxins, insecticides, and diethylstilbestrol (DES). There is some evidence that agents such as aflatoxins increase the incidence of liver cancer in certain developing countries.[1] However, we know of no evidence that man's exposure to DDT or DES, as present in food, has led to an increased

360

risk of cancer. An increased risk could indeed not be expected on the basis of the concentrations to which man is exposed by consuming foods contaminated with DDT or containing DES.[2, 3] Time and space restrictions preclude a detailed discussion of this topic within this communication.

Epidemiology and geographic pathology have increased what we know about the relationship of environmental factors and cancer. Although the relative risk of developing a specific cancer is quite different in Japan than in the United States, both societies use similar food additives, colorants, or contaminants. This epidemiologic evidence suggests that these are not implicated in disease development. We would like to caution those who are responsible for evaluating food additives and the role of food contaminants to consider the dosage required to induce carcinogenic effects in experimental animals, to determine whether such a dose has any meaningful relationship to human exposure, and to investigate whether man's liver or other tissues are as susceptible to these agents as

TABLE 1

DIETARY FACTORS AND CANCER

1. Food Additives and/or Contaminants.
2. Specific or General Nutritional Deficiencies or Imbalances.
3. Specific or General Nutritional Excesses or Imbalances.

TABLE 2

SUGGESTED ASSOCIATIONS: NUTRITIONAL DEFICIENCIES OR IMBALANCES

Iron	(Plummer-Vinson)	Upper G.I. Tract
Iodine	(Goiter)	Thyroid
Vitamin B$_2$	(Alcoholism)	Upper G.I. Tract
Vitamin A	(Low Fat)	Cervix, Stomach
Pyridoxin		Liver

those of the rodent. The fact that knowledge has increased about contaminants is testimony to the development of refined, precise analytical technology. In considering the prohibition or relative safety of specific food additives or contaminants, we must also consider the costs and benefits of such actions. We are pleased to note that the National Cancer Institute has established a National Clearinghouse for Environmental Carcinogenesis that will deal with these and other issues in the future.

Deficiencies

The second area relates to nutritional deficiencies (TABLE 2). Epidemiologic evidence suggests that the reduction of gastric cancer, particularly in developed countries, relates to various nutritional modifications. Such dietary changes include a decreased intake of carbohydrates with a concomitant increase of fresh fruits and vegetables and, particularly, an increase of vitamin C. It

TABLE 3

EFFECT OF A MIXED WESTERN HIGH-MEAT DIET OR A NON-MEAT DIET ON FECAL
β-GLUCURONIDASE ACTIVITY IN MAN

Analysis	Activity of β-Glucuronidase	
	High Meat	Non-Meat
	Bacterial pellet	
Protein	285±25*	127±17
(per mg)		
Dry feces	20±2.5*	5.6±0.98
(per mg)		
Daily total	3440±408*	1198±229
($\times 10^{-2}$)		
	Supernatant	
Protein	84±3.8*	42±3.8
(per mg)		
Dry feces	15±1.8*	3.6±0.41
(per mg)		
Daily total	2610±295*	770±99
($\times 10^{-2}$)		

* Significantly different from non-meat group. $p < 0.01$.

has been suggested that a high vitamin C intake is likely to prevent the possible formation of nitrosamides.[4]

In epidemiologic studies, vitamin A deficiency has been linked to the development of cancer of the cervix. A partial explanation for this relationship is that high vitamin A intake strengthens the integrity of the mucous-producing epithelium which, in turn, protects the cervix.[5] Among smokers, alcohol has been established as a promoting factor for cancer of the upper alimentary tract and the larynx.[6, 7] However, present evidence suggests that there is nothing carcinogenic in alcohol *per se*. The promoting effect appears to be related either to the way alcohol acts as a solvent on tobacco carcinogens or to nutritional deficiencies commonly existing in chronic alcoholics. It may also modify enzymic capabilities so that carcinogens from tobacco are metabolized to active forms. We believe that the effect of riboflavin deficiency, not uncommon among alcoholics, may be similar to the effect that long-term chronic iron deficiency has on the development of Plummer-Vinson's disease.[8, 9] Plummer-Vinson's disease is known to increase the risk of cancer of the upper alimentary tract among women, who are more prone to this condition than men.[10, 11] The importance and usefulness of preventive medicine was demonstrated by the sharp decline in Plummer-Vinson's disease and upper alimentary tract cancers in women after World War II with the introduction of supplementary iron and vitamins in Swedish flour.[11]

So far, the epidemiological leads linking alcohol to cancer of the upper alimentary tract in man have not been properly pursued by experimentalists. In our laboratory we are currently exploring the effect of riboflavin deficiency on mitochondrial activity. McCoy has successfully isolated functional mitochondria from the squamous epithelium of the cheek pouch of hamsters.[12] Difficult as this biochemistry may be, it will give us insight into the biology and biochemistry of the squamous cell, a cell in which cancer occurs so much more commonly in man than in the liver cell. It is important that we follow the leads that nature provides for us rather than pursuing those roads that, as chemists or biologists, we find to be the easiest.

Excesses

As expected, dietary excesses play a particularly important role in developed societies. Nutritionally related cancers are much more common in developed than in developing countries and in Japan where dietary intake significantly differs from that of Western countries (FIGURE 1).

A number of cancers have been shown to be linked to overnutrition (FIGURE 2). As used in this context, overnutrition relates more to an excess of specific macronutrients, especially fat and fat-related variables, than to obesity. In fact, only two cancers, cancer of the endometrium and cancer of the kidney in women, have been linked to obesity.[13, 14] Thus, the epidemiology of excess nutrition in relation to cancer appears similar to that of the epidemiology of arteriosclerosis, in that the correlation applies more to the type of diet consumed than to excess weight.

It appears that cancer in the large bowel, in endocrine-controlled tissues such as the breast, prostate, ovary, endometrium, and perhaps kidney and urinary bladder stem from nutritional causes. The present discussion is limited to a description of two cancer sites for which we have evidence that nutritional factors are implicated in their etiology. Evidence will be presented that permits us to conclude that overnutrition is causally related to the development of these cancers. When we use the term causal, we do not necessarily mean that specific

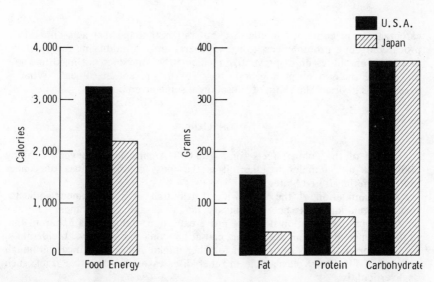

FIGURE 1. Comparison of per capita consumption of calories and nutrients in the U.S. and Japan. (From National Nutrition Survey, Japan, 1969; National Food Situation, U.S.A., 1968.)

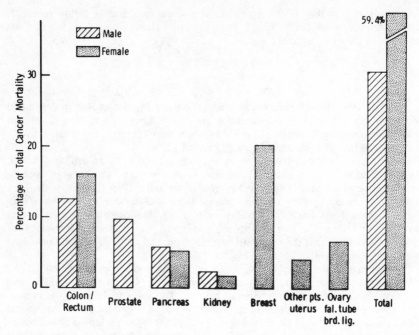

FIGURE 2. "Over-nutrition"-related cancer deaths by sex, U.S., 1968. (Source: U.S. Vital Statistics, 1968.)

carcinogens are contained in the diet, but rather that the diet acts either as a procarcinogen, a promoter, or, to use a general term, a modifying factor. It is, of course, an old lesson of preventive medicine that one does not need to know the precise method of pathogenesis in order to prevent an illness. What is necessary is to break the chain of causation at some given point.

COLON CANCER

Cancer of the colon affects some 100,000 Americans each year. Taking both males and females together, it is the most common cause of cancer mortality in the United States.

An examination of the worldwide distribution of colon cancer indicates that a correlation exists between dietary fat intake and colon cancer (FIGURE 3). Obviously, correlation does not prove causation, though it is apparent that in the absence of such an association, causation would be unlikely. Incidentally, no such correlation has been shown for fiber intake and colon cancer, although absence of fiber may play a role in other diseases of the digestive tract, such as diverticulitis.

The correlation should be viewed as part of the logical progression toward a causative concept. It appears logical that diet affects fecal constituents and that fecal constituents, in turn, play a role in colon carcinogenesis. Diet can also affect plasma constituents, which can reach the colon mucosa independently of the gut contents.

Migrants from low-risk to high-risk countries (e.g., Japanese to the U.S.) soon develop the risk for colon cancer approximating that prevalent in the new country (FIGURE 4).[15] This suggests that some modification in life-style of these migrants increases their risk for this disease. With specific reference to the Hawaiian data, it has been shown that Japanese tend to modify their dietary habits, approximating those of Americans.[16] These migrants eventually have higher serum cholesterol levels (a major risk factor in coronary disease) and develop more of the cancers related to overnutrition, including that of cancer of the colon, than the Japanese in Japan.

We will next consider classical case-control studies. Unfortunately, such studies are not very illuminating when only American populations are studied, in part because dietary histories cannot be adequately obtained in a population where "overeating" is the norm.[17] Since a significant quantitative error appears when one is asked what was eaten only yesterday, a determination of what was eaten two to four decades ago seems an impossible task. In Japan, we have found that patients with colon cancer tend to consume a more Westernized diet than controls,[17] and their recently reported increase in the incidence of colon cancer is consistent with a general increase in the Westernization of the Japanese diet.

Our studies have shown no correlation between weight or constipation and colon cancer. The latter finding indicates that differences in transit time, at least as they relate to constipation, do not play a role in colon carcinogenesis.

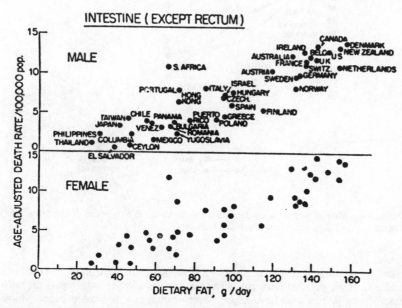

FIGURE 3. Positive correlation between per capita consumption of fat and age-adjusted mortality from cancer of the intestine (except rectum). (From Carroll & Khor.[32] By permission of S. Karger Inc.)

With the exception of ulcerated colitis, familial polyposis, and adenomatous polyps, we found no other colonic diseases related to cancer.

We have investigated the metabolic epidemiology of fecal constituents of individuals from high- and low-risk populations and the fecal constituents from patients with colon cancer. We have found, as have our colleagues Hill and Williams in England, that individuals at high risk have a higher concentration

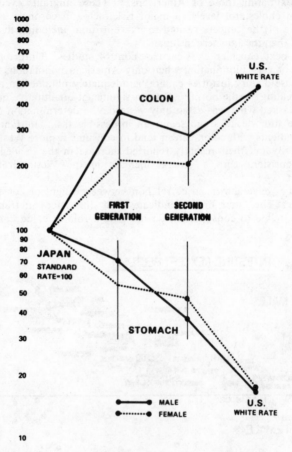

FIGURE 4. Mortality trends of Japanese migrants to U.S. (From Haenszel et al.[16] By permission of *Journal of the National Cancer Institute*.)

of neutral steroids and bile acids in their stools than controls [18, 19] (FIGURES 5 and 6). Also, patients with colon cancer, and to a lesser extent patients with adenomatous polyps who have higher than normal risk for colon cancer, have more neutral steroids and bile acids in their stool than the respective controls (FIGURE 7). These findings strengthen the concept of a causative association between these stool constituents and colon cancer. Recent studies conducted

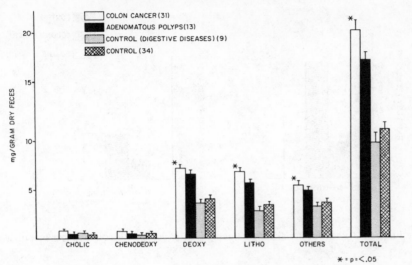

FIGURE 5. Fecal bile acid patterns in patients with colon cancer.

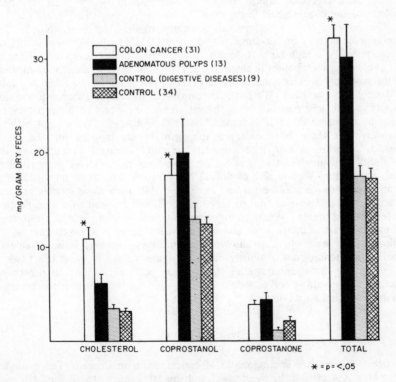

FIGURE 6. Fecal neutral steroid pattern in patients with colon cancer.

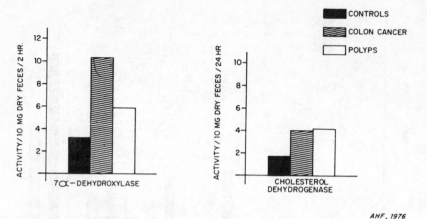

AHF, 1976

FIGURE 7. Fecal bacterial enzyme activity in patients with colon cancer or polyps.

by Reddy on patients with familial polyposis showed an increase in unmetabolized cholesterol in the stool and no changes in bile acids. On the other hand, patients with ulcerated colitis showed an increase in neutral steroids (both cholesterol and coprostanol) in the stool.[20]

The possible role of dietary fat in animal models was also studied. The carcinogenic activity of 1,2-dimethylhydrazine (DMH) for the colon in the rat is enhanced by a high-fat diet. Such rats excreted higher levels of bile acids and cholesterol metabolites in their stools. The carcinogenic activity of MNNG on the colon of rats was enhanced when certain bile acids were applied topically to the colonic mucosa.[21] We have demonstrated, therefore, a tumor-promoting activity of bile acid metabolites in the rat. Thus, the effect of high dietary fat might be mediated through increased bile acids in the gut. We do not believe, however, that these bile acids are the primary carcinogens for the colon mucosa. Martin in our laboratory is currently engaged in exploring the possibility that an oxidative product of cholesterol may exhibit such carcinogenic properties. We are also exploring the suggestion by Wilk that a reactive form of cholesterol may be formed in vivo.[22] Although these studies are still in progress, it is apparent that dietary modifications can lead to a modification of fecal constituents. When monitoring individuals who change from high fat to a low fat diet, we have shown that when using β-glucuronidase as an indicator, the metabolic capability of the intestinal contents is modifiable; a modification that would obviously have its greatest effect early in life (TABLE 3).[23] Among the specific studies that appear necessary is one to determine whether adenomatous polyps would regress when an individual is placed on a low-fat, low-cholesterol diet.

BREAST CANCER

Breast cancer is a leading cause of cancer death in women. The evidence suggests a correlation between diet and breast cancer, based on evidence similar to that presented for colon cancer (FIGURE 8). Again, we must make the same qualifications that we presented previously. While showing some increased risk associated with factors such as late pregnancy and late menopause, studies by us and other groups have not revealed any variables that could explain the sizable differences in incidence between Japanese and U.S. women, pre-menopausally, and particularly post-menopausally (FIGURE 9).[24, 25] In our population, we found no correlation with weight, height, or nursing practices. Again, we have to look at metabolic epidemiology. MacMahon and his group in Boston suggested that some differences in urinary estrogen output, as a reflection of dietary factors, were likely to be of etiological significance, with estriol acting as a protective agent.[26] This view has recently been challenged, and in fact, studies on plasma estrogens between high- and low-risk populations, both by Bulbrook in England and Hill in our group, have not revealed any major differences in estrogen content of the plasma.[27, 28] In fact, both groups indicated that some low-risk groups tended to have a higher level of the experimental carcinogenic estradiol in their plasma. Hill has suggested that perhaps a high amount of androgens in the plasma of high-risk groups might be of etiological significance, especially in post-menopausal women.[29] In general, however, it may be concluded that differences in estrogens and androgens in high- and low-risk groups, if they do exist, cannot account for the major differences in incidence rates between high- and low-risk countries.

We, like others, have become interested in assays of prolactin levels in the serum, not just during the day but especially at night, since much of the prolactin is produced and released during deep sleep and since the half-life of prolactin in the plasma is short. We showed that the production of prolactin at night is significantly reduced when women are placed on a low-fat diet (FIGURE 10).[30]

Prolactin, and specifically a high prolactin/estrogen ratio, has been shown to play an important role in the development of breast cancer in the rat

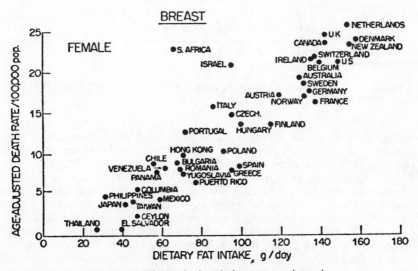

FIGURE 8. Dietary fat in relation to tumorigenesis.

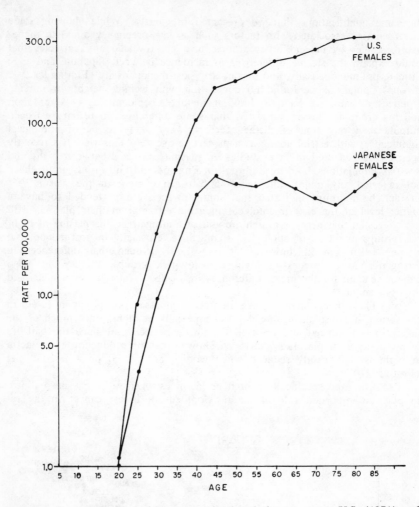

FIGURE 9. Age-specific incidence rates for female breast cancer, U.S. (1971) and Japan (1973).

model. Both Chan and Cohen of our Institute and other investigators (particularly Carroll and his group) have shown that a high-fat diet accelerates tumor formation in the rat when initiated either by DMBA or NMU (FIGURE 11).[31-33] This increase in tumor incidence is concomitant with an increase of prolactin, as induced by a high-fat diet (FIGURE 16). These data, both in women and in rats, provide an interesting correlation and a demonstration of yet another biological and physiological parameter influenced by dietary fat.

It is our current hypothesis that hormones, and specifically the prolactin/estrogen ratio, relate to the promotion of breast cancer. Stimulated by the work of Petrakis, we began to look into breast fluid as a possible source of carcinogens.[34] We have found appreciable amounts of cholesterol in the breast fluid, as well as the presence of prolactin.[35] We are currently following women who secrete breast fluid to determine whether we can alter the cholesterol and other constituents of their breast fluid by dietary modifications. We suspect, as in the case of colon carcinogenesis, that some metabolite of cholesterol may play a role in carcinogenesis within the breast ducts and that the breast fluid plays a vital role in the initiation and probably also the prevention of breast cancer.

While these studies are in progress, it may be asked what preventive measures women should engage in to lessen their chances of developing breast cancer. This, of course, is of particular interest to women known to be at

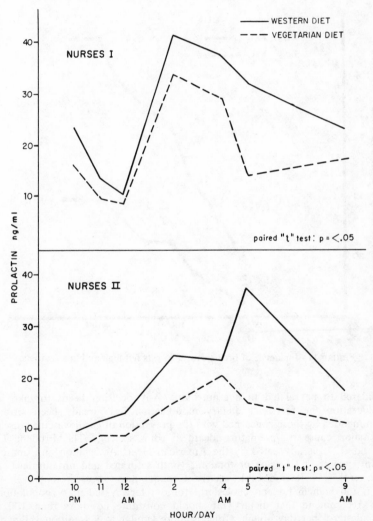

FIGURE 10. Release of prolactin by time of day in four women, by type of diet.

particularly high risk, such as women with benign diseases of the breast, and especially those with a family history of breast cancer. It seems a prudent measure to undertake dietary modification in terms of lower fat and lower cholesterol intake .

PRUDENT DIET

In view of the data presented, it may be asked what course our society should take to help eliminate, or at least decrease, the incidence of cancer

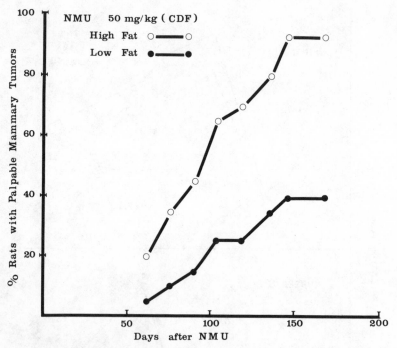

FIGURE 11. Incidence of breast cancer in rats fed high and low fat diets.

considered to be related to overnutrition. Any decision needs to take into consideration the fact that dietary modification has already been strongly recommended by those concerned with the prevention of cardiovascular disease, the major cause of premature death in our society. The Prudent Diet (FIGURE 12), as advocated by the American Heart Association and our own group, suggests a lowering of total fat (both saturated and unsaturated) and cholesterol.[36, 37] It is possible, as the Connors have stressed, that even this diet is too high in fat and cholesterol for our largely sedentary population.[38] They recommend that dietary fat should constitute no more than 100 mg of cholesterol per day. Such a diet is more similar to a traditional Japanese diet (FIGURES 13 and 1). It has also been suggested that dietary modifications

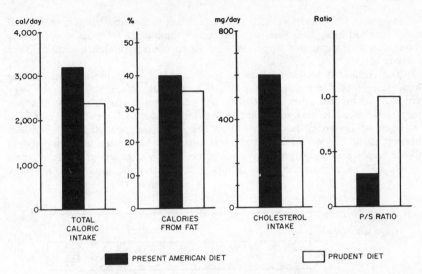

FIGURE 12. Prudent diet and present American diet.

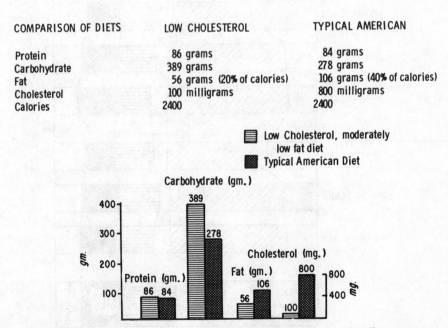

COMPARISON OF DIETS	LOW CHOLESTEROL	TYPICAL AMERICAN
Protein	86 grams	84 grams
Carbohydrate	389 grams	278 grams
Fat	56 grams (20% of calories)	106 grams (40% of calories)
Cholesterol	100 milligrams	800 milligrams
Calories	2400	2400

FIGURE 13. Composition of the low-cholesterol, moderately low fat diet as compared with the American diet.

be instituted very early in life, not only because dietary habits are formed early in childhood, but also because certain biological feedback mechanisms have their beginning, and apparently adjust to control reference settings, very early in life.

The American people need to be re-educated about a diet that on the one hand is optimal for proper physical and intellectual development of the very young, and on the other one that is optimal for a useful longevity. In this respect we need to recognize that in the long history of preventive medicine the greatest drawback has always been the individual, who tends to consider himself to be "immortal." The greatest successes have been accomplished in the area of managerial preventive medicine, which changed products at their source. We need to reduce the fat content of our milk, attempt to see how

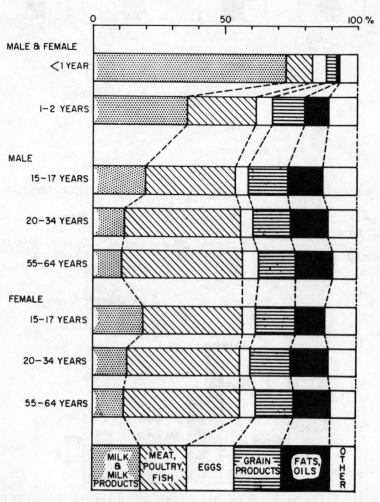

FIGURE 14. Fat from food eaten in one day—contribution of food groups.

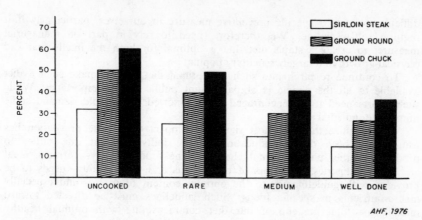

FIGURE 15. Percentage of fat content of various forms of beef, on dry matter base.

the cholesterol content of eggs could be reduced, and reduce the fat content in meat. The contribution of milk and meat to total fat intake at various ages is well demonstrated in FIGURE 14. The fat content of meat is far greater in corn-fed cattle than in range-fed cattle. It would, therefore, appear that eating range-fed beef is healthier, although perhaps not as tasty nor as economical. The institution of corn feeding of cattle is a modern byproduct that relates negatively to optimum health. The full medical impact of high-fat corn-fed meat and the high fat content of hamburgers has, perhaps, not as yet been seen. In this respect, it is also noteworthy that meat prepared "well-done" is lower in fat calories than rare meat (FIGURE 15).

It would seem that our national diet has to be re-engineered. We should convene a National Commission on this subject, a commission that would have a far greater impact on the health of our country than the many advisory groups that have been convened to deal with possible hazards due to specific food additives and contaminates. We need to develop a national diet that is tasteful, that our country can produce, and that is consistent with the development and maintenance of optimal health. Such a national diet is one of the birthday presents this country could and should give itself in this Bicentennial year.

CONCLUDING REMARKS

From what has been said previously, it seems evident that nutrition, principally its deficiencies and excesses, significantly affects human carcinogenesis as well as numerous other diseases and disorders. While deficiency-related cancers tend to decrease in the industrialized world, cancers related to excesses have been shown to increase. Both agricultural and food industries and the general population need to ask what type of diet is optimal for the proper mental and physical growth of our children and the useful longevity of our adult populations. We tend to become used to and, therefore, continue to eat those foods that are available and affordable. As individuals, we find it difficult to relate a specific preventive measure to ourselves, particularly if it requires self-discipline. We, therefore, need to rely in part on managerial measures to create a staple diet that is optimal for both the intellectual and physical growth of a largely sedentary population.

To continue research into such an optimal diet and to make such a diet available to all the people is of paramount public health importance. While such efforts need to be encouraged and supported, we should demand some immediate remedial action.

We recognize that the most significant impact on disease prevention has usually not been due to education of the individual but due rather to product or other environmental changes. The food industry—farmers, meat and dairy industries, producers of baby foods and snack foods—needs to be provided with guidelines as to the optimal content of micro- and especially macro-nutrients in specific foods. Such guidelines must be directed toward making the total makeup of our diet commensurate with optimal healthy growth and development.

As stated, today's diet does not appear to be optimal for a largely sedentary population. Its deficiencies and its excesses adversely affect the health of our young and adult population. We suffer, as so aptly put by René Dubos, simultaneously from a malnutrition of the poor and a malnutrition of the affluent. If we would give as much attention to the major components of the average American diet as we do to minor food additives and contaminates, we could streamline the American diet into one that our bodies could appropriately metabolize and, subsequently, have a lower risk of chronic diseases.

Obviously, nutrition has a profound effect on human health. Recognizing this plus the fact that food modification is possible, we expect that during our third century, we could modify our foods to such an extent that nutritionally related diseases could be eliminated. If we succeed in this endeavor, those diseases that are related to diet would disappear, as have many of the diseases of previous centuries.

If asked what I would wish for our country as a Bicentennial present, it would be a healthier society—one in which we could not only be fully productive but also fully enjoy life's many blessings. To accomplish such a goal, optimal nutrition plays a decisive role.

ACKNOWLEDGMENTS

I want to express my appreciation to Drs. Peter Hill, Bandaru Reddy, and John Weisburger for their collaboration in this work and to Margaret Mushinski and Joan Spivak for technical assistance in the preparation of this manuscript.

REFERENCES

1. WOGAN, G. N. 1975. Dietary factors and special epidemiological situations of liver cancer in Thailand and Africa. Cancer Res. 35(11): 3499–3502.
2. JUKES, T. H. 1973. The Delaney "Anti-cancer" clause. Prev. Med. 2: 133–139.
3. FLAMM, W. G. 1976. The need for quantifying risk from exposure to chemical carcinogens. Prev. Med. 5: 4–6.

4. MIRVISH, S. S. & P. SHUBIK. 1974. Ascorbic acid and nitrosamines. Nature **250:** 684–689.
5. WYNDER, E. L. 1976. Epidemiology of carcinoma *in situ* of the cervix. Obstet. Gynecol. Surv. **24:** 697–711.
6. ROTHMAN, K. J. & A. Z. KELLER. 1976. The effect of joint exposure to alcohol and tobacco on cancer of the mouth and pharynx. J. Chron. Dis. **25:** 711–716.
7. WYNDER, E. L. & K. MABUCHI. 1972. Etiological and preventive aspects of human cancer. Prev. Med. **1:** 300–334.
8. WYNDER, E. L. & U. E. KLEIN. 1965. The possible role of riboflavin deficiency in epithelial neoplasia: I. Epithelial changes in mice in simple deficiency. Cancer **18:** 167–180.
9. WYNDER, E. L. & P. C. CHAN. 1970. The possible role of riboflavin deficiency in epithelial neoplasia: II. Effect on skin tumor development. Cancer **26:** 1221–1224.
10. WYNDER, E. L., J. HULTBERG, F. JACOBSON & I. D. J. BROSS. 1957. Environmental factors in cancer of the upper alimentary tract: A Swedish study with special reference to Plummer-Vinson (Paterson-Kelly) syndrome. Cancer **19:** 470–487.
11. LARSSON, LARS-GUNNER, A. SANDSTROM & P. WESTLING. 1975. Relationship of Plummer-Vinson's disease to cancer of the upper alimentary tract in Sweden. Cancer Res. **35**(11): 3308–3316.
12. McCOY, D. Manuscript in preparation.
13. WYNDER, E. L., G. C. ESCHER & N. MANTEL. 1966. An epidemiological investigation of cancer of the endometruim. Cancer **19:** 489–520.
14. WYNDER, E. L., K. MABUCHI & W. F. WHITMORE. 1974. Epidemiology of adenocarmcinoma of the kidney. J. Natl. Cancer Inst. **53:** 1619–1634.
15. HAENSZEL, W. & M. KURIHARA. 1973. Studies of Japanese migrants: I. Mortality from cancer and other diseases among Japanese in the United States. J. Natl. Cancer Inst. **51:** 1765–1779.
16. HAENSZEL, W., M. KURIHARA & M. SEGI. 1972. Stomach cancer among Japanese in Hawaii. J. Natl. Cancer Inst. **49:** 969–988.
17. WYNDER, E. L., T. KAJITONI, S. ISHIKAWA, H. DODO & A. TAKANO. 1969. Environmental factors of cancer of the colon and rectum. II: Japanese epidemiological data. Cancer **23:** 1210–1220.
18. REDDY, B. S. & E. L. WYNDER. 1973. Large bowel carcinogenesis: Fecal constituents of populations with diverse incidence rates of colon cancer. J. Natl. Cancer Inst. **50:** 1437–1442.
19. HILL, M. J., B. S. DRASAR, V. ARIES, J. S CROWTHER, G HAWKSWORTH & R. E. O. WILLIAMS. 1971. Bacteria and aetiology of cancer of the large bowel. Lancet **2:** 95–100.
20. REDDY, B. S. & E. L. WYNDER. 1977. Metabolic epidemiology of colon cancer: Fecal bile acids and neutral steroids in colon cancer patients with adenomatous polyps. Cancer. In press.
21. REDDY, B. S., R. NARASAWA, J. H. WEISBURGER & E. L. WYNDER. 1976. Promoting effect of sodium deoxycholate on colon adenocarcinoma in germ-free rats. J. Natl. Cancer Inst. **56:** 441–442.
22. WILK, M. & W. TAUPP. 1969. Dehydrierung des cholesterins ein aktiviert adsorbierten zustand unter normal-bedingungen, ein Beitrag zur Frage der Endogenese carcinogener, polycyclischer kohlenwasserstaffe. Z. Naturforsch. (B) **24:** 16–23.
23. REDDY, B. S., J. H. WEISBURGER & E. L. WYNDER. 1974. Fecal bacterial β-glucuronidase: control by diet. Science **183:** 416–417.
24. MACMAHON, B., P. COLE & J. BROWN. 1973. Etiology of human breast cancer: A review. J. Natl. Cancer Inst. **50:** 21–42.
25. WYNDER, E. L., I. D. J. BROSS & T. HIRAYAMA. 1960. A study of the epidemiology of cancer of the breast. Cancer **13:** 559–601.

26. MACMAHON, B., P. COLE, J. B. BROWN, K. AOKI, T. M. LIN, R. W. MORGAN & N. C. WOO. 1974. Urine oestrogen profiles of Asian and North American women. Int. J. Cancer. **14:** 161–167.
27. BULBROOK, R. D., M. C. SWAIN, D. Y. WANG, S. KUMAOKA, O. TAKATANI, O. ABE, M. UTSUNO & J. IYA 1976. Breast cancer in England and Japan. Eur. J. Cancer **12:** 725–735.
28. HILL, P., E. L. WYNDER, P. HELMAN, R. HICKMAN, G. RONA & K. KUNO 1976. Plasma hormone levels in different ethnic populations of women. Cancer Res. **36:** 2297–2301.
29. HILL, P. 1976. Androgen production in post-menopausal women. Presented at 5th International Congress of Endocrinology. Hamburg, Germany.
30. HILL, P. & E. L. WYNDER. 1976. Diet and prolactin release. Lancet **1:** 806–807.
31. TANNENBAUM, A. 1942. The genesis and growth of tumors: III. Effect of a high fat diet. Cancer Res. **2:** 468–475.
32. CARROLL, K. K. & H. T. KHOR. 1975. Dietary fat in relation to tumorigenesis. *In* Progress in Biochemical Pharmacology: Lipids and Tumors. K. K. Carroll, Ed. : 308–345. S. Karger. New York, N.Y.
33. CHAN, P. C. & L. A. COHEN 1974. Effect of dietary fat antiestrogen, and antiprolactin on the development of mammary tumors in rats. J. Natl. Cancer Inst. **52:** 25–30.
34. PETRAKIS, N. L., L. MASON, L. ROSE, B. SUGIMATO, S. PAWSON & F. CATCHPOOL. 1975. Association of race, age, menopausal status, and cerumen type with breast fluid secretion in nonlactating women, as determined by nipple aspiration. J. Natl. Cancer Inst. **54:** 829–833.
35. HILL, P. Unpublished data.
36. BENNETT, I. & M. SIMON. 1973. The Prudent Diet. David White. New York, N.Y.
37. American Health Foundation. 1972. Position statement on diet and coronary heart disease. Prev. Med. **1:** 255–286.
38. CONNOR, W. E. & S. L. CONNOR 1972. The key role of nutritional factors in the prevention of coronary heart disease. Prev. Med. **1:** 49–83.

DISCUSSION PAPER: PREVENTION OF ATHEROSCLEROSIS BY A FAT-MODIFIED DIET

Haqvin Malmros

University Hospital
Lund, Sweden

Already 9 years ago the National Board of Health and Welfare of Sweden and the Medical Board of Finland issued an official statement recommending that the entire population of these countries change their diet in an effort to prevent atherosclerosis.[1] The total consumption of fat, especially all kind of saturated fats, ought to be reduced. Instead of saturated fat, polyunsaturated fat could be used.

Practical experience from Sweden over the last few years has shown that it is rather difficult to persuade the general public to change their food habits and particularly to reduce the consumption of fat. We noticed at first a small reduction of the fat consumption, but later on we found a new increase, probably a consequence of subsidized low prices on meat and cheese.

Initially, the emphasis was placed mainly on reduction of the total consumption of fat, and little attention was given to the types of fat that were used. The food industry, however, proved interested in the problem, and in recent years they have placed quite a number of new products on the market. In Sweden we have for some years had a low-fat milk with only 0.5% fat. It tastes much better than no-fat milk and contains the same amount of vitamins as standard milk. We also have a butter made rich in linoleic acid by addition of 20% soybean oil and different types of linoleic-acid-rich margarine, such as liquid margarine with 60% linoleic acid. It tastes better than pure oil and shortening and is better to use for frying because one notices more easily whether the temperature is too high—the color turns dark brown, just like real butter. A so-called imitation- or margarine-cheese, made from skim milk and sunflower seed oil and containing 40% linoleic acid instead of about 3% in ordinary cheese, is also becoming increasingly popular; it is now also exported to U.S.A.

In order to find out if it would be possible to persuade the general public to change the type of fat and to use polyunsaturated fat instead of saturated fat, I have performed a dietary trial with some people living in a district in Lund, the same town in the south of Sweden where I live. I informed the public as well as the school children of the significance of the diet for good health and invited all those interested to take part in a dietary trial. To begin with we took blood samples for cholesterol determination on 650 persons of all ages, also some children 11-13 years old. In total it was about 10% of the inhabitants living in the district. The two grocers' shops had in the meantime ordered and received new food products with modified fat composition, and the dietary trial could start.

This public has from the very beginning been very interested in the new types of food products with high linoleic acid and low saturated fat content, and their interest has been sustained. After half a year, 1 year, and 2 years we have again determined the blood cholesterol in those persons who volunteered—mostly people who have carefully followed the dietary prescriptions.

The control examination 6 months after modification of the diet showed much lower cholesterol levels in most people. Especially when the initial value was high the effect of the diet was striking; in many cases the cholesterol value fell 75–100 mg/100 ml (FIGURE 1). It was very encouraging to note that also in some cases with familial hypercholesterolemia that we have found among the participants in the trial, modification of the diet induced a distinct drop in the blood cholesterol. Some children who at the first examination were found to have a low cholesterol value—below 200 mg/100ml—had nevertheless kept to the diet because the whole family had changed their dietary habits. In many such cases a further, although modest, reduction of the cholesterol value occurred. In one of these cases the level was extremely low—99 mg/100 ml. No undesired side effect of such low cholesterol values could be observed. The blood cholesterol was again determined after 1 and 2 years. The values then were still much lower than before the diet with modified fat was started.

Such fat-modified dairy products are now quite popular, particularly in the south of Sweden. About 30% of the milk consumed in Sweden is now low-fat milk, with 0.5% fat. It is used by the school children and also in most hospitals.

The Swedish food industry so far used sunflower seed oil imported from Russia or other countries when replacing saturated fat by polyunsaturated in some dairy products. We have, however, now started growing suitable oil-plants in Sweden, viz. sunflower that flourish in our climate and white poppies. At the plant genetic center in Svalöv Nyman and Hall[2] have succeeded in obtaining a new papaver-variant that scarcely forms any morphium and gives

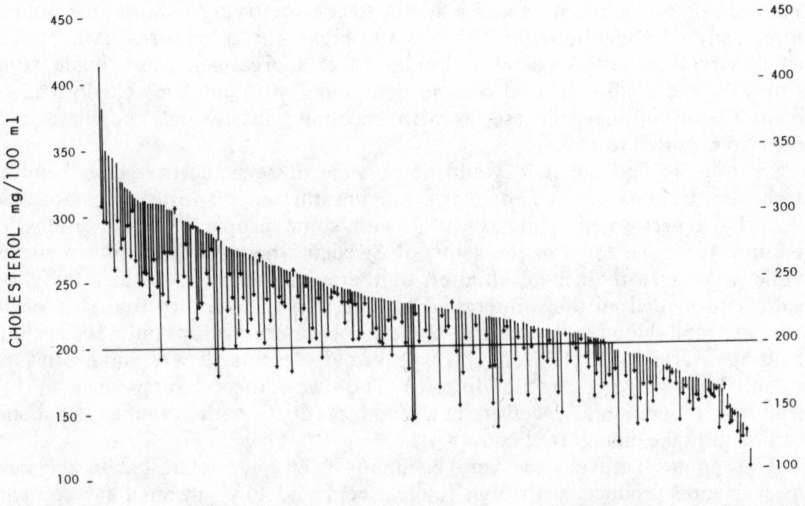

FIGURE 1. Serum cholesterol in the individual cases before the start of the trial and after a year on a diet with low saturated and high polyunsaturated fat content.

TABLE 1

WORLD PRODUCTION OF FATS AND OILS *

	Production 1970	Projection 1980
Grand Total Edible Fats	39,416	53,000
Butter	4,974	5,400
Lard	4,963	5,900
Tallow	4,591	5,900
Marine oil	1,317	1,300
Coconut oil	2,079	2,900
Palm kernel oil	492	900
Palm oil	1,661	3,700
Soft Vegetable Oils		
Soybean oil	6,068	8,200
Sunflower seed oil	3,575	5,100
Cotton seed oil	2,781	3,300
Groundnut oil	3,222	4,700
Rapeseed oil	1,897	3,000
Olive oil	1,279	1,900
Sesame seed oil	617	700

* Source: F.A.O. (U.N.) Agricultural Commodity Projections 1970–1980 (1971). Rome.

an oil containing more than 70% linoleic acid. We hope to start growing these new oilplants on a large scale next year.

From a global point of view it is, of course, of paramount importance to try to produce such fat as is wholesome and not simply a source of calories—and profit. So far a large part of the world production of fats consisted of saturated fats (TABLE 1). A considerable part of the liquid vegetable oils used to be hydrogenated, which does not improve the situation. In recent years large areas of land have been planted with oil palms, financed by development funds. The yield of palm kernel fat is about 25% of the total yield of palm oil. The chemical composition of palm kernel oil is roughly the same as that of coconut fat, i.e. it consists almost entirely of saturated fatty acids. The import of coconut oil this year in the U.S.A. is likely to be about twice what it was last year—calculated to be at least 1 billion pounds.[3]

It is possible to grow sunflowers in many parts of the world, both in the East and West, in the North and South. The center of production has, however, been the U.S.S.R. and some other countries in eastern Europe (TABLE 2). Until now, only small quantities of sunflower seed and oil have been exported to other countries. Undoubtedly it would be worthwhile to grow sunflower instead of other oilplants, which produce fat of inferior quality.

Since the food industry now has the opportunity to produce new food products with modified fat composition, it is, of course, very important to secure an ample supply of linoleic acid-rich vegetable oils. There is no reason to continue the use of food containing large amounts of saturated fat if other products, made for instance with sunflower seed oil, are available.

TABLE 2

SUNFLOWER SEED AND SUNFLOWER SEED OIL PRODUCTION AND EXPORT, 1974
IN THOUSAND TONS *

	Production	Export	
	Seed	Seed	Oil
Bulgaria	400	14	17
Hungary	150	23	29
Rumania	671	2	120
Turkey	425	3	
U.S.S.R.	6760	75	430
Yugoslavia	298	12	
Western Europe	412	15	
U.S.A.	291	182	
South America	1083		2
Africa	380		
Australia	76	33	
China, Mainland	180		
World Total	11110	405	696

* Source: F.A.O. Production yearbook. 1974. 28: 1.

REFERENCES

1. Official Collective Recommendation on Diet in the Scandinavian countries. 1968.
    Nutr. Rev. **26:** 259.
2. NYMAN, U. & O. HALL. 1974. Breeding oil poppy (Papaver somniferum) for low
    content of morphine. Hereditas **76:** 49–54.
3. Fats and Oils Situation, 1976. **282:** 11–12 U.S. Department of Agriculture.

GENERAL DISCUSSION

Jonathan E. Rhoads, *Moderator*

Hospital of the University of Pennsylvania
Philadelphia, Pennsylvania 19104

UNIDENTIFIED SPEAKER: Are height and weight reasonable indexes for effects of malnutrition when you're talking about a wide range of individual differences? How do you parcel out the effects contributed by malnutrition?

DR. BRASEL: Well I think most people who are following children who have been chronically malnourished would agree that weight at the time you weigh a child is apt to reflect more precisely present nutritional status, other factors being equal. Obviously this may not be true if there is superimposed other serious disease that will contribute to weight when the child is seen. But someone who has had significant chronic malnutrition in the past will usually demonstrate short stature at a later date. That is if it occurs at the growing age. So height in later childhood and in adulthood can be a reflection of past nutritional status and will be significantly altered if there has been significant chronic malnutrition. So that is one public health measure of assessing what past nutritional status in a community has been. You're quite right though that growth and development can be affected by any number of facts, and if one has a history of other things that might alter growth and development in addition to nutrition, it will be very difficult to assign the shortening or change in weight status simply to nutrition alone. However, it is still considered by most workers in the field as a valid reflection at least to some degree of past nutritional status. If someone has been well nourished throughout his or her life then he is not going to be short unless he has other problems on top of it which you should discover by historical information. In this series it was only used to get some idea how severely affected the children might be, because it was about the only kind of data available on the orphanage charts that could be reliably used to assess their nutritional status between a year and 18 months of age. This was the age when most of them entered the orphanage.

DR. J. E. RHOADS: I wonder if everybody here can define a stanine. Perhaps Dr. Brasel would define it for me.

DR. BRASEL: It is really a means of normalizing data that are recorded in different types of parameters and you want to compare one group to the next. In this case it was achievement scores versus I.Q.'s. If one takes the normal distribution of the data and divides it into blocks of nine, one that has nine stanines, and stanine number nine is the highest one-ninth of the data and stanine number one is the lowest one-ninth of the data, and stanine number five is that part of the data which hovers around the mean. One can then convert anything to these numbers and then look at everything in stanines instead of trying to compare an I.Q. of 102 versus an achievement score that might be expressed in terms of mental age or something else. It's just a way of normalizing the data for comparison purposes.

DR. RHOADS: Most of them have been developed by somebody with nine digits?

DR. BRASEL: I expect so, although if you did it by tens where would the mean be? That struck me in looking at this that at least they have got a number in the middle, five, that is used in the middle for looking at the mean data.

UNIDENTIFIED SPEAKER: The intake of meat in the United States is a factor in the causation of heart disease, in my estimation. You may disagree, but since we know that meat is approximately 60% fat I think it's an important factor. As you did mention, those people who eat less meat eat more fiber. Don't you think that as we eat less meat and perhaps less cheese and other fatty foods that we will decrease the incidence of coronary heart disease?

DR. KRITCHEVSKY: Meat doesn't have to be 60% fat. It depends on how you treat the meat, and it also depends whether you like to eat all of it. There is an old literature relating the intake of animal protein to the possible susceptibility to heart disease. I think, yes, if we decreased the general intake. However, you asked specifically if we just decreased meat and cheese. I think that the answer to a lot of this is a generally moderate diet, and if you eat fewer calories everything else is liable to take care of itself. There are really a lot of people who think that one way of taking fewer calories is taking a lot of fiber. A lot of people have suggested that this inhibits energy, but this is something that still has to be definitely proven.

MR. BOB RESPINO (Temple University, Philadelphia, Pa.): Miller and Miller, in a recent review article on carcinogenesis, endorse the theory of electrophilic attack by some compounds on free radicals and also on certain other compounds. You said in your presentation that dietary fibers in some cases bind and protect these compounds from attack. I am wondering first of all specifically about anything other than bile-acids; has it been proven that anything other than bile-acids have been shown to bind?

DR. KRITCHEVSKY: Yes. I would direct you to the work of Martin Iselet, who has published extensively on the cationic binding of many substances by these various kinds of food products.

MR. RESPINO: You state that they bind trace metals. Is magnesium also bound?

DR. KRITCHEVSKY: Yes.

MR. RESPINO: Wouldn't that tend to destabilize the DNA then?

DR. KRITCHEVSKY: I don't know. Many absorption studies are designed to obtain information on one particular nutrient. Most of these studies are bizarre because they are specifically designed to prove a point. The data that are available from Iran are just natural. The kids eat a lot of crude fiber, and they are all zinc deficient.

DR. MAX RUBIN (University of Maryland, College Park, Md.): Would you connect the formation of cholesterol gallstones with the biosalt fiberchrome?

DR. KRITCHEVSKY: Again there are a couple of papers in the literature that would indicate first that a low fiber diet will lead to gallstone formation. As you know Enric Dam published extensively on a diet which was mostly simple carbohydrate and salt, and VanLinden and Borgmann separately showed that in animals in which cholesterol gallstones are established the addition of either a drug such as cholestyromine or actin to the diet will decrease formation of gallstones. So again what we're talking about really is the very widely integrated network of dietary interchange, and when you try to single out one component or another you are always liable to fall into a trap. But in general I would say yes—in animal studies it would appear as if the fiber-free diet and one that is high in saturated fat and simple carbohydrates is what leads to formation of cholesterol gallstones.

UNIDENTIFIED SPEAKER: Dr. Kritchevsky, I have two items I would like to address myself to. As a result of the fiber fad we've had recently, a number of new products have been introduced on the market. There are the high-bran breads which contain 2, 3, 4 and sometimes 5 times as much bran as whole wheat bread and the cellulose breads. Papers have been published on the negative effects of cellulose or potential negative effects of cellulose. A paper was published in 1974 on the uptake of ingestive microcrystalline cellulose in the blood of dogs, rats, and pigs. G. Sweiber published a couple of papers on the uptake in the blood and urine of humans of ingested diet cellulose. I think it's understood by most of the people here that the high cellulose parts are very good for label claims in terms of crude fiber. I would just like your comments on the industry's response to the fiber fad and how you feel about these products.

DR. KRITCHEVSKY: What has been the industry response? I really can't say. I would imagine most of these things had been tested. You know the studies that were done on the type of cellulose uptake and crystalline cellulose weren't done by making it into a bread, and as you well know you can alter how a material is handled merely by how it's fed. I don't know if they should be indicted any more than the health food stores that will sell you all the bran you want to sprinkle on your food. I think that you said there were no data on the response of fecal bulk. As a matter of fact, Hippocrates comments on the fact that whole grain bread is better, and I think it is also well to point out that although in ancient Rome they had bakeries that baked white bread, the gladiators were fed dark bread because they fought better. The people who watched the gladiators ate the white bread. Maybe there is a lesson there. In any event I think that it's incumbent on the industry to be sure that the material they feed is in a form that is not going to show up in the blood. There is no question that Olmstead and Williams showed this in the 30's. They fed high doses of bran and got increased fecal excretion. So this has been studied for a long time, and it's incumbent on these people and I guess on the regulatory agencies to make sure they don't do it. I can't go out and police them.

DR. S. S. FLASCHEN (*IT&T Corp., N.Y., N.Y.*): I had a question for you Dr. Kritchevsky but before I ask it I would like to make a plea for the profession to properly define its terms. The previous speaker spoke about cellulose in bread and then related studies done on microcellulose and dietary cellulose. They are completely different products—as different as salt is from sugar. So once again we've fallen into the trap of lumping a generalized term and proving our arguments by taking different parts of the definition. Dr. Kritchevsky, based upon your experiences and observations to date, have you changed your diet in any significant way?

DR. KRITCHEVSKY: No.

MR. RALPH FLOOD (*New York, N.Y.*): You mentioned the effects of social class on obesity and pointed out that low social classes are associated with obesity. Did you study the diet of poor people? I have spent a good deal of time among the rural poor, and there is a high percentage of obesity there too. I think it was Dr. Timmer who on Wednesday spoke of the diet of Irishmen in the 19th century as composed of up to 10 to 12 pounds of potatoes a day and a pint of milk. What kinds of diets do the poor people have now that cause obesity?

DR. STUNKARD: We really don't know that, and if it were diet alone my impression would be that it might go the other way in that the upper classes have higher fat diets and that may be more conducive to obesity than even concentrated carbohydrates, although that would probably be number two on the list. This very powerful social class influence isn't really well understood, and I think probably dietary and home studies would be very much in order to try to find out how it works.

DR. E. M. WIDDOWSON: I would be very interested in relating what you have told us Dr. Stunkard with what Dr. Brasel told us earlier today, and it's so evident that we have to take into account mental stimulation when we want to rehabilitate a malnourished child. The same thing appears when you go to a meeting on lactation. Behavior side is so much more important than anything else. I think that pure nutritionists have to realize that they haven't got the whole story, and I think this relation between behavior and food is terribly important and we're appreciating this nowadays.

DR. STUNKARD: Thank you. You know the Heart and Lung Institute has gotten quite interested in this and has sponsored two workshops on nutrition and behavior. There are really quite up to date discussions of this inter-relationship between nutrition and behavior.

MR. ALLAN GRIFF: All that you talked about is a one-to-one or patient-to-himself relationship, so to speak. Is there a place for getting at intermediaries? I'm particularly thinking of parents who are not necessarily obese at a very early age when the child is one, two, three, four or five, and teaching them how to teach their children to eat.

DR. STUNKARD: Yes, very definitely. Actually the Weight Watchers is a mediated one where you have groups of up to 50 people. But just let me read the list of the groups that I think can have an influence—religious, fraternal, recreational, health, youth, educational, government, media and programs in the work setting. I think all of these are very much in line for the future, including parents.

DR. ANITA BAHN (*University of Pennsylvania School of Medicine, Philadelphia, Pa.*): As an epidemiologist I have a question. I'm all for the reduction of intake of improper food for coronary heart disease because I think it has been shown on an individual basis that there is a relationship between cholesterol intake, obesity, etc. However, in the area of colon cancer I think we're still at the ecological level where we were looking at countries and their dietary patterns and colon rates. Now a lot of things go on in countries as they become Westernized and urbanized besides diets, and there are many other factors that go on in lifestyle, and to attribute a change in colonic cancer, breast cancer, to dietary habits, is a big jump. For example, how do you put into a unifying theory of cancer of the colon the fact that there is a consistent difference within a country such as the United States? Higher rates of cancer of the colon in urban areas than in rural areas, or nonurban areas? Are the differences in diet that great to explain that? How does that fit in with your theory of diet?

DR. WYNDER: The evidence of colon cancer and diet goes beyond association with countries. As we have shown, differences in fecal constituents between high and low risk populations and between colon cancer and control patients do exist, and have in the formal comparison been linked to dietary differences. Also, dietary changes have been shown to lead to changes in the fecal constituents. An effect of diet on colon carcinogenesis has also been demonstrated in various experimental animals. In terms of recommending dietary changes, we need to consider the "prudent" diet. We might be more conservative if we did not have evidence that a prudent diet is already indicated to replace the leading cause of death in the Western world, coronary artery disease. From a public health point of view, a prudent diet for coronary disease prevention might have a possible additional benefit and would carry no known risk. A research study to see whether dietary intervention would cause polyps to regress would be of interest. I have been asked to what extent I have changed my own diet. I drink very little whole milk, I eat less red meat than before. I do this not only because I would like to live as long as I can, but because I believe we as physicians must be an example for our patients and for the rest of society.

DR. GLASSMAN: I just want to mention one or two points first. We know that in certain countries—specifically Japan and other areas—that people have a low-fat diet and seem to have a low incidence of coronary heart disease. I believe Dr. Wynder mentioned that he feels we should be on 20% fat, and now we know it's approximately 40%. I believe the American Heart Association wants to reduce this to 25% to 30%. There is an organization called the Longevity Foundation in California. Their philosophy is that the American diet should be 10% fat. Since we know that certain societies do better as far as incidence of coronary artery disease, why do you say 20% fat and how do you really feel about this, or are you afraid that the American public won't go along? This question is addressed to Dr. Wynder and to Dr. Krehl.

DR. WILLARD KREHL: First of all I think we do have to face the practicalities of the American public. I do not believe that large numbers of people are going to suddenly change their diet. I think Dr. Wynder pointed out that those of us who are going to work every day, seemingly enjoying life, don't really feel that this is a major problem for us. It's only when we begin to identify the problem, by identifying risk factors, that we become possibly concerned, and yet how many will change? I think the American Heart Association's goals and objectives are to try to perhaps modify this. Speaking of Japan, by the way, I was extremely interested in noting last summer that even the school children there are now developing a Westernized diet. They feed them hamburgers, and they did not have rice or anything characteristic of the culture of Japan. In fact, death from atherosclerotic coronary heart disease is accelerating very rapidly in Japan today, simply because they are moving toward what we feel we should not have. Now I don't know if I fully answered your question. I don't know of any evidence of any population group in the world living perhaps on 10% to 15% of their calories from fat who are suffering any nutritional deficiencies that relate to fat. They may have poor diets from other points of view. But their serum cholesterols are well down in the 150 to 175 range, and I would agree with Dr. Wynder that I think we should be shooting in our own society for certainly less than 200. If I have a patient who is 250 I must tell him that that's high. He should lower it. So I think we do have to do this.

DR. WYNDER: I think that in life I always try for the ideal, but I realize I have to settle for what's realistic. One of the things that I think is realistic, and Dr. Taylor referred to it, is the importance of dietary changes very early in life. We heard earlier about the importance of malnutrition in the early part of life, and I believe that this has an effect not only in fat cells but also in brain cells. Also cholesterol metabolism is very much affected by the supplemental feeding that we give our children. I think therefore that a particular emphasis must be placed on feeding our children not only *in utero* but particularly in the postnatal period. Preventive medicine, therefore, has its beginning in all areas as early in life as we can get in these children. For that reason, Dr. Krehl, I appreciate your reference to the comment that Dr. Williams made.

UNIDENTIFIED SPEAKER: I direct my question to Dr. Wynder again. In your talk you considered the direct causal relationships between diet and cancer. Would you now comment on the more indirect effects of general nutrition, or specifically the effects of vitamin A, vitamin E, and vitamin C on the susceptibility of a person to chemical carcinogens or carcinogens in the environment and the progress of tumor development?

DR. WYNDER: Nutrition is a modifying rather than causative factor. We have not yet identified, for colon cancer or breast cancer, the specific direct carcinogen, and I indicated that I believe it may be a cholesterol byproduct but we still have to prove it. In preventive medicine if you change an exposure and you reduce disease you don't really care whether it was a direct or indirect cause. You referred specifically to vitamin A. Our friend from the National Cancer Institute, Dr. Sporn, has done a great deal of work in vitamin A. In terms of epidemiology it really doesn't fit with colon cancer and lung cancer, but it does fit with cancer of the cervix. It is quite possible that our poorer people who have more cancer of the cervix because of poor hygiene also have a low vitamin A intake, which really interferes with the integrity of mucous-producing epithelium. So it's quite possible that if we would supplement them with vitamin A we could reduce the incidence of cervical cancer. In an experimental study where vitamin A was given to a hamster that was also being given carcinogens to the cervix the vitamin A was found to be protective.

UNIDENTIFIED SPEAKER: I would like to direct this to Dr. Brasel or any of the panelists who want to answer it. Is there any evidence in children that low cholesterol diet is detrimental?

DR. JO ANNE BRASEL: The only diets that might be considered very low cholesterol diets that children have been put on recently in an attempt to prevent obesity are the skim milk diets that some pediatricians are instituting at 4 to 5 months of age, and most pediatricians feel that that is not proper practice, not because of concern about the lack of cholesterol but because the diets provide inadequate calories for normal growth at that age. There are other ways of handling the problem of excessive weight gain in early infancy, under a year of age, without starting a skim milk diet or a very low fat diet. Now someone else on the panel, Dr. Kritchevsky or someone else might want to speak to the issue, but I'm not aware of even those infants who have been on that diet having any problems with cholesterol.

DR. KREHL: I would like to add one comment to your point, namely that I believe now we have very well demonstrated LDL receptor mechanism at the cellular membrane level, which I think rather effectively regulates serum and cellular cholesterol levels. I think that the biosynthetic mechanisms that we have endogenously, certainly help in this matter. I personally do not know of any evidence in any underdeveloped country where—presuming that there is a reasonable caloric intake and other balanced nutrients—that a low blood cholesterol per se has any adverse effect whatsoever in the physical or mental development of children.

DR. KRITCHEVSKY: I can't dispute that. My patients range from mice to baboons. But I would like to comment on one study that has been published and another that has been confirmed in two other laboratories but not published, and this is done in rats who are either permitted to be weaned on mother's milk or were given a soybean formula. They grew very well. When they were about 120 days old they were challenged with cholesterol. The rats who had been weaned on mother's milk were able to get rid of that cholesterol. The rats who were not were not able to get rid of it. Now maybe this is true just with rats, but I think that you have to balance all these things. I believe Dr. Wynder is correct in saying that moderation starts early, but we cannot go overboard. Children may need those calories, and they may be at an age where they can handle them.

Ms. SALLY MCLAUGHLIN: Dr. Henkin, I am interested in your remarks on zinc therapy. I would like to ask you if the primary objective is the return to normalcy, how can you recommend zinc deprivation for weight loss?

DR. R. I. HENKIN: The point being that obesity is a very severe disease, and as you saw in a picture that Dr. Krehl showed of a 16-year-old boy, something has to be done to take care of that patient, both acutely and chronically. There have to be various kinds of therapies that one can use, both immediate and long-term. One way of doing that has been handled by the surgeons, who actually remove large parts of the bowel and run into great side effects. What I am suggesting is an alternative and a useful method of beginning the onset of anorexia and hence the beginning of the onset of weight loss, and that has some usefulness in this whole story. It's one among many various processes that I think should be considered as a possible source of beginning the weight-loss process.

Ms. MCLAUGHLIN: Does it have any long-range success in your opinion?

DR. HENKIN: I don't think that we have had enough experience in terms of years. In my experience we handled this over a period of weeks or months. When we've done that, each patient has to be carefully controlled. This is a big gun. This is a drug that has serious side effects unless it is carefully monitored. But obesity has in itself an inherent risk, and with those patients who are at risk, we should go ahead and handle it in a way that any physician would handle any other serious disease.

DR. MICHAEL RABIN: I will address my remarks to Dr. Wynder. The data we have seen are very impressive, but on the basis of my own practice I haven't found that to be quite so. As a matter of fact, people are wondering what it is that was changed in the diet from what people ate 40 to 50 years ago when we didn't have so much degenerative diseases of all kinds. It's been suggested by responsible investigators that reduction in intake of the refined carbohydrates, notably white flour and sugar, seems to have been effective in reducing cholesterol on an individual basis, supplemented by blood tests that tell us whether these things are really happening. Would you care to comment?

DR. WYNDER: If I understand your question, in areas of preventive medicine that relate to a complicated thing like diet can we work effectively as individuals or must we work with society? Obviously in any chronic disease there are those factors, many of which we do not understand and probably will never understand. In carcinogenesis we deal with factors that may be only a statistical probability. And while I am always in favor of doing more and more work in host defences I believe that in preventive medicine, the approach to the total population is what we need. The other day I said that in a population where 40% of us die of one disease, in this case cancer or heart attacks, it is clear that all of us are diseased. We have 100,000 new cases of colon cancer a year. It means that all of us are targets for cancer of the colon. Why some of us can metabolize cholesterol differently when we are on the same diet is a problem that may take many years to resolve. But I believe that this whole problem of chronic disease etiology that led to these lifestyle variants in which diet plays such a complicated role can only be changed by what I call managerial medicine. The example that Dr. Malmros just gave us from Sweden is a case in point. Sweden has reduced disease not only by diet, but by adding iron and vitamins to flour. Sweden is an example for all of us to follow. People may say many unkind things about Swedish social democracy, but one thing you can say very positively is that it's a function of our society to see that we live a life and have an environment that is as healthy as possible because, as I've stressed, we as individuals will always have to have a problem. We think it cannot happen to us, but society and politics must give us an environment that is healthy, in which we can enjoy a useful longevity, and I would certainly agree with Dr. Watkins when he says that to reach a society is a job for our governments.

DR. RHOADS: I have one announcement and one gratuity. After a wonderful morning of learning how we should live, I can't help thinking of a previous rebellious younger generation whose spokesman was Edna St. Vincent Millay. She wrote "My candle burns at both ends, and will not last the night; but ah my foes and oh my friends, it gives a lovely light." To those of you here, for I know that most of you burn your candle at both ends, I hope that you will go out and enjoy your lunch without too much attention to what's been heard.

CONTRIBUTIONS OF AMERICAN INDUSTRY TO THE IMPROVEMENT OF AMERICAN NUTRITION

William O. Beers and John F. White

Kraft, Inc.
Glenview, Illinois 60025

In order to assess any contributions to improved nutrition, it obviously is first necessary to define the term "good nutrition" itself. Here we have a dilemma, for there are probably nearly as many definitions of "good nutrition" as there are nutritionists. However, I think most will agree that a balanced selection from a variety of food products, all consumed in moderation, is a reasonable base for a nutritious diet.

American industry's greatest contribution in this area has been that of making a wide selection of food products which are consistent in quality and reasonable in price, available on a year-round basis. This may sound somewhat prosaic, especially after the sophisticated, scientific, and technological reports presented here. However, the food-processing and supply chain that has been established by industry in the United States is a tremendous accomplishment, unmatched anywhere else in the world.

Certainly, there are specific contributions in the areas of enrichment, fortification, restoration, and supplementation to which industry can point with pride. Elimination of certain deficiency diseases is an important accomplishment as well. Also, the wide range of product types, with varying caloric and fat content, different degrees of processing, all contribute to the basic achievement of providing choices for the consumer.

In the kind of food distribution system we have established and hope will continue to function, freedom of choice is inherent. This freedom puts the responsibility for choice squarely on the consumer. However, industry recognizes its responsibility to help educate each consumer on how to make the best possible choice. The food industry also recognizes its continuing responsibility to provide new and modified products as progress is made toward a better understanding of human nutrition.

At this Bicentennial Conference, which observes the beginning of American political independence, we would like to draw your attention to the bicentennial of another event which significantly influenced the way in which the food industry has been able to affect American nutrition during these past 200 years. We refer, of course, to the publication of *The Wealth of Nations,* in which Adam Smith defined the basic laissez-faire capitalist economic system. This is essentially the same system under which the American food industry operates today. His classic analysis of the processes of the marketplace, and his observations concerning the conditions under which companies produce and sell goods and services are, in many respects, as valid today as they were in 1776.

Before discussing specific contributions of American industry to the improvement of public nutrition, I would like to comment briefly on the circumstances in which a food manufacturer must operate within our economic system, beginning with the dynamic relationship between scientists, food manufacturers, and consumers.

In effect, the relationship works as follows: On one hand is the scientific and academic community telling consumers what they *should* eat; on the other are the consumers telling one and all what they *want* to eat. In between is the food industry, trying to satisfy both groups and itself as well.

The interaction between these three is the determining factor in the improvement of American nutrition. The key to cooperation and mutual understanding is full and open communication.

In discussing the function of research and development for a large food manufacturing corporation, it is important to emphasize the developmental aspects of this activity. Research and development programs throughout the food industry serve as bridges, bringing the results of basic research to the public, whose needs we all serve. In fact, the entire food industry—and that includes the farmer, the processor, the distributor and the retailer alike—is needed to provide the transition from nutrition theory to nutrition practice. Until businessmen actually implement a nutrition concept by carrying it through the necessary stages into a marketable food product, there is little chance of that concept ever leaving the laboratory.

A requirement of the process is that a product must be marketed profitably. Business must produce significant, practical results, generally in the form of profits, or it cannot survive. Because of this imperative, an understanding of profit system is essential to the cooperation needed in working toward our common goal. That goal is an adequate, satisfying, and nutritious diet that all can afford.

Although the role of corporate profit is frequently misunderstood in this country, its importance cannot be overstated. Profit enables a company to maintain and expand its business, to conduct research, to provide jobs, to be responsive to investors, and to contribute to the general welfare through taxes and voluntary gifts. Profit, literally, is the vital commodity on which everything else business hopes to achieve must depend.

The very system by which food is gathered, prepared, and distributed to consumers throughout the United States and other developed nations, by any standard a major achievement, is fueled by profit. Thus, profit is an integral aspect of the food industry's ability to improve public nutrition.

I believe that the providing of a wide range of products within the framework of free competitive enterprise is an essential feature of efforts to improve nutrition. This process is further enhanced by the feedback which consumers continually provide to industry through their purchases. Not all people will adopt a diet simply because they have been told it is good for them, nor can they be regimented to adopt a diet except under extreme circumstances.

In an article published last year, two eminent nutritionists wrote: "While scientists may be uniquely qualified to define nutritional targets and goals, they sometimes are strangely unsophisticated in discussing the means to be used in reaching these objectives. Their models seem almost uniformly to be based on considerations that are applicable only under conditions of total war and are carried out by a well-informed government, a large and well-organized bureaucracy, and a highly disciplined population (such as in Britain during World War II)." [1]

Such schemes, which are based on prolonged nationwide rationing, are not satisfactory models for peacetime food and nutrition policies in any country, wealthy or poor, the authors point out. The key to ultimate breakdown of rationing is the consumer, who may be willing to endure inconvenience during war or revolution, but is loath to do so indefinitely. Regardless of which economic or political system is involved, the same authors go on to say: "It is a misconception to believe, incidentally, that the centrally planned economies of Eastern Europe and Asia have succeeded in implementing nondemand nutrition policies while the capitalistic countries have lagged behind. . . . It is a gross oversimplification to believe that a centrally planned socialistic economy means that problems of demand have been eliminated and that supply is automatically adjusted 'to each according to his needs.' " [1]

This is an accurate observation, and its message is familiar to businessmen. The message is this: The success or acceptability of any product is determined not in the laboratory but in the marketplace. Kraft products alone are purchased by an estimated 80 million consumers every week. For us, and for other food processors as well, the jury is always out.

It is industry's responsibility to provide new or improved food products that fill the consumer's needs and wants. There is an important difference between need and want. In fact, consumers need the best possible nutritional value in the foods they buy, but what they want is often quite different. Nutritional value is but one aspect of the consumer's wants; the other criteria include taste appeal, convenience, and cost. Also, food purchasing decisions are strongly influenced by habit, custom, and tradition.

The market is an impartial referee, without favorites among competing companies. Given the need to succeed in the marketplace and consumer reluctance to change established eating habits, it is easy to understand the high failure rate for new products. Some surveys will show that the average conversion rate of new food product ideas to successful new food product introductions can be as low as 4 percent, or less. This low success rate places a heavy burden on the research and development function. To improve these heavy odds, food companies employ marketing research techniques to reduce guesswork by determining in advance which ideas are likely to succeed before money is spent to develop them into products.

To summarize then, the guidelines that have a major influence on the food industry's efforts to improve nutrition are, first the need to earn a profit; second, the consumer's frequent reluctance to change his eating habits; and third, the generally low success rate for new products. Does this mean that the task is hopeless, that programs within the private sector to improve nutrition cannot succeed? Quite the contrary is true, for business has been, and quite likely will continue to be, the chief agent of progress in this vital area.

Now let's look at some of the ways by which U.S. food companies have improved nutrition in the past, and mention some current programs that offer promise for the future.

The food industry had its origins in the period when America ceased to be a nation of rural communities and began the shift to urbanization. To use a contemporary term, the food industry came into being as a result of a basic change in our nation's life-style.

From the beginning, the food industry applied basic scientific knowledge to its products. As knowledge of food and nutrition expanded through research, industry kept pace by incorporating the results into new and exciting products. Similarly, as American life-styles continued to change, industry met that challenge as well. A single illustration will make this point clear.

A critical nutritional problem in our country is that of obesity. We are told by health authorities that fully 25 percent of all Americans are significantly overweight. We no longer require the large intake of calories that were needed in earlier times, when physical labor was common. The food industry has responded to this change with a variety of new products that contain fewer calories and lower levels of fats and carbohydrates. This pattern of successful problem solving, followed by the emergence of fresh challenges from previous solutions, has been repeated often within the food industry.

Since the 1930's, industry has fortified and enriched conventional foods by the addition of essential nutrients. There is no question of the value of these efforts in substantially reducing the incidence of many deficiency diseases, including beriberi, ariboflavinosis, pellagra, and endemic goiter. The last-named offers a classic example. Once the relationship between goiter and iodine deficiency was diagnosed, it was relatively simple to fortify our salt supply. Again, industry involvement was the key to the distribution of this important addition to the consumer's diet.

Freezing has long been recognized as an excellent way of preserving food, leaving much of its original nutritional value intact for prolonged periods of time. The application of this technology to fruits and vegetables is a direct result of the pioneering efforts of the Birdseye organization, beginning as far back as 1929. Since World War II, the frozen food industry has assumed major importance in the eating habits of the American consumer.

To step outside the United States for a moment, several recent studies have called attention to the fresh vegetable deficiency in the average Canadian's diet. Kraft has done extensive consumer education in that country, with informational advertising that urged the consumer to use fresh vegetables. For us, of course, our corporate goal was the increased use of our salad dressing products. We believe our efforts have contributed to the 17.3 percent increase in apparent consumption of fresh vegetables during a recent 2-year period in Canada.[2]

It is fair to say, we believe, that food technology is an area that falls within the expertise of the food industry. Beyond the actual manufacturing of food itself, industry utilizes technology in other areas, including transportation, distribution, packaging, and the various marketing skills that are essential in our economy.

Within the field of applied science, which is a major part of corporate technology, opportunities for nutrition advances can be developed through new uses for byproducts. At Kraft, for example, the disposal of whey is a formidable task. From our own cheese manufacturing operations alone, we produce more than 3 billion pounds of whey annually. This amount would fill 20,000 railroad tank cars, making up a single train more than 265 miles long. Whey is rich in lactose, minerals, and vitamins. It contains lactalbumin—a biologically superior form of protein—and traces of fat. These are important nutrients, which could be lost unless ways are found to utilize their value to the company and to the consumer.

Whey has been an important ingredient in animal feed supplements for years; lately, it has been adapted for human consumption in a variety of forms. Yeast grown on whey to produce single cell protein may become a significant alternate raw food material. Other uses have been found for whey, usually in combination with other ingredients, until finally, that 265-mile-long train has been dramatically shortened.

Notwithstanding the best efforts of the scientific community and industry to improve our nation's nutrition, the final responsibility rests with the individual consumer. Delegation of this responsibility to agencies of the government is not consistent with a belief in the authority of the individual. Also, from a purely pragmatic point of view, as we indicated earlier, there is some question as to whether nutrition programs imposed by government decree can permanently succeed.

As an example of the wide variety of products that industry can offer the consumer from which to choose, our company sells a broad line of milk and dairy products, each with its own nutritional characteristics. Some are strictly traditional, while others are reduced in fat content. Offering the consumer this variety to choose from is a fundamental principle of the marketplace. It also is part of the concept of liberty in a free society.

In return, however, the food industry's standards must equal or exceed those of the public agencies that seek to regulate it. Because it is closer to the production, preservation, and distribution of our nation's food supply, industry must shoulder the responsibility for its quality. A company's franchise in the market is based on a balanced scale: public confidence in the company's products and the company's continued respect for the consumer's judgment.

This does not, however, preclude us from guiding the consumer in appropriate ways to what we believe are sound and healthy eating habits. In general, we advocate the use of our products in balanced combination with other foods. Consumer education programs have been a major thrust of food companies for many years, and we will cite several examples later.

It is encouraging to note growing interest among consumers in the nutritional values of their food. The nutrition labeling program, which was initiated by industry in recent years, has been a step in the right direction, but we still need much better methods for conveying essential information in terms the consumer can understand and use. The listing of ingredients without explanatory or supporting data has been compared to announcing the score of a ball game without telling the listener which teams played and who won. We think the caloric values, which currently appear on food labels, represent the only information which consumers can use effectively.

Where do consumers turn for nutrition information? A nationwide study, published by the U.S. Department of Agriculture, revealed a number of sources from which respondents learned about nutrition. These sources included, in descending order of importance, high schools, newspapers and magazines, mothers or grandmothers, and grade schools.[3] Only 7 percent named doctors or other professional sources. It is surprising that America's physicians are generally a poor source of nutritional counseling for their patients, but this seems to be true. It has been estimated that only about half of the nation's medical schools offer nutrition training that might be considered adequate.[4]

Clearly, consumer information and education programs are important aspects of the overall task and are recognized as such by many companies and industry associations. For Kraft, these efforts are largely a matter of enlightened self-interest, for by helping consumers to eat properly, we help ourselves. We do not wish to hold our own company up as a model, because other food manufacturers are making valuable contributions to the total effort, but let us indicate what Kraft is doing.

We mentioned service advertising as a vehicle for nutrition education. To supplement this outreach, Kraft has a school program, now in its 17th year. This program provides a wide variety of materials for teachers of nutrition, consumer education, home economics, and related courses. A series of comprehensive teaching kits and films have been produced and made available to the nation's schools. Through these media, facts on food production and quality, nutrition, packaging, labeling, and home preparation are presented. It is estimated that we contribute to the knowledge and training of more than half of America's 25 million teenagers.[5] And, our high schools, as mentioned earlier, are the nation's chief source of nutrition knowledge.

As a result of an industry-associated activity beyond our company, milk consumption rose dramatically among a group of teenagers after special training by the Dairy Council of California. Working through junior high school teachers, the Council introduced a program to instruct teenagers on how to balance their diets nutritionally, regardless of where they eat—at home, in school, or at a fast food outlet. Tests show that exactly 75 percent of the students increased their consumption of milk and dairy foods to the recommended level of four servings a day. Further, they were almost unanimous in their approval of the program.[5]

Efforts such as these, and there are many equally commendable, can succeed in transforming established eating preferences into individual programs of sound nutrition.

To substantiate the observations made earlier, we would like to summarize the conclusions reached in a comprehensive report on the food industry that was prepared for the United States Senate Select Committee on Nutrition and Human Needs.[6] The report notes that the food industry is the sole provider of a large variety of fresh, frozen, canned and dry-packaged foods available in population centers that are located far from sources of the raw food materials, both geographically and seasonally. This, in fact, is the enduring basis of industry's contribution to improved nutrition. Within its complex structure, the industry performs basic functions of maintaining supplies of safe, high-quality food to meet continuing consumer demands. As we have said, a wide variety of foods is essential to good nutrition, and the committee noted that it is the exception rather than the rule when problems develop in connection with the availability of this diverse food supply.

Finally, while we strive to attain perfect knowledge about nutrition, we must work cooperatively to make effective use of what we have already learned. To that end, industry will continue to support scientists and researchers in their basic laboratory work and in speaking out on their findings. And within our own corporations, we will continue to make use of advances in nutrition knowledge in producing improved food products and promoting their use. This has been the pattern of the past and it will continue.

REFERENCES

1. DWYER, J. T. & JEAN MAYER. 1975. Beyond economics and nutrition: The complex basis of food policy. Science : 566.
2. Statistics Canada Catalog No. 32–226.
3. U.S. DEPARTMENT OF AGRICULTURE. 1976. Homemakers' Food and Nutrition Knowledge, Practices and Opinions. Home Economics Research Report No. 39. Government Printing Office. Washington, D.C.
4. 1976. Recommendations for raising national nutrition and health levels. Food Prod. Dev. : 54.
5. 1976. Teenagers, learning nutrition skills, drinking more milk. Am. Dairy Rev. : 8–9.
6. U.S. SENATE SELECT COMMITTEE ON NUTRITION AND HUMAN NEEDS. 1974. National Nutrition Policy: The Food Industry—Its Resources and Activities in Food Production and Nutrition, a working paper prepared by Cynthia B. Chapman. Government Printing Office. Washington, D.C.

ADDITIVES IN OUR FOOD SUPPLY

Sanford A. Miller

Department of Nutrition and Food Science
Massachusetts Institute of Technology
Cambridge, Massachusetts 02139

For a civilization to flourish, it must, in some way, establish and maintain control over the environment in which it exists. One of the major factors in the environment is food.

Food has always been a determinant of civilization. The first need mankind had to satisfy, even before shelter, protection and defenses, was his need for food. Eight thousand years ago, Neolithic man was able to develop the arts of masonry, pottery, and weaving *only* after he had become a food cultivator rather than a hunter and food gatherer.

But mankind had to move a step further before his culture could truly begin the long march to civilization. For farming alone did not remove all of the uncertainties of a food supply. Insecurity of weather, agricultural pests and diseases and,most of all, the lack of a stable distribution system and an inability to store food against the future still kept man locked to the soil, existing from year to year with no sense of future security. More importantly, this sustenance level of food production could not permit any significant number of people to do anything but produce food.

The first step to modify this situation was in the area of crop improvement. Plant varieties such as wheat and barley, foods that were readily stored and transported, were developed not by pure chance alone but, conceivably, as a means of protecting against future famines and freeing man's mind from the drudgery of the soil.

The introduction of processing techniques such as drying and baking were also important contributions to the process of increasing storage life, permitting development of reserves and allowing transportation of food over significant distances. The discovery that the addition of several chemical materials such as salt or vinegar would also permit longer storage and better distribution was one of the most significant contributions to this process. The result of these developments in storage and distribution was the rise of the great civilization of the past, for when all men did not have to raise food for individual needs, when only a part of the population was required to maintain a consistent food supply, the remainder were free to use their minds for other purposes, to congregate, interact, and found cities.

Thus, early in his existence on this planet, man had learned a fundamental rule of reciprocity still in existence today: as man is able to control the production, storage, and distribution of foods, so is he able to enhance the arts and sciences. And as he advances the arts and sciences, so is he able to control better his food supply by improving the production, storage, and distribution of foods.

The capacity to produce "surplus" food and to store and transport it, and the need to supply increasing "urban" populations led to the development of and increasing dependence on a third party in the food chain, intermediate between producer and consumer. Originating as millers and transporters of grain, the food processing industry really became of significance with the introduction of new preservation methods and the discovery of chemical additives. With these, greater variety and amounts of food could be supplied over a greater distance, providing for the consumer potentially more nutritious and more easily handled products. Thus it is not surprising that the first great merchants of the past were millers and later brokers of food. Even more importantly, the control of this aspect of the food system was earlier, and, in the middle ages played a major role in the religious communities.

Thus it seems clear that the introduction of chemical additives was not only an important step in man's attempts to control his environment and thus a contribution to the growth of civilization but was also an action that was almost

TABLE 1

CONTROL OF THE FOOD ENVIRONMENT
PRESERVATION TECHNIQUES

	Time for General Introduction
A. Past	
1. Drying	Centuries
2. Smoking	,,
3. Fermentation	,,
4. Salting	,,
5. Pickling	,,
6. Spices	
B. Present	
1. Canning	Decades
2. Refrigeration and Freezing	,,
3. Synthetic Additives	,,
4. Packaging	
C. Future	
1. Radiation	Years
2. Fabricated Foods	,,
3. New Additives	,,

as old as mankind itself. As shown in TABLE 1, early man had several options open to him. For example, he could preserve his flesh foods by smoking, thus introducing a whole series of organic materials to his food. He could dry the product or add alcohol by fermentation or add salt or vinegar. In the classical period, the use of spices and herbs to prevent spoilage and improve palatability added new dimensions to his armamentarium of approaches.

In more modern times, the development of thermal processing techniques at the end of the 18th century gave new impetus to the drive to control this aspect of the environment. With the later introduction of economical and reliable refrigeration and freezing techniques, the capacity of the industry to store and distribute food products expanded enormously and led, in part, to the increasing movement of people to the cities as well as increasing dependence of people on the industry to provide them with this most basic of needs. On the part of industry, these new techniques demanded new means of preserving quality or improving efficiency. With the rise in organic chemistry, new additives became available for this purpose in response to the need.

In the future, techniques already in the lab or pilot plants offer not only the possibility of even greater available food supplies but also the need for even more additives of new capability.

The rise in the capacity of the food industry to do its job is unquestionably one of the most dramatic examples of technologic success. But this success itself has given rise to the set of problems faced by the industry today. In general, these problems are concerned with the questions of safety and wholesomeness of foods. The public is beginning to question its food supply based on an increasing feeling of uncertainty. Are the "chemicals" we add to our "pure" food safe? they ask. Will they cause cancer, produce monsters or, perhaps, cause my hair to fall out? The result of this uneasiness has been the rise of consumer activist activity and increasing demand for greater control over industry.

Is there reason for this concern? Or, more importantly perhaps, why has the perception of food and its associated industry fallen in the precipitous manner it has? Several factors may have contributed to the problem.

First is the question of time. As shown in TABLE 1, the introduction of new techniques and, more importantly, new additives, took centuries in the past. Thus, society had extensive experience with them, and since few were introduced at a time, dislocation in prejudice was relatively slight. Even more importantly, greater experience in terms of hazard was possible, based on direct human experience. Thus, relatively few people were harmed by an acutely toxic product, and thus it could be removed before general introduction.

In more recent times, the time scale of introduction has been contracted even further. Decades or less are all that is necessary for the exposure to new materials to become widespread. The time for experience has become short, too short to be used as a basis for judging hazard. These perceptions of the problem led, in my opinion, to the establishment and proliferation of the food regulations in this country and to the development of the concept of toxicity testing in animals. It is important to note, however, that the testing approach was originally designed to deal with acute effects and, even today, is concerned with the elucidation of clearly definable toxic responses.

The problem will become even more acute in the near future when the time of introduction becomes even shorter as a result of better communications and distribution. Under these conditions, no reliance can be placed on "experience" since before any such "experience" can be obtained it is probable that major portions of the population will be exposed to the new material. Moreover, the nature of these new products, for example fabricated foods, offers increasing problems of combination and amounts of additives that have not been considered in the past.

Second is the problem of the exponential rise in numbers and diversity of such additives. For the first 90% of the time of their use, the number of additives generally in use probably did not exceed 50, including spices and flavorers. Today there are over 2000.[1] Their variety and functional use is legion; and, of equal importance, they represent an enormous volume of use (TABLE 2). Thus, the number and quantity of such materials has increased so enormously that actual levels of exposure become important criteria in determining safety, based

TABLE 2

MAJOR CLASSES OF FOOD ADDITIVES (1967) AND THEIR USE IN U.S.*

Item	Quantity Lb./Millions	Value $ Million
Preservatives	37.0	14.9
Antioxidants	15.5	20.5
Sequestrants	0.3	0.1
Surfactants	162.5	46.6
Stabilizers—thickeners	306.5	86.9
Acidulants	101.5	25.0
Leavening agents	113.0	8.6
Food colors	81.1	19.4
Nutrient supplements	19.4	10.1
Flavoring materials	174.5	140.0
Flavor enhancers—potentiators	43.8	22.5
Basic taste modifiers	2.7	5.0
Enzymes	N/A	19.7
Functional protein additives	222.0	37.1
Miscellaneous (including sorbital, anticaking agents, yeast foods, and dough conditioners)	68.7	16.0
Total	1,348.5	472.4
Average/Lb.		35¢

* ADL estimates based on field interviews.

not only on a single use of the substance but on multiple uses in multiple products.

The third problem is concerned with the perception of the concept of "toxicity." In general, the industry and the public tend to view toxicity of additives in the pharmacologic sense, i.e., a substance that demonstrates potential to adversely affect health.[2] The problem lies in the definition. For the professional and the industry, this is related to a clearly definable abnormal response capable of being quantitated and compared statistically. For the public, this may mean something considerably less precise, more associated with a feeling of well being rather than with any specific pathologic lesion. This is largely the result of our increased lifespan and control over some aspects of our health environment. The general availability of food, the decreasing lack of danger from acute environmental hazards such as infectious disease, have led to a decrease in concern over lifespan and an increase in demand for a better way of life in which health and happiness are equated. When this concern is extended "even unto the future generation," the problem facing the development of model systems to test these possibilities becomes awe inspiring. It is this difference in the perception of safety that, I believe, lies at the root of the problem dividing professional and public. The professional offers safety from hazards he can measure based upon traditional approaches to *relatively* acute known pathology; the public demands safety so that their life and that of their descendants can be healthy, happy, and complete. For them the question is not whether they will live to 90 but rather *how* they will live to 90.

The matter is made even more complex by the phenomenally rapid development of knowledge in molecular biology and other areas associated with the exploration of life processes. These have, in part based upon the incompleteness of our knowledge, given rise to fears and questions concerning the subtle effects of additives in food on these most basic aspects of life without offering reliable methods of studying these effects and predicting accurately their importance to human welfare. Thus, it presents another amorphous contribution to the disquiet of the consumer.

In large measure then, the public is asking for measurements of safety that begin to approximate the noise level of the system itself, that is, levels equivalent to and perhaps surpassing the toxicity of naturally occurring materials. That these substances themselves can be diverse and widespread is suggested by the list shown in TABLE 3, itself representative and by no means complete. Nearly every food has in one way or another a toxic substance. It must be pointed out, however, that these are generally of low activity in their respective classes and that they are often inactivated or removed by processing. What is important, however, is that, for the public, they represent a basal level of acceptable risk and for the toxicologist should represent a goal towards which technology should strive.

The traditional approaches to the judgment of safety of food additives are shown in TABLE 4. With few exceptions, it is the list of techniques used to evaluate new substances. It is clear, I believe, that they do not completely approach the question raised by consumers concerning their perception of safety. Accepting this, one may ask if their application over the past several years has offered any degree or assurance of the safety of food additives at any levels.

For the past 5 years, the Select Committee on GRAS Substances of the Federation of American Societies for Experimental Biology has, under contract from FDA, been reviewing the safety of GRAS substances. These compounds designated as "Generally Recognized as Safe" occupy a unique position in the list of food additives and are among the most commonly used of these substances. The result has been the most comprehensive review of the safety of any group of environmental compounds yet performed and has offered to the Committee members a unique experience in this field. One result of this review was the development of a document outlining areas of concern and suggestions

TABLE 3

NATURALLY OCCURRING TOXIC SUBSTANCES

Substance	Food
A. Goitrogens	Turnip, Rutabaga, Cabbage
B. "Estrogens"	Palm Kernel
C. Tumorigens and Carcinogens	
1. Ergot (*C. purpurea*)	Rye
2. Yellow Rice (*P. islandicum*)	Rice
3. Aflatoxin (*A. flavus*)	Peanuts
4. Safrol	Sassafras
D. Hemagglutins	Legumes
E. Stimulants and Depressants	Nutmeg, Coffee, Tea, Tobacco
F. Pressor Amines	Cheese, Pineapple Juice, Plantains, Bananas
G. Cholinesterase Inhibitor	Eggplant, Valencia Orange
H. Seafood Toxins	Many

for future actions based on this experience.[3] Some of these conclusions bear on the questions raised earlier in this report.

First, there is no evidence of acute, major toxicological problem associated with the use of any of the additives reviewed by this Committee. This is not to say that questions were not raised about several of these substances, but rather, in each case, the problem was not knowing rather than conviction of hazard. Since, in the general opinion of the Committee, a conservative approach was prudent, suggestions were made for limitation of use of such substances or, in a limited number of cases, elimination from the diets of special groups in the population.

Yet, in spite of this extensive review, many questions remained. In part these were generally associated with the lack of information on several substances. For example, the number of references associated with specific compounds ranged from 20 or less in the case of carnauba wax to over 20,000 in the case of vitamin A and glutamic acid.[3] More importantly, important areas were not covered for many compounds, particularly the so-called natural products or derivatives. Information was deficient concerning fetal exposure, for example, for more than four-fifths of the substances reviewed. This was a

TABLE 4

TYPICAL TOXICOLOGICAL EVALUATION

1. Acute (7 days—high single dose)
2. Chronic (lifetime—continuous exposure)
3. Reproduction (2–3 generations—continuous exposure)
4. Mutagenesis (special protocols involving both *in vitro* and *in vivo* testing—(?))
5. Teratogenesis (exposure during critical periods of fetal development)
6. Carcinogenesis (related to mutagenesis studies but also special tissue examination during chronic studies)

particularly important consideration in view of the probability that most GRAS substances are consumed by at least some pregnant women. The matter is made more complex by the fact that most traditional multigenerational studies designed to test such compounds do not permit the observation of long-term effects in succeeding generations, inasmuch as the test animals are usually killed when they are 6 months of age.

Information concerning the hazard to the neonate and infant was also lacking for nearly all substances. The neonate stands peculiarly at risk when exposed to substances that may offer only minimal hazard to the adult. For many xenobiotic substances, major shifts in toxicity have been found between neonate and adult.[4] In addition to the fact that many such substances pass readily into milk,[5] the modern tendency to early weaning and the introduction of the infant to table foods during the first months of life [6] has increased the urgency with which studies of the direct effect of such additives on the neonate must be performed.

The problems of evaluating carcinogenicity hazard are another major area of concern. Not only is there lack of agreement among professionals concerning the adequacy of test protocols, but more importantly there is a central conceptual issue concerning the threshold effect for such substances. Is there a "no effect" level for carcinogens as there is for other substances, or are these unique in that the presence of any number of such active molecules offers danger to cellular organization? Thus the conclusion of carcinogenesis is a difficult judgmental matter in which the lack of agreement among "experts" has led to increasing public concern.

Although practically all guidelines for toxicological testing for food additives call for teratologic observation (TABLE 4), the translation of results from experimental animal to human experience is still in a primitive state. For example, in a recent compilation of over 600 agents producing congenital abnormality in animals, only about 20 are known to cause human defects.[7] Not only do different species react differently, but even different members of the same litter are dissimilar in reaction. When these uncertainties are combined with the newly awakened public concern over the welfare of future generations, the question of teratogenic hazard becomes an important and significant contribution to uneasiness.

Additional questions may be raised about many other issues, such as the problem of estimating exactly how much of each additive the public is exposed to, what margin of safety is to be used, and so on. In each case, however, these all are important in the evaluation of two essential points. First, how much risk is the consumer assuming by the use of the substance and for what benefit? This concept of risk-benefit ratio has become an institutional magic phrase that appears to suggest some quantitative way of automatically determining whether or not a substance should be used in food. While of great value in assessing the use of therapeutic and prophylactic agents, its application to the problems of food additives is much more difficult. The fact that the levels of hazard in the use of such materials are so low, and, for many substances, information is lacking, and the fact that there are no good techniques for evaluating health as the public probably views it, make the assignment of an order of magnitude for risk difficult. On the other hand, agreement on the relative value of the various benefits resulting from the use of such substances is also difficult to attain. Thus, the establishment of adequate quantitation of each of the terms of such an equation is really not likely at the present time. The acceptance of the concept in general terms does provide a framework, however vague, for judgmental considerations.

The second point concerns the question of how much regulation is required for the industry. In the first place, the unique position of the food industry as a principal maintainer of urban civilization and concomitant dependence of the public on its activity makes the need for public control of its actions unquestionable. In addition, this increasing dependence, coupled with decreasing freedom of choice on the part of consumers in excluding particular ingredients in their food, also supports the argument for governmental control of the industry. In contrast to these arguments is the danger that increasing restriction of options for the industry leading to rigorous control will also lead to reduction in innovation, a commodity much in demand in this world of increasing population and limited food. It should also be pointed out that, for biological systems, the ultimate in rigor is death. The determination of the proper amount of regulation to satisfy both of these needs requires accurate estimates of hazard to man. Without them, prudent bureaucracy will respond properly with greater and more severe restriction.

Even if all these questions were answered or answerable, and even if the public and professional agree on the definitions of risk, benefit and hazard,

404   Annals New York Academy of Sciences

there would still exist a major problem of credibility of the industry. Beginning from a position of the highest status and one in which public trust was implicit, the industry today occupies a position in which few of its claims are accepted by the public. Moreover, this reputation has so spread that individuals associated with or supported by the industry come under suspicion. Perhaps, the problem began at the turn of the century, when it became more important to determine what to say about a food product rather than to become concerned about what was in it or for what it was to be used. The growth of merchandising and marketing influence on food company policy has, in my opinion, led to many of the problems of trust and confidence that the industry faces today.

The current public concern over the use of additives in our food supply is then based upon several considerations. The reduced time for introduction, the increased number and amount of each in use, the growing dependence on the industry and the concurrent reduction in freedom of choice, the change in emphasis from questions of survival to those of a better life not only for ourselves but for future generations, the lack of information on many materials, and the lack of agreement among experts all contribute to the problem. To argue that many of these are based on public ignorance or "activism" begs the issue. In the end, it is the public that must decide its future and its needs, and it is the responsibility of the industry and the professional to satify these requirements. The public must also decide whether it wants to pay directly or indirectly for the development of techniques adequate to fulfill its expectations and desires and, if so, to insist that its legislators honor this request.

The problem of industry credibility is also one of concern. To solve it, the industry must begin to develop a greater sense of its own responsibility and importance to the community. The question must not only be one of satisfaction of legal requirements but more of satisfaction of public responsibility not only in toxicity testing but also in advertising, merchandising, and public information.

The fact is that the provision of a safe, constant, and highly acceptable food supply requires the conscientious efforts of both public and industry working together as partners, not adversaries. We have perhaps permitted legalistics to interfere too often with this natural alliance of consumer and industry. The establishment of a center, operated by a board of trustees consisting of industry, government, academic and legislative and consumer representatives, whose function would be to establish and perhaps perform new, unique, and innovative evaluation of the safety of food additives, could go a long way towards solving these problems of mutual trust. Moreover, such a center supported by both government and industrial funds, staffed by the best people in the field, whose entire activity was public, could provide a new basis for ensuring the future of our food supply. In the end, it is this last goal that may prove to be the most important sustainer of our civilization.

REFERENCES

1. NATIONAL RESEARCH COUNCIL, Food and Nutrition Board. 19655. Chemicals Used in Food Processing, Publ. 1274, National Academy of Sciences, Washington, D.C.
2. CHRISTIANSEN, H. E. & T. T. LUGINBYHC. 1975. Registry of Toxic Effects of Chemical Substances. Contract No. CDC 99–74–92. Dept. Health, Education, & Welfare. Government Printing Office. Washington, D.C.
3. SELECT COMMITTEE ON GRAS SUBSTANCES. 1977. Evaluation of health aspects of

food additives: Lessons learned and questions unanswered. Fed. Proc. In press.

4. GOLDENTHAL, E. I. 1971. A compilation of LD$_{50}$ values in newborn and adult animals. Toxicol. Appl. Pharmacol. **18:** 185–207.
5. CATZ, C. S. & G. P. GIACOIA. 1972. Drugs and breast milk. Ped. Clin. N. Am. **19:** 151–166.
6. FOMON, S. J. 1974. Infant Nutrition. 2nd edit. Saunders. Philadelphia, Pa.
7. SHEPARD, T. H. 1973. Catalog of Teratogenic Agents. John Hopkins Univ. Press. Baltimore, Md.

GOVERNMENTAL REGULATORY DIFFICULTIES

John E. Vanderveen

Division of Nutrition
Bureau of Foods
Food and Drug Administration
Washington, D.C. 20204

The Food and Drug Administration under the Federal Food, Drug, and Cosmetic Act and at least nine other laws has the mandate to regulate the nutritional quality of the national food supply and to protect consumers by assuring that food products under FDA's jurisdiction are safe and conform to labeled claims. These objectives are achieved through the following regulatory activities:

1. Setting standards for product composition, manufacturer, and labeling.
2. Conducting inspections, surveys, and analyses to monitor compliance with statutory requirements and administratively set standards.
3. Initiating enforcement action where necessary to effect compliance with the laws and implementing regulations.
4. Informing and educating industry and consumers about the requirements of our laws and regulations.

Food is just one of a vast number of products regulated by the FDA. Other products include human drugs including vaccines, blood and its derivatives, medical devices, radiation-emitting instruments, animal drugs and feeds, and, of course, cosmetics. The problems facing the agency in regulating all these products are many and very complex. This presentation is limited to those problems associated with the regulation of the nutritional qualities of foods. The scope of this activity is massive, for foods make up annually more than three-fourths the $145 billion of products FDA regulates. This regulatory authority extends far beyond the producers, manufacturers, and distributors of food and includes concern over other types of products, such as chemicals that have the potential for contaminating foods through air pollution, water pollution, interaction with packaging material, and other means. For example, lead, cadmium, and other heavy metals from industrial activity can enter the food supply and have an impact on the nutritional quality of foods.

Obviously, such vast breadth of responsibility presents many critical pathways for the evolution and enforcement of regulations. These include the availability of scientific and technical information, knowledge about consumer needs and desires, efficient and productive means for rule-making, ability to enforce the laws and regulations, and resources to conduct all of the associated activities. All of these factors are at some time or other difficulties in governmental regulatory activity.

Perhaps the most fundamental deficiency in carrying out the mandates for assuring the nutritional quality of the food supply is the lack of scientific and technical information. In order to regulate the nutritional quality of the food supply, nutritional regulatory policy has to be established, and in order to establish nutritional regulatory policy, knowledge about both the nutritional status of the population and the nutrient quality of the food supply must be known. To meet these requirements the Food and Drug Administration has depended heavily and has become the primary government user of such surveys as the USDA Household Food Consumption Survey and the Health and Nutrition Evaluation Surveys (HANES). We also use data from commercial sources, such as the Market Research Corporation of America and others. We also have funded the creation of the National Nutrition Data Bank, and we conduct substantial intramural research to provide critical data. Despite this level of activity, FDA frequently lacks sufficient data to clearly define appropriate regulatory policy. Added to this dilemma is the fact that frequently consumer activists, scientists, and manufacturers overextend the use of data beyond scientific merit. Consequently, many times demands for regulatory action are generated, when sufficient information for sound regulation does not exist. The solution to this problem can only come through an increase of research activity to provide scientific and technical data. The cost of obtaining such data is high. Safety testing for food additives now cost in excess of one-half million dollars. The cost for such studies is generally paid by the petitioner, who expects to recover his investment by selling the product to the consumer. In some areas such as foods for special dietary use, the prospects for a manufacturer recovering the large developmental and testing cost are small. To fill consumer needs for such products, support for development and testing will likely have to be derived from the public as well as the private sector.

Recently, the FDA has encountered concerns relative to the integrity of some data submitted in response to a food additive petition. Congress has responded to this problem by providing the agency with increased resources to inspect laboratories which submit data to FDA. However, it is unlikely that any reasonable level of inspection will assure absolute integrity of data. What is needed is that scientific societies, industrial societies, and other professional organizations initiate procedures to set standards, conduct inspections, and level sanctions for those who repeatedly fail to meet acceptable levels of performance. Unfortunately, there has been a significant loss in public confidence as a result of what might have been and hopefully was a very rare exception to the way that testing and evaluation has been conducted in this country.

Perhaps the most significant problem for any regulatory agency is to be capable of changing policy when circumstances surrounding establishment of such policy change. This is particularly true for FDA in the food area. Food habits of the population are changing. We can expect changes in the food supply which are partly brought on by consumer demands and partly by economic considerations which result from such things as the energy crisis and the increased world population. The regulatory process must, therefore, be flexible so that regulations will be relevant and responsive to societies' needs.

Many of FDA's least productive proceedings have been the result of the cumbersome and unwieldy statutory framework within which we must operate. Perhaps the most flagrant examples of agency action being needlessly delayed or frustrated have involved "rule-making on the record" proceedings subject to Section 701(e) of the Federal Food, Drug, and Cosmetic Act. That provision requires that agency rules promulgated under seven different sections of the act undergo an incredibly lengthy process before they become final. The process is divided into several parts.

First, a notice of proposed rule-making, setting forth the proposed rule and providing an opportunity for interested persons to comment in writing is published. After considering the comments, the commissioner publishes an "order" in the *Federal Register*, acting upon the proposal. Up to this point, the procedure resembles informal rule-making. This order may not be final, however, because any person adversely affected by it may file objections, and the filing of objections operates to stay the portions of the order objected to. If no objections are filed, or if the objections filed are legally insufficient to warrant a hearing, a notice to that effect can be published and the order then becomes effective. Most rule-making proceedings under Section 701(e) end at this stage.

Where legally sufficient objections to an order are filed, however, the agency must conduct a formal adjudicatory proceeding on the stayed portions of the order before an administrative law judge. Any interested person may appear and participate either in person or by representative. Sworn testimony is taken, either in writing or orally, and under certain circumstances, witnesses are subject to cross-examination by any participant. A stenographic transcript is prepared. The presiding officer then prepares a report to the commissioner complete with findings of fact and conclusions of law—in other words a recommended or initial decision.

On the basis of the record thus developed, the commissioner issues a tentative order, complete with detailed findings of fact and conclusions of law on which it is based. Any party on record may object to the tentative order and may request oral argument before the commissioner. After any oral argument, the commissioner publishes his final order containing the findings of fact on which the order is based. This order is reviewable in a court of appeals under the substantial evidence standard.

An example of this lengthy procedure can be found in the vitamin and mineral proceedings.

The "Food for Special Dietary Uses" proceedings grew out of FDA efforts to establish standards of identity and labeling requirements for vitamin and mineral products. The original notice of proposed rule-making was published in June of 1962, triggering over 50,000 comments. The vast majority of these were form letters from various health food groups; nevertheless, some offered important or serious suggestions and criticisms.

Had the proceeding been subject to notice and comment rule-making, the commissioner would have considered and analyzed these comments, and then issued his final order, terminating the administrative phase of the proceeding.

However, because the action fell under Section 701(e), the final order, which appeared in June of 1966, was stayed by objections by nearly 100 parties. Simultaneously, a lawsuit was brought by the Pharmaceutical Manufacturers Association, seeking to require that the entire action be reproposed. The Court of Appeals dismissed the suit in June of 1967.

The trial-type hearing required by Section 701(e) began in May of 1968. More than 100 independent parties, many with different and conflicting interests, filed notices of intent to participate. Despite efforts by the hearing examiner to bring some order to the chaos which inevitably occurs in any proceeding of that size, the hearing proved almost unmanageable. Witnesses were subjected to lengthy repetitious cross-examination by a myriad of parties, and many experts simply refused to testify for the Government because of the commitment of time.

By the time the hearing closed in 1970, more than 32,000 pages of testimony had been assembled. It is fair to say that little of this testimony was of use to the agency in promulgating the final regulation.

The hearing examiner issued his opinion in 1971. Opportunity then had to be given to the parties to object to the various findings. The FDA's final order appeared in August 1973. The order was appealed to the Court of Appeals, and in August 1974, the Second Circuit ruled in favor of FDA on most of the issues. However, it remanded the case to the Agency for the purpose of permitting further cross-examination of one of the 162 witnesses who had appeared. The hearing was reconvened in November 1975, and seven additional days of hearings were held merely to cross-examine one witness.

The administrative law judge issued his opinion on February 20, 1976. Parties then had an opportunity to submit exceptions to the ruling, and the final regulation was issued on October 19, 1976.

The Consumer Food Act of 1975 (S.641), currently before Congress, would revise the Section 701(e) procedures with the objective of minimizing the possibility of another vitamin-hearing debacle. It would reduce the current multistep procedure to a two-step one in which FDA would first publish a proposal, then receive comments and concurrently hold a hearing only on disputed factual issues, after which it would issue its final order. Furthermore, at the hearing, parties could be grouped according to their interests.

In the enforcement area there are two main difficulties. The first deals with analytical problems. As you are aware, food presents unique analytical problems not common to other biological materials. The state of current methodology prohibits differentiation between natural sources of material such as sugar versus that added. Similarly, it is difficult to differentiate between sources of protein or fat; without such methodology, regulations have little practical effect. Yet there are reasonable demands on the part of consumers for accurate information based on allergy or other considerations.

Resources are always a problem for any organization. The FDA is a small organization, and it operates on a small budget. However, our most serious problem is to get qualified people. It is important that the Agency maintain an ability to conduct good scientific research so that our scientists can avoid becoming perfunctory and we can continue to attract talented people. I might also add in this regard that current criticism of people entering the Agency from industry adds to the difficulty of attracting good people. True, there is the possibility that the consumers' interest may be compromised by the revolving-door phenomenon; however, in terms of individual integrity, I find it difficult to differentiate between employees having come from industry and those who have not had industry experience. On the other hand, the abilities of employees from industry are frequently superior to those who do not have industrial experience.

Although a recent poll shows that the FDA rates high with consumers (80% were generally familiar with the FDA, and 60% viewed the Agency favorably), we need more information about consumers. We need better assessment of their knowledge of nutrition, and we need to understand what information would be useful to them. The science of assessing consumer needs is yet in its infancy. Our ability to measure the consumer's capacity to process and use information is limited and complicated by restrictions on survey research. Yet we recognize that most information put on food labeling adds to the cost of the product. The Agency has initiated several programs designed to inform consumers, such as nutrition labeling. Several knowledgeable individuals have questioned the effectiveness of these programs because consumers may not have the knowledge with which to apply the information. This criticism may be valid for current condi-

410 Annals New York Academy of Sciences

tions; however, the Agency must also attempt to assess future conditions. In some instances, the consumer education process cannot occur unless the information is made available. In other situations, the information may be relevant to only a small percentage of consumers, but for these individuals the need is urgent.

Finally, there is the ever increasing complexity of the decision-making process. Because the food supply has and continues to become more complex, the regulatory process has become more complex. In the past, Congress has clearly implied that the regulatory decisions were to be made entirely on the basis of scientific fact (i.e., the Delaney Amendment of the Food, Drug and Cosmetic Act). The controversy over saccharin, however, has raised the prospect of the gradual adoption of the concept of risk/cost benefit in the FDA regulatory process. In the event that such a change occurs, the criteria for making risk/cost benefit decisions must be defined. The question of what is an acceptable risk must also be defined.

Part of a decision-making process is the need to establish appropriate levels of action. The Agency must be sure that the action taken to protect consumers will serve their interest in the long term as well as the immediate. For example, too narrow a regulatory posture may result in curtailment of future food development or product improvement, or too stringent standards may curtail production and raise food cost; whereas too broad a regulatory posture or too lax a standard will not protect the consumer. Quite literally, overregulation of the food supply can lead to consumers' detriment, just as can insufficient regulation. Therefore, despite the fact that we are a consumer organization and have no mandate to look after the interest of any segment of agriculture, fishing or industry, we have a continuing problem of making certain that in the process of protecting and serving the consumer we do not needlessly harm the economic environment necessary for food production.

THE U.S. SCHOOL FOOD SERVICE PROGRAM—SUCCESSES, FAILURES AND PROSPECTS

Paul A. Lachance

Department of Food Science
Rutgers—The State University of New Jersey
New Brunswick, New Jersey 08903

INTRODUCTION

Early in this century, Robert Hunter [1] and John Spargo [2] directed attention to the folly of a society assuming the responsibility of education for the young, without assuming the responsibility that the children are fit to receive that education—including the need to provide meals to children, especially those of poor families. The relationship between the economically deprived child and the educationally needy child was self-evident.

For most proud and strongly individual Americans this viewpoint prevails today. We have yet to recognize that the more important relationship is between health and performance and that it transcends the issue of economic status. The fact is that all children are needy. While the economically disadvantaged are at a greater health risk, the well-to-do American does not stand out as having attained ideal health and longevity. The advantage that the affluent have is that of being able to afford better environments, thus decreasing the risks of disease exposure, as well as being able to afford more rapid, personal, and better quality medical care *after* illness strikes. Both the needy and the affluent have a right to programs that assure health and thwart illness. The situation in the U.S. is that we have the promulgation of health education and sound nutrition resulting from diet, but a separate promulgation of school food service—the laboratory of food experience. This is as unrealistic for the rich as for the poor.

A BRIEF HISTORY

Local organizations and governments financed school lunch through the 1920's and 30's. Federal loan assistance was provided to defray labor costs. With the advent of the Surplus Relief Corporation in 1933 and the Works Project Administration in 1935, surplus commodities and no-cost labor stimulated the expansion of the school lunch concept. The first legislation was enacted in 1946—the National School Lunch Act, providing the first long-term commitment of cash and commodities and establishing nutritional guidelines, non-profit operation, and free or reduced price meals for the economically deprived. In 1962, the law was amended to allocate a greater share of the funds to areas with lower per capita incomes. The Child Nutrition Act of 1966 authorized funds for a pilot breakfast program, meal service for preschool programs and funds for food service equipment and to defray administrative costs. The Act also centralized in the USDA several related activities that existed in other agencies.

The inquiries of the Senate Select Committee on Nutrition and Human

411

Need, and the backwash of the 1969 White House Conference on Food, Nutrition and Health resulted in several further amendments leading to a rapid expansion of the program. Today, school food service is the second largest away-from-home food market, with a value of $7 billion, with the Federal share being 30 percent. Approximately 25 million children are served daily; approximately 33% of meals are free or at reduced price. In this Bicentennial year, school food service is an established nationwide program that reflects a sense of societal responsibility that remains ill-defined in significance but has contributed substantially to the alleviation of hunger. The future challenge is its integration into a nationwide health assurance system.

Effective school food service (SFS) requires the almagamation of a well-managed food delivery system, an effective nutrient delivery system, and a systematic food, nutrition, and health education system.

SCHOOL FOOD SERVICE AS A FOOD-DELIVERY SYSTEM

There are several major methods for preparing and serving food in schools. Neither Congress nor the USDA has dictated the choice of method, provided a certain array of foods are served. Many large school districts use a combination of methods.[3] The choice of systems is invariably predicated upon the extent and quality of the existing school facilities. Practically all school districts have a food service facility at the high school level, whereas the elementary schools may have either (1) a complete kitchen, (2) a PTA kitchen or (3) no facilities. The typical situation in the southeast United States is complete kitchens in each school, whereas the situation in the northern United States—particularly the larger and older cities—is a complete kitchen at the high school level and a mélange of adequate to no facilities at the elementary school level. The extent of facilities at the elementary school level is related to the year the school was constructed and whether it was constructed as a neighborhood school. Until the early 70's the management and operation of a school food-service facility by a contract food service company was not allowed. Today, the SFS system in some districts is completely managed by a contractor. The traditional system, however, remains that operated by the school district, but it may also include contractor services for one or two schools in addition to the district satelliting meals (to receiving schools) from its high school (or sending school) facility. Several major school districts have constructed manufacturing kitchens in order to satellite meals to all schools in the district.

Because of the management alternatives, which are largely dictated by school district economics, and depending on the quantity and quality of the existing food service equipment, school districts may use several food service methods: bulk preparation with cafeteria service at the high school, with or without bulk transport to receiving schools. By operating the bulk production facilities during non-school hours, additional meals can be prepared and chilled either in bulk or preplated. If the bulk production facilities are limited, the district may contract for preplated chilled or prefrozen meals for delivery to outlying elementary schools. These are reconstituted on site in a convection oven situated in a PTA kitchen or a suitable corner of the building. The beverage and bread component (and foods eaten cold) is served separately.

Meals are invariably eaten in a common eating room: a cafeteria at the high school level, a multipurpose room at the elementary school level. A number of the older schools have no available space, and meals are eaten in the classroom. Teacher contracts are increasingly specifying freedom from lunchroom duty, and so teachers are replaced in the common eating rooms by volunteer or paid lunchroom aides.

A number of problems should be self-evident:

1. The attitude of the business manager, and the school board at the district level, and the school principal at the individual school level, substantially dictates the choice and operation characteristics of the food service program and the educational priorities that the program receives. The decision to use contract food service management companies reflects emphasis on the economical, convenience, and service role of food and de-emphasis of the educational and health role of food in daily life.

2. The variable nature of school facilities has required diverse food service systems to be used, which complicates both the management and the economics of the program. The realization of optimal food service preparation conditions is substantially denied by the low educational priority of school food service.

3. The psychological role of the eating environment has been completely overlooked.[4] The decor of most lunchrooms is drab and often reflects the colors and odors to be expected from active gymnasiums. Further, the noise level is invariably high.

A national trust fund to rebuild decayed U.S. schools that would include suitable and distinct food service dining rooms and separate physical education facilities is needed.

SCHOOL FOOD SERVICE AS A NUTRIENT DELIVERY SYSTEM

The nutrient delivery system is dependent upon food quality, menu planning, food merchandising, and food acceptance. The nutrient balance of school meals is related to the federal specifications which have existed since 1946 for school lunch (Type A) and subsequent food combination specifications for other meals (e.g., breakfast) (TABLES 1 & 2). Contrary to the food delivery system options, federal regulations dictate what must be served and to some degree who must be served, i.e., free and reduced price meals for qualified students. On a national scale approximately 33% of school lunches are served to needy children, whereas 80% of breakfast meals are served to needy children in 10% of schools across the nation.

Three separate studies have demonstrated that the Type A pattern does not provide the nutrient delivery advantages of a nutrient-defined menu-planning approach.[5-7] It is very likely that the regulation pertaining to the Type A pattern will be modified in the near future. The thrust of the regulations will be to coincide portion-size requirements with age level. The Type A pattern also needs modification because it fails to consider changing food preferences. The advent of nutritional labeling provides a simple and unique opportunity to plan and display the nutrition profile of recommended components and meals.[8]

The SFS program represented a convenient, economical method for handling surplus commodity food. The foods involved also coincided with the Type A pattern. The commodity program is now limited because surpluses are less frequent and legislation has had to be enacted to provide cash for the Secretary of USDA to purchase preferred commodities and also to provide cash in lieu

TABLE 1

REQUIREMENTS FOR THE STANDARD "TYPE A" LUNCH *

1. One-half pint fluid milk.
2. Two ounces of protein, such as lean meat, poultry, fish or cheese (or an egg, ½ cup of cooked beans or peas, 4 tablespoons of peanut butter).
3. Three-fourths of a cup serving of two or more vegetables or fruits, or both (⅓ may come from juice).
4. A slice of bread or cornbread or a roll or muffin made of whole grain or enriched flour.

* Offer vs. serve in senior high school permits 3 or more items to be considered compliance. A proposed revision will adjust serving sizes to elementary, junior high, and senior high intakes.

of commodities. The availability, quality, and kind of commodities available also affect the program. If the supply of commodity foods is not predictable or cannot be expected when anticipated, both menus and local budget allocations are dislocated. A huge surplus of a food (e.g., cranberries in 1974 and 1976) can result in inordinate menu frequency for the product. The challenge with ingredient type commodities (e.g., flour, rice, oil) is to incorporate such items in various recipes. The director/supervisor with suitable facilities is able to do this, but a number of school districts do not have this capability. This can leave schools with limited facilities at a disadvantage. This problem has been ameliorated by (1) permitting contract vendors to accept commodities and decrease food cost to the schools they serve, and (2) the institution by state agency of contract arrangements with food companies to process the commodities into readily useable or shelf-stable products such as bread, pasta, and mayonnaise.[9] Administratively, the commodity program is invariably handled at the state level by a different agency than that which administers school food service in general. It should be very evident that there is no food and nutrition policy in general, or for school food service in particular, at the district, state, or national level.

Food quality relates to nutrient content from field through processing to preparation and to the recipient. With diverse food sources, donated commodities, and delivery systems, consistent nutrient delivery is difficult to optimize, and one has to marvel at the effectiveness that has been realized. However, knowledge of menu preferences, menu planning, and food merchandising determines food acceptance and plate waste. Acceptable food represents nutrients delivered, and plate waste represents nutrients wasted. The preexisting food

TABLE 2

SCHOOL BREAKFAST PROGRAM—MINIMUM FOOD REQUIREMENT

1. One-half pint of fluid milk as beverage and/or on cereal.
2. One-half cup of fruit or full strength fruit or vegetable juice.
3. One slice whole grain or enriched bread or an equivalent serving of corn bread, biscuits, rolls, muffins, etc. (or) ¾ cup or 1 ounce whole grain cereal, or enriched or fortified cereal.

habits and developing independence of children in food choices appear to
override the effect of promoting good food choices by serving idealized choices,
but benefits in terms of nutrients received from foods that would not otherwise
be consumed evidently occur (TABLE 3).[10] This is a respectable accomplishment in view of the law prohibiting "any requirement with respect to teaching
personnel, curriculum, instruction, methods of instruction, and materials of
instruction in any school." *

The singular advantage of a cafeteria facility is the opportunity to offer and
meet alternate preferences, whereas the principal disadvantage of preplated
meals is the inability to offer on-the-spot alternatives and to control portion
sizes. Experience in airline food service demonstrates the advantage of presenting alternate choices in meeting most passenger preferences. Arguments as to
the nutrient quality superiority of on-site cooked meals versus frozen preplated
meals are contrary to scientific evidence.[11] Freezing is an optimal method of

TABLE 3

NEW JERSEY DAIRY COUNCIL SURVEY (1973–75)

9,097 Fifth Graders in 119 Schools
 484   Teenagers in 1 High School

Criteria: 24-Hour Conformance to Basic Four (Recall Method)	Fifth Graders	Teenagers
Complete Conformance	10%	5%
Poor Conformance		
(a) Eat primarily meat & cereal	64%	68%
(b) Omit green & yellow vegetables	56%	61%
(c) No fluid milk consumption	9%	22%
No Conformance		
All snack diet	2%	13%

Participated in School Lunch (2,559 Fifth Graders)	Yes	No
Ate three or more food groups at lunch	77%	49%

nutrient retention. Improper preparation and holding of either frozen or non-
frozen foods can be detrimental.

Simple methods for school food service directors to measure food acceptance
and plate waste have only recently been introduced.[12] This is important because
limited data [13] indicate differences in what students perceive as problems and
lunch supervisors perceive as problems, in spite of the fact that the suggestions
of both groups for increasing participation coincide: more flexibility in menu
planning, student participation in menu planning, more cheerful and less hurried
lunchroom atmosphere, and more educational material as to why some seemingly interchangeable foods are nutritionally different. For the child who has
been identified as eligible for free SFS, at least 30% and up to 66% of the
daily RDA is provided by SFS meals.

* Child Nutrition Act of 1966, Sec. 11a; and National School Lunch Act, Sec. 12c.

Nationally, the breakfast program has been hampered by the negative attitude of school administrators who feel that breakfast is and should remain a family responsibility. However, different studies [10, 14] have shown that 37–50% of children have no breakfast or a very inadequate one. At least 30% of mothers have nothing to do with a child's breakfast. Recently the Commission on Manpower Policy revealed that women comprise 40% of the national labor force, in contrast to 33% in 1960. Very often when a breakfast program is initiated the special milk program (mid-morning break) is dropped.

Many students do not participate in SFS programs everyday. There is an apparent relationship to economic need (high participation), grade level (lower participation at secondary school level), and food preferences and acceptance (higher participation for a la carte foods).

The nutritional impact of school food service has never been systematically measured, but many studies conducted at various university experiment stations have supported the premise that nutrients delivered benefit the general performance of the child.[15] The specifics are not clearly delineated. The Iowa Breakfast Studies were extensive and demonstrated improvements in attitude and attention span. A study of milk consumption on intellectual achievements conducted in Holland [16] demonstrated some positive benefits. The fact is that all such studies have over time demonstrated equivocal or positive results, and therefòre, the consistent, coherent evidence has been positive. In biochemical, physiological, and psychological terms, all children are needy. The parents have transferred their responsibility to the educational institutions to include an assurance of mental as well as physical health development, therefore the responsibility must be met.

PROBLEMS AND PROSPECTS

1. Federal menu-planning guidelines that constrain food acceptance and nutrient balance must be broadened. The recent acceptance of the nutrient standard menu-planning approach by state directors gives promise to meeting preferences, optimizing nutrient delivery, and decreasing food waste; however, a simplified system [8] is necessary and must be used in conjunction with a food pattern. Selective nutrification of foods such as cereal food products [17] would substantially aid the assurance of a balanced array of ingested nutrients.

2. The commodity food program needs to be reexamined to provide users with clear and consistent alternatives. The concept of processing commodities into acceptable and shelf-stable products could be operated on a regional rather than state-by-state basis. Distribution could be optimized by means of computer-analyzed routing schemes.[18] In other words, the commodity program activity should serve as a centralized broker for school districts on a multi-state regional basis.

SCHOOL FOOD SERVICE AND FOOD, NUTRITION AND HEALTH EDUCATION DELIVERY

Given the distinct definitions of food, nutrition, and health and their interrelationship, it should be evident that education about one facet, i.e., health, does not necessarily and adequately guarantee consideration of other facets, i.e., nutrition and food.[19] Much has been said and written about nutrition education, but very little about food education. Since food is the input to nutrition, it should not be surprising that the cost effectiveness of nutrition education, in the absence of food education, has been very poor. The school is the site of compulsory education for 12 to 13 years of a child's life, yet the relationship of food-delivery programs to food and nutrition education, and the significance of nutrient-delivery programs to educational performance and health benefits has rarely been recognized and never systematically considered as significant in American education planning.

The responsibilities for food, nutrition, and health continue to be disseminated throughout the Federal Government, with health being emphasized primarily as the study of disease, e.g., the various National Institutes of Health. The deficiencies perceived at the local level are in fact due to limitations stemming from the very uncoordinated structure of the Federal programs. America has failed to perceive, in spite of history to the contrary, that the solution to diseases resides in basic research that is not compartmented by disease, and that solutions to national food, nutrition, and health education issues reside in coordinated and systematic programs irrespective of given commodities, regulatory agencies, or research institutes. The education aspects of food and nutrition have not been a mandate of the enabling School Lunch Act and Child Nutrition Act legislation, and the school food service director has not been considered a member of the teaching faculty but rather a member of the service staff. Under the circumstance it is naive to have expected a greater effectiveness. The irony is that at the State level, the school food service office is a bureau of the State Education Department. Again, however, the role is viewed by the State as a service function rather than a leadership and educational function.

Very recently at least two [20, 21] K-12 curricula for nutrition (and some food) education have been developed; however, there is no program to insure their implementation. School districts have had the option of rejecting implementation of SFS. In recent years several States (Massachusetts and New Jersey) have mandated SFS in all public schools. Other States are likely to follow these legal precedences.

CONCLUSION

In reality, the prospects of school food service transcend the mere service of food to needy children. The child must be viewed as a human resource critical to the nation, and the health of all citizens should be of utmost concern since the productivity of the nation is related to the productivity of its people. A health assurance delivery system should include concern for food, nutrition and health maintenance. Whereas many communities do not have hospital facilities, and many do not have resident physicians, it is noteworthy that each community has a school district, with a school food service program and health education responsibilities. Further, the community invariably has public health, senior citizen, Woman Infant and Children, and other health assurance delivery programs. All these programs should be coordinated from one site—the school district.[22]

REFERENCES

1. HUNTER, ROBERT. 1905. Poverty : 382. The Macmillan Co. New York.
2. SPARGO, JOHN. 1906. The Bitter Cry of The Children: Grosset and Dunlap Pub. New York.

3. BARD, BERNARD. 1968. The School Lunchroom: Time of Trial. John Wiley & Sons, Inc. New York.
4. RENDON, R. J. 1976. The School Lunchroom in The Experience of Grade School Children—A Case Study. M.A. dissertation. Goddard College, Vermont.
5. LACHANCE, P. A. 1972. Balanced nutrition through food processor practice of nutrification. Food Technol. 26(6): 30–40.
6. OSTENSO, GRACE. 1972. New concepts in child nutrition programs: Nutrient standard menu planning, computer-assisted menu planning. In Proceedings of The National School Food Service Conference : 45–53. Rutgers University. New Brunswick, N.J.
7. JANSEN, G. R. & J. M. HUDSON. 1974. Nutritional aspects of nutrient standard menus. Food Technol. 28(1): 62–67.
8. LACHANCE, P. A. 1977. Simple techniques for school food service: The nutritive profile of meals. J. Sch. Foodserv. 31(2): [41]
9. CASTILLO, JUAN DEL & ELSWORTH RIES. 1972. Processing contracts for donated commodities. In Proceedings of The National School Food Service Conference : 136–140. Rutgers University. New Brunswick, N.J.
10. LOVE, MARTHA & LORRAINE SHAEFER. 1973. Food Choices of 2,559 Fifth Grade Students in Middlesex County, New Jersey. Report of the Dairy Council of Northern New Jersey. East Orange, N.J.
11. HARRIS, R. S. & E. KARMAS, Eds. 1975. Nutritional Evaluation of Food Processing. AVI Pub. Co. Westport, Conn.
12. LACHANCE, P. A. 1976. Simple research techniques for school food service. Part I: Acceptance testing. J. School Foodservice 30(8): 54. Part II: Measuring plate waste. J. Sch. Foodserv. 30(9): 68.
13. PRICE, D. W., D. Z. PRICE & JASPER WOMACH. 1975. Problems in The Management of the National School Lunch Program in Washington School Districts. Washington State Univ. Agric. Exp. Sta. Pullman, Wash. Bull. 817.
14. LACHANCE, P. A. 1973. The vanishing American meal. Food Prod. Dev. 7(9): 36–40.
15. MARTIN, H. P. 1973. Nutrition: Its relationship to children's physical, mental and emotional development. Am. J. Clin. Nutr. 26(7): 766–775.
16. DEFARES, P. B., G. N. KEMA & J. J. VAN DER WERFF. 1967. Schoolmilk and Intellectual Achievements: The Effect of School Milk Consumption on Intellectual Achievements. Van Gorcum Ltd. Netherlands.
17. FOOD AND NUTRITION BOARD. 1974. Proposed Fortification Policy for Cereal-Grain Products. National Academy Sciences. Washington, D.C.
18. SCHNEIDER, L. D. 1971. Truck Routing Model for The Delivery of USDA Surplus Commodities to New Jersey Public Elementary School Districts. M.S. Thesis. Rutgers University. New Brunswick, N.J.
19. LACHANCE, P. A. 1971. Nutrition Education—A Point of View. J. Nutr. Educ. 2(2): 52–53.
20. NATIONAL DAIRY COUNCIL. 1977. Curriculum Materials for K-12. 6300 N. River Road, Rosemont, Ill. 60018.
21. SOCIETY FOR NUTRITION EDUCATION. 1976. Curriculum Materials for K-12. 2140 Shattuck Avenue, Suite 1110, Berkeley, Calif. 94704.
22. LACHANCE, P. A. 1975. School foodservice at the crossroads. J. Sch. Foodserv. 29(8): 29–32.

NUTRITIONAL NEEDS OF SPECIAL POPULATIONS AT RISK

Arnold E. Schaefer

Swanson Center for Nutrition, Inc. and
University of Nebraska Medical Center
Omaha, Nebraska 68132

The population groups most vulnerable to problems of malnutrition are the hard-core poor, migrant workers, and Native Americans. Within these groups priority for prevention of malnutrition (over and under nutrition) must be given to the pregnant, preschool-age children, the aged, and adolescents. The findings of the 10-State Nutrition Survey of 1968–70 clearly reveal consistent socio-economic effects on size, growth, and development.[1]

Ten States were selected to provide geographic representation of the major regions of the country and to reflect a broad diversity of economic, ethnic, and sociocultural characteristics, high-risk vulnerable groups, and to include States wherein participation in food donation and welfare programs was rated poor and good.[2] The random sample was selected from one-quarter of the population of each State living in census tract or enumeration districts having the largest percentage of families with incomes, as of the 1960 census, below the poverty index ratio (PIR). At the time of the study, this was, for example, an urban family of four, with a male as head with an income of less than $3,335 per year or $2,345 for a farm family.

The data were biased and do not represent the entire population of the states nor certainly the United States as a whole. However, the characteristics of the sampled population groups—income, housing, education, age, sex, family composition, ethnic origin, participation in food or welfare programs—enable one to predict the kinds of problems to be expected in population groups with similar characteristics. Numerous other studies were launched in various vulnerable population groups, and although usually done in populations with greater overall poverty problems, the same kinds of nutrition problems were found— usually at a much higher prevalence and of more severe nature.

The methodology employed and the guidelines for interpretation of the biochemical, dietary, and anthropometric data were defined in the HEW publication.[2] The five States categorized as "Low Income," i.e., having the greatest percentage (from 46 to 63%) of families below the poverty index ratio (PIR), were Texas, Louisiana, South Carolina, West Virginia, and Kentucky. The remaining States—Michigan, New York, Massachusetts, Washington and California—categorized as "High Income," had from 18 to 33% of the families living below the PIR.

This first attempt at a comprehensive survey of the American population included over 86,000 individuals, of which 40,847 were studied from an anthropometric, biochemical, dietary, medical (including dental), socioeconomic, and cultural point of view. Of this sample nearly 16,000 participants were in the pediatric age group, with over 7,800 pre-school age children.

419

OBESITY

Although the published report of the 10-State Nutrition Survey [2] ignored the problem of obesity, the recent report by Dr. Stan Garn et al.[1] clearly defines the magnitude of obesity and the need for updating our standards or guidelines for interpreting anthropometric measurements. Some of the key findings were that the poor are leaner, and those at median incomes are fatter. This holds in general for males at all ages and for females through early adolescence. However, poor girls were leaner during adolescence and end up fatter than those of higher incomes, who end up leaner. With increased income, children were fatter and heavier, had greater head circumference, more advanced skeletal and dental maturity, and higher hemoglobin levels. Children of obese parents were three times as fat as those of lean parents. When both parents were lean, the children tended to be lean. When both parents were obese, the children tended to be obese. Dr. Garn stated "These findings suggest that the level of fatness may be more acquired because of family eating and exercising habits than genetically inherited."

The survey revealed that black boys and girls tended to be taller, had a larger skeletal mass, greater bone density, and skeletal and dental advancement over white boys and girls, thus indicating a need for appropriate, adjusted anthropometric standards for black children.

GROWTH RETARDATION

Height and weight retardation, as evaluated by the Stuart-Meredith norms (which underestimate the problem in black children), was evident in an excess of 15 to 33% for height and 12 to 20% for weight at age 6 (TABLES 1 & 2). This retardation was noted in all ethnic groups irrespective of whether the children were from the "high" or "low" income states.

The growth data of Spanish-American children from Texas—data which for an unexplained reason were omitted, by the Center for Disease Control of HEW, from the official 10-State Nutrition Survey Report—revealed that the mean height for the 0 to 6 year olds followed the 16th percentile standard growth curve. By age 4 there was an average growth retardation of 6 to 9 months.

One of the population groups most vulnerable to malnutrition in the '60s and early '70s were the Native American Indians. Dr. Jean Van Duzen's [3, 4]

TABLE 1

PERCENTAGE BELOW 15TH PERCENTILE FOR HEIGHT OF STUART-MEREDITH STANDARD

Age (Years)	Percent of Children			
	Male		Female	
	White	Black	White	Black
2	42	46	46	37
4	39	34	44	36
6	37	30	38	32

TABLE 2
PERCENTAGE BELOW 15TH PERCENTILE FOR WEIGHT OF STUART-MEREDITH STANDARD

Age (Years)	Percent of Children			
	Male		Female	
	White	Black	White	Black
2	26	34	31	27
4	22	22	33	33
6	27	27	35	37

study and documentation of calorie-protein malnutrition in Navajo Indian children clearly emphasizes that kwashiorkor and marasmus do occur in this population. During the period 1963–73, Dr. Van Duzen, working in the Public Health Service Indian Hospital in Tuba City, Arizona, documented the prevalence and severity of the problem.

A comparison of two 5-year periods, 1963–67 and 1969–73, revealed an 18% reduction in total number of patients under 5 years of age admitted to the hospital and a 39% reduction in the number of patients admitted with deficits in weight for their chronological ages. The height and weight data on 1,462 Head-Start children, measured in 1973, revealed that when compared with data obtained in 1967, there was still a significant deviation from the Boston growth curves; however, a definite improvement did occur, especially in height. Thirty percent of the boys and girls fell below the 3rd percentile of the Boston growth standard, and in 1973 these figures were 11% in girls and 16% in boys.

During these two 5-year periods, admissions to the Tuba City Indian Hospital of children less than 5 years old with malnutrition were reduced from 616 to 377. A total of 15 cases of kwashiorkor and 29 of marasmus were admitted in the 1963–67 period, compared to 9 kwashiorkor and 8 marasmus during 1969–73.

The cases of marasmus decreased despite the trend away from breast feeding to early weaning. This is attributed to the fact that infant formula has been made available to most Navajo infants under 1 year of age. Although much of the success in reducing infant malnutrition can be credited to the greatly expanded and improved food donation and mother and infant health programs, some of the improvement is obviously the result of better housing and sanitation. The battle to eradicate malnutrition is, however, far from over and requires continued, expanded programs for self-help, economic viability, and improved health delivery systems.

VITAMIN A STATUS—PRESCHOOL CHILDREN

The percent serum vitamin A levels of less than 20 mcg per 100 ml for the entire population fail to identify the vulnerable groups.

The vast majority of the "unacceptable" and "deficient" levels of vitamin A were contributed by the 0–5 year-old age groups. In Texas 40% of all pre-school age children had values of less than 20 mcg and 80% less than 30 mcg of vitamin A per 100 ml serum. In South Carolina 26% of the pre-school children had less than 20 mcg, 34% less than 22 mcg, and 45% less than 25 mcg (TABLE 3). In the black population of Michigan and Kentucky 20% had unacceptable levels of vitamin A.[2]

It must be remembered that in the early stages of the surveys (Texas, Louisiana, Michigan, Kentucky, and New York State) the vast majority of skim milk powder distributed by U.S.D.A. in the Food Distribution Program for the poor had not been enriched with vitamins A and D. The Department of Agriculture, in November 1968, issued a directive requiring the enrichment of all skim milk distributed through the food donation program with vitamins A and D. While the Nutrition Survey was in progress numerous research investigators not only substantiated the survey findings with reference to vitamin A but identified an even more serious problem in selected poverty population groups.

TABLE 3

SERUM VITAMIN A DISTRIBUTION AND MEAN VALUES

	Percent Prevalence less Than *				Mean Value (mcg per 100 ml)
	10	20	25	30	
		(mcg per 100 ml)			
Texas	2.0	17	Na †	41	31.6
South Carolina	0.6	10	22	36	34.1
Louisiana	0.9	8	Na †	15	47.2
Kentucky	3.6	9	19	31	40.1
West Virginia	0.0	8	18	28	37.7
Michigan	0.1	4	16	24	40.4
New York City	1.5	3	9	13	44.9
Massachusetts	1.0	10	17	25	44.4
Washington	6.0	23	36	38	31.1
California	0.1	1	3	6	57.8

* <10 mcg per 100 ml: "deficient"—severe risk group.
  <20 mcg per 100 ml: "unacceptable level"—moderate risk group.
† Values not available for this summary.

High,[5] from Meharry University, reported that of 178 pre-school children studied in the Bluffton and Hilton Health Areas of South Carolina, 30% had less than 20 mcg and 8% less than 10 mcg vitamin A per 100 ml serum. Hepner, of the Community Pediatric Center, University of Maryland, Baltimore,[5] reported that 14.5% of the 4–5 year olds had less than 15 mcg. Unglaub,[5] of Tulane University, reported a prevalence of 16–35% in 900 Head Start children studied in Alabama, Louisiana, and Mississippi with levels of less than 20 mcg per 100 ml serum. Chase,[6] of the University of Colorado Medical Center, reported a prevalence of 20% in 300 pre-school children in 1969, with serum levels of less than 20 mcg. Zee,[7, 8] of St. Judes Children Research Hospital, Memphis, Tennessee, reported a prevalence in pre-school children of 44% with less than 20 mcg per 100 ml serum.

TABLE 4

UNACCEPTABLE HEMOGLOBIN VALUES—PERCENTAGE OF TOTAL POPULATION

Low-Income States		High-Income States	
Texas	20	Michigan	19
South Carolina	38	New York State (upstate)	10
Louisiana	42	New York City	16
Kentucky	18	Washington	10
West Virginia	13	California	10
		Massachusetts	9

While the physical-clinical evidence did not suggest a severe medical problem, the biochemical findings did indicate a serious degree of risk that warranted preventive action.

ANEMIA

Population groups having hemoglobin values of less than the "acceptable" levels defined in the guidelines for interpretation [9] constituted the most prevalent nutritional problem next to obesity. The prevalence of unacceptable hemoglobin values varied from 40% in South Carolina to 10% in Washington, New York, California and Massachusetts (TABLE 4). However, in these later States the prevalence in blacks was over 20%. Likewise, the "poor" having a PIR of less than one-half usually had twice as many unacceptable hemoglobin values as did individuals from families with an income of twice the PIR.

Unacceptable hemoglobin levels, i.e., less than 11 gm/100 ml, were found in approximately 20% of children 2–5 years of age ranging in various ethnic, sex, and State groups from 8 to 49%. Deficient levels of hemoglobin of less than 10 g per 100 ml were much less frequent, with a prevalence, however, of 11% in black children from the low-income States (TABLE 5). The anemia was primarily an iron deficiency. Sixty-four percent of the 2 to 5-year-old children with hemoglobins of less than 10 g per 100 ml had a transferrin saturation index of less than 20%.

Since anemia can be caused by a deficiency of several nutrients besides iron, especially folic acid, special studies on subsamples were performed for the Public Health Service by the U.S. Army Medical Research and Nutrition

TABLE 5

HEMOGLOBIN VALUES IN LOW-INCOME STATES

Hemoglobin (g/100 ml)	% of Children 2–5 Years of Age		
	White	Black	Spanish American
<10	3.2	11.2	5.7
<11	13.1	34.0	9.5

Laboratory at Fitzsimmons General Hospital (now designated the Letterman Army Institute for Research). All blood samples identified as "unacceptable" according to their hemoglobin values were then analyzed for serum iron transferrin saturation index, serum folic acid and red blood cell folate. In addition, these samples were matched with samples by age and sex having "acceptable" values.

A comparison of the red blood cell folate and transferrin saturation index findings in the States of Washington and South Carolina indicates that the major cause of anemia ("low" hemoglobin values) is that of iron deficiency (TABLE 6). However, the suboptimal red blood cell folates (less than 140 Ng/ml) indicate that some of the anemia may well be due to inadequate folate nutrition.

The hemoglobin, iron, and folate data revealed that the risk of mild anemia (low hemoglobins) was virtually as high in males as in females. The serum iron values and transferrin saturation index in males clearly implicate an insufficiency of dietary utilizable iron for males as well as females. For example, in the Navajo Indian study (data omitted by HEW from the 10-State Nutrition Survey Report) the percentage of "unacceptable" serum irons in all males above age 12 years was 19% and for females above age 12 was 29%. The unacceptable transferrin saturation index for males age 12 and above was 25% as compared to 38% for females.

A review of red blood cell folate values in Kentucky, for example, showed that among males above age 16, there were 22% with "deficient" values (less than 140 Ng/ml) and 37% with "unacceptable" values of less than 160 Ng/ml. The prevalence in females was 13% "deficient" and 23% with "unacceptable" values.

The age-old question as to the over or underestimation of problems of malnutrition inadvertently resides in "what standards or guidelines are used to interpret the data." This is especially true in definition of or willingness to recognize the problem of "anemia," be it mild, moderate, high, low or severe. The recent data of the Central America Nutrition Surveys, which utilized the same methodology plus additional hematology, have provided a new guideline for interpretation of anemia.[10] Do females in the United States differ from females in Central America in that they *do not* require an equivalent level of hemoglobin? The hemoglobin values indicative of a risk of anemia in males are indeed very similar to the U.S. interpretive guidelines used in the 10-State Nutrition Survey; however, the guidelines used to interpret "low" and deficient levels for females are approximately 1 to 2 g of hemoglobin lower than the

TABLE 6

| | Percent with "Deficient Levels" | |
	Transferrin Saturation *	rbc Folates †
South Carolina	52	27
Washington	28	21

* Less than 20% transferrin saturation index for males and 15% in females.
† Less than 140 Ng/gm red blood cells.

TABLE 7

BIOCHEMICAL FINDINGS IN PREGNANT AND LACTATING MOTHERS
IN THE 10-STATE NUTRITION SURVEY

	Percent of Population Groups	
	Hemoglobin < 11 gms/100 ml	Serum Albumin < 2.8 g/100 ml
White		
Low-income states	13.6	10.0
High-income states	7.9	8.5
Black		
Low-income states	37.6	13.6
High-income states	19.6	4.0
Spanish-American		
Low-income states	13.3	10.7
High-income states	20.4	5.0

newly defined level for females in Central America. Thus, the 10-State Survey
Report underestimates the anemia problem in females.

PREGNANT AND LACTATING MOTHERS

The vast majority of the data collected on pregnant and lactating mothers
has not been analyzed by the Center for Disease Control of HEW. With the
transfer of the Nutrition Program to Atlanta in 1970, the nutrition staff was
dissipated, funding shifted to other programs, and no effort made to complete
the analysis of the data collected. However, the available data on hemoglobin
and serum albumin indicates that nutritional risk problems do exist, especially
in the black population. Irrespective of race or whether from "high" or "low"
income states, the data support the need for the current expanded Women,
Infants and Children (WIC) feeding program (TABLE 7). Even though in
pregnancy serum albumin values are normally lower, one cannot accept a
prevalence of 5 to 14% having a serum albumin of less than 2.8 g per 100 ml.
The prevalence of hemoglobins of less than 11 g per 100 ml in 8 to 33% of
those studied dictates the need for concern and initiation of prevention programs.

MIGRANT WORKERS

In addition to the Migrant Workers studied in the Texas Nutrition Survey,
the Nutrition Program of the Public Health Service along with the Office of
Economic Opportunity supplemented a project by the University of Colorado
Medical Center under the direction of Dr. Peter Chase, to evaluate the nutritional status of pre-school Mexican-American migrant farm children and to
develop and evaluate a health and nutrition program.[6]

The findings were similar to those noted in the Spanish-American populations studied in Texas. Vitamin A deficiency was a major medical problem.

Fifty-seven (20%) of 288 children had serum vitamin A values of less than acceptable (20 mcg per 100 ml). Thirty-six percent of the children were below the 10th percentile for triceps skin-fold measurements. Height attainment was low in 54 of 300 children. This group had a high infant mortality of 63 per 1,000 live births.

VULNERABLE GROUPS

If one reviews the prevalence of "unacceptable" biochemical values, the most vulnerable population groups defined on the basis of age, race, and economic status would be black, pre-school age children from families with incomes below the poverty index. Close to them would be migrant workers and Native American Indians. As an example, if one reviews just the prevalence of "unacceptable" hemoglobin values for New York State (minus New York City), one could readily assign priorities for action; namely, black and Spanish-Americans having incomes below the poverty index, with the highest prevalence in pre-school age children and the aged (TABLE 8).

TABLE 8

PERCENTAGE "UNACCEPTABLE" HEMOGLOBIN VALUES FOR NEW YORK STATE
(NOT INCLUDING NEW YORK CITY)

< 6 years of age	20.2	White	8.0
6–16 years	6.8	Black	21.7
17–59 years	9.6	Spanish Am.	16.1
> 60 years	13.2	Above poverty level	9.3
		Below poverty level	15.4

SUMMARY

The nutritional needs of special populations at risk require a *concerned government, a concerned bureaucracy* which funds and operates health, welfare and food-delivery systems. Equally, if not even more important, is the concern and involvement of citizens at the "local-state-county-city" level. Some of the vulnerable groups, such as the migrant workers and the Native Americans, are the responsibility of the Federal Government. This does not mean that State and local citizens should do nothing, which by and large characterizes what has happened. The solution to provide optimum nutrition for the *entire U.S.* population is not merely a recitation of: food production figures, food costs, documentation of how much the Government spends on feeding people, how many free or reduced school lunches are served, how good or bad the problem is.

We need to *update* and monitor programs that deal with the delivery of health, welfare and food; nutrition education for educators, Congress, doctors, and the public; food enrichment and fortification; nutrient analysis of foods; and nutrition research.

REFERENCES

1. GARN, S. M. & D. C. CLARK. 1975. Nutrition, growth, development and maturation: Findings from the Ten-State Nutrition Survey of 1968–70. Pediatrics 56(2): 306–319.
2. U.S. DEPARTMENT OF HEALTH, EDUCATION AND WELFARE. 1972. Ten State Nutrition Survey 1968–70. Atlanta, DHEW Pub. No. (HSM) 72–8130, Center for Disease Control, Vol. 1–5.
3. VAN DUZEN, J., J. P. CARTER, J. SECOND & C. FEDERSPIEL. 1969. Protein and calorie malnutrition among pre-school Navajo Indian children. Am. J. Clin. Nutr. 22(10): 1362–1370.
4. VAN DUZEN, J., J. P. CARTER & R. VANDERSWAGG. 1976. Protein and calorie malnutrition among pre-school Navajo Indian children, a follow-up. Am. J. Clin. Nutr. 29(6): 657–662.
5. Personal communication.
6. CHASE, H. P., V. KUMAR, J. M. DODDS, H. E. SAUBERLICH, R. M. HUNGER, R. S. BROCTON & V. SPALDING. 1971. Nutritional status of pre-school Mexican-American migrant farm children. Am. J. Dis. Child. 122: 316–324.
7. ZEE, P., T. WALTERS & C. MITCHELL. 1970. Nutrition and poverty in pre-school children. J. Am. Med. Assoc. 213(5): 739–41.
8. ZEE, P. & H. G. KAFATOS. 1973. Nutrition and Federal food assistance programs: A survey of impoverished pre-school blacks in Memphis, Tennessee. Fed. Proc. 32(3).
9. O'NEAL, R. M., O. C. JOHNSON & A. E. SCHAEFER. 1970. Guidelines for classification and interpretation of group blood and urine data collected as part of the National Nutrition Survey. Pediatr. Res. 4: 103–107.
10. VITERI, F. E., F. DETUNA & M. A. GUZMAN. 1972. Normal hematological values in Central American populations. Brit. J. Haemat. 23: 189–197.

GENERAL DISCUSSION

N. Henry Moss, *Moderator*

*Temple University Health Sciences Center and
Albert Einstein Medical Center
Philadelphia, Pennsylvania 19141*

DR. GLASSMAN: I wonder in your nutrition information that you hand out to the schools what is the recommended fat content in the diet, and can you tell me what Kraft Company is doing to reduce the fat content of their various cheeses?

MR. WHITE: As I've indicated in the talk I'll answer the first question last. We make available cheese and all of the other products that we produce that contain significant quantities of fat in a wide range of levels. We are not putting one product out and telling the consumer this is what we expect you to use. We give the consumer the choice from the full fat of the conventional cheese to much reduced fat content. In the information on the amount of fat in the diet we tend to use the concept of the prudent diet, talking about, as Dr. Wynder mentioned this morning, the necessity of lowering the total fat content and in general lowering our intake of calories.

MR. ARTHUR MILLER: Sir, I wonder if you could reflect upon two statements that I have heard time and time again, one from the industry and one from consumers. The industry's statement, which is too prevalent, is that we give people what they want primarily in the marketplace. The consumers, on the other hand, say people eat what industry gives them. I would like to hear your opinion.

MR. WHITE: Well, I almost wish that the latter were true; then we could really push the high-profit products. But the statement that is made that industry, whether it's a food industry or any other consumer goods industry, pushes products down consumers' throats is just a lot of nonsense because in the society that we live in and the kind of competitive situation that we have people aren't forced to take any one particular product. They will pick and choose, and as I indicated in the discussion the jury of consumers is making its decision every time a food product is purchased.

DR. ASBURY: If I understood you correctly you said calories were the only thing that the consumer really needed to know. In that case why wouldn't you eat sugar all the time and get the most calories for the money?

MR. WHITE: No, what I said was that calorie information is really the only thing that we feel is being absorbed by the consumer today. We do not say that's the only thing they need. They need much more. What we need, and I think what industry needs, is for the government to help them find a way to make all the additional information that is needed comprehensible to the consumer. If you look at the nutrition information on a can of peas or a can of beans, even for someone who is trained in nutrition and is skilled in making diet choices, it becomes a fairly complex task. How then are you going to get someone who has difficulty even reading to understand what they need to know about nutrition in the content of the foods they buy to make up an adequate diet. That's where the problem exists.

DR. ASBURY: I agree with that, but I would just like to add in closing that you could use your television ads to teach them instead of enticing them to something else.

MR. WHITE: It is very difficult to teach much in 30 seconds in a commercial.

DR. GENE CALVERT: What should be the role of industry in developing and implementing national nutrition policies?

MR. WHITE: I think that there has to be at least a joint program on anything that's going to be a national policy, and as such, it is obviously going to have to come from the government. But industry should have, and I think *is* having a part in establishing that policy, or at least in establishing the groundrules that go to make it up.

DR. R. HENDERSON (*Olin Corp., New Haven, Conn.*): I don't understand why we have this great emphasis on animal testing, and the lists you have here could have been written 20 years ago in spite of the biochemical advances that have been made since then. Why can't we have some sort of biochemical input into these processes because one of the first questions to be posed is, "Are any of these additives metabolized?" Those things that are readily metabolized into simple sugars or fatty acids or other normal metabolites certainly can't be considered any real problem, whereas those that are not metabolized or that are metabolized into potentially toxic intermediates certainly have more complicated possible effects. I just want to ask why there hasn't been any biochemical input into toxicological testing schemes like this.

DR. SANFORD A. MILLER: In all fairness I suppose I really ought to say that there is. There is always a significant amount of this done in any kind of toxicological testing. There are really two sets of problems. Number one, the answer is really not as simple as saying a substance that's oxidized is in fact a safe substance. Such oxidations will lead to other products which are sometimes difficult to define. Even when they don't, the question of the physiological state of the organism during the course of the oxidation, the maximal level capable of being oxidized, the possibility of long-term accumulation, and rather small amounts of these materials all lead to enormous amounts of difficulty in trying to translate the kind of response that one gets from a biochemical testing, to practical solutions to safety questions. This testing, by its nature, must be simplistic in order to get reasonable answers compared to the complexities of doing it in the real world. Now having said that, there is no question that the future of toxicity testing has to be in that direction or even in the direction of cell culture techniques. The problem has been that the amount of money available over the past 50 years for the development of new techniques in toxicological evaluation has been essentially zero. As far as I know most of the work has been offshoots of other kinds of work. But I agree with you wholeheartedly, and this is exactly the point that I was trying to make, that such innovative approaches to evaluate toxicity are absolutely required. Current techniques just don't answer the questions that need to be answered. That's all there is to it.

UNIDENTIFIED SPEAKER: I think a final comment on the last question ought to be that pharmacokinetics is still only in the kindergarten state, and that's not sufficient. But I would like to make a comment to Dr. Miller and ask him a question as a result. I find it surprising for an MIT professor to suggest that a poor structure of self-interest any more than the free market will produce necessarily a balance in forces. It seems to me that there ought to be some recognition and that there are some condensation processes which leads the center of balance somewhat askew. Would you care to comment on that?

DR. MILLER: In the first place no one should ever be surprised at anything an MIT professor does. I suppose it's the thing that keeps us young. However, in answer to your question, of course what you're saying is absolutely correct. But the fact of the matter is that other kinds of idealistic approaches to the problems of this area have proven to be unsuccessful. I'm perfectly willing at this stage to get into the problem that even a congregation of thieves can end up doing something worthwhile for mankind. Enlightened self-interest I've always felt has been one of the prime movers of man's activities, and it hasn't been tried yet in this area simply because there seems to be this continuous antagonism between the various forces that are involved. Neither of the activists (right or left) is "right." The academics aren't right. Industry isn't right. The legislatures are rarely right. The result of all this is that each one is approaching the problem in its own way and it has thus far failed. As far as I am concerned this is the only simplistic solution I could think of that would go along this way. I would be glad to listen to anything else. At this point I would admit I'm rather desperate myself. I'm sorely afraid that the food industry can be bound so vigorously by regulation that innovation will die, and if it does die I think that the possibility of future development of food products is also going to die. This is not to say that the industry did most of what it has done because it originally intended to do so. A lot of what has happened has resulted from pressure from the outside. However, once industry gets started on these things, it has improved and expanded the original thought and has gone a long way to solving many of our problems. I don't want to see that particular flexibility lost.

DR. B. L. OSER: I'd like to make a comment on one particular slide of Dr. Miller's because it contains the sort of information that I believe adds unnecessarily to public concern. That is the slide that showed the number of food additives and the pounds of food additives produced annually. I think that this is not only meaningless, but also misleading, when it refers, for example, to 1500 additives used in a total amount of 1348.5 million pounds per year. This is like saying we eat 200 billion pounds of food a year without reference to whether the foods are nutritious, safe, or wholesome. We must consider the various types of food additives, both regulated and exempt ("generally recognized as safe" [GRAS]), as defined under the law. For example, they include many nutrients, mineral salts, vitamins, amino acids, pH regulators, etc. They also include a large number of natural products, such as spices, flavoring substances, and so-called "synthetic" products, which may actually be chemicals derived from natural sources, as well as synthetic compounds which are the analogues of naturally occurring substances. The largest single category of food additives is flavoring substances, about 75 percent of which are used at average levels not greater than 0.001 percent in food. The annual production of about 75 percent of synthetic flavors corresponds on a compound basis to a daily per capita intake of 0.1 micrograms per kilogram of body weight. In the light of these facts I believe that simply to report that 1500 or 3000 or 5000 additives are in use surely needs clarification.

DR. MILLER: In the first place the table didn't only list the total. It listed about 15 different categories of food additives, indicating the distribution among the poundage used for each of these. In the second place the function of the table was to give an idea of the increasing use of additives. The fact of the matter is that there are a lot of additives used in our food, and you can't get away from this fact whether they are nutrient supplements or whether they are natural ingredients. By the way I don't buy the argument that because a substance is a natural ingredient it's safe. The table in no way was meant to indicate that this use was safe or unsafe. It is simply a fact, and a fact that has to be considered in my opinion in the overall estimation one makes concerning the hazard of these materials. The table also suggests more of the variety of additives used, which as far as I am concerned is a much more important factor than is the actual amounts that are being used. The function of the table is to indicate the variety of additives and the fact that there are many.

DR. MICHAEL RABIN: When there is a difference of opinion in the personnel and the agency with regard to the safety of some measure or some findings, must it be submitted to superiors before publication? Is it true that if they do not approve it it cannot be published? I have friends in the agency and at NIH and I understand this is so. The reason that people are asking this is they are concerned there is censorship that goes on that prevents some of these findings from becoming public, and I would cite the case of the firing of Tony Mores in the case of the swine flu vaccine.

DR. VANDERVEEN: Of course I'm not in the position to tell you if indeed this is or is not fact. From my vantage point I have never been subjected to any undue pressure to change my stand or to not speak out on an issue which I feel I need to speak out on. I can also say that that's true of any of my people because we have had some times when disagreement was apparent between us at our level and supervision at higher levels. And it's true that many times what we propose for a final regulation does not meet the goals of the Commissioner. However, the law in this regard says that the Commissioner must make the decision. So, as you know, the Commissioner makes the decision and he's subject to the scrutiny of Congress and whoever else wants to review that process. We have the ability to talk out on any issue. I think in the case that you mentioned there was clear insubordination. I don't think he was fired because he spoke out. He was fired because he did not do what he was supposed to do as the record reads. I can't say that to be absolute fact because I did not investigate the situation. The board did and said that they didn't agree with his firing, but they did agree that he should have been reprimanded, and it was the Commissioner's decision as to what penalty should be paid for his insubordination.

DR. GENE CALVERT: What should industry's role be in developing and implementing national nutrition policies?

DR. VANDERVEEN: I find it difficult to say that we can sit down and draw a policy and it's going to solve all our problems at this point in time. I view policy as a changing situation. I think the important aspect of policy is that the machinery to formulate policy be established, and we have not done that either on the side of industry or government, or for that matter in terms of the public. The public has not been concerned about policy in terms of nutrition through the years. They are becoming aware. There are some people out there now who are really talking about it, but we as a society have to be concerned about policy. Now I would like to say that within certain government agencies policy has been a function for a long time. Agriculture has had policy on how to improve production, how to deal with the economic issues, and so that is part of this overall policy. The F.D.A. obviously has to have a means of arriving at policy for regulation of food additives, etc. And that's another segment of this policy. And I think that it has to be a combined activity involving a total society. It's got to change. The food supply is changing, our values are changing. It's got to be a continuous effort. I think the description that was read last night had those elements. I find difficulties with listing a whole series of items and saying this ought to be our policy because it's only going to be short-lived if we do that type of thing.

DR. DANIEL ROSENFIELD (*Miles Laboratories, Inc., Elkhart, Ind*): Why not move the school lunch program in local neighborhoods out of departments of education and into a department of Human Resources or something like that? In other words, just because people vote in a school does not mean that the Board of Education controls the voting system. Just because a school lunch program feeds children in a school does not mean that the school district should run it because, as you well know, the best thing about the school lunch program is that there were no fights that day and nobody fell down the stairs. So if you say put it on the school district you should go 180 degrees the other way and say that the school lunch program should be taken out of local boards of education and put into a department of Human Resources.

DR. LACHANCE: I can't say. I believe that that's an alternative, but one would have to sit down and trade that off. I would like to try to work with at least what we have and just modify it a little bit.

DR. H. MALMROS: I just wondered why milk/butter and peanut butter are fed to the children. If you want to prevent arteriosclerosis you have to start early and you have to start it in children. You could use low fat products with plenty of polyunsaturated fatty acids in the preparation of such food. But don't use peanut butter.

DR. LACHANCE: The point here is that we do not specify the kind of milk any more. We used to specify whole milk. We now allow skim milk, we allow buttermilk, we allow any kind of milk. The state can overrule that. If they want to ban chocolate milk they can. Even school districts do it nowadays. You can double milk consumption with chocolate milk incidentally. I've demonstrated that. The other point is that we don't require butter anymore. Margarine is an optional thing. Most of the time it is margarine. Peanut butter is a protein source. It is not looked at from the fat point of view. Generally speaking these meals from a nutrient profile point of view are not too bad with respect to saturated fat content and the like. Incidently, I don't think you are going to change anything in this country relevant to peanuts for four years at least.

DR. Z. W. WILCHINSKY (*Exxon Chemical Co., Linden, N.J.*): Dr. Lachance, could you give an estimate of the average cost of a meal?

DR. LACHANCE: That varies very much by the county. Throughout the country, on the average I have to use a number like $.85. There are areas like New York City where, because of the total business of featherbedding and a few other things, meals are probably a dollar, but it's still a very economical meal. You can't do that in any other kind of setting. It's really a very efficient system, and I can't really put down how effective this school food service has been in terms of that kind of economics, at any rate.

DR. D. M. WATKIN: Dr. Lachance, you commented that school lunch services were in certain specific instances receiving advice from student members who were recipients of the school food service. In view of the fact that many young people have a concern for the quality of nutrition, and in view of the fact also that in our symbiotic relationship between the nutrition program for the elderly and the school lunch program through the donated food distribution system we have had some difficulty in limiting the salt content of our foods, not because of any theoretical objection but because the people in charge of school lunch programs throughout the country have said students wouldn't eat it if it didn't have a high salt content; also in view of the fact that we have had a great deal of opposition from school health authorities about instituting a nutrient standard, I'm wondering if in your experience with these isolated episodes you referred to you find that the students are able to bring some good nutrition principles into the conduct of school lunch program activities?

DR. LACHANCE: In every instance that I'm familiar with the answer is yes. They are obviously not running their own show alone. One of the important recommendations I've made is that each school have a committee which consists of a school teacher or two, particularly a school nurse, one of the phys. ed. teachers, and an interested teacher, the school food director, and two or three students, depending on what grade levels are involved. They debate these issues. They learn from them. They come up with a program of not only teaching certain foods in the classroom but also displaying those foods and not making people eat them. They try to teach them new recipes. Then you turn them on and you do Chinese cookery for example, and the kids begin to appreciate foods. So young people have contributed in this respect. Now as far as nutritive planning of meals, I think that that is more possible than we've given it a chance to be. I'll have an article in the *Journal of School Food Service* in February showing how to do this just using nutritional labeling information. People will quibble about how good that is, but it's certainly in the right direction and it can be done. And you also can educate with this. You can place histograms in the room showing the nutritive profile of the meal and whether it adds up to a third of an RDA or not or whatever standard you want to set. With cake or pie the histogram reveals that you have nutrients in it, but the calorie bar is so much higher than all the other nutrients that the message comes across, and even the janitor says, gee whiz, I didn't know that.

UNIDENTIFIED SPEAKER: If obesity is too detrimental to health and if at age 40 twice as many females are obese than males then why do women outlive males by at least seven years on a national average?

DR. SCHAEFER: It's a good question. I'm not sure that I have all the answers, but by the same token I wouldn't encourage obesity. I just don't have the final answer. There is an increasing evidence of diabetes in that obese group.

DR. S. S. FLASCHEN (*International Telephone & Telegraph Corp., N.Y., N.Y.*): The F.D.A. acts to ban or limit the sales of products suspected of being a hazard to the health. What further evidence is required by the F.D.A. to ban or limit the sale of cigarettes?

DR. J. E. VANDERVEEN: I believe the regulation of tobacco is not directly under our jurisdiction, and I really have to plead ignorance on exactly where it fits in the scheme of things. The decision to label cigarettes came under the Surgeon General of the Public Health Service. I do know that tobacco is regulated by a commission on tobacco, alcohol and firearms. We do not consider tobacco a food. We do consider alcohol a food, and we have a labeling requirement proposal out for alcohol. I think we're not going to win on that one, but we feel they ought to label the ingredients.

SUMMATION AND PERSPECTIVE

Magnus Pyke

British Association for the Advancement of Science
London, England

We are all indebted to The New York Academy of Sciences for having organized this conference. In opening it, Dr. Henry Moss, past-president of The Academy and Bicentennial Chairman, pointed out the way in which it differed from most Academy conferences. It was not a specialist conference for the presentation of detailed research findings. Rather it has been planned to examine a number of different points of view by which understanding and knowledge can be brought to bear on the production and distribution of food for the greater benefit of mankind at this present confused period of the world's history, 200 years after the founding of the United States of America as an independent developing nation.

To what extent may we conclude that the five objectives of the conference, as listed by Dr. Moss, have been achieved? They were to consider the world's food and the contribution of the United States to its provision, to reflect on the proper uses of technology in producing food, to assess the level of malnutrition in the world, and to try to outline a plan for nutrition for the United States where such does not exist at present. The fifth objective was to provide a place where people of diverse interests could come together to discuss all these matters profitably.

To deal with these aims there have been contributions of three sorts: (1) Those concerned with the adequacy of the food supply, the nutritional status of different communities and with forecasts, either gloomy or cheerful, of how things may change in the future. (2) Then there have been reviews by expert commentators of the state of the scientific knowledge that is known as well as a look at some of the areas of scientific ignorance. (3) Lastly, there are those communications—the nub of the conference and the main justification for holding it—to discuss in the light of current knowledge of agriculture, food science and nutrition, what can be done to improve the human condition.

THE PROBLEM TO BE SOLVED

It is salutary for those who have long been concerned with worldwide problems of food and nutrition to compare the present assessment with that of nearly half a century ago. In 1936, John Boyd Orr published his study of the diets of working-class families in Great Britain under the title of "Food, Health and Income." He showed, almost for the first time in terms of specific nutrients, what had been known throughout history, that an inadequate income is associated with an inadequate diet. A generation later, as the first Director General of the Food and Agriculture Organisation of the United Nations, Orr found that the same principle that affected British workmen and their families applied worldwide, for of such is the "world food crisis." And in 1976 it is still with us. But if a crisis is a continuing state of affairs, should it be defined as a crisis, or is it the normal—if regrettable—state of affairs?

434

A crisis may be taken as something that can be solved, a state of affairs, something that can perhaps be ameliorated. Wallace Aykroyd entitled his recent historical review of the food shortages by which mankind has been dogged since time began, "The Conquest of Famine." Jean Mayer, in the opening paper to this conference, reviewed evidence to show that the application of scientific knowledge, the growth, albeit slowly, of international goodwill, a change in the demographic outlook, and some spread in understanding all provide support of a measure of prudent optimism. The conference started out, therefore, in the first aspect of its work, on a line of thinking refreshingly different from the apocalyptic gloom which has been the fashion of the age.

NEW KNOWLEDGE FOR SOLVING PROBLEMS

In its second aspect, to delineate new knowledge, other new things were brought to light. Dr. Sylvan Wittwer's paper again drew attention to what other observant nutritionists had deduced before, namely that the production of food poses no worldwide problem. While this can seem strange to concerned Americans, any strangeness the idea might once have had has long worn off for Europeans, all too well aware of the readiness with which mountains of butter, beef, and dried milk and lakes of wine can appear if farm prices are pitched too high so that the cost of food limits the amount that the inhabitants of the European Economic Community can afford to eat. Dr. D. J. Greenland's paper was fresh to many of his listeners detailing information new to them about the possibilities of tropical agriculture, as also was Dr. R. W. F. Hardy's account of basic studies of nitrogen fixation, photorespiration, and the maximization of the harvested parts of particular crops. Then there were contrasting contributions from Dr. Elsie Widdowson and Dr. Clement Finch describing what is known about prenatal nutrition and some of the incompleteness of our knowledge about iron nutrition. Dr. Kritchevsky debated the knotty question of fiber, and Dr. Henkin discussed the diverse factors affecting appetite.

These were only some of the contributions delineating the onward march of knowledge by which man the scientist controls his own destiny. It was therefore salutary that the organizers of the conference had arranged for Dr. Reid Bryson to draw attention to the evidence suggesting that during the honeymoon years of the scientific ascendancy, when each year's harvest was larger than the last, the climate was—taking a more extended time-scale—exceptional. More than this, when the long-range situation is reviewed, it is clear that abrupt climatic changes can occur. And if they do in our times, and the ice returns or the rains fall in a different place, all our self-confident plans will be in vain. Can it be that Man, with all his scientific cleverness, is not God after all?

HOW PROBLEMS ARE SOLVED

Most scientific conferences are concerned with the discussion of new knowledge. This one was different. It aimed to study how scientific understanding could be brought to bear to improve the state of society. Dr. V. Ramalingaswami described how knowledge was applied to a real community so that 100,000 children each year who live their lives blind through lack of vitamin A may not do so. Dr. Walter Mertz detailed the way in which the need for the supplementation of American foods could be sensibly assessed and appropriate amounts of vitamins and minerals incorporated in them for the good of the community. This and other papers gave rise, however, to prolonged discussion of the basic issue of how a nutrition policy for the United States, so long lacking, could be brought into being.

There is no difficulty in defining the target. Everyone would like to see clean air, pure water, a beautiful land and nourishing food, with social justice prevailing so that all would benefit both in the United States and, because of the matchless productivity of the land and the generosity of the people, in the whole world too. But if this is the target, how is it to be attained? If scientists believe that they know best what the community should eat and what should be done to produce it, they cannot claim autocratic authority to impose their knowledge on their fellow citizens. At best, they can use their knowledge to reinforce their powers of persuasion within the political system by which their community is organized. To do so, they can work to educate that community and in doing this—for thus it emerged in the debate—the scientists themselves may become better educated. Even now they do not always show that they understand that the function of food is more than nutrition. It also serves aesthetic and social ends. Christmas pudding, Thanksgiving turkey, and wedding cake possess attributes other than nutritional. Butchers are only partly in the nutrition business, they are in the entertainment business as well. And food must be considered fit to eat. In wartime Great Britain under rationing a proposal to use pet food to increase poultry production and sacrifice the dogs to the war effort as sausages received short shrift.

In organizing the Conference on Food and Nutrition in Health and Disease in the way that it did, The New York Academy of Sciences demonstrated the variety of sciences affecting the diverse operations of food production, transport and processing, the understanding of dietetics and medicine, the intricacies of biochemistry. Dr. Stunkard introduced psychology in a discussion of obesity, Dr. Brasel considered nutrition and brain growth. But no matter how widely the disciplines extend, the special contribution that the scientist can make to the debate as a whole is through his adherence to rationality. A scientist, striving to elaborate a national nutrition policy, may need emotion—he can have fire in his belly—but his special claim to attention is knowledge based on the rational principle of assessing facts from which conclusions may be drawn. Only on this basis can such policy as may be elaborated be submitted, perhaps to the Office of Science and Technology Policy or whatever other mechanism may be designed to advise the President in the midst of his various terrifying responsibilities, so that the policy targets can be translated into action.

WHY ARE WE ALL HERE?

Why was this conference gathered together, and why was it appropriate for it to be in Philadelphia? Perhaps it is fitting that the great compliment of being invited to sum up was paid to me, a foreigner in this city and an Englishman to boot. The reason why we seek good nutrition for the people of the United States and for the wider brotherhood of man is because 200 years ago wise and humane men established a nation on the basis of certain ideals. During the conference we looked at Professor Garrett Hardin's solution to America's problems by limiting the lives of redundant populations elsewhere and we recoiled. *Your* population explosion may be *my* children!

We have sought further knowledge at this conference and means to share it with fellow citizens in the United States and abroad for the same purpose as that which was articulated 200 years ago in this place, namely to improve the human lot. It is for this that a humane society, if it can justly be so designated, exists. And with these words I would like in your name to terminate the conference.

Author Index

Italicized page numbers refer to Comments in Discussions

Asbury, D., *428–429*

Bahn, A., *386*
Barbero, V., *268*
Baum, E., *174*
Beers, W. O., 391–396
Behar, M., 176–187, *246, 248*
Bolaffi, A., *170*
Brasel, J. A., 280–282, *383–384, 388*
Brin, M., 239–250 (Moderator), *239, 242–244, 246, 250*
Bryson, R. A., 40–53, *54–55, 100–101*

Calvert, G., *16, 101–102, 248, 429, 431*
Cantor, S. M., 262–263, *267, 270, 274–276, 279*
Chafkin, S. H., *7–10, 13, 15*
Clapham, W. B., Jr., 228–238

Dobbins, C. N., Jr., 148–150, *171–172*
Doyle, M., *271*
Duke, R. C., *10–13, 15, 16*

Ellis, R., *54*

Finch, C. A., 221–227, *242, 250*
Flaschen, S. S., *385, 433*
Flood, R., *109, 385*

Gat, J. R., 33–39, *55–56*
Gilman, G., *275*
Glassman, D., *387, 428*
Goldblith, S. A., 161–166, *167–175* (Moderator), *172, 174–175*
Goodwin, M., *249–250, 270*
Gordon, W. W., *54*
Granbert, S., *277*
Greenberg, S., *169*
Greenland, D. J., 112–120, *167–169*
Griff, A., *386*

Hamilton, D., *174–175*
Hardin, G., 87–91, *99–100, 106–107*
Hardy, R. W. F., *168*
Henderson, R., *429*
Henderson, T. R., *277*
Henkin, R. I., 321–334, *389*
Homer, C., *106, 108*

Iacano, J., *266–267*
Iberall, A., *15*
Ifekwunigwe, A. E., 69–86, *104*

King, G., *103*
Krehl, W. A., 335–359, *387–388*
Kritchevsky, D., 283–289, *384–385, 388–389*

Lachance, P. A., *246–247*, 411–418, *432–433*
Latham, M. C., *105–106*, 197–209, *248–249*
Leveille, G. A., 259–261, *267–272, 277*

Malmros, H., 379–382, *432*
Marshall, B. H., *167–168*
Mayer, J., *5–7, 14, 16*, 54–56 (Moderator), *55*
McLaughlin, S., *389*
Mertz, W., 151–160, *173–174, 244, 271*
Miller, A., *170, 428*
Miller, S. A., 397–405, *429–431*
Milner, M., *110–111*, 129–147, *169–171, 242–243, 268*
Moss, N. H., 1–2, *278–279, 428–433* (Moderator)
Mossef el Man, *169–170*
Murray, J., *242*

Nicholson, T., *271–272*

Oppenheimer, J. R., *101, 168*
Oser, B. L., *275, 430*

439

Pimentel, D., 26–32, *54–55*
Pottman, A., *54, 273–274*
Pyke, M., *108*, 434–437

Rabin, M., *171, 173–174, 249, 269, 389, 431*
Ramalingaswami, V., *15*, 210–220, *245–246*
Raphael, D., *247–248*
Rawlins, S. L., *55*, 121–128, *168–169*
Rensberger, B., *98–100, 103–104*
Respino, B., *384*
Revelle, R., 57–58, 96–111 (Moderator), *97–100, 102, 104, 106–110*
Rhoads, J. E., 383–390 (Moderator), *383, 390*
Rosenfield, D., *276–277, 432*
Rothschild, E., *96, 99, 111*
Rubin, M., *384*

Sarett, H. P., *172–173*
Schaefer, A. E., *55, 419–427, 433*
Schneider, H., *14*, 251–254, 266–279 (Moderator), *266–269, 274, 277–279*
Scrimshaw, N. S., 129–147

Seeley, R. D., *171*
Shaughnessy, D. E., 92–95, *102–104, 107–108*
Stillings, B. R., *240–244*
Stunkard, A. J., 298–320, *386*

Teply, L. J., *239–240*
Timmer, C. P., 59–68, *97–98, 102–103*

Vanderveen, J. E., 406–410, *273, 431–433*

Wang, D. I. C., 129–147
Watkin, D. M., *13–14, 169*, 290–297, *432–433*
White, J. F., 391–396, *428–429*
Widdowson, E. M., *173*, 188–196, *246, 386*
Wilchinsky, Z. W., *432*
Wilcox, W. W., 255–258, *268, 269*
Winick, M., 280–282
Winikoff, B., *96–97, 99–100, 104*
Wittwer, S. H., 17–25, *54*
Wynder, E. L., 360–378, *386–390*

Subject Index

Page numbers in italics refer to material in figures or tables

Acidulants, *400*
Actin, 384
Acupuncture, *323*
Additives; *see* Food additives
Adenine, 142
Adenomatous polyps, 366
Affluence
  cardiovascular diseases and, 338, 340
  obesity and, 264, 302, 321, 351
Afforestation, 38; *see also* Deforestation
Aflatoxins and cancer, 360, *401*
Africa
  breast feeding in, 118, 198
  drought in, 5, 13, 70
  fiber intake in, 284
  food situation in, 6–7
  no-till agriculture in, 112
  plant diseases in, 114
  population distribution in, 112
  starvation and drought scenario for, 234–235
  women's rights in, 10
"Agent for change," 94
Aging, 290–296
Aging-nutrition-health triad, 290–296
Agricultural experimental stations, 106, 130, 137, 138, 139
Agricultural policy and production, 93–95, 98, 240–241, 253–254, 256–257; *see also* Public Law 480
Agricultural research institutions, 107, 112–113, 243; *see also* Agriculture—colleges and universities; State agricultural institutions
Agricultural Research Service, *24*, 266–267
Agriculture
  breakthroughs in, 9, 59
  colleges and universities of, 107, 129–130, 138, 141, 142, 252; *see also* Agricultural experimental stations
  enrollment in, *24*
  data collection of, 73–75
  development increase of, 7, 17
  in deserts, 34, 36–38
  energy-intensive, 240–241
  export figures for, *24*
  Federal funding of research in, *24*
  food needs and, 17–25, 164
  genetic protein improvement by, 133–134

Green Revolution and, 59–65, 68
  gross income of, *24*
  inputs of, 164
  in lowland humid tropics, 112–119, 167, 241, 435
    pests and plant disease in, 114, 117–118
  major U.S. events of food and, *24*
  national parks and, 89
  National Science Foundation funding of, 129–130, 143, 147
  Nigerian gains in, 113–117, 167
  particulate pollution from, 47
  productivity gains in, 59–60
  profit incentive in, 58, 62–65
  programs in China, 13, 98
  research in
    animal protein, 137
    cereal protein technology, 135
    first application of basic, 17
    fundamental mission-oriented, 143–146
    NSF and, 242
    nutritional overview in, 66–68
    production incentives of, 65
    tropical production, 113–115, 435
    U.S. decline in, 257
  "slash and burn" method of, 26, 47
  U.S. subsidies, scenario of, 233
  U.S. supply prospects in, 130–131
Agriculture and Consumer Protection Act of 1973 (U.S.), 255–256
Agronomy, N-fixing systems in, 134
Agung volcano (Bali), 46
AID; *see* Draper World Population Fund
Aid intervention
  in Asia, 107
  agricultural failure of, 107–108
Alabama, Vitamin A levels in, 422
Alameda County (Cal.), 1965 health survey in, 294
Albumin in zinc metabolism, 325
Alcoholics, nutrition of, 362
Alcoholics Anonymous, 387
Alcoholic beverages
  cancer and, 362
  regulation of, 433
Alcohols in SCP production, 140
Alfalfa (dietary), protein in, 141–142
  atherosclerosis and, 286
  toxins and, 287
Alfisols, 112, 115

441

Algae, single cell protein production from, 141, 146
Alkaline phosphatase, Zn metabolism and, 333
Almonds, toxins in, 132
Alps, Little Ice Age of, 43
Aluminum deficiency in tropical soils, 116
Amaranth, 287
American Cancer Society and weight control, 317–318
American Heart Association
    cholesterol education programs, 102
    Prudent Diet, 372–375, 387
    recommended dietary fat, 387
    Selected Heart Facts, 337
    weight control programs, 318
Amino acids
    chemical synthesis of, 142
    in fetal blood, 190–192
    limiting factors of, 184
    in potatoes, 40
    protein improvement of, 133–134, 184
Anemia, 151, 207
    in Central America, 424–425
    child blindness and, 210
    detection of, 225
    explanations for, 224
    incidence of, 9
Animal agriculture, 148–150
Animal feed production, 171–172
Animal health
    studies of, 18
    trypanosomiasis and, 118
Animal products
    consumption of, 5
        income and, 68
    reclamation of, 170
Animal protein; see also Protein production; Protein resources
    American addiction to, 343–344
    colon cancer and, 285–286
    lipid risk levels of, 343
Animals; see Livestock; Poultry
Anorexia
    defined, 322
    production of, 322, 389
    sensory dysfunctions of, 322
    zinc deficiency and, 324–325, 328, 329, 330, 331, 389
Anorexia nervosa, 322
Antarctic, krill fishing in, 139–140, 145
Anthropometry, NDRO unit testing with, 76
Anthropologists
    breast-feeding and, 248
    in famine relief, 79

Antioxidants, 171, 174, 265, 400
Anti-tryptic activity, 165
Aphrodisiacs, 262
Appetite, 321–333
    centers of, 193
    control of, 193, 321–322
    methods of altering, 322, 323, 389
Aquatic proteins
    culturing and harvesting of, 145
    potentials and research needs of, 139–140
    U.S. resource study of, 129–130
Arava Valley, 34
Arcus corneai, 347
Arid zone, water potentials of, 33–38
Arizona
    calorie-protein malnutrition in, 421
    growth retardation in, 421
Atherosclerosis, 379–382; see also Cardiovascular diseases
    blood cholestrol in, 379–380
    carbohydrate theory in, 345–346
    dietary agents and, 341, 355–356
    dietary fiber and, 286
    exercise and, 351, 356
    fat-modified diet and, 379–382
    Framingham study and, 342–343
    genetic role in, 346–348, 355
    lipid biochemistry of, 349–351
    macro and trace metals and, 352–354
    pediatrics and, 348, 356
    risk factors for, 337–338
    selected heart facts on, 337
Artificial flavoring, 262
Ascariasis, 212
Ascorbic acid; see Vitamin C
Asia
    caloric intake in, 60, 61, 70
    climate change in, 41, 101
    Club of Rome policy study of, 228–229
    future food production scenario of, 232
    malnutrition scenario in, 231–233
    population density of, 112, 228
    rice agriculture in, 125, 126
    rice consumption in, 112
    soybean breeding and, 135
    vitamin A deficiency in, 80
Asian Development Bank, 126
Atlantic Ocean, climate over, 42
Atlas Mountains, water sources of, 35
Atmosphere
    over Bali, 46
    industrial pollution of, 47, 55
    transparency of, 48, 49
    variations of, 45–47

ATP
  in N-fixation systems, 134
  synthesis of, 142
Australia
  breast-feeding in, 198
  harvests in, 5
  rainfall in, 49–50
Austria, molybdenum deficiencies in, 152

B vitamins, 158, *323,* 361–363
Baby foods, 207, 376; *see also* Weaning
Bacteria, SCP processing of, 145
Bacteriological warfare, 83
Bali, atmosphere in, 46–47
Bananas, 18
Bangladesh, 99
  Birot's spots in, 213
  crunch situation in, 90
  famine in, 70, 111
  income distribution in, 96
  keratomalacia in, 212
  nutrition in
    knowledge of, 11
    situation of, 6, *11,* 212
  vasectomies in, 12
  vitamin A dosing in, 215
Bangs disease, 171
Barley, 18, 20, 397
  protein improvement of, 133–134
Basic food groups
  number system of, 259–260
  school systems and, 103–104
Beef
  colon cancer and consumption of, 286
  fat content of, *375*
  management systems for, 23
  production of ground, 170
  protein energy costs of, 30, *55*
  U.S. consumption of, 29
"Behavioral Control of Overeating" (Stuart), 304
Behavior modification, 303–310, 319
  in health, 316
BHA, 162
Biafra
  church aid in, 76
  famine causes in, 70, 73
  multipurpose clinic in, 81–82
  orphanages and family in, 84–85
Bile acids, fiber and, 286, 384
Bioassay, research and reviews of, 135
Biomass, livestock and human, *29*
Bioregulators, 21
Birdseye frozen foods, 394
Birth rates, drop of, 109–110

Birth weights, 189–191
  in Europe, 188–189
  fetal growth curves from, 189
  in Japan, 189
  nutrition and, 246–247
  in Shetland horses, 190–191
Bitot's spots, 215, 249
  xerophthalma and, 213
Blindness in childhood, 210–217
Blockades, famine and, 69–70, 82–83
Blood, 190–192
  in birth, 190–192
  carbon monoxide in, 192
  pressure of
    atherosclerosis and, 342, 556
    selected heart facts on, *337*
    sugar and, 346
Blood sugar, 191, 193; *see also* Diabetes; Hyperglycemia
Bluffton and Hilton Health Areas (S.C.), 422
Bottle-feeding, 198–208
  commerciogenic nutritious foods and, 204–205
  costs of, 202–204
  malnutrition and, 68, 199
  results of shift to, 202
Botulism, 163, 175
Bowel cancer; *see also* Cancer—colon
  dietary fiber and, 162–163, 284–286
Boy Scouts of America and health, 318
Bran
  as dietary fiber, 285, 385
  hypocholesteremic properties of, 287
Brazil
  blindness and vitamin A in, 210
  drought in Nordeste, 36
  frost in, 49
  maize yields in, 112
  nutrition situation in, 6–8
  soybean production in, 8, 131
Bread; *see specific types*
Breakfast cereals, 103–104
Breast-feeding, 197–208
  bottle-feeding vs.
    adverse results of, 202
    countries, 198–201
    reasons for increase of, 200–201, 247
  results of shift to, *201,* 202, 249
  economics of, 202–204, 247–248
  human milk production in, 197–199
  Native Americans and, 421
  protection provided by, 212
  reasons for weaning from, *201,* 247–249
  self-determination in, 248

Breast fluid, carcinogens in, 370–371
Brillat-Savarin, Anthelme, 164
British Association for the Advancement of Science, 108
Broad beans, 132
Brookings Institute, 268
Burkitt's Syndrome, 162, 174
Butter
  linoleic acid in, 379
  mountains of, 435
  soybean oil in, 379
  world production of, *381*
Butylated hydroxytoluene (BHT), 162
Butz, Earl, 111, 256

^{14}C, dating groundwater with, 35
Cabbage, *401*
Cachexia
  defined, 322
  treatment of, 322
Cadmium, atherosclerosis and, *353*
Calcium
  atherosclerosis and, 352, *353*
  phosphorus ratio with, 157
  in prenatal blood, 191
  in tropical soils, 116
Calcutta (India), bottle-feeding costs in, 203
Cali (Columbia), 281
California
  anemia in, 423
  poverty index ratio of, 419
Calories; *see also* High-protein calorie diet
  adequacy of, 20–21
  cardiovascular diseases and, 341
  in Dutch war rations, 188
  excess of, 321–323, 343
  fat levels and, 343
  fiber and, 384
  intake of
    Asian total, 60, *61*, 70
    from cereals, 29–39, *61*
    from cocoa, *61*
    from corn, *27, 29*, 30
    from fat, 387
    from nuts, *61*
    from pulses, *61*
    Russian total, 5
    world total, 60, *61,* 62–65, 70
  label information of, 395, 428
  micronutrients and, 153
  PCM epidemiology of proteins and, 176
  protein affect on, 132
  restrictions of, 293

sugar and, 428
total distribution of, 97
Cambodia, atmospheric smoke in, 54
Camels, relief operations using, 76
Canada
  salad dressing industry in, 394
  temperature change in, 101
Canadian Department of Health and Welfare, Long-Range Planning Committee of, 312
Cancer, 360–376
  additives related to, 360
  breast, 363
    androgens and, 369
    breast fluid and, 370–371
    cholesterol and, 370–371
    dietary correlation to, 368
    dietary fats and, 369–372
    nursing practices and, 369
    plasma estrogens and, 369
    prolactin and, 369–371
    urinary estrogen and, 369–370
    vitamins and, 388
    weight/height correlations to, 369
  cervix, *361, 362*
    vitamin A and, 388
  colon, 364–368
    bile acids in, 366, *367, 368*
    constipation and, 365
    dietary fat and, 364, 386
    1, 2-dimethylhydrazine (DMH) in, 368
    diseases related to, 366
    fecal constituents and, 366–368, 386–387
    fiber and, 284–286, 364
    incidence of, 389–364
    among Japanese migrants, 365
    MNNG in, 368
    neutral steroids in, 366, *367*
    transit time and, 365
    weight and, 365
  contaminants related to, 360
  of endometrium, 363
  epidemiological evidence on, 360–361
  of kidney, 363
  liver
    aflatoxins and, 360
    pyridoxin and, *361*
  mortality from, 389–390
  nitrates and, 175
  nitrosamides and, 362
  nitrosamines and, 163
  nutritional excess and, 363–364, 375
  obesity and, 321, 363–365

Cancer—*Continued*
  stomach
    vitamin A and, *361*
    vitamin C and, 361–362
    taste acuity in, 330, *331–332*
    of thyroid, *361*
    of upper GI tract, *361,* 362
    vitamin deficiencies and
      riboflavin, 362
      vitamin A, 362
      vitamin C, 361–362
Cannibalism, 10, 262
Canning, *398*
Carbohydrates, 89, 343
  atherosclerotic factor of, 345–346, 389
  fiber and, 384–385
  impaired tolerance of, 342
  U.S. consumption of, 276
Carbon dioxide in plants, 168–169, 321
Carbon fixation in grain crops, 135, 140
Carbon monoxide, 142
Carcinogenesis, 360–376; *see also* Cancer
  electrophilic theory in, 384
  food additives and, 389, 402–403
  nutrition and, 163, 175, 360–375
Cardiovascular diseases, 335–356; *see also*
      Atherosclerosis; Coronary artery
      disease; Ischemic heart disease;
      Stroke
  diet and, 338, 345–349, 354–356, 372;
      see also Diet—cardiovascular dis-
      eases
    agents of, 341
    habits of, 338, 340, 341
  genetics and, 348
  health education and, *311*
  host factors in, 340–341
  lipid theory in, 341–342
  low-fat diets in, 343
  mortality from, 5
  nutritional epidemiology studies of,
      335, *336,* 340–344
  obesity and, 316, 321–322
  prevention and treatment of, 335, 337
  "risk factors" of, 335, 337
  selected heart facts on, *337*
  U.S. decrease in, 354–355
  worksite programs for, 316
Caritas Internationalis, 76
Carnauba wax, 302
Carotenoids, 211, 214
Carrying capacity, 51–53, 88–91, 96, 99–
      101, 106
  and quality of life, 99, 107
Carter, Jimmy
  administration of, 255, 256, 258
  candidacy of, 105, 278

Case Reserve University, Club of Rome
      computer-based program at, 228–
      229, 231–237
Casein, *287*
Cassava, 18, 20, 112–118
  high-yield cultivars of, 117
  mycorrhiza and, 115
  toxins in, 132
  yields of, 112–113
Cassava bacterial blight (CBB), 114, 117
Cassava mosaic disease (CMD), 114, 117
Cattle
  dairy management systems of, 23
  desert water sources for, 33–34
  dust pollution from, 54
Cattle industry; *see also* Livestock
  economics of production, 13–14
  management systems in, 23
Cells
  lipid biochemistry and, 349–350
  toxicology and, 429
Cellular biology, 19, 23
Cellulose
  in dietary fiber, 283, 287, 385
  world production of, 22
Central America, vitamin A fortification
      in, 216
Cereal crops
  cattle production and, 13–14
  studies of, 18–19
Cereals, 60–65
  antioxidants and, 174
  bile acid binding by, 286
  diverse breeding of, 170
  for famine relief, 80
  food legumes combined with, 136
  Green Revolution and, 60–65
  protein resource studies of, 129, 135,
      242
  U.S. energy intake from, 153
  weaning foods from, 204, 207
Cereal grains, *see* Grain crops
Cereal proteins
  intergenetic crossing for, 131
  technology of, 144
  U.S. resource study of, 129–130
  use and value upgrading of, 135
Cervix; *see* Cancer—cervix
Charity and food aid, 91
Cheese
  automated production of, 137
  heart disease and, 385
  Kraft's, 394
  Scandinavian consumption of, 379
  toxins in, *401*
  vegetable extenders in, 270

Chemical synthesis
  potentials and research needs of, 142, 146
  U.S. protein resource study on, 129–130
Chemicals; *see also* Food additives—chemicals
  cancer caused by, 161, 163
Chicken; *see also* Poultry
  paraffin synthesis in, 142
  U.S. consumption of, 29
Childhood blindness and vitamin A deficiencies, 210–217
Chile
  breast-feeding in, 199
  cholesterol levels in, 346
China
  agricultural production in, 98
  aid to, 91
  birth in
    control of, 7, 13
    rate of, 109
  breast-feeding in, 198, 200
  caloric intake in, 30, *31*
  development in, 88
  drought in, 50, 70
  food in
    distribution of, 96–99
    harvests of, 5
    priorities of, 62
    reserves of, 6
  Green Revolution impact on, 61–62
  malnutrition in, 63
  nitrites in, 163
  obesity in, 302
  population control in, 88–89
  rice preparation in, 98
  sun in, 45–46
  work site training and, 317
Chinese food, 270
Chinese Revolution, 97
Chocolate milk, 432
Cholesterol, 379–382
  in American males, 14
  atherosclerosis and, 286–287, 355, 379–381
    risk of, 337–338, 341–344
  in breast cancer, 370–372
  coronary risk factor, 365
  copper deficiency and, 154–155
  in colon cancer, 368, 386
  dietary low, 388–390
  exercise and, 351
  fiber and, *285*
  genetics and, 346–348
  lipid theory of, 341–344, 355
  meat prices and, 102–103

  metabolism of, 349–351, 355–356, 387–388
  nutritional studies on, 137–138
  obesity and, 310, 386–390
  optimum levels of, 354
  pediatrics and, 348, 388–389
  polyunsaturated fats and, 344–345, 379–381
  in Prudent Diet, 372, *373,* 387
  selected heart facts on, *337*
  7-country study of heart disease and, 344
  sugar and, 345–346, 389
  Swedish surveys of blood, 379–380
  white flour and, 389
Cholesterol esters, 350
Cholesterol gallstones, 384–385
Cholesterolemia, polyunsaturated fats and, 344
Cholestyramine, 347, 384
Cholinesterase inhibitors, *401*
Chromium
  biological availability of, 156
  dietary deficiencies of, 154, 158
  food fortification with, 155, 173
  heart disease and, *353*
Chylomicronemia, 347
Cigarette smoking
  and atherosclerotic risk, 337–338, 341
  FDA regulation of, 433
  mycardial infarction and, 345
CIMMYT (Mexico), 197
Clean air, policy/goal of, 14, 101–102
Climate
  changes of, 40–53, 100–101, 435
  farm systems for, 23
  food and nutrition policies and, 105
  modification of, 97
  in North America, 40–45, 49–50
Climatologists, 257
Club of Rome, The, 109, 228–237; *see also* Computer-based policy planning
CO_2
  atmospheric incidence of, 47, *48, 49,* 55
  crop productivity with, 22
  water transportation and, 168–169
Cocoa, 114
  caloric intake from, *61*
Coconut oil, *381*
Coconuts, 18
Coffee
  coronary atherosclerosis and, 341, 354
  toxins and, 401

Colon
  cancer of; *see* Cancer—colon
  fiber and, 284–286, 288
  sigmoid volvulus of, 288
Colorado, vitamin A levels in, 422
Colorado River, 168
Colorants and cancer, 361
Colombia
  pre-Head Start Program in, 281
  weaning in, *201,* 248–249
Commission on Manpower Policy, 416
Commodity market production, 95
Communism, food distribution under, 97
Community Pediatric Center (University
  of Maryland), 422
Computer-based policy planning (The
  Club of Rome), 228–237
"Conditioning" infections, NDRO field
  assessment of, 79
Congo, atmospheric smoke in, 54
Conjunctival xerosis, 213
"Conquest of Famine, The" (Aykroyd),
  435
Constipation, dextromaltose and, 249
Consumer Food Act of 1975, 409
Consumers
  acceptance by
    education and, 10–13, 174
    food additives, 339–404
    novel protein foods, 13
  FDA and
    alleged data misuse of, 407
    informing by, 406, 409–410
    research restrictions of, 409
  government regulation and, 406
  informing the, 273, 399–404, 406, 409–
    410
Consuming Passions (Pullar), 262
Consumption, over- and under-, 59; *see
  also* Overconsumption; Overnutri-
  tion; Undernutrition
Contraception, 11–12
Convenience foods, 164
Cooling, The, 40
Cooperative State research service, *24*
Copper
  biological availability of, 156
  dietary deficiencies and, 154
  food fortification with, 154–155, 172,
    244, 277
  molybdenum-rich soil and, 152
  RDA of, 244
  in tropical soils, 116
  -zinc antagonism, 157, 241, 244, 330
Corn (maize), 18
  Chinese preparations of, 98
  climate and, 44–45

comparative cost rise of, 131
energy inputs in production of, 26–29
  in Mexico, *27*
  in U.S., *29*
fed to livestock, 29–30, 55, 148–150,
  240–241, 375
hybrid development of, 23–24
Green Revolution yields of, 60
input conditions of, 169
management systems of, 23
mycorrhiza and, 115
NPU of, 148
opaque-2 genetic type of, 20
price of, *24*
protein improvement of, 133–134
as silage, 171
tropical yields of, 112
tropical diseases of, 114
Tzb cultivar of, 113
waste feed compared with, 149, 242
yield/energy outputs of, *29*
zero tillage of, 22, 116–117
Corn and beans diet, 179–183
Corn belt, temperature changes in, 40,
  44–45, 49
Corn-fed beef
  energy conversion in, 29–30, 55
  high-fat content of, 240–241, 375
  rising costs of, 131
Corneal epithelium, 246
Corneal lesions, 210–213
Coronary artery disease; *see also* Cardiovascular diseases; Coronary heart
  disease
  fats and, 387
  obesity and, 322
Coronary heart disease; *see also* Atherosclerosis; Cardiovascular diseases;
  Heart attack; Ischemic heart disease
  blood pressure and, 355
  dietary links of, 108, 344, 355–356,
    365, 384, 386
  genetic role of, 348, 355
  health education and, *311*
  in Japan, 387
  lipoproteins and, 350–351, 355
  meat and, 102–103, 384
  nonlipid dietary studies in, 137–138
  obesity and, 337–338, 341–344, 365,
    384, 386
  pediatrics and, 348
  polyunsaturated fats and, 344–345
  risk factors for, 337–338
  saturated fat and, 384
  selected facts on, *337*

Coronary heart disease—*Continued*
  sugar and, 345–346, 354–356
  U.S. incidence of, 335, *337*
Coronary Risk Handbook, 343
Cotton, 23
Cottonseed oil, 20, *287*
  world production of, 381
Cottonseed protein, 135
Cowpeas, 18
  tropical yields of, 113, 115, 118
Cranberries, aminotriazole in, 162
Cropping by animal power, 149
Crops; *see also* Food production
  climate change and, 51
  destruction of, 69–70
  failure of, *40*, 51–52
  improving yields of, 21, 397
Crunch, defined, 90, 99
C.S.M. (corn-soya-milk), 80
Cuba
  food distribution in, 97–98
  revolution in, 97
Cultivation, shifting basis of, 112
Cyclamates, 162, 287
Cystic fibrosis, 280

Dairy Council of California, 396
Dairy industry, U.S. Senate and, 14
Dairy products
  per capita consumption of, 137
  potentials and research needs of, 137–138
  technology needs of, 145
  U.S. protein resource study of, 129–130
DDT and cancer, 360–361
Death rate and Zero Population Growth, 88
Defoliation and famine, 69–70, 82–83
Deforestation, 90, 107
Delaney Amendment (Federal Food, Drug and Cosmetic Act), 410
  aminotriazole in, 161–162
  "scientific fact" in, 410
Demographic transition theory, 88–89, 109
Dendritic arborization, 280
Dental health and fluorine, 152
Depressants, *401*
DES (diethylstilbestrol) and cancer, 360–361
Deserts
  defined, 33
  groundwater recharge in, 34–36
  irrigated agriculture in, 34

salinity of, 38
sources of water in, 33–38
Developing countries
  aflatoxin in, 360
  birth in
    rate drop of, 109
    weights of, 188–193, 246–247
  breast-feeding in, 188–193, 246–249
  centralized food programs in, 10
  food/family planning in, 12
  programs in, 10
  protein-calorie deficits in, 176–187
Development theory, 88
Dextromaltose, 249
Diabetes, 162
  fiber and onset of, 285
  hypertriglyceridemia and, 347
  in livestock, 171
  obesity and, 285, 321
Diarrhea
  in pigs, 171
  preceding xerophthalmia, 212
  protein-calorie malnutrition and, 181
Diet; *see also* Food—fortification
  adequacy research on, 66–67
  behavior changes and, 151–152, 311, 316–317, 372, 386–387, 379, 407
  cardiovascular diseases and
    carbohydrates in, 345–346
    cholesterol in, 351, 372–375, 386
    coffee in, 354
    eggs in, 375
    glucose in, 337–338
    intake habits in, 340, 386
    lipids in, 341–345
    obesity in, 338, 386
    sodium in, 351–352
    trace metals in, 352
    triglycerides in, 347
  fat modification of, 379–382
  fiber in; *see* Fiber
    in food/appetite control, *323*
  gastric cancer and, 361–362
  harm in, 59–60, 102, 374
  high-protein calories as, 26, 30
  income and, 434
  in pediatrics, 348–349
  to prevent cancer, 372, 386
  prudential modification of
    cholesterol in, 372, *373*
    fat in, 372, *373*
    management of, 374, 387
  recommendations of, 153, 173–174, 372–376
  rice and fruit as, 351–352

Diet foods
    FDA rule on, 408
    fiber and, 385
    obesity and, 312–313
Dietrary allowances, see Minimum Daily
    Requirement (MDR); Recom-
    mended Dietary Allowance
    (RDA); U.S. Recommended Daily
    Allowances (U.S.RDA)
"Dietary Goals for the U.S." (U.S.
    Senate), 306
Dietetic food, 162, 312–313
Diethylstilbestrol (DES) and cancer,
    360–361
1,2-Dimethylhydrazine (DMH), 368
Dinicotinic acid chromium complex, 156
Disease control, 18
    children and, 185
    of food legumes, 136
    of livestock, 23
    of potatoes, 140
2,5-Di-t-butylhydroquinone (DBH), 287
Diverticular diseases, 284–285
DNA, 19
Draper World Population Fund, Agency
    for International Development
    (AID), 11–12, 15
Drought, 40, 123
    in Africa, 5, 13, 36–37
    in China, 50
    in Corn Belt, 45–49
    in Europe, 49
    famine and, 69–70, 73
    food system scenario of, 231–233
    in India, 50–51
    in Mexico, 121
    in U.S., 19, 45
Drug therapy, 249
Drugs, FDA regulation of, 406
Dubos, René, quoted, 376
Dysgeusia in Zn metabolism, 330
Dystrophic conjunctival, 246
Dysosmia in Zn metabolism, 330

Earthquakes
    aid after, 90
    famine and, 69–70, 73
ECG abnormalities, 338
Ecology, 165
    food systems and, 229
EDTA, 158–159, 222
Education programs, 10–13, 15, 16, 67,
    293, 374
Eggs, 148–150
    cholesterol in, 379–375

consumption of, 6
    U.S., 29
    fossil energy ratio and, 30
    grain required for, 148
    NPU of, 148
    potentials and research needs of, 138–
    139
    production/policy effects in, 138
    required U.S. production of, 26
    technology needs for, 145
    U.S. protein resource study of, 129–
    130
Eggplant, 401
Eggyolk and non-heme iron, 158
Egypt
    desert waterlogging and salinity in,
    122, 168
    water in, 33, 37
El Salvador, 212
    vitamin A dosing in, 215
Electrophilic attack, 384
Endemic goitre, 211
Endometrium, cancer of, 363
Endomycorrhizae, 21
Energy
    food system and, 246
        requirements of, 30
        world model of, 229
    from grain, 59, 60, 61, 101
    -intensive agriculture, 240–241
    labor and use of, 26–27, 124–125
    meat and eggs cost of, 138
    protein intake of, 178–179
    resources of, 26–32, 54
Energy (chemical), food production and,
    26, 28, 29
Energy (fossil), 29
    agricultural research on, 54, 124–125
    beef protein from, 30, 55
    food systems and, 26–28, 30–31
    irrigation systems and, 124–125, 127–
    128
    squandering of, 252
    work and, 153
Energy (labor)
    food systems and, 26–28, 127–128
    inputs in Mexico of, 27
Energy (solar); see Solar energy
England
    arterial disease in, 345
    wheat price in, 51
Enriched flour, trace elements in, 157
Enrichment
    and food carriers, 156–157
    and fortification of food, 151–153

Environment
  cancer and, 361
  disease prevention and, 376
  in food systems, 263
  improvement of, 165
  issues of, 138
  malnutrition and, 280–281
Environmental Protection Agency (EPA),
  131, 256–257
Equatorial Highlands, 107
Ergot, 43, *401*
Ethiopia, drought in, 5, 70
Ethio-Swedish Pediatric Unit (Addis
  Ababa), 206
Europe
  agriculture in, 43, 51
  breast-feeding in, 198
  demographic transition in, 88
  drought in, 49, 232
    scenario for starvation and, 232, 234
  standard of living in, 54
  undernutrition in, 188–189
European Economic Community, 435
Evapotranspiration in rice crops, 125
Exercise
  cardiovascular diseases and, 338, 340,
    351
  obesity and, 314, 315, 351
Eye diseases, 210–217; *see also specific*
  diseases

F amilial polyposis, colon cancer and,
  366, 368
Family, disruption of, during famine
  disaster, 79–80, 82
  reunion after, 84–85
Family planning, 10–13, 16, 67
  scenario analysis of, 236–237
Famine, 69–91
  ad hoc assistance in, 71
  defined, 69
  disaster-prone areas, 73–77
  disasters causing, 69–76
  food distribution system and, 69–86,
    397
  media and, 94
  NDRO operations during, 71–86
  poverty circle in, 70, 177
  predictions of, 7
  protein-calorie malnutrition and, 177–
    178
  relief for, 71–82
    emergency shelter, 75, 79, 82
    food and nutrition, 80–81, 111
    food availability data for, 73–75, 79
    food in operations of, 80–81

  health and medical, 81–82
  national policy provisions of, 72–73
  organization for, 71
"Famine Code" (India), 77
FAO/WHO, protein recommendations
  of, 132, 246
Farmers, incentives for, 18
Fats, 379–382; *see also* Cholesterol; Lipids; Oils; Polyunsaturated fats;
  Saturated fats
  benefit-risk evaluation of, 272
  calories in, 387, 432
    child hyperlipidemias and, 349
  cancer and
    breast, 369–371, 372
    colon, 285–287, 364, *365*, 386–387
  cardiovascular diseases and, 341–346,
    355, 372
  in cheese, 429
  from daily diet, *374*, 387
  in meat, *375*, 384, 386–387
  in Prudent Diet, 372–375
  quality of, 275
  Scandinavian consumption of, 379–381
  in school lunches, 432
  urban consumption of, 252, 264, 276
  world production of, 380
Fatty acids, 429; *see also* Polyunsaturated
  fats
  synthesis from carbon monoxide, 142
Favism, 132, 165
Federal Food, Drug and Cosmetic Act,
  406–407
  Section 701 "rule-making on the
    record" of, 407–408
  Delaney Amendment of, 161–162, 410
Federal Insecticide, Fungicide and Ro-
  denticide Act, 256, 257
Federal Register, rule-making and, 408
Federal Trade Commission, 316
Federation of American Societies for
  Environmental Biology, 401
Feed, 13–14, 55
  single cell proteins for, 140
  U.S. animal consumption of, 148–149
Feed grains
  animal production from, 140–141
  animal ration percent of, 148
  reserves (1976), 256
Feeding, studies of practices of, 16
Fermentation, *398*
Ferric compounds, listed, *156*
Fertility rate
  food supply and, 88
  population growth and, 109

Fertilizers, 164
crop yields and, 51–53, 89, 113
energy inputs, 125, 135
in food systems, 263
influence on yields, 51–53, 89, 113
investment in, 121–122
irrigation and, 124–125, 128
potatoes and, 140
recovery of, 19, 21, 23
reduced need for, 143
in tropical agriculture, 113–114, 167–168
Fetus
blood supply of, 190–192
exposure to toxins of, 402
growth of, 189–192
Fiber, 102, 283–288
availability of trace elements and, 158, 173
bile acid binding in, 286, 384
bowel cancer and, 162–163
calories and, 384
carbohydrates and, 384–385
colon cancer and, 284, 285–286, 364–365
defined, 283
deleterious effects of, 288–289
diabetes and, 285
diseases and, 284
electrophilic attack and, 384
fad in, 385
gallstones and, 384–385
heart disease and, 286, 384
hypocholesteremic properties of, 287
toxic materials affected by, 287
Weende method of analysis of, 283–284
Fiberchrome, 384–385
Finland
atherosclerosis in, 379
Medical Board of, 379
Fire, famine and, 70
Fish
colon cancer and consumption of, 286
for famine relief, 80
food engineering of, 139
listed for polyculture, 139
NPU of, 148
U.S. annual consumption of, 29
Fish protein; see also Aquatic proteins
energy costs of, 55
as livestock feed, 30
sources of, 139–140
Fisheries, research and development of, 129, 139–140
Fitzsimmons General Hospital, 424
Flatus, oligosaccharides and, 136

Flavor enhancers, 400
Flavorings, 399, 400, 430
artificial, 262
Floods, 40, 90
in East Asia, 50
famine and, 69–70, 73
Flour; see Cereals; Enriched flour; White flour
Fluorine, 152
Folic acid, 172
in U.S. risk populations, 423–424
Food; see also Food additives; Food industry—regulations; Government regulation; specific foods
advertising of
nutritional, 277
socioeconomic forces in, 311
of affluence, 338, 340, 349, 354–356
charity and, 90–91
chemicals in, 398–404
combining of, 395
legume utilization research in, 136
under Communism, 97
contaminants of
advisory groups and, 375
attention to, 376
cancer and, 360–361
distribution of
adequacies of, 69–70, 97–98
computer-based policy in, 288–237
famine and failures of, 69–70
free choice in, 391
policy in, 57, 62, 68, 94–95, 228–229, 237, 397
production and, 97–98, 434
storage and, 397
systems of, 263
enrichment carried by, 157–159, 391
in famine relief, 73–75, 79–81
5-Fs of, 270
fortification of; see also Iron; Trace elements; specific trace elements
availability in, 155–156
benefits in, 151, 173–175, 391, 394
carrier in, 157–159
dietary imbalances in, 157
Food and Nutrition Board guidelines for, 154–155, 174
human requirements in, 154–155
needs and constraints in, 154–159
policies in, 151–152
problem areas in, 154–159
programs of, 172, 244
protein supplements in, 172
government and
priorities of, 8–9
regulations of, 131, 406–410

Food—*Continued*
  marketing of, 392–393
    acceptance in, 263, 270, 312–313
  policy of; *see also* Agricultural policy;
    Food and nutrition policy; Junk
    foods
  recommended allowances in, 102
  preservation of, 397, 398
  processing of; *see* Food processing
  production of; *see* Food production
  regulations of, 165
    FDA, 131, 406–410
  research on; *see also* Nutrition—re-
    search; Nutritional surveillance
    human milk supply, 197
    FDA, 406
    protein production recommendations
      and priority determinants for,
      130–132
  reserves of, 6, 14, 57–58; *see also*
    Food — stockpiling; Food — stor-
    age; Food—world
  in restaurants, 313
  safety of, 110–111, 129–130
  in schools, 315
  shortages of, 87–91, 98, 188–193
    future scenario on, 228–237
  spoilage of, 397–398
  stockpiling of, 76
  storage of, 69–70, 397–399
  supply of
    chemicals in, 162–164
    homogenization of, 270
    improvement of, 165
    quality of, 166
  technology of; *see* Food technology
  trends and preferences in, 153
  waste of, 13, 22–23
  wholesomeness of, 399
  world
    problems of, 5, 66–68
    reserves of, 6, 14, 101, 252
Food additives, 397–404
  abuse of, 163, 174–175
  advisory groups and, 375
  cancer and, 360–361, 399, 402–403
  consumers and, 399–400, 401–404
  diversity of, 399, 401, 429
  exposure to, 402–403
  historical development of, 397–398
  introduction time of, 398–399
  metabolism of, 429
  preservation with, *398*
  research in, 66, 429
  risk/benefits of, 6, 165, 174–175
  safety of, 399–402, 406–407

toxicity testing of
  biological input and, 429
  cost of, 407
  fetal exposure and, 402
  GRAS substances and, 401, 402
  information in, 402
  natural materials and, 401
  proliferation and, 399, 430–431
  safety time in, *402*
  techniques of, 401, 429
  teratology of, 403
Food aid
  direct operation of, 106–107
  for famine, 80–81, 99, 111
    multi- or bilateral, 93
  intervention of, 106–108, 241
  protein production and, 129
  U.S. policy of, 111
  to U.S. risk populations, 419, 421
Food and Drug Administration (FDA)
    (U.S.)
  Federal Food, Drug and Cosmetic
    Act and, 406–407
  "Food for Special Dietary Uses" rule
    of, 408–409
  nutrition regulation by, 406–410
  objectives of, 406
  policy of, 431–432
  recruitment problems of, 408
  tobacco and, 433
  thalidomide and, 316
  U.S. RDA used by, 259
Food and nutrition policy; *see also* Agri-
    cultural policy
  alternatives in, 255–256
  Congress and, 105, 110–111, 253, 255–
    257, 266–269, 278
  delivery of, 94–95, 252–253
  distinction between, 102
  distribution and, 97–98
  economics and, 329–343
  industry and, 429, 431–432
  intervention in, 106–108, 241
  media and, 94–95, 103–104
  national goals of, 101–105, 252–254
  nutrient planning and, 93–94, 110
  nutriment history and, 251–252
  politics of, 92–95, 97–98, 105, 108
  private sector in, 94, 104
  production and, 95, 98, 102, 111, 240–
    241
  public health impacts on, 110–111
  on U.S. grain stocks, 256
  vitamin A deficiencies in, 214–215
Food Balance Sheets, 197
Food colors, *400*
Food crunch, 90, 95

Food faddism, aging and, 293
Food for Peace, *see* Public Law 480
"Food, Health and Income" (Orr), 434
Food industry, 391–396; *see also* Agriculture—research; Food production—constraints; Food production—future needs; Food technology
 boasts of, 394–396
 diet foods and, 312–313
 free enterprise and, 253–254, 391, 429–430
 lobbies of, 108
 nutrition information from, 395–396, 428–429
 nutrition policy of, 429, 431–432
 obesity and, 311–312
 profit motive in, 392–393, 428
 regulation of
  credibility and, 403, 404
  FDA and, 406–409
  innovation and, 403, 430
  self-, 307
 research and development of, 392
 school program of, 395–396
Food processing, 104, 241, 391, 262–265, 270–271, 397; *see also* Food technology
 acceptability of, 393
 biological availability of Fe and, 156, 165–166
 chemical additives and, 398–404, 406–409
 diet deficiencies and, 173–174
 protein resources and, 129–130
 regulation of, 92, 102, 131, 406–410
 techniques of, 397
Food production, 93, 161–166; *see also* Food processing
 aid intervention and, 106–107, 253, 256
 biological process of, 19
 carrying capacity and, 100
 climatic impact on, 40, 43, 45, 47, 49–51, *52*, 53, 69–70, 101
 commercial weaning foods in, 204–205
 constraints on, 113–115
 controls on, 102
 cost increases of, 70
 dietary supplements in, 152
 disincentives of, 106
 drought and starvation scenario of, 232–237
 energy and
  inputs in, 124–125
  resources and land constraints of, 26–31, 138, 240

fossil fuel and, 27, 124–125, 240
frontiers in, 19-21
future needs of, 17–19, 112, 134–142, 144–145, 232–237
grains in, 26, 59–61, 62–65, 95
high-priority research in, 257
human milk research in, 197
indentification of research topics of, 66–68
inadequacies of, 69–70, 95
income/temperature change of, 101
irrigation and, 121–125
in lowland humid tropics, 112–119
 small plots, 240–241
major crops listed, 18–19
management of, 21–23
marketing and processing of, 391–395
 systems of, 23, 30, 211, 263
population density and, 112
studies of, 18
Food programs, *see* Food aid
Food stamps, 5, 15, 92, 253, 256–257, 266
Food systems, 262–265
 agricultural production and, 263
 consumption in, 263
 described, 229
 distribution in, 263
 human behavior in, 263
 ideals and realities in, 262–265
 industrialization in, 264
 market-domination of, 265
 nutrition in, 264
 processing in, 263
 scenario analysis of, 231–237
Food technology, 93
 different viewpoints on, 161
 industry and, 393–4
 utilization of, 96–97, 100
 uses and abuses of, 164–165
Forages
 production of, 22–23
 studies on, 18
 utilization of, 137, 148–150
Ford, Gerald A., 130, 256
Ford Foundation, 107
Foreign Assistance and Food Emergency Act (1975), 243
Foreign policy, grain sales and, 90–91; *see also* Food and nutrition policy
Forests, regeneration of, 113–114; *see also* Deforestation
Formosa; *see* Taiwan
Formula feeding, 183–184, 203–208, 249–250; *see also* Weaning foods
Fortification; *see* Food fortification
Fossil fuel, 28, 31, 49

4-H Clubs, *318*
Framingham study (Kannel and Gordon), 300, 335, 342
  dietary lipid profile in, 342–343
Frozen foods, 262, 415
France, foreign aid by, 107
Franklin, Benjamin, 251
Freedom of Information Act, 273
Freezing, *398; see also* Frozen foods
Frosts, 40, 121
Fruits
  juices of, 187
  studies of, 18
Fuel; *see also* Energy
  beef protein conversion of, 30, *55*
  estimated world consumption of, *28,* 30
  food production systems and, 124–125, 127–128
  price index of, *24*
  U.S. corn production from, *29*
  work energy of gasoline, 27
Fungicides, 132
Furness, Betty, 265

Gallstones, 284, 384–385
Gandhi, Indira, 12
Gastrointestinal infections, bottle-feeding and, 199, 208
Genetic improvement, 164
  of animals, 18
  of plants, 19–20
Geochemical environment, 152
Germany, birth weights in, 189
Girl Scouts of America, health and, 318
Glucose
  cardiovascular diseases and, 338
  chromium and, *353*
  fiber and, *285*
Glutamic acid, 402
Gluttony, 321, *323*
Goiter (goitre), 151, 211
Goitrogens, 132
Gossypol, 132
Government, welfare concerns of, 426
Government regulation; *see also* Food industry—regulation; *specific legislative acts*
  Food and Drug Administration, 131, 406–410
Grain; *see also* Wheat
  climate and yields of, 40–41, 43, 45, 49, 51
  ergot blight on, 43
  foreign policy and, 91
  iron sources from, 223–224

1972 U.S. shortfall of, 57–58, 255, 259
  per capita protein available from, 60
  phytic acid in, 287–288
  PL 480 and export of, 93, 253, 268
  production of
    cattle industry and, 13–14, 29–30, 55, 148–149
    Chinese, 62
    protein priorities in, 148
  reserves of, 255, 257
  required U.S. production of, 26
  stocks of, 55
  soybean protein availability of, 148–149
  surpluses absorbed, 14, 55
  world production of, 59, 95
Grain crops
  genetic diversity of, 134–135
  improving protein quality in, 133–135
  new development of, 131, 134–135, 170–171
  protein resources of, 144, 170–171
  U.S. protein resource study of, 129–130
Grain legumes, 21, 113–114, 118
GRAS (Generally Recognized As Safe), 401–402
Grasses, nitrogen fixation in, 134
Grazing land, South American availability of, 13
Great Britain
  foreign aid by, 107
  dietary studies in, 434
  National Milk Formula of, 207
  petfood in, 436
Great Depression, 253
Great Plains, temperature change in, 101
Green Revolution, 53, 60–61, 107, 121–128
  energy inputs of, 125
  generational problems of, 61
  high-frequency irrigation and, 121–128
  market effects of, 63
  nutritional impact of
    direct and indirect, 61–63
    roundabout, 63–64
    "way out," 64
  technology package described, 121, 125
Gross National Product (GNP)
  climate change and, 51
  consumption needs and, 265
  rise in U.S. of, 231
  temperature variants and, 101
Groundnut oil, *381*
Groundwater, recharge mechanisms of, 34–38

Growth
  fetal, 189–192
  prenatal catch-up, 192
  retardation of, 420–421
Growth limits, 88
Guatemala
  birthweights in, 188
  calorie-protein malnutrition in, 180–181
  INCAPARINA in, 183–184
  malnutrition studies in, 280
Guinea-Bissau, breast-milk substitutes in, 202
Gustin, Zn metabolism and, 330, 333

Haemagglutinins, 165
Haiti, keratomalacia in, 212
Hamburger, 170, 375, 387
HANES survey (HEW), 261, 407
Hay, animal ration percent of, 148
Head-Start program, 421, 422
Health
  breakthroughs in, 9
  continuum of, 290–296
  goal/policies of, 101–102, 110–111, 152,
  meat and, 138
  NDRO data collection on, 75, 79
  role of food in, 263–264
  services of food in, 182–183, 411–417
Health and Nutrition Evaluation Surveys (HANES), 261, 266, 407
Health care
  aging/nutrition continuum of, 290–296
  costs of, 295–296
  right to, 10
  voluntary agencies for, 317–318
Health clubs, 313–314
Health insurance, changing contingencies of, 314
Health restaurants, 313
Health spas, 314–315
Health food stores, 385
Heart and Lung Institute, 386
Heart attacks; see also Atherosclerosis; Cardiovascular diseases; Coronary heart disease; Hypertension
  dietary agents and, 389
  selected facts on, 337
Heavy metals, 406; see also specific metals
Hemagglutins, 401
Hemicellulose, 283
Hemoglobin values
  for New York State, 426
  in U.S. risk populations, 423–424

Hepatomegaly, 347
Herbicides, 29, 116, 118, 164, 167–168
HEW; see U.S. Department of Health, Education and Welfare
High-protein calorie diet, energy and, 26, 29–30, 132
High-technology living and cardiovascular diseases, 338, 340
Hippocrates, quoted, 251, 284, 385
L-Histadine, 323
  anorexia induced by, 329
  brain barrier and, 333
  Zn metabolism and, 325–326, 327, 328–330, 333
Histamine, 323
Histograms, 433
Hoarding and famines, 69, 72
Holland
  birth weights in, 188–189
  wheat price in, 51
Holmes, Oliver Wendell, 161
Hong Kong
  birthrate drop in, 109–110
  breast-feeding in, 198
  nutrition progress in, 6
Hookworm, iron loss from, 225
Hormones
  neural, 280
  vitamin A deficiency and, 249
Hothouse Earth, 40
Human Lactation Center (Conn.), 247
Human milk and food production research, 197–198, 247; see also Breast-feeding
Hunger
  elimination of, 59
  famine defined as, 69
  meat diet and, 148
  politics of, 59–60, 62, 64, 66–68, 69
Hurricanes and famine, 69–70, 73, 75
Hyderabad mix, 204
Hydrology of deserts, 33–38
Hypercholesterolemia, 154
  an atherosclerotic risk, 337–338
  fiber and, 287
  genetics and, 346–347
  incidence of, 346–347
  LDL receptor model and, 349–350
  in lipid theory, 342–343
  pediatrics and, 348
  in Sweden, 380
Hyperglycemia, fiber and, 285; see also Blood sugar
Hyperinsulinemia, 347

Hyperlipidemia
an atherosclerotic risk, 337–338
dietary factors of, 341
genetics and, 346–348
Hyperlipidemias, 340–341
characteristics of, *356*
genetic role of, 346–348, 356
obesity and, 351
pediatrics and, 348–349
Hyperlipoproteinemia
genetic role of, 348
in lipid theory, 342–343
Hypertension
atherosclerotic disease and, 337–338, 341, 351
cadmium and, *353*
control of, 6
diet and, 354
incidence of, 335
mortality and treatment of, 354
obesity and, 321
"rice diet" and, 351–352
selected facts on, *337*
sodium and, 351–352
sugar and, 346
triglycerides and, 347
work site programs for, 316
Hypertriglyceridemia
genetic role of, 347–348
in lipid theory, 341
Hyperzincuria in Zn metabolism, 325, 330
Hypogeusia in Zn metabolism, 324, 330, *331*
Hyposmia in Zn metabolism, 330

I ce Age and climate, 40, 43–44, 50
Iceland, climate changes in, 42–43, *44*
ICNND Nutritional Program, 345–346
Immigration, U.S., 89–90
Immunization, 215
nutrition and, 245–246
Imperial Valley (Cal.), irrigation in, 34
INCAP (Instituto de Nutrición de Central America y Panamá), 179, 216, 239
pregnancy study by, 246
INCAPARINA (Incaparina), 183–184
use of, 184, 239
Income
birthrate and, 109
diet and, 434
distribution of, 60
figures for bread, *24*
Green Revolution and, 62, 64–65
gross agricultural figures for, *24*

India
aid to, 91
intervention, 91, 107
birth control in, 7
blindness and vitamin A in, 210
breast-feeding in, 198
climate change in, 41–42, *43*
cotton hybrids in, 20
drought in, 50–51
farming changes in, 64
5-year plan of, 93
food in
harvests of, 5
intervention and, 91, 107
legume decline and, 63
reserves of, 6
rice preparation, 98
land of
salinity of, 122
waterlogging of, 122
nitrites in, 163
Planning Commission in, 239
recall type survey in, 267
population capacity of, 90
vasectomies in, 12
vitamin A and disease in, 213, 215
weaning foods in, 204–205
Indian Council of Agricultural Research, 107
Indians (North America); *see* Native Americans; Navahos
Individualism and population, 89
Indonesia, 100
AID program in, 12
vitamin A dosing in, 215
Indus Plain, water table of, 122
Industrialization
aid intervention and, 107
food systems and, 264
overconsumption and, 264
particulate pollution from, 47
Infants
formula foods for, 249–250
elimination of, 249
toxicity testing of, 402
undernutrition of
bottle-feeding and, 203–204
lifestyle diseases and, 293
water requirements of, 205–206
Infarction, calcium and, *353*
Infectious diseases
iron deficiency and, 242, 245
malnutrition and, 81–82, 199, 206–208, 245
PCM and, 181, 247
Inflation, chronic food shortage and, 70
Injected sclera, 249

Insecticides
cancer and, 360
energy inputs of, 29
Insects
control of, 21, 23, 137, 140
in tropical agriculture, 114, 117–118
Instant aging, 295–296
Institute of Tropical Agriculture, Ibadan
(IITA) (Nigeria), 113, 117, 169
Grain Legume Improvement Program
of, 118
Insulin, 285
hypertriglyceridemia and, 347
Intercropping, 117–118
International Commission on Irrigation
and Drainage, 122
International Cooperative Study on the
Epidemiology of Cardiovascular
Disease, results of, 345
International Disaster Relief Organiza-
tion (IDRO), 71
International Institute for Tropical Agri-
culture 113, 117, 169
International Planned Parenthood Fed-
eration, 11
International Rice Institute (Nigeria),
169
International Vitamin A Consultation
Group (IVACG), 212–213
Intervention, food and nutrition pro-
grams of, 106–108, 241; see also
Food aid; PL 480
Intrauterine anorexia, 191
Intrauterine device (IUD), 11, 202
Iodine, dietary deficiencies of, 151–152
Iodized salt, 152
Iowa Breakfast Studies, 416
IQ, stanines and, 383–384
Iron, 221–226
biological availability of, 221–222, 244
ascorbic acid and, 156, 158, 223, 226
food processing and, 156
nutrient depressants of, 158
values of, 155
body content of, 222
deficiencies of, 153–155
explanations for, 224, 250
implications of
infectious diseases and, 242
PCM and, 207
Plummer-Vinson's disease and, 362
in U.S. risk populations, 423–424
dietary supplies of, 221–222
leafy green vegetable, 212
requirements of, 221, 222, 271
supplementation of, 225
food effects on, 157–158, 222–224

fortification with
cereal product, 156, 250
discussion of, 172–174
infant formula, 249–250
RDA of, 155
technology of, 240
value of, 155–156
heme, 221, 156
loss of, 221
non-heme, 155, 157–158, 173, 221–223
in N-fixation, 134
IRRI (Philippines), 197
Irrigation, 121–128
aid intervention in, 107
corn production by, 29
costs of, 127–128
full-scale systems of, 121–122
of potatoes, 140
surface distribution systems of, 122–
123
waterlogging from, 122–123
world production under, 121
Ischemic heart disease, 286, 341
Isolationism, compared to mutualism, 90
Isotropic dating of desert water, 35–36

Jamaica, weaning in, 201, 248–249
Japan
birth weight in, 189
colon cancer in, 365
energy and protein intake of, 178
foreign aid by, 107
fat (dietary) in, 372, 387
heart disease in, 334, 353, 387
krill fishing by, 139
rice production in, 125, 126
serum cholesterol in, 387
Jefferson, Thomas, 251
Jericho, oasis of, 34
Journal of School Food Service, 433
Junk foods
5-Fs and, 270
in schools
lunches, 315
vending machines, 104
sugar and, 275
TV commercials and, 10–11, 103, 174

Kalahari Desert, water-source dating
in, 35
Kerala, 15
Kentucky
blood folate levels in, 424
poverty index ratio of, 419
vitamin A levels in, 422

Kenya
  bottle-feeding costs in, 203
  corneal lesions in, 212
  weaning foods in, 205
Keratomalacia, 211–217
  collagenase and protease in, 217
  control of, 213–214
  PCM and, 213, 215
  transport proteins and, 217
Kidney
  atherosclerosis, 335
  cancer, 363
Kirchner Marsh (Minn.), climate of, *41, 42*
Kissinger, Henry, 130
Korea
  birthrate drop in, 109–110
  food aid intervention in, 107
  study of malnourished orphans from, 280–281
Korean War, 90
Kraft, Inc., 393–395, 428–429
Krill, protein from, 129, 139, 145
Kwashiorkor, 176, 179, 185, 188
  milk and, 206–207
  among Native Americans, 421
Kwashiorkor Food Mix (K-Mix), 80

Labelling of nutrients, 6, 259–261, 269–270, 275, 395, 428
  cost of, 409–410
  FDA and, 406, 409–410
  School Food Service and, 413, 433
Labor
  energy use and, 26–27
  farm systems of, 23
  in irrigation, 127–128
  primary agricultural resource of, 21–22
  tropical agricultural constraints of, 114–115, 118
Lactalbumin, 394
Lactation
  decline in humans, 197–208
  in U.S. risk populations, 425
Lactose, infant intolerance for, 206–207
Laissez-faire
  economics of, 391
  population and, 88
Lamb, U.S. consumption of, 29
Land
  arable resources of, 30–31, 54, 112–113
  farming limits of, 65
  life support of, 90
    primary resource of, 21–22
    set-aside figures for, *24*
Lard, *381*
Lathyrism, 132
Latin America
  breast-feeding in, 198
  food production in tropics of, 112–119
  harvests in, 5
  protein-calorie malnutrition in, 178
  rice production in, 112–113
  vitamin A deficiency in, 80
LDL (low density lipoproteins), 346–347, 348–356, 388
Leaf protein
  toxicology studies on, 133
  U.S. resource study on, 129–130, 141, 142
Leavening agents, *400*
Left ventricular hypertrophy, 338
Legumes
  biological N-fixing in, 134
  cereals vs., 65
  as dry mulch, 118
  for famine relief, 80
  improving protein in, 20, 134
  land use and, 63
  major crop listing, 18
  for N-fixing, 115
  production and marketing of, 136
  research area in, 144
  resistant varieties of, 117
  toxins and, 401
    inhibiting, 132–133
  U.S. protein resource study of, 129–130
  weaning foods of, 204, 207–208
Leningrad, 188
Letterman Army Institute for Research, 424
Leucoma, 214
Libyan desert, water in, 37
Life, quality of, 7, 12
Life cycle, role of nutrition in, 293–294
Lifeboat ethics, 105
Lifespan and toxicity, 400–401
Lifestyle
  aging and improvement of, 291–296
  cardiovascular diseases and, 338, 340, 343
  colon cancer and, 365, 386
  diseases of, 293, 338, 340, 348, 360, 386
  nutrition related to, 294
  obesity and, 311, 386
  premature aging and, 294
Lignin, 283, 284, 286; *see also* Fiber

Lima beans, 118
toxins in, 132
Lime, 116
Linoleic acid, 381
Lions Clubs and health care, 317, *318*
Lipids; *see also* Cholesterol; Fats; Fatty
acids; Polyunsaturated fats; Saturated fats
in atherosclerotic epidemiology, 341–
352, 354–356
biochemical aspects of, 349–357
profile of Framingham study on, 342–
343
transport of, 349–351, 356
Lipoproteins
biochemical aspects of, 349–350
exercise and, 351
low density (LPL), 346–347, 349–356
very low density (VLDL), 346, 348
Lipoproteinemia, genetic role of, 347–
348
Liquid margarine, 379
Lithium
hard water and, 353
heart diseases and, *353*
Little Ice Age, 43–44
Liver
B₆ and, 361
susceptibility to cancer of, 361
Liverpool (England), infant feeding in,
199
Livestock
alternative food sources for, 137, 149
biomass in U.S. of, *29*
by-products from, 149
degenerative diseases in, 171
forage diet of, 149
grain stocks and production of, 255
land utilization and, 13, 18
meat NPU of, 148
potentials and resource needs of, 137
productivity of, 18, 22–23
advances in, 137, 149
ration components of, 148
research on
area of, 144–145, 148
strategy for, 24, 144–145
soybean feed for, 20, 148
U.S. protein resource studies of, 129–
130
wastage for, 144–145, 148
Locke, John, 89
Locusts and famine, 69–70
London (England), obesity surveys in,
300, 301
"Longage" of people, 87–88, 90

Longevity, 5, 411
obesity and, 433
optimal diet for, 374–375
Longevity Research Institute (Santa
Barbara), 355, 387
Los Angeles (Cal.), 104
TV weight loss program, 315
Louisiana
poverty index ratio of, 419
vitamin A levels in, 422
Low-calorie drinks, 313
Luxury-energy and population, 89
Lysine, 179, 184

Macronutrients, food concentrates of,
376
Magnesium
atherosclerosis and, 352–354
fiber binding of, 384
Maharashtra, weaning foods in, 204–205
Maize; *see* Corn
Malabsorption and undernutrition, 322
Malaria, 242
Malnutrition, 280–282; *see also* Protein-
calorie malnutrition; Undernutrition
achievement and IQ tests in, 281
aging and, 293
Asia future scenario of, 231–237
bottle-feeding and, 68, 199
causes of, 57, 59–60, 68, 73
determination of, 76, 79, 228–233
food and
relief priority of, 81
supplements and, 152–153
growth in
behavior and, 280
development and, 280–281
nutrition and, 383, 386, 434
human costs of, 66
infectious diseases and, 81–82, 181,
208, 383
iron deficiency in, 207
rehabilitation in, 386
severe form of, *see* Protein-calorie
malnutrition
solutions to, 179
U.S. and
risk population groups in, 419–426
role in, 228, 233–237
vitamin A deficiency in, 207–208
war and, 73
Manhattan, socioeconomical status and
obesity in, 298–300
Manila (Philippines), protein malnutrition in, 11

Manure, refeeding of, 141, 149
Marasmus, 176
  milk and, 206
  among Native Americans, 421
Margarine
  linoleic acid in, 379
  liquified, 379
  palm oil, 20
  in school lunches, 432
Margarine-cheese, 379
Marine oil, *381*
Market Research Corporation of Amer-
  ica, 407
Marxism, 90–91
Massachusetts
  anemia in, 423
  poverty index ratio of, 419
Massachusetts Institute of Technology
  (MIT), 129–130, 429–431
  Department of Nutrition and Food
    Science of, 129–130
  publication policy at, 431
Mauretania, drought in, 5
Mauritius, birthrate drop in, 109–110
Measles, vitamin A and, 212
"Measly eye," 212
Meat
  anemia and osteoporosis from, 244
  cost rise of, 131
  colon cancer and consumption of, 286
  fats in
    content of, *375*, 384
    reduction of, 375, 387
  health and palatability of, 138
  heart disease and, 384
  iron sources of, 223–224
  nitrite-cured, 163
  NPU of, 148
  potentials and research needs of, 137–
    139
  Swedish consumption of, 379
  in U.S.
    consumption, 29, 102–103, 148
    production, 26, 29
    protein resource study, 129–130
  technology needs for, 145
Meat analogs, 144
Meat anemia, 244
Media and weight reduction, 314–315
Meharry University (S.C.), 422
Menopause, colon cancer and, 369
Medical nutrition education, 279, 395
Medical quackery and aging, 293
Medicine, relief work in, 77–79, 81–82
Mental illness, Midtown Study of epi-
  demiology of, 298–300

Mesquite, 20
Metrecal, 312–313
Mexico
  breast-feeding in, 199
  food situation in, 121
  foreign aid by, 107
  Green Revolution in, 121
  high-yield agriculture in, 169
  protein-calorie malnutrition in, 181–
    182
Micronutrients in food fortification, 151–
  154, 157–159, 376
Michigan
  poverty index ratio of, 419
  vitamin A levels in, 422
Middle East, war in, 5, 7
Midtown study, 298–300, 302
  status and obesity in, 298–299
Migrant workers, nutritional status of,
  425–426
Milk, 148–150, 183, 379; *see also* Human
  milk
  calcium source of, 137
  commerciogenic nutritious forms of,
    204
  consumption of, 6, 29, 270, 385, 395
  fat reduction of, 374–375, 432
  for famine relief, 80
  grain required for, 146
  NPU of, 148
  processing research on, 137
  production figures for, *24*, 137
  in U.S.
    consumption, 29, 137
    required production, 26
Millet, 18, 20
Mineral deficiencies, 152–159, 164
  of "newer trace elements," 155
Mineral supplements
  for famine relief, 80
  FDA ruling on, 408
Minerals
  food fortification with, 151–159
  soil deficiencies and, 152
Minimum Daily Requirement (MDR),
  described, 260; *see also* Nutrition
  —norms; Recommended Dietary
  Allowance (RDA); U.S. Recommended Daily Allowances (U.S.
  RDA)
Minimum daily requirements, 173, 271,
  277
Minimum human requirements, 153–155,
  277
Minnesota
  climate record in, *41*
  temperature change in, 40

Mississippi, vitamin A levels in, 422
Mixed cropping vs. monoculture, 117–
    118; *see also* Multiple cropping
MNNG and colon cancer, 368
Molybdenum
    anionic form of, 152
    in N-fixation, 134
Mondale, Walter, 105, 278
Monoculture, mixed cropping and, 117–
    118
Monogastric livestock, listed, 23
Monosodium glutamate (MSG), 162,
    207–208
Monsoons, 41–42, *43*, 50–51
Mormons, *310*
Multiple cropping, 128, 140; *see also*
    Mixed cropping
Mung beans, 18
Muslims, reproduction rate in U.S.S.R.
    of, 109
Mutualism, compared to isolationism, 90
Myocardial infarction
    smoking and, 345
    sugar and, 345
Mycorrhiza, 115
Mycorrhizal fungi, 21, 115
Mycotoxins, 133, 165
    cancer and, 360
Myelination, brain growth and, 280
Myocardium, *353*

N abateans, control of water supply by,
    33
National Academy of Science, 172
    Food and Nutrition Board of
        food fortification guidelines, 154–
            155, 174, 241
        RDA established by, 259
        scientific understanding forums at,
            274
    presidential study request to, 130
    scientific delegation to China of, 62
    World Food and Nutrition Study
        National Research Council and, 18,
            132
        Nutrition Overview Study Team
            and, 59–60
National Accelerated Food Production
    Program (Nigeria), 113
National Association of State Universities
    and Land Grant Colleges
    Agricultural Research Policy Commit-
        tee of, 130
    formula funding of, 243
National Cancer Institute, 361, 388

National Clearinghouse for Environ-
    mental Carcinogenesis (National
    Cancer Institute), 361
National Disaster Relief Organization
    (NDRO), 71–86
National Heart Association, cholesterol
    intake and, 102
National Heart Institute, 108
National Institute of Dental Health, 108
National Institutes of Health (U.S.), 417
National Research Council, U.S. RDA
    of, 259
National Science Foundation (NSF)
    beef production study by, 170
    MIT protein resource study by, 129–
        130, 135, 137–141, 147
Native Americans
    breast-feeding among, 421
    corn farming by, 44–45
    malnutrition of, 420–421
    nutritional status of, 419–421, 426
    obesity study of, 302
Navahos, 302, 420–421
NDRO, *see* National Disaster Relief Or-
    ganization
Negev desert
    climate of, 34
    potable water in, 33–34
    water yield in, 36–38
Negev-Sinai aquifer, 37
Net Protein Utilization Value (NPU),
    148
New Jersey Council Survey (1973–75),
    415
New Valley (Sahara Desert), aquifers in,
    34
New York Academy of Sciences, Con-
    ference on Food and Nutrition in
    Health and Disease
    criticism of, 8, 57
    Nutrition Forum, 251–254
    objectives of, 1–2, 434–437
New York City; *see also* Manhattan
    teenage pregnancies in, 11
New York State, poverty in
    anemia and, 423, 426
    index ratio of, 419–423
    survey of, 422
New Zealand, selenium deficiencies in,
    152, 173
Niacin, 172
Nigeria
    cassava production in, 113–114, 117–
        118
        blight and, 114, 117
    crop yields in, 112, 169
    eye glasses in, 212

Nigeria—*Continued*
  Federal Department of Agriculture of, 113
  income in, 167
  nutrition level in, 167
  population density of, 112
  rice yields in, 169
  "road to health chart" in, 207
  root crops in, 118
  shrubs and soil management in, 116
  weaning in, *201*, 248–249
Night blindness, 213, 215, 249
Nile Valley, irrigation projects in, 34
Nitrification, 21, 116, 135
Nitrates, 163, 174
Nitrites, 163–164
  benefit-risk evaluation of, 272
  in meats, 163, 174–175
Nitrogen
  energy of
    quality and, 28
    U.S. corn production inputs in, *29*
  loss of, 21, 124
  sources in plants, 20
  in tropical soils, 115
  uptake and translocation of, 135
Nitrogen fixation, 115, 130, 321, 435
  in cereals, 144
  enhancement of, 19–21, 134–135, 143, 240, 435
  rhizobia and, 115
Nitrosamides, 362
Nitrosamines, 163, 175
No-till agriculture, 167–168
Non-fat solids, consumption of, 6
Non-nutrients, 66–68
Non-protein nitrogen, utilization of, 137
North Africa
  desert water in, 33, 37
  food distribution in, 57
North America
  breast-milk production in, 198
  caloric supply in, 70
  climate change in, 40–50, 101
  drought and starvation scenario for, 232–233
  rainfall in, 41
Northern Hemisphere, temperature changes in, 45, *46*
NPU (Net Protein Utilization value), 148
NSF; *see* National Science Foundation
Nucleic acids, 145; *see also* RNA
Nutmeg, *401*
Nutrient-nonnutrient interactions, 59
Nutrient-host interactions, 66

Nutrient Film Technique, 22
Nutrients; *see also* Labelling; Micronutrients; Nutrition
  additives and, 430–431
  history of, 252
  requirements of, 151, 154–155, 259
Nutriment, 251–252
Nutrition
  -aging-health triad, 290–296
  biological era of, 252
  biomedical aspects of, 59
  birth weights and, 108–109, 191, 246–247
  chemical-analytical period of, 252–253
  component complexity of, 255
  Congress and, 110–111
  deficiencies of, 152–159
  education in
    aging and, 293
    breast-feeding, 207
    consumers' sources of, 395
    Dairy Council of California and, 433, 396
    elementary levels of, 165–166
    FDA role in, 406
    food groups in, 260
    Kraft's school program, 395–396
    mass media for, 104
    obesity and, 307–309, 315–316
    protein-calorie malnutrition, 185
    programs of, 16
    right to, 10–13
    schools and, 103–104
    unworkable, 102–103
  famine relief and, 81
  food intake in, 264
  Green Revolution's impact on, 61–63
  harm from, 59–60
  health and progress in, 5–7, 17
  history of
    food and nutrition policies and, 252–254
    phases in, 251–252
  human requirements for protein in, 132
  improvement of, 18, 23, 102–103, 151–160
  industry and, 312–313, 315, 391–396, 428–429
  iron in, 221–226
  MIT study of protein production and, 132
  NDRO data collection on, 76, 79
  norms of
    basic four food groups as, 259–260
    Minimum Daily Requirement and, 260

Nutrition—*Continued*
  norms of—*Continued*
    Recommended Dietary Allowance (RDA) as, 259
    reviewed, 259
    U.S. Recommended Daily Allowances as, 259
  nutriment phase of, 251–252
  planning in, 93–94, 101–102, 151
  policy of, 151; *see also* Agricultural policy; Food and nutrition policy
    food policy distinguished from, 102, 104
  politics of, 59–60, 62, 92–93, 129, 228, 429, 436
  protein evaluation in, 132
  research in
    Decennial Survey of, 268
    FDA's, 406
    health survey in, 267–268
    programs of, 59–68, 159, 228–237, 259
    recall-type survey in, 267–268
    USDA's, 138, 260–261, 266–268, 295
    U.S. 10-State survey of, 419–422, 424–425
  status in
    aging lifestyle and, 291–296
    surveys of, 291, 419–426
  in United States
    policy, 1, 9–10, 92–93, 101–102, 129, 151–153, 228, 237, 436
    risk populations, 419–426
  vitamin A in, 210–217
Nutritional epidemiology, 335–356
  biochemical enrichment in, 349–351
Nutritional excesses; *see* Overnutrition
Nutritional surveillance, 110, 266–268; *see also* Food—research; Nutrition—research
Nuts, caloric intake from, *61; see also specific nuts*

Oatmeal bread, 164, 174
Oats, 18
Obesity
  affluence and, 264, 302, 321
  age and, 298, 300–302
  atherosclerotic risk of, 338, 341, 386
  behavior modification for, 303–310, 319
  cancer and, 363
  cholesterol and, 310
  diabetes and, 433
  diet foods and, 312–313

  dietary iron and, 153
  ethnicity and, 299–300
  future influences on
    education and, 315
    government and, 315–316
    media and, 314–315
    voluntary agencies and, 317–318
    work site training and, 316–317
  generation in U.S. and, 299
  hazards of, 322, 389
  hyperlipidemias and, 351
  hypertriglyceridemia and, 347
  incidence of, 322
  industry influence in
    direct service, 312
    health spas, 313–314
    life and health insurance, 314
  in Manhattan, 298–300, 302
  mechanisms of, 9, 321
  media campaigns, 310
  medical programs and, 309–310
  nutrition education and, 307–309, 315
  out-patient treatment of, 303–306
  overnutrition and, 302
  permutations and combinations of, 318
  self-help groups and, 306–308
  socioeconomics of
    class in, 385–386
    forces in, 311–312, 321
    status in, 298–302, 319–321
    surveys of, 298–302
    therapy as, 303
  TOPS (Take Off Pounds Sensibly) and, 305, 307–308
  undernutrition and, 302
  U.S. income and, 420
  Weight Watchers International and, 309–313, 386
  in Western U.S., 302
Oil palm and soil erosion, 114
Oil-producing nations, 5, 7, 91
  Nigeria, 167
Oils (edible)
  hydrogenated vegetable, 381
  world production of, *381*
Oilseed proteins; *see also* Soybeans
  food processing and utilization of, 133, 149
  listed, 135
  potentials and research needs of, 135–136
  research area in, 144
  toxic inhibitors in, 132–133
  U.S. protein resource studies of, 129–130
  utilization of, 133, 149
  weaning foods of, 204

Oligosaccharides, flatus production of, 136
Olive oil, *381*
Oral contraceptives, 342
Osteoporosis, 244
OTA; *see* Office of Technology Assessment
Ovary, cancer of, 363
Overconsumption, 102
  diet histories in, 365
  food behavior and, 265, 321–322
  mass markets and, 264
  stress-related diseases and, 264
Overgrazing, 150
Overnutrition, 321–323; *see also* Overconsumption
  cancer and, 363
  carcinogenesis and, 360, 363–365, 372–376
  under- and, 323
Overpopulation, 90
Oxidation of toxins, 429
Oxisols, 112, 115
Oxygen in iron transport, 225

Pakistan
  contraception in, 11
  crop improvement in, 13
  food aid intervention, 107
  nutrition in
    knowledge of, 11
    situation of, 6
Paleowaters, desert sources of, 35–38
Palestine, famine causes in, 70
Palm kernel, *401*
Palm oil
  in shortenings, 20
  yields of, *381*
Palmyra, oasis of, 34
Panels, Food, Nutrition and Population Interactions, 5–16
Parasitism, food shortages and, 90, 106
Parenteral alimentation, 153–154
Pastures, animal ration percent of, 148
Patent flour, *157*
PCM; *see* Protein-calorie malnutrition
Peanut butter, 452
Peanuts, 18, 135, *401*
Pectin (dietary)
  arteriosclerosis and, 286
  hypocholesteremic properties of, 287
  in plant cells, 283
  toxins affected by, 287
Pellagra, 151
Permanent Advisory Commission on Human Nutrition, 278

"Perspective on the Health of Canadians" (Lalonde), 312
Pest control; *see* Insects—control
Pesticides, 164
  in animal feed production, 172
  essential energy inputs of, 26
  in Green Revolution, 121, 125
  toxicity of, 132
Pet feeding, 145
pH, 430
Pharmaceutical Manufacturers Association, 408
Pharmacokinetics, 429
Philippines
  breast-feeding in
    foods to wean from, 205
    income and, 203–204
    weaning from, *201, 248–249*
  nutrition in, 207–208
  obesity in, 302
  vitamin A fortification in, 193–194, 207–208, 214
Phosphorus
  -calcium ratio, 157
  in fetal blood, 191
  marginal soil and, 21
  in tropical soil, 115
  U.S. corn production energy inputs of, *29*
Photosynthesis, 115
  improving efficiency of, 19, 23
Phthisis bulbi, 214
Phytic acid, effect on trace minerals of, 287–288
Pickling, *398*
Pigs
  garbage for, 171
  growth factors in, 192–193
Pineapple, 168–169
Pineapple juice, 401
Pizza, 270
Placenta
  blood flow in, 191–192
  growth rate of, 191
  weight of, 191
Plant disease in tropical agriculture, 114
Plantains, *401*
Plant protein
  animal proteins converted from, 29–30
  genetic improvement of, 133–134
  meat compared with, 148
  molecular research on, 146
Plasma
  cholesterol and, 349
  fetal and maternal forms of, 190–191
Plummer-Vinson's disease, *361,* 362
Poliomyelitis, 312, 316

Pollutants, atmospheric forms of, 47, 55
Polyculture as aquatic protein resource, 139, 145
Polyps, 366, 387
Polysaturated fatty acids, 159
Polyunsaturated fats; see also Fats; Polysaturated fatty acids
  in lipid theory, 341–345
  Prudent Diet and, 372
  role of, 344–345
  saturated and, 344–345, 379–381
Poppyseed oil, Swedish production of, 380–381
Population
  carrying capacity of, 51–53, 88–91, 99–101
  climate and increase of, 44, 47, 50–51, 52, 53, 100–101
  energy consumption and, 27
  famine and, 70
  food and
    production of, 112, 150
    systems of, 26, 228, 407
  land system and, 229
  limits to, 89, 101
  limits in desert of, 34n
  of livestock, 22, 29, 54
  U.S. nutritional needs of, 419–426
  world
    estimates, 28
    food system model input, 229
    increases, 5–7, 54, 229
  zero growth of, 88–90, 109
Population growth, 16, 87–90, 107, 436–437
  aging and, 291–292, 295
  reproduction rate of, 109–110
Potassium
  atherosclerosis and, 352
  energy inputs in U.S. corn production of, 29
  in fertilizer, 21
  in fetal blood, 191
  in tropical soils, 115
Potato crisps, 164
Potatoes, 98, 140
  Irish diet of, 385
  protein levels of, 140
Potatoes (sweet), 118
Poultry; see also Chicken
  colon cancer and consumption of, 286
  food resources from, 23
  NPU of, 148
  technology needs and, 145
  U.S. protein resource study of, 129–30
  waste feed for, 149, 171
Poverty and chronic food shortage, 70

Poverty index ratio (PIR)
  anemia and, 423
  of U.S. states, 419
Pre-albumin, 217
Precipitation; see Rainfall
Pregnancy
  colon cancer and, 369
  placental growth during, 191
  undernutrition during, 188–190
  in U.S. risk populations, 425
Prenatal nutrition, 188–193, 246–247, 425
Prenatal care, 68
Pressor amines, 401
Preventative medicine, drawbacks and successes of, 374–376
Pritikin diet, 355
Processed feed, animal ration percent of, 148
Processing; see Food processing
Prolamine, 134
Prostrate, cancer of, 363
Protein
  balanced diet and, 20–21, 60
  calories affecting, 132
  colon cancer and dietary, 285–286
  commerciogenic nutritious forms of, 204
  deficiencies in, 11–12, 21–22
  forms of, 204
  distribution of, 97–98
  fossil energy converted to beef, 30, 55
  innovative technology and, 133, 143, 146
  intake of energy and, 178–179
  lysine supplementation of, 184
  in malnutrition, 280
  molecular research of, 146
  nitrogen-fixation enhancement and, 19–21
  nutrition evaluation of, 143
  PCM epidemiology of calories and, 176
  production of; see Protein production
  resources of; see Protein resources
  retinol and, 215, 217
  sources of, 129–147, 170–171
  toxicology of, 132–133, 143
  U.S. consumption of, 5, 29, 55
Protein-calorie malnutrition (PCM), 176–185
  causes of, 179–182
  childhood blindness and, 211–214, 217, 242
  corn/bean diets and, 179–181
  described, 176, 207
  keratomalacia and, 213
  lactose intolerance and, 206–207

Protein-calorie malnutrition (PCM)—
    Continued
  low birthrate and, 176, 179
  mental development in, 177, 280–281
  of Native Americans, 420–421
  non-food factors in, 181–182, 185
  physical work output in, 177
  prevention of, 176, 179, 182–185
  resistance to infections in, 177, 181,
      245, 247
Protein-energy malnutrition; *see* Protein-
    calorie malnutrition—described;
    Energy—protein intake
Protein production
  conversion of vegetable to animal in,
      29–30, 148–150
  domestic needs of, 129
  export demands of, 129
  from grain, 60, 63, 129–131, 133–135,
      169, 255
  ground-beef studies in, 170
  MIT study of, 129–147
    conclusion of, 147
    determinants for, 130–132
    organization of, 130
    potentials and research needs in,
        134–142
    problems and issues in, 132–134
    research recommendations of, 143–
        147
  research funding for, 130
  specific resources of, 129, 134–142
  U.S. resources studies in, 129–130
Protein resources
  aquatic forms of, 139–140, 145
  cereal technology in 118, 135, 144
  by chemical synthesis, 142, 146
  grain crops for food and feed as, 134–
      135, 144, 240–241, 255
  of human milk, 197–199
  of leaves, 141–142, 146
  of legumes, 65, 134, 136, 144
  livestock animal production as, 18,
      137–138, 144–145, 148–150, 172,
      240–241
  nonconventional technologies and,
      170–171
  oil seed as, 132–133, 135–136, 144
  of potatoes, 140
  of roots and tubers, 118
  of single cell proteins (SCP)
    nonphotosynthetic, 141, 145–146
    photosynthetic, 140, 146
  of soybeans, 135, 172
Proteinex, *204*
Prudent Diet, The (American Heart
    Association)

cholesterol levels in, 372
fat levels in, 372, *373*
managerial preventive medicine in, 374
present American diet and, *373*
Public health issues, 110–111, 249
Public Health Service; *see* U.S. Public
    Health Service
Public Law 480 (Food for Peace), 93,
    253, 256; *see also* Agricultural pol-
    icy; Cereals; Food aid; Food and
    nutrition policy; Grain crops; Nu-
    trition—politics
  adverse effects of, 268
  Brookings Institute Seminar on, 268
  grain export under, 256
Puerto Rico, obesity in, 302
Pulses
  caloric intake from, *61*
  cereal profits and, 63
Pyloric stenosis, 280
Pyridoxin; *see* Vitamin B₆

Quality of life, 89, 96
  carrying capacity and, 99, 107

Radiation and preservation, *398*
Rainfall; *see also* Drought
  in deserts, 33–37
  distribution of, 47, 49
  famine and, 70, 73
  in humid tropics, 112, 114
  in India, 41–42, *43,* 50–51
  in Israel, 34
  storage of, 123–124
  in United States, 40–41, 43–45
Rapeseed oil, *381*
Rapeseed protein, 135
RDA; *see* Recommended Dietary Allow-
    ance
Recommended allowances (diet); *see*
    Minimum Daily Requirements
    (MDR); Nutrition—norms; Rec-
    ommended Dietary Allowance
    (RDA); U.S. Recommended
    Daily Allowances (U.S. RDA)
Recommended diet, 60, 151, 153, 173–
    174, 181, 372–378; *see also* Rec-
    ommended allowances
Recommended Dietary Allowance
    (RDA); *see also* Minimum Daily
    Requirements (MDR); Nutrition
    —norms; U.S. Recommended
    Daily Allowances (U.S. RDA)
  described, 260, 259
  healthy population and, 174

Recommended Dietary Allowance (RDA)—*Continued*
  iron in, 153, *155*
  in School Food Service, 415, 433
  standard abuse of, 259–260
Refined foods, 284–285, 389
Refrigeration, *318*
Relief workers, 77, 81–82, 86; *see also* Famine—relief; Famine—national policy provisions; Relief organizations
Research stations; *see* Agricultural experimental stations; Agricultural research institutions
Research and development
  in agriculture, 17–18
  capabilities of protein productivity by, 130–131
  obesity control and, 312
  protein resources and, 129–131, 242–243
Resource development, world-model input of, 229
Resource management, 21–25
  studies of, 18
  systems of, 23, 54
Restaurant foods, 313
Retinol, 215, 217
Retinol Binding Protein (RBP), 217
Retinyl palmate, 215
Revolution and famine, 69–70, 72–73
Rhizobia, N-fixation from, 115
Riboflavin (B₂), 172
  mitochondrial activity and, 362–363
  upper GI tract and, *361*, 362
Rice, 18, 20, 55, 118
  amino alteration of, 134, 184
  Asian dependence on, 112–113
  exported from Pakistan, 13
  Green Revolution and, 53, 60, 62
  high-yield production of, 169
  hypertension diet of, 351–352, 354–355
  milling of, 98
  NPU of, 148
  price decrease of, 2
  toxins and, *401*
  tropical diseases of, 114
Rickets, 151
Riots and famine, 69–70, 72–73
Riverside (Cal.), 127
RNA
  placenta growth and, 191
  removal from SCP, 141
"Rockefeller Diet," 312
Rockefeller Foundation, 107
Rocky Mountains and Little Ice Age, 43
Roosevelt, Franklin D., 316

Roosevelt, Theodore, 162
Root hydraulics and irrigation, 123–124
Roots and tubers
  study of, 18
  in tropical agriculture, 113, 118
Rowett Laboratories (Scotland), 324
Royal Society (England), 251
Rubber trees, 114
Ruminants
  listed, 23
  populations of, 148
  studies of nutrition of, 18
Runoff farming, desert schemes of, 36–37
Russia, 109; *see also* Soviet Union
Rutabaga, *401*
Rye, 18
  animal ration percent of, 148
  toxins and, *401*

Saccharin, 162
Saccharine Disease, The (Cleave), 284
Safrol, *401*
Sahara, 100
  food distribution in, 57
  water sources in, 33–35, 56
Sahel
  atmospheric dust in, 54
  drought in, 13, 36–40, 70
St. Vincent, weaning in, *201*
Salination of soil, 122, 125, 128, 168
Salmonella, 171
Salt, 158–159
  abuse of, 164
  as additive, 430
  cardiovascular diseases and, 341
  hypertension and, 351–352
  iodization of, 152–165, 211, 217, 352
  obesity and, 310
Saltsjobaden (Sweden), Symposium in, 71, 83
Sanitation control, 185
Saponins, 132
Saturated fat
  atherosclerosis and, 341–346, 347
  consumption of, 6
  exercise and, 351
  in lipid theory, 341–345
  obesity and, 318
  polyunsaturated and, 344–345, 379–381
  Prudent Diet and, 372
Sassafras, *401*
Saudi Arabia
  water sources in, 37
  wealth of, 96
"Scaled neutral" in agriculture, 25, 54

Scandinavia, reproductive rate in, 109
School food programs, 15, 67, 432; *see also* U.S. School Food Service
Scleroderma, 325
SCP; *see* Single cell proteins
Seafood, 401
Secretary of Agriculture (U.S.), 252–253, 256
Seed legumes, studies of, 18
Select Committee on GRAS Substances (Federation of American Societies for Experimental Biology), 401
Selected Heart Facts (AHA), 337
Selenite, 156
Selenium, 152–157
    biological availability of, 156
    decontaminating property of, 157
    food fortification with, 155, 173
Selneno methionine, 156
Sequestrants, *400*
Serum ferritin method, 226
Sesame, 135
    seed oil of, *381*
Seventh Day Adventists, Smoking Cessation Clinics of, 317, *318*
Sewage, SCP resources of, 145; *see also* Wastes
Shelf life of food, 263
Shetland horses, birth weights of, 190–191
Shortage of food, 87
Shortening, 20, 379
Shrimp, energy production cost of, *55*
Shriners and health care, 317, *318*
Silage, 171
Silicon metabolism, 156
Simet (Mexico), 169
Sinai Desert, water sources in, 35, 37–38
Singapore
    birthrate in, 109–110
    breast-feeding in, 198–199
    nutrition progress in, 6
Single cell proteins (SCP), 263
    potentials and research needs of, 140–141
    protein resources of
        nonphotosynthetic, 141, 145–146
        photosynthetic, 140, 146
    toxicology studies on, 133
    from whey, 394
Skim milk diets, 388
Skim milk powders, *204*
"Slash and burn" agriculture, 26, 47
Small pox, 245, 294
Smell
    dysosmia in, 330
    sensory dysfunction of, 321–322

Smoking
    cancer and, 362
    clinics to stop, 317
    obesity therapy and, 304
    video influence on, 315
Smoking for preservation, *398*
Smoking Cessation Clinics (Seventh Day Adventists), 317
Snack foods, 376
Social Security, retirement age and, 295
Social Security Administration (U.S.), 295
Social stratification and food systems, 229
Sodium and atherosclerosis, 352
Sodium sulfite, 175
Soil; *see also* Irrigation
    in deserts, 33–38
    erosion of, 31, 90, 114–117
    fertility of, 112, 115–117
    intercropping on, 117–118
    irrigation effects on, 122–123
    lowland humid tropics and, 112–117
    mineral deficiency of, 152
    rainfall and, 123–124
    salination of, 122, 125, 128, 168
    waterlogging of, 122
Solar energy
    biological conversion of, 19, 28, *55*
    food systems of, 26, 28
Sorbitol, *400*
Sorghum, 18, 20, 24
    protein improvement of, 133–134
    toxins in, 132
South America, grazing land in, 13
South Carolina
    anemia in, 423–424
    poverty index ratio of, 419
    vitamin A levels in, 422
South Korea, education programs in, 12
Soviet Union
    drought and starvation scenario for, 232, 234
    feedgrain storage in, 14
    food harvests in, 5
    krill fisheries of, 139, 145
    molybdenum excess in, 152
    reproduction rate in, 109
    sunflowerseed oil exports from, 380
    wheat failure in, 40, 49
Soy protein, 179
Soya, 174
    engineered foods from, 164
Soybean oil
    in butter, 379
    in margarine-cheese, 379
    world production of, *381*

Soybeans; *see also* Oilseeds
  comparative rise in cost of, 131, 170–171, 242
  foliar nutrients and, 21
  haemagglutinins in, 165
  in infant formulas, 389
  management systems for, 23
  NPU of, 148
  oil crop of, 20
  prices of, *24*
  production in Brazil of, 8
  protein source of, 135
  rising demand for, 131
  toxic inhibitors in, 132
  waste feed compared with, 149
  yield increases of, 134–135
Stabilizers, *400*
Spanish-Americans
  growth retardation among, 420
  vitamin A levels among, 425–426
Spices for preservation, 398–399
Sri Lanka
  birthrate in, 109–110
  food aid intervention in, 107
Standards of nutrition, 259–261
Stanford Heart Disease Prevention Program, 309
Stanford Three-Community Study, 314
Stanine, defined, 383–384
Staphyloma, 214
Stark, William, 346
Starvation, 12–13, 17, 87; *see also* Malnutrition; Undernutrition
  scenario of future in Asia of, 231–234, 236
  U.S. role in, 228, 233–237
  world ban on, 83
State agricultural institutions, protein research at, 130, *135, 136, 137*, 139; *see also* Agricultural research institutions; National Association of State Universities and Land Grant Colleges
Stimulants, *401*
Stomach, *see* Cancer—stomach
Stomates and plant respiration, 168–169
Storage life, 397
Stress, 341
Stroke; *see also* Arteriosclerosis; Cardiovascular diseases
  dietary agents and, 341
  epidemiological evidence of, 360
  hypertension and, 354
  pediatrics and, 348
  risk factors for, 337–338
  selected heart facts on, *337*

Sugar, 89, 211, 216
  analytical methodology and, 409
  cardiovascular diseases and, 341, 349
  coronary heart disease and, 345–346
  crop studies of, 18
  dental disease and, 108
  dietary fiber effect on, 287
  fast foods and, 174, 264
  price of calories from, *24,* 153, 346, 428
  replacement factor of, 275–276
  western disease and, 284, 389
Sugar beets, 18
  management systems for, 23
Sugarcane, 18, 21, 114
Sunflower protein, 135
Sunflower oil, 20
  import or, 380
  in margarine-cheese, 379
  world production of, 381, *382*
Sunlight and volcanic dust, 46–47, *49, 50, 54–55*
Surfactants, *400*
Surgeon General (Public Health Service), 433
Surplus Commodities in school lunches, 413–414, 416–417
Sweden
  atherosclerosis in
    fat consumption and, 379–381
    water hardness and, 353
  dairy products in, 380
  energy and protein intake in, 178
  National Board of Health and Welfare of, 379
  vegetable oil production in, 380–381
  vitamin fortification in, 390
Swedish Nutrition Foundation, 71
Sweet potatoes, 18, 20
Swine, feed effects on, 171

T aiwan (Formosa)
  birthrate drop in, 107, 109–110
  food aid intervention in, 107
  nutrition program in, 6
Tallow, *381*
Tannic acid, 158
  iron availability and, 222
Tanzania, bottle-feeding costs in, 202–203
Taste
  appeal of, 393
  control of, 321
  dysfunction of, 322, 324
  dysgeusia in, 330
  gustin in, 330, 333
  modifiers of, *400*

Taste—*Continued*
  thresholds in cancer, *331–332*
  zinc loss and, 324–333
Tax exemption and famine disasters, 72
Tea, 158, *401*
Technology
  agricultural application of, 6, 17–18
  areas of adaptability of, 23–24
  farming systems and, 23–24
  food and
    production of, 240–241
    system factors of, 229
  politics of, 93, 228–229
  "scaled neutral" adaptations of, 25, 54
  science and, 161
  uses and abuses of, 1, 161–166
Temperature; *see also* Climate; Drought
  in corn belt, 40, 44–45, 49
  in Minnesota, *41–42*
  in North America, 45, *46*
  sunlight and, 47, 49
  wheat prices and, 51, 101
Ten-State Nutrition Survey (1968–70),
    419–422, 424–425
Tennessee, vitamin A levels in, 422
Texas
  growth retardation in, 420
  nutrition survey in, 425
  poverty index ratio of, 419
  vitamin A deficiency in, 421–422
Texas Nutrition Survey, 425
Textured vegetable protein, 263
Thailand, vitamin A deficiency in, 213
Thiamine, 172
Thyroid hormone, *323*
Tidal waves and famine, 69–70, 73
Timber, 90
Title 12, food and agricultural policy
    council under, 243
Tobacco
  protein from, 142
  toxins and, *401*
Tobago, birth rate in, 109–110
Tomatoes, 165
TOPS (Take Off Pounds Sensibly), 305,
    307–308
Tortillas, 179
  fortification of, 247–248
Toxicity, concept of, 40; *see also* Food
    additives—toxicity testing; Toxi-
    cology; Toxins
Toxicology; *see also* Food additives—
    toxicity testing
  additive metabolism and, 429
  food-safety problems in, 132–133, 399–
    404
  protein production and, 132–133, 136

Toxins
  food testing for, 399–404
  in legumes, 136
  of plants, 132–133, 136
Trace elements; *see also specific elements*
  food fortification and, 152–159, 173
  ratio to iron of, *157*
  requirements for, 261, 271
  in tropical soils, 115
Trace minerals, RDA for, 271; *see also*
    Trace elements
Trade, in Club of Rome study, 230, 233–
    234
Transit time
  constipation and, 365
  dietary fiber and, 284–285
  stool weight and, *284*
Transpiration in plants, 168–169
Tree crops, 114, 168
Triage, 100, 105
Triglycerides
  in atherosclerotic diseases, 341–344,
    348
  fiber and, *285*
  fructose and, 346
  genetics and, 347–348
Trinidad, birthrate drop in, 110
Triticale, 20
Tritium, dating ground water with, 35
Tropics
  food production in, 112, 119, 167
  lowland humid defined, 112
Trypanosomiasis, 118
Tuba City Indian Hospital (Ariz.), 421
Tuberculosis, 212
Tulane University, 402
Tumors, development of, 388
Turkey, U.S. consumption of, 29, 436
Turnip, *401*
"Tween 20, 60," 287
Twinkies, 175
Typhoons, *see* Hurricanes

Uganda, 188
  maize yields in, 113
Ulcerated colitis and colon cancer, 366
Ultisols, 115
Undernutrition; *see also* Malnutrition
  anorexia in, 322
  birth weight and, 188–190, 192–193,
    246–247
  blood pressure and, 190
  cachexia in, 322
  defined, 322
  factors in, 322–323
  poverty and, 70

Undernutrition—*Continued*
pregnancy and, 188
trace elements and, 152
Uniprotein, *204*
United Nations
Disaster Relief Coordinator Office (UNDRO), 71
Food and Agriculture Organization (FAO)
crop monitoring by, 73
Director General of, 434
errors in data of, 87
food energy and protein data of, *178*
U.S. support of, 132
Fund for Population Activities, 11
7th Special Session on New Economic Order, 109
World Health Organization (WHO), 132, 212–213, 352
iron fortification program of, 226
United States
agricultural and food events in, *24*
anemia in, 423–425
breast-feeding in, 200
climate changes in, 40, 44–45
consumption levels in, 5
food aid by; *see also* Food aid; PL 480
intervention of, 106–108, 241
policy of, 111
food production in, 17–18, 22
policies of, 255–258, 410, 436
prospects of, 130–131, 147
food reserves in, 6
foreign aid by, 107
goiter in, 151
heart disease statistics (1958–1967) of, 344, 355
immigration into, 89–90
irrigation systems in, 127
Korean orphans studied in, 280–281
nutrition in
calories and, 70
deficiencies of, 151–152, 154–155, 158
food policies and, 92–93, 96, 110–111, 129–131, 147, 253, 255–257
iron fortification, *156*
junk food, 10–11, 103–104, 174, 270, 275
standards of, 127, 295–296
selenium and, 152
surveillance of, 266–268
obesity in, 298–302, 420, 436
pre-agricultural hunters in, 26
protein resources and needs of, 129
standard of living in, 54

vitamin deficiency in, 421–423
water and heart disease in, 353
Weight Watchers International in, 309
WIC program of, 207
U.S. Army Medical Research and Nutrition Laboratory 423–424
U.S. Congress, 105
food and agriculture research and, 243, 266–269, 278
nutrition and
policy of, 110–111, 253, 255–257
surveillance of, 266–268
Wampler Bill in, 243, 257, 269
U.S. Child Nutrition Act (1966), 411, 415*n*, 417
U.S. Federal Trade Commission, 316
U.S. Food and Drug Laws, 161
U.S. Department of Agriculture (USDA), 130–131
animal protein research of, 138, 139
cereal protein research of, 135
Child Nutrition Act and, 411
"consumption" information of, 264–265
dairy research by, 138
Economic Service survey by, 268–269
Food Distribution Program of, 422
Health and Nutrition Evaluation Surveys (HANES), 407, 261
Household Food Consumption Survey (1965) of, 260–261, 266
leaf protein research by, 142
livestock research by, 137
nitrite authorized by, 163
nutritional surveillance by, 266–267
School Food Service and, 412–414
Science and Education Staff of, 295
on sugar consumption, 276
traditional research of, 143
waste reclamation research by, 169
on world crop yields, 51, *52,* 55
U.S. Department of Health, Education and Welfare (HEW)
Center for Disease Control of, 420, 425,
Health and Nutrition Evaluation Survey (HANES), 261, 266, 407
Ten-State Nutritional Survey, 419–422, 424–425
U.S. Food and Drug Administration (FDA); *see* Food and Drug Administration
U.S. Head-Start program, 421, 422
U.S. National School Lunch Act (1946), 411, 415, 417
"U.S. Nutrition Policy," a partial proposal, 278–279

U.S. Office of Economic Opportunity (OEO), 425
U.S. Office of Management and Budget, 267
U.S. Office of Science and Technology Policy, 278, 436
U.S. Office of Technology Assessment, 110, 243
 Food Advisory Committee of (OTA), 18, 268, 269n
U.S. Public Health Service
 anemia studies by, 423–424
 Indian Hospital (Ariz.), 421
 nutrition programs, 425–426
 tobacco regulation and, 433
U.S. Recommended Daily Allowances; see also Minimum Daily Requirements (MDR); Nutrition—norms; Recommended Dietary Allowance (RDA)
 of copper, 244
 described, 259
 nutrition labelling of, 260
U.S. School Food Service (SFS), 411–417, 432, 433
U.S. Senate Select Committee on Nutrition and Human Needs (1974)
 on food industry, 396
 report on diet and disease, 295
 School Food Service and, 411–412
 on U.S. dietary goals, 316
U.S. Social Security Administration, 295
U.S. Surplus Relief Corporation (1933), 411
U.S. Women, Infants and Children (WIC) program, 92, 425
U.S. Works Progress Administration, 411
University of Colorado Medical Center, 425
University of Georgia Extension Veterinary Department, 149
University of Maryland Community Pediatric Center, 122
University of Nebraska, 170
University of Southern California, 355
University of Wisconsin, 142
Urbanization, 164–165
Urea
 in animal diets, 149
 nitrification with, 116
Uric acid, atherosclerotic risk of, 338
Urinary bladder, cancer of, 363

V accinations, 12, 406
Valencia orange, 401
Vanadium, 353

"Vanishing zero," 161
Variola (smallpox), 245, 294
Vasectomy, 12
Veal consumed in U.S., 29
Vegetable oil
 for famine relief, 80
 products of, 165
Vegetable protein products, 153, 164–165
Vegetables
 cereal profits and, 63
 for famine relief, 80
 gastric ulcer and, 361
 leafy green varieties, 212
 protein analogues from 137–138
 studies of, 141–142
 as weaning foods, 207
Vegetarian diet
 energy and labor input of, 26, 27
 evaluation of, 21
 sigmoid volvulus and, 288
 transit time of, 284
Venezuela, cholesterol levels in, 346
Verdanization, 38
Vietnam War, 90
Vinegar, 397–398
Vikings, 42
Vitamin A
 cervix cancer and, 362, 388
 control of, 213–216, 245, 249, 425–426
 deficiency of, 210–217, 435
 discovery of, 210
 dosage levels of, 216–217
 effect on carcinogens, 388, 362
 epidemiology and natural history of, 212–214
 family income and, 208
 for famine relief, 80
 fortification with, 207–208, 214
 massive dosing of, 214–217, 402
 Philippines study on, 193–194, 208
 U.S. risk populations and, 421–422
Vitamin A Consultation Group, International (IVACG), 212–213
Vitamin B (riboflavin), 361–363
Vitamin B_6, 158
 food and appetite control and, 323
 liver cancer and, 361
Vitamin C
 effect on carcinogens by, 361–362, 388
 effect on non-heme iron by, 156–158, 223, 226
Vitamin D, 158, 422
Vitamin E, 159, 215
 carcinogens and, 388

Vitamins
  chemical synthesis of, 142
  deficiencies of, 152–153, 164
  for famine relief, 80
  FDA rule on, 408–409
  fortification with, 151, 158–159
VLDL (very low density lipoproteins),
    346, 348
Volcanos and sunlight, 46–47, 49–50,
    54–55

Wadi beds, desert hydrology of, 35–36
Wadi Feiran (Sinai Desert), oasis in, 35
Wampler Bill, 243, 257, 269
War and famine, 69–70, 72–73, 82–83
Warren Report, 87
Washington (state)
  anemia in, 423–424
  poverty index ratio of, 419
Wastes, 13, 22, 149
  farm systems and, 23
  reclamation of, 131, 169
  recycling of animal, 137
  production of feed from, 149
Water
  cardiovascular deaths and, 353
  desert sources of, 33–38
  energy inputs of, 125, 128
  farm systems of, 23
  in food systems, 263
  infant requirements of, 205–206
  irrigation supplies of, 121–122, 128,
    168–169
  NDRO field assessment of, 79
  quality in deserts, 38
  resources of, 54, 68
  salinity of, 168
Waterlogging, 122–123, 125, 128
Wealth of Nations, The (Smith), 391
Weaning; see also Formula feeding
  foods for, 183–184, 247–250
    alkaline elimination in, 249
    commerciogenic nutrition and, 203–
      205, 207–208
    dextromaltose in, 249
    undernutrition and, 40, 48–50
Weather
  agriculture and, 19
  management of, 100
Weed control, 21
  in tropical agriculture, 113, 116, 117,
    118, 167–168
Weight control, 303–319, 389; see also
    Behavior control; Obesity
Weight Watchers International, 309–313,
    386

Weizmann Institute (Israel), 169–170
West Bengal, blindness in, 213
West Virginia, poverty index ratio in, 419
Wheat, 18, 20, 165; see also Grain
  animal ration percent of, 148
  comparative cost rise of, 131
  development of, 397
  Green Revolution yields of, 52, 60, 62,
    107, 121
  input conditions for, 169
  in India, 41
  NPU of, 148
  price of, 24, 51
  protein improvement in, 134–135, 169–
    170, 184
  reserves (1976) of, 256–257
  wild relatives of, 169–170
Wheat belt and climate, 45, 101
Wheat gluten, separation of, 135
Whey
  lactalbumin in, 394
  protein from, 165, 394
  research on, 138
  single cell protein from, 344
White bread, 164, 174, 273
  in ancient Rome, 385
White flour
  disease and, 284, 389
  nutrients in, 153, 164
White House Conference on Food and
    Nutrition in Health, 105
White House Conference on Nutrition
    and Human Needs (1969), 275,
    412
WHO; see United Nations World Health
    Organization; FAO/WHO; WHO/
    USAID
WHO/USAID Meeting, 212–213
Whole grain in School Food Service, 414,
    416
Wholewheat bread, 164, 174, 273, 385
WIC program, 92, 207, 425
Wiley, Harvey, 162, 175
Winged bean, 20, 118
Women, knowledge rights of, 10–13, 15
Women, Infants and Children program
    (WIC), 92, 207, 425
Wood in food systems, 30
World Bank, 107
World Council of Churches, 76
World Food and Nutrition Study (NAS),
    59
  Summary of Research by the Nutrition
    Overview Team of, 66–68
World food bank, 90
World Food Conference, 6, 106, 130
  on world grain reserve, 257–258

World War I, 90
World War II, 90, 207, 262, 335, 362, 392, 394
WPA (U.S. Works Progress Administration), 411

Xanthelasmas, 347
Xanthomas, 347
Xanthomatosis, 347–348
Xerophthalmia, 210–214, 216–217

Yam (white), 118
Yeasts
    chromium in, 156
    SCP processing of, 145
Yeast foods, 400
Yellow rice, 401
Young Men's Christian Association and health behavior, 317–318

Zaire, cassava blight in, 114
    cultivars resistant to, 117
Zero Population Growth
    achievement of, 88–90
    in Germany, 109
Zinc
    appetite and, 323, 324
    -copper antagonism, 157, 241, 244, 330
    deficiency of, 153–154, 244
    depletion studies in, 324–330
    deprivation of, 389
    fiber and, 385
    food fortification with, 154–156, 173–174, 241, 244, 277
    metabolism of, 323–333
        biological availability in, 156–158
        controlled body depletion in, 328
        protein transport in, 325
        serum concentrations in, 325–326
        weight loss in, 330
    recommended allowances for, 271
    taste system and, 333
    in tropical soils, 116